ENDOMETRIOSIS - BASIC CONCEPTS AND CURRENT RESEARCH TRENDS

Edited by **Koel Chaudhury**
and **Baidyanath Chakravarty**

Endometriosis - Basic Concepts and Current Research Trends
Edited by Koel Chaudhury and Baidyanath Chakravarty

Published by InTech

Janeza Trdine 9, 51000 Rijeka, Croatia

Publishing Process Manager Bojan Rafaj

Technical Editor Teodora Smiljanic

Cover Designer InTech Design Team

Additional hard copies can be obtained from orders@intechopen.com

Endometriosis - Basic Concepts and Current Research Trends,
Edited by Koel Chaudhury and Baidyanath Chakravarty
p. cm.
ISBN 978-953-51-0524-4

For EU product safety concerns:
IN TECH d.o.o., Prolaz Marije Krucifikse Kozulić 3, 51000 Rijeka, Croatia,
info@intechopen.com or visit our website at intechopen.com.

Meet the editor

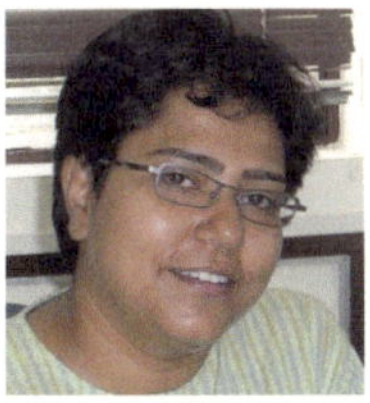

During the early part of her career, Dr. Koel Chaudhury, Ph.D worked extensively on the development of a non-hormonal injectable male contraceptive, RISUG which is presently in Phase III clinical trials. Her present research focus is on Women's Health which includes clinical proteomics and metabolomics based biomarker discovery in endometriosis and gestational hypertension, understanding endometrial receptivity and pathogenesis of endometriosis at a molecular level and role of oxidative stress in infertility. She has successfully established the threshold level of reactive oxygen species beyond with IVF/ICSI outcome is not favourable. Dr. Chaudhury has several projects funded by the Government of India and has a large number of international publications to her credit. She is also a peer reviewer of reputed journals. She is presently working as an Associate Professor in the School of Medical Science and Technology, Indian Institute of Technology, Kharagpur, India.

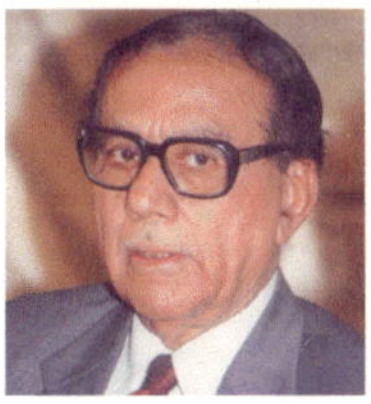

Dr. Baidyanath Chakravarty, F.R.C.O.G, D.Sc. (Hon) is presently the Director of the Institute of Reproductive Medicine, Salt lake, Kolkata, India. Dr. Chakravarty, known for his brilliant teaching skills, retired as a Professor of Obstetrics and Gynecology from NRS Medical College, Kolkata, India in 1986. Amongst other stalwarts, Dr. Chakravarty was instrumental in proving that India was one of the first countries to pioneer the IVF-ET technology. He, along with his close associate and inspiring team-member, Dr. Subhash Mukhopadhyay, created the world's second and India's first IVF baby in 1978 and has successfully delivered 3385 IVF babies so far. Apart from being an eminent clinician, his contributions towards infertility-related research deserve a special mention. He has successfully developed cost-effective ovulation induction protocols for women with repeated IVF failure. He has also investigated the genetic basis of various infertility related disorders, role of oxidative stress in male and female infertility, and endometrial receptivity in endometriosis and recurrent spontaneous miscarriage. Dr. Chakravarty has published over 275 scientific papers and 26 book chapters on obstetrics and gynecology, infertility and ART. He has received several prestigious awards for his immense contribution in the field of reproductive health. He remains an active clinician, with particular interest in advanced research for improved patient care.

Contents

Preface

Dedication

We dedicate this book to thousands of women all over the world suffering from endometriosis

Endometriosis is a progressive debilitating disease affecting the physical, social and psychological aspects of normal life quality in nearly 1 of 7 women of reproductive age. Endometriosis is considered to be an enigmatic disease owing to the lack of specific set of symptoms, poorly understood pathogenesis, complexity in diagnosis and limited therapeutic options available for management of the disorder. The last three decades we have witnessed a significant volume of research related to endometriosis. We felt the need to bring together contributions of experts working on pathophysiology, diagnosis and therapeutic aspects of endometriosis. We genuinely hope that the readers will enjoy reading these informative articles contributed by eminent clinicians and scientists. We, as editors, would sincerely feel rewarded if the readers put to use the contents of the book to alleviate the pain and misery of women suffering from endometriosis, a disease which still remains a challenge.

We sincerely appreciate the valuable contributions of all the authors who have put in considerable effort to make the book a success. We are grateful to Dr. Ashalatha Ganesh for providing her expert opinion and valuable suggestions. We are most thankful to InTech publisher for providing us with an opportunity to edit a book of such great clinical relevance. Finally, our sincere thanks to Bojan Rafaj, Publishing Process Manager for the excellent support extended to us throughout the editing process.

Koel Chaudhury (Editor)
Associate Professor
School of Medical Science and Technology
Indian Institute of Technology, Kharagpur
India

Baidyanath Chakravarty (Co-editor)
Director Institute of Reproductive Medicine
Salt Lake, Kolkata
India

Section 1

Endometriosis

1

Endometriosis

Mohammad Reza Razzaghi[1],
Mohammad Mohsen Mazloomfard[2] and Anahita Ansari Jafari[2]
[1]*Chairman of Urology Department,*
[2]*Medical Laser Application Research Center,*
Urology Department of Shohada Tajrish Hospital,
Shahid Beheshti University (MC), Teheran,
Iran

1. Introduction

Endometriosis is classically defined as the growth of endometrial glands and stroma at extra-uterine sites, most commonly implanted over visceral and peritoneal surfaces within the female pelvis (1). Though endometriosis has been described for the first time in 1690 by the German physician, Daniel Shroen, researchers remain still unsure as to the definitive cause of this disease (2). The most widely accepted theory for the pathogenesis of endometriosis (retrograde menstruation/transplantation), proposed in the 1927 by Sampson (3). Although a great deal has been learned about endometriosis since Sampson's land mark studies, there is still a lot about it that is unclear and controversial. It remains an enigmatic disorder in that the cause, the natural history, and the precise mechanisms of its presentation are not known (4).

Endometriosis is most commonly found on the pelvic peritoneum but may also be found on the ovaries, rectovaginal septum, ureter, and rarely in the bladder, pericardium, and pleura. More rarely, colon, small intestine, appendix, umbilical scar and even sites not closely contiguous to the pelvis (e.g., lung and brain tissue) may also be involved (5). It is a leading cause of disability in women of reproductive age, responsible for dysmenorrhea, pelvic pain and subfertility. The most common symptoms for women who have endometriosis are pelvic pain and infertility; both adversely affecting the quality of life. The pregnancy rate in women with endometriosis is about half of women with tubal factor infertility and is negatively correlated with the severity of disease. The cause of reproductive failure may be due to poor oocyte development, implantation or embryogenesis. In addition to infertility, a strong cause–effect relationship between endometriosis and pelvic pain is commonly observed (6, 7). Dysmenorrhoea is associated with cyclic recurrent microbleeding within various entities of ectopic endometriotic implants and consequent inflammation. Endometriosis-related adhesions and compression or infiltration of nerves in the subperitoneal pelvic space by ectopic lesions also cause painful symptoms (8, 9).

In the last few years, there is a growing interest in endometriosis, because of the large number of women it affects (about 3–10% of the female population in the reproductive age, and up to 40–80% of women complaining of pelvic pain) and the significant morbidity associated with this disease, mainly with regard to the possible consequences on reproductive function and on the risk of developing gynecologic tumors, such as ovarian cancer (10-12). The prevalence in women without symptoms is 2-50%, depending on the diagnostic criteria used and the populations studied (9). The incidence of endometriosis is difficult to quantify, as women with the disease are often asymptomatic, and imaging modalities have low sensitivities for diagnosis. The primary method of diagnosis is laparoscopy, with or without biopsy for histologic diagnosis (13, 14). Using this standard, investigators have reported the annual incidence of surgically diagnosed endometriosis to be 1.6 cases per 1,000 women aged between 15 and 49 years. The incidence is 40-60% in women with dysmenorrhoea and 20-30% in women with subfertility. The severity of symptoms and the probability of diagnosis increase with age. The most common age of diagnosis is reported as around 40, although this figure came from a study in a cohort of women attending a family planning clinic (15).

The clinical picture of endometriosis is widely heterogeneous. A correct diagnostic work-up of these patients can sometimes be very difficult, since there are a number of gynecological, intestinal and systemic diseases mimicking endometriosis, as well as other conditions that could be associated with or area consequence of this disorder. Therefore, multidisciplinary care should been courage to ensure correct evaluation and improve the management of these patients (16).

2. Prevalence

Although endometriosis was originally felt to be a disease only seen in women who had undergone a minimum of 5 years of ovulatory menstrual cycles, it is now well-documented that endometriosis can be seen as early as the premenarchal age group, in girls who have initiated thelarche (63). Prevalence is estimated to be 6–10% in the general female population and 35–50% of the patients experience pain and/or infertility. The prevalence in women without symptoms is 2-50%, depending on the diagnostic criteria used and the populations studied (9). The true incidence of endometriosis in adolescents is difficult to quantify and estimates vary among different studies. The incidence of endometriosis is difficult to quantify, as women with the disease are often asymptomatic, and imaging modalities have low sensitivities for diagnosis. Using this standard, investigators have reported the annual incidence of surgically diagnosed endometriosis to be 1.6 cases per 1,000 women aged between 15 and 49 years (64). The incidence is 40-60% in women with dysmenorrhoea and 20-30% in women with subfertility. According to the Endometriosis Association, 66% of adult women with endometriosis report the onset of pelvic symptoms before age 20, and those who seek care for symptoms as a teen see on average 4 or more physicians before receiving a diagnosis (15).

3. Classification

The primary method of diagnosis is visualization of endometriotic lesions by laparoscopy, with or without histologic confirmation. Since the extent of endometriosis can vary widely between individuals, attempts have been made to develop a standardized classification to objectively assess the extent of endometriosis. Sampson, Acosta et al., and many other investigators developed staging systems that have all been criticized for multiple reasons, including their inability to predict clinical outcomes, especially pregnancy rates (PRs) in infertile patients. In 1979, the American Fertility Society (AFS) (now the American Society for Reproductive Medicine, or ASRM) first proposed a classification system. This was extensively evaluated, modified in 1985, and is still used today. Despite these revisions the currently used revised AFS system has serious limitations, including not effectively predicting the outcome of treatment.

Endometriosis fertility index surgery form.

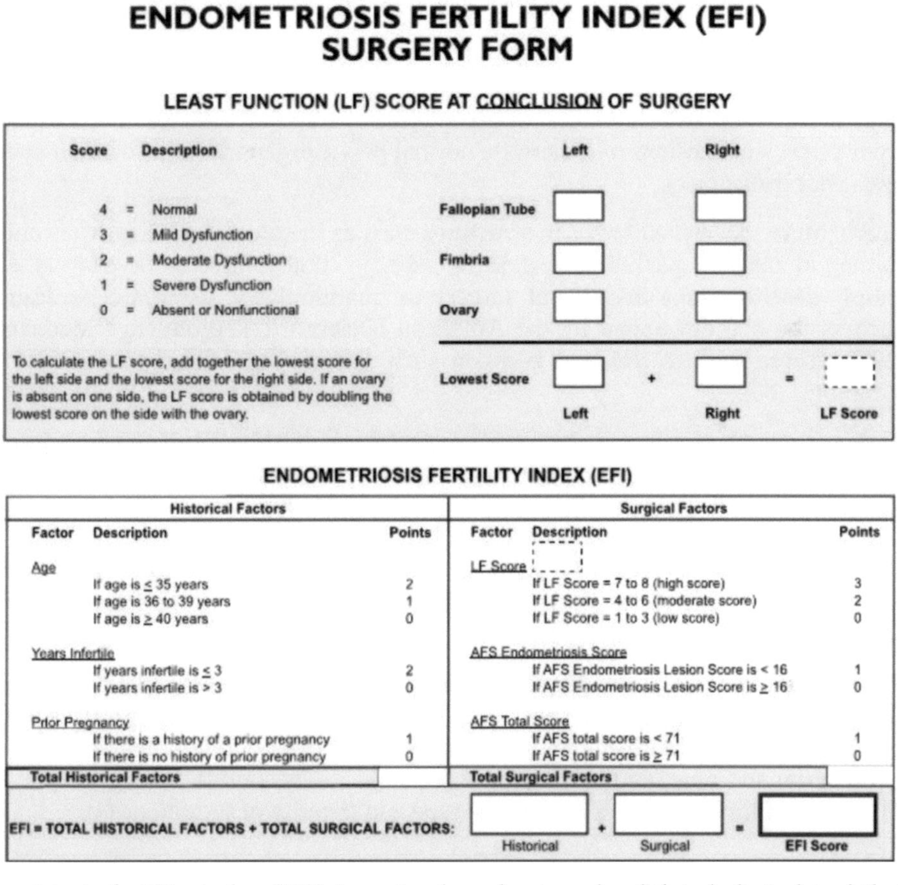

ENDOMETRIOSIS FERTILITY INDEX (EFI) SURGERY FORM

LEAST FUNCTION (LF) SCORE AT CONCLUSION OF SURGERY

Score	Description		Left	Right
4	= Normal	Fallopian Tube		
3	= Mild Dysfunction			
2	= Moderate Dysfunction	Fimbria		
1	= Severe Dysfunction			
0	= Absent or Nonfunctional	Ovary		

To calculate the LF score, add together the lowest score for the left side and the lowest score for the right side. If an ovary is absent on one side, the LF score is obtained by doubling the lowest score on the side with the ovary.

Lowest Score: Left + Right = LF Score

ENDOMETRIOSIS FERTILITY INDEX (EFI)

Historical Factors			Surgical Factors		
Factor	**Description**	**Points**	**Factor**	**Description**	**Points**
Age			LF Score		
	If age is ≤ 35 years	2		If LF Score = 7 to 8 (high score)	3
	If age is 36 to 39 years	1		If LF Score = 4 to 6 (moderate score)	2
	If age is ≥ 40 years	0		If LF Score = 1 to 3 (low score)	0
Years Infertile			AFS Endometriosis Score		
	If years infertile is ≤ 3	2		If AFS Endometriosis Lesion Score is < 16	1
	If years infertile is > 3	0		If AFS Endometriosis Lesion Score is ≥ 16	0
Prior Pregnancy			AFS Total Score		
	If there is a history of a prior pregnancy	1		If AFS total score is < 71	1
	If there is no history of prior pregnancy	0		If AFS total score is ≥ 71	0
Total Historical Factors			**Total Surgical Factors**		

EFI = TOTAL HISTORICAL FACTORS + TOTAL SURGICAL FACTORS: Historical + Surgical = **EFI Score**

The endometriosis fertility index (EFI) is a simple, robust, and validated clinical tool that predicts PRs for patients after surgical staging of endometriosis (see figure below). The EFI score ranges from 0–10, with 0 representing the poorest prognosis and 10 the best prognosis. Half of the points come from the historical factors and half from the surgical factors. Uterine abnormality was not included in the score. The EFI is very useful in developing treatment plans in infertile patients with endometriosis. The EFI is useful only for infertility patients who have had surgical staging of their disease. It is not intended to predict any aspect of endometriosis-associated pain. It is required that the male and female gametes are sufficiently functional to enable attempts at non-IVF conception. One factor found to predict pregnancy that is not included in the EFI is uterine abnormality. Sensitivity analysis showed that even with substantial variation in the assignment of functional scores the EFI varies very little (65).

4. Anatomic sites

Endometriosis may develop anywhere within the pelvis and on other extrapelvic peritoneal surfaces. Although the condition is usually limited to the ovaries, uterosacral ligaments, and Douglas' pouch, it has been reported in almost every organ of the body. Extra-pelvic endometriosis refers to endometrial implants found elsewhere in the body, including the skin, central nervous system, gastrointestinal tract, urinary tract, lungs, and heart. Macroscopically, three forms of endometriosis are described: superficial peritoneal (or ovarian) endometriosis, endometriotic cyst of the ovary or ovarian endometrioma, and deep infiltrating endometriosis (DIE).(4)

The most commonly affected sites are the pelvic organs and peritoneum, although other parts of the body such as the lungs are occasionally affected. The extent of the disease varies from a few, small lesions on otherwise normal pelvic organs to large, ovarian endometriotic cysts endometriomas).

There can be extensive fibrosis in structures such as the uterosacral ligaments and adhesion formation causing marked distortion of pelvic anatomy. Disease severity is assessed by simply describing the findings at surgery or quantitatively, using a classification system such as the one developed by the American Society for Reproductive Medicine (ASRM) (1997). There is no correlation between such systems and the type or severity of pain symptoms (66).

Endometriosis typically appears as superficial "powder burn" or "gunshot" lesions on the ovaries,serosal surfaces and peritoneum-black, dark-brown, or bluish-puckered lesions, nodules or small cysts containing old haemorrhage surrounded by a variable extent of fibrosis. Atypical or "subtle" lesions are also common, including red implants (petechial, vesicular, polypoid, hemorrhagic, red flamelike) and serous or clear vesicles. Other appearances include white plaques or scarring and yellow-brown peritoneal discoloration of the peritoneum (66, 67).

Endometriomas usually contain thick fluid like tar; such cysts are often densely adherent to the peritoneum of the ovarian fossa and the surrounding fibrosis may involve the tubes and bowel. Deeply infiltrating endometriotic nodules extend more than 5mm beneath the peritoneum and may involve the utero-sacral ligaments, vagina, bowel, bladder or ureters. The depth of infiltration is related to the type and severity of symptoms (4).

5. Pathophysiology

5.1 Etiology

Despite extensive research, its pathogenesis still remains elusive and the disorder is considered to be 'enigmatic'. Endometriosis is a multi-factorial disease with multi-faceted features. The theories that have withstood the test of time and remain in vogue include retrograde menstruation, coelomic metaplasia, and endometrial stem cells. All the theories on its pathogenesis must be taken complementary to one another and by no way are mutually exclusive. The most widely accepted theory is the implantation of viable endometrial tissue onto peritoneal visceral structures from retrograde menstrual flow into the pelvic cavity (17). However, the origin is multifactorial, also having hormone, immune, and genetic components. The relationship of endometriosis to estrogen is well-established. Two thirds of women with a diagnosis of endometriosis report having a family member with endometriosis. A large percentage of women with endometriosis have other co-morbidities such as fibromyalgia, chronic fatigue syndrome, hypothyroidism, allergies, asthma, and auto-immune disorders. The associated risk factors are directly related to low body mass index (BMI), and family history and are inversely related to exercise (18).

5.2 Retrograde menstruation

The earliest and most widely accepted theory relates to retrograde menstruation through the fallopian tubes with subsequent dissemination of endometrial tissue within the peritoneal cavity. Sampson's theory of endometrial implantation, offered in the 1927, proposes that retrograde menstruation through the fallopian tubes was responsible for endometriotic lesions. Three prerequisites are necessary for Sampson's theory: (1) retrograde menstruation, (2) viability of menstrual endometrial cells, and (3) implantation of endometrial cells onto the peritoneal/ovarian surfaces (3). Since the introduction of his theory, retrograde menstruation has been confirmed at laparoscopy, and it appears to occur in the vast majority of women. Keettel and Stein in the 1950s demonstrated the viability of shed menstrual endometrial cells by invitro culture of menstrual endometrium (19). The viability of retrograde menstrual endometrium has been shown by Mungyer et al by culturing endometrial glands and stroma collected from peritoneal lavage (20). In addition to these invitro studies, Ridley and Edwards injected menstrual blood into the skin of women scheduled for a laparotomy in the next 3 to 6 months. On excision of this tissue, several women had endometriotic lesions at the injection site. Further circumstantial evidence supporting Sampson's theory is the increased risk of endometriosis in women with Mullerian anomalies and other outflow tract obstructions (21).

Refluxed endometrial fragments adhere to and invade the peritoneal mesothelium and develop a blood supply, which leads to continued implant survival and growth. However, this theory fails to explain the presence of endometriosis in such remote areas outside the peritoneal cavity, as the lungs, skin, lymph nodes, and breasts. Moreover, the presence of the disease in early puberty and exceptionally also in newborns further contrasts the validity of the theory (22).

5.3 Coelomic metaplasia

The coelomic metaplasia theory claims that formation of endometriomas in the ovary or recto-vaginal endometriosis is caused by metaplasia of the coelomic epithelium, perhaps induced by environmental factors (23). Because the ovary and the progenitor of the endometrium, the müllerian ducts, are both derived from coelomic epithelium, metaplasia may explain the development of ovarian endometriosis. In addition, the theory has been extended to include the peritoneum because of the proliferative and differentiation potential of the peritoneal mesothelium.

This theory would explain why most women have some degree of retrograde menstruation but only a little percentage has endometriosis and the presence of the disease in absence of menses. However, the absence of endometriosis in other tissues derived from coelomic epithelium argues against this theory (22).

5.4 Induction theory

The theory of endometrial stem cells or transient amplifying progenitor cells claims that circulating stem cells originating from bone marrow or from basal layer of endometrium could differentiate into endometriotic tissue at different anatomical sites (24). In vitro studies have demonstrated the potential for ovarian surface epithelium, in response to estrogens, to undergo transformation to form endometriotic lesions. Although many putative factors have been identified, their propensity to cause endometriosis in some women but not in others demonstrates the still unidentified etiology of this disease (25).

5.5 Lymphatic or vascular spread

Evidence also supports the concept of endometriosis originating from aberrant lymphatic or vascular spread of endometrial tissue. Findings of endometriosis in unusual locations, such as the perineum or groin, bolster this theory. The lymphatic and hematogenous spread of endometrial cells can explain the presence of endometriosis in the pelvis or elsewhere. However, in the last few years, strong evidence indicates the possible role of immunologic factors and the lack of adequate immune surveillance in the pathogenesis of endometriosis (26, 27).

5.6 Hormonal effect

Endometriosis is an estrogen-dependent disorder. Aberrant production of estrogen by endometriotic stromal cells is indispensable for the development and maintenance of endometriosis especially during the period of menstruation when no ovarian estrogen is available. This notion was supported by identification in endometriotic stromal cells of the presence of all proteins/enzymes required for denovo synthesis of estrogen:steroidogenic acute regulatory protein (StAR), P450 side-chain cleavage enzyme (P450scc), 3b-hydroxy steroid dehydrogenase (3b-HSD), 17 a-hydroxylase 17,20 lyase, P450 aromatase and 17b-HSD type1. Among these enzymes, StAR and aromatase control the first and last committed steps in the biosynthesis of estrogen. StAR transports cholesterol across the mitochondrial membrane to the inner mitochondrial leaflet, where the first enzymatic reaction occurs. Aromatase catalyses the conversion of androstenedione to estrone. Estrone is further converted to 17b-estradiol (normally referred to a sestrogen) by 17b-HSD type1, whereas 17b-HSD type2 reverses this process. In disease-free uterine endometrium, no StAR or aromatase are detected but there are increased StAR and aromatase levels in extra-ovarian endometriotic implants and endometriomas. In addition, the absence of 17b-HSD type2 in pelvic endometriotic implants further favors an increase in the local concentration of estrogen (28-30).

5.7 Steroid receptor genetics

Endometriosis is an estrogen-dependent disease. The action of steroids such as estrogen, progesterone and androgen are mediated through their respective receptors (SRs). SRs are ligand (hormone)-dependent transcription factors. Upon activation with the specific hormone they can interact with hormone response elements in the promoter of target genes. Since the action of steroids such as estrogen, progesterone and androgen are mediated through their respective receptors - Estrogen Receptors (ER), Progesterone Receptors (PR) and Androgen Receptors (AR) - these receptors must be and have shown to be intimately involved in the pathogenesis of endometriosis. ERs, PRs and AR, along with glucocorticoid receptor and mineralocorticoid receptor, form the steroid receptors (SRs) family, which is one of three members of the nuclear receptor (NR) superfamily of transcription factors. Besides the SR family, other members of the NR superfamily, such as vitamin D receptor, retinoic acid receptor, and peroxisome proliferator-activated receptor may also be involved in endometriosis (31).

5.8 Immunologic factors

There is ample evidence indicating that alterations in both cell-mediated and humoral immunity contribute to the pathogenesis of endometriosis. Increased number and activation of peritoneal macrophages, decreased T cell and natural killer (NK) cell cytotoxicities are the alterations in cellular immunity, yielding diminished removal of ectopic endometrial cells from the peritoneal cavity. In addition, increased levels of several proinflammatory cytokines and growth factors produced by immune and endometrial cells are likely to be involved in facilitating implantation and growth of ectopic endometrial cells by promoting proliferation, inflammation and angiogenesis (32).

There is evidence that TNF-α promotes the adherence of stromal cells to the mesothelium and stimulates proliferation of endometriosis stromal cells. Both of these may be important mechanisms in the pathogenesis of endometriosis, and it has been suggested that TNF-α is one of the essential factors for the pathogenesis and maintenance of endometriosis. Concentrations of TNF-α in peritoneal fluid are higher in women with endometriosis than in patients with normal pelvic anatomy and peritoneal fluid TNF-α concentrations correlate with the stage of endometriosis. Serum TNF-α levels also are significantly increased in patients with endometriosis, especially in early stages of the disease. Also, TNF stimulates the expression of prostaglandin synthase-2, which in turn increases the production of prostaglandins E2 and F2a, an indirect mechanism by which TNF may cause inflammatory pain (33-37).

Endometriotic implants contain both estrogen and progesterone receptors and respond to changes of hormonal levels with bleeding or production and release of inflammatory mediators, especially prostaglandins E2 and F. For a long time, it has been thought that prostaglandins are involved in endometriosis-related severe dysmenorrhea, and probably dyspareunia and nonmenstrual pelvic pain. Some of the data suggest that endometriotic lesions actually may produce greater amounts of prostaglandins than does eutopic endometrium. In fact, prostaglandins in endometriosis were produced mainly by Cox-2 (38-40). Matsuzaki et al. found higher levels of Cox-2 in the epithelium and the stroma of endometriosis than in normal endometrium from controls without endometriosis. They also found higher levels of Cox-2 in the stroma of eutopic endometrium of women with endometriosis than in the stroma of women without endometriosis (41). Ota et al. have published similar results, showing higher levels of Cox-2 in endometriosis than in endometrium from controls. These data support the conclusion that Cox-2 is induced by endometriosis and leads to higher levels of prostaglandins (42).

5.9 Clinical association between endometriosis and autoimmune diseases

Clinical conditions associated with endometriosis by patients, providers, and researchers alike have included headaches, arthralgias and myalgias, allergies, eczema, hypothyroidism, fibromyalgia, chronic fatigue syndrome, and susceptibility to vaginal candidiasis. These often ill-defined entities carry an allure of mystery, paralleling many nonspecific symptoms encountered by patients with known autoimmune disease. Because of this parallelism, and with no alternative explanation for a patient's extraperitoneal symptoms, patients and health care providers may suspect an immunopathologic mechanism. The potential link between autoimmune disease and endometriosis has been studied from a number of perspectives. Some investigators have reported common clinical elements among patients with endometriosis and patients with various autoimmune processes, whereas others have reported interesting serologic parallels (43-46).

6. Risk factors

6.1 Genetic factors

Endometriosis regarded as a genetic disease due, apparently, to its reported familial aggregation. Yet even the reported familial aggregation, when examined closely, may be debatable and there has been little progress regarding the identification of genetic variants that predispose women to endometriosis. First degree relatives of patients with endometriosis have a 6.9% incidence of endometriosis in comparison with a 1% risk in controls (47).

There is a prevailing view that endometriosis is a polygenic disease and, as such, genetic polymorphisms that predispose women to endometriosis can be identified through linkage or association studies. In the last decade, numerous large-scale gene expression profiling studies have demonstrated, unequivocally, that many genes such as oncogenic K-ras are deregulated in endometriosis. Yet despite many publications, seemingly little headway has been made in elucidating the specific genetic factors that have a major impact on the risk of developing endometriosis. Few, if any, positive findings from genetic association studies have been replicated, and those who tried to replicate previously reported positive findings often end up with negative results. Not surprisingly, three meta-analyses on association of endometriosis and some genetic polymorphisms coding for dioxin detoxification enzymes, sex steroid biosynthesis and their receptors found no evidence of association even though meta-analyses known to have upward biases in risk estimates, especially the 'winner's curse' of first reports (48-49).

6.2 Environmental factors and dioxin

Environmental factors, such as dioxin, might interact with multiple genetic susceptibility loci to produce the phenotype of endometriosis. Most of these environmental contaminants exhibiting estrogenic effects will lead to endocrine disruption through various environmental media such as food and water. Dietary intake of dioxin-like compounds with biological activity will increase the body burden (the total amount of these chemicals that are present in the human body at a given point in time), which might contribute to the pathogenesis of endometriosis. In addition, these chemicals can pass through the placenta to affect fetal environment. In a prospective cohort study, the rate of laparoscopically confirmed endometriosis was 80% greater among women exposed in utero to diethylstilbestrol (a synthetic estrogen originally prescribed in pregnancy to prevent miscarriage) after 10 years of follow-up. However, the relationship between endocrine disrupting chemicals and endometriosis remains controversial because of lack of studies with sufficient statistical power (50-54).

Several excellent reviews have been published characterizing dioxins. Chemically, dioxin, an abbreviation of 2, 3, 7, 8-tetrachloro-dibenzo-p-dioxin, or TCDD, is a polycyclicaromatic agent with chloral substituent. Dioxin is a lipophilic material that could accumulate in tissues with a high fat content. There is insufficient evidence at this moment in support of the hypothesis that dioxin exposure may lead to increased risk of developing endometriosis in women. Dioxins may act similarly to estrogen in estrogen-target tissues such as endometrium (eutopic or ectopic), promoting proliferation. However, it should be noted that in the presence of Aryl hydrocarbon Receptor (AhR) agonists, the function of liganded ER is attenuated. Since the local estrogen production is increased in endometriosis due to aberrant regulation of aromatase and of type $_2$ 17 b-hydroxy steroid dehydrogenase, it is unclear what the net effect of AhR agonists such as dioxins is on ectopic endometrium (55-57).

6.3 Anatomic defects

Reproductive outflow tract obstruction can predispose to development of endometriosis, likely through exacerbation of retrograde menstruation. Accordingly, endometriosis has been identified in women with noncommunicating uterine horn, imperforate hymen, and transverse vaginal septum. Because of this association, diagnostic laparoscopy to identify and treat endometriosis is suggested at the time of corrective surgery for many of these anomalies. Repair of such anatomic defects is thought to decrease the risk of developing endometriosis (58, 59).

A number of Mullerian anomalies, most importantly those associated without flow tract obstruction, are associated with endometriosis. In a series by Schifrin et al. 15 patients (40%) younger than 20 years of age with endometriosis had a genital tract anomaly (60). This is opposed to findings by Goldstein et al who noted congenital anomalies in only 11% of 74 teenagers with endometriosis (61). The clinical course of endometriosis associated with reproductive tract anomalies is quite different from that in the adult. Sanfilippo et al described a series of patients with extensive endometriosis in association with outflow tract obstruction (62). Once correction of the outflow tract occurred, there was virtually 100% reversal of intra-abdominal endometriosis on follow-up laparoscopy. It is thought that the pathophysiology of the disease process is different in the adult as compared with adolescents with an outflow tract obstruction. Interestingly, the fact that many adolescents without flow tract obstruction show significant endometriosis at the time of laparoscopy does support the theory of retrograde menstruation as an etiology for development of endometriosis. However, given that endometriosis resolves without further treatment after correction of the outflow tract abnormality suggests that retrograde menstruation, in and of itself, is not sufficient to induce a state of progressive endometriosis. Other factors besides retrograde menstruation, such as immune system defects, may be fundamental to creating an environment for induction of progressive endometriosis (63).

7. Patient symptoms

Although women with endometriosis may be asymptomatic, symptoms are common and typically include chronic pelvic pain and infertility. As previously stated, the current ASRM classification of endometriosis, which describes the extent of disease bulk, poorly predicts symptoms. Thus clinically, women with extensive disease (stage IV) may note few complaints, whereas those with minimal disease (stage I) may have significant pain or subfertility or both (68, 69).

The following symptoms can be caused by endometriosis based on clinical and patient experience:

- Severe dysmenorrhoea;
- Deep dyspareunia;
- Chronic pelvic pain;
- Ovulation pain;
- Cyclical or perimenstrual symptoms (e.g. bowel or bladder associated) with or without abnormal bleeding;
- Infertility;
- Chronic fatigue.

However, the predictive value of any one symptom or set of symptoms remains uncertain as each of these symptoms can have other causes. A large group of women with endometriosis is completely asymptomatic. In these women endometriosis remains undiagnosed or is diagnosed atlaparoscopy for another indication. A subset of women with more advanced disease, ovarian or deep invasive rectovaginal endometriosis, is asymptomatic as well. This makes the development of guidelines for the diagnosis and the therapy rather cumbersome. Endometriosis should be suspected in women with dysmenorrhoea, deep dyspareunia, acyclic chronic pelvic pain and/or subfertility.

8. Physical examination

Physical examination of the pelvis is useful for the diagnosis of deep infiltrating lesions or endometriotic cysts. The examination may be normal. It is more reliable when carried out during the menstrual period. Examination of the retrocervical area using the speculum, by vaginal and (possibly) rectal examination, is recommended. Examination of the vagina and cervix by speculum examination often reveals no signs of endometriosis. Occasionally, bluish or red powder-burn lesions may be seen on the cervix or the posterior fornix of the vagina. Pelvic organ palpation often reveals anatomic abnormalities suggestive of endometriosis. Uterosacral ligament nodularity and tenderness may reflect active disease or scarring along the ligament. In addition, an enlarged cystic adnexal mass may represent an ovarian endometrioma, which may be mobile or adherent to other pelvic structures (15, 63).

9. Differential diagnosis

The symptoms of endometriosis are nonspecific and may mimic many disease processes. Because endometriosis is a surgical diagnosis, several other diagnoses may be considered prior to surgical exploration. Since there is such an extremely variable presentation, an accurate differential diagnosis should always be performed in patients suspected of endometriosis. First of all, other gynecological disorders, such as ovarian and tubal diseases, pelvic inflammatory disease and ectopic pregnancy, should be excluded (16). Then a series of gut disorders should be considered; among these conditions, irritable bowel syndrome

(IBS) is worthy of particular attention (70). Crohn's disease should also be considered in the differential diagnosis of endometriosis, since this condition shows several similarities regarding both the locations and the anatomo-pathologic pattern (71). Although rare, familial Mediterranean fever (FMF) should be considered in the differential diagnosis of endometriosis (72). Rarely the presence of parasitic infestations has been reported in women with symptoms suggestive of endometriosis (73).

10. Laboratory testing

To exclude other causes of pelvic pain, laboratory investigations are often undertaken. Initially, a complete blood count (CBC), urinalysis and urine cultures, vaginal cultures, and cervical swabs may be obtained to exclude infections or sexually transmitted infections that may cause pelvic inflammatory disease (63).

Although concentrations of the cancer antigen CA125 are slightly raised in some women with endometriosis, the test neither excludes nor diagnoses endometriosis and is not considered useful in establishing the diagnosis. The threshold for surgery is unlikely to be influenced by the CA125 concentration and the guidelines from the Royal College of Obstetricians and Gynecologists described CA125 as having only limited value as either a screening or a diagnostic test (15).

11. Imaging and endometriosis

Endometriomas are uncommon in the adolescent population, and information regarding the adnexa can be obtained noninvasively with a pelvic ultrasound. Ultrasound as the primary imaging investigation can aid in its diagnosis. Transvaginal ultrasound (TVUS) with color flow Doppler can detect endometriomas with a high degree of accuracy. Ultrasound is limited in its ability to detect small peritoneal implants and adhesions (74).

MRI is an excellent imaging modality for the evaluation of patients with deep pelvic endometriosis, showing high accuracy in the diagnosis and prediction of disease extent. The MRI diagnosis of deep pelvic endometriosis is based on the conjoint presence of signal intensity and morphologic abnormalities in the anterior and posterior compartments of the pelvis and the presence of surrounding fibrosis. The use of endovaginal and rectal contrast is useful to better delineate the anatomy and map out the extent of disease. Atypical locations of deep pelvic and extrapelvic endometriosis have been presented and grouped under the term anterior endometriosis. An accurate diagnosis therefore resides in clinical awareness and systematic review via MRI. A key finding of malignant transformation is the presence of enhancing nodules in the endometrial cyst on T1-weighted images (74, 75).

12. Laparoscopic findings

Laparoscopy is the gold standard for the diagnosis and staging of endometriosis and allows for curative surgical resection at the same time. Patients found to have endometriosis at the time of laparoscopy should either be treated through surgical ablation, resection, or laser treatment. In addition, biopsy is recommended, as lesions of endometriosis in adolescents often take on a different appearance as compared with the typical powder-burn lesions seen in adults. Interestingly, clear or red endometriotic lesions are much more commonly seen in the adolescent population (76).

13. Histological confirmation

Histologic confirmation is essential in the diagnosis of endometriosis. The utility of peritoneal wash cytology for diagnosis of endometriosis has been reported. In most cases, only hemosiderin-laden macrophages are identified. The presence of endometrial cells is more specific but less sensitive than hemosiderin-laden macrophages for the diagnosis of endometriosis. The endometrial cells have been reported in 25%–52% of peritoneal washes done in endometriosis. However, recognition of endometrial cells as well as hemosiderin-laden macrophages is essential for diagnosis on morphological basis alone. Histologic examination of the tissue confirmed for endometriosis by the presence of both endometrioid glands and stroma (15).

14. Treatment

Treatment must be individualized, and the effect of the kind of treatment on quality of life must be considered. There is not any confidence that a uniform therapeutic way be enough and successful, however in the most of the patients there is not a curative treatment. The choice of treatment is based on various factors such as size, location and extent of the disease, type and severity of the symptomatology, wish for pregnancy, and age of the patient. (77) Planning for the treatment is based on two important symptoms: pain and infertility. All the therapeutic ways divide to two main surgical and medical treatments.

14.1 Medical treatment

1. Selective progestron receptor modulators, progestogens and anti progestins (Androgens)
2. Gn-RH agents
3. COC (Combined Oral Contraceptives)
4. Aromatase inhibitor & NSAIDs and cox2- inhibitors
5. Chinese Medications
6. Angiogenesis inhibitor
7. Gene Therapy
8. Modulation of Cytokines , inhibition of Matrix Metalloproteinase

I. Selective progestron receptor modulators, progestogens and anti progestins

a. Progestogens
   1. Medroxyprogestrone acetate / 30 mg / po / daily
   2. Megestrol acetate / 40 mg / po / daily
   3. Lynoestrenol / 10 mg / po / daily
   4. Dydrogestrone / 20-30 mg / daily

The role of the LNG IUS (Levonorgestrel intra uterin system) in management of this common and troublesome disorder has been evaluated by multiple studies.(78-80)

A pilot study examined the role of LNG IUS as a postoperative adjunct to surgical ablation for endometriosis. When compared with expectant management, the LNG IUS recipients had a reduced rate of recurrence of pelvic pain (2/20 compared with 9/20) and an increased rate of satisfaction (15/20 compared with 10/20). (81) The LNG IUS offers several advantages for control of pelvic pain associated with endometriosis, including effective contraception, minimal systemic effects, and up to 5 years of benefit, as compared with 6 months, typical of GnRHa treatment.

Dienogest (DNG), a progestin of 19-nortestosterone derivative, has good oral bioavailability and is highly selective for progesterone receptors. Owing to its antiovulatory, antiproliferative activities in endometrial cells, and its inhibitory effects on the secretion of cytokines, DNG is expected to be an effective treatment for endometriosis. Progesterone receptor-binding affinity is higher for DNG than for progesterone.

- DNG has moderate affinity to the progesterone receptor. DNG shows low binding to the androgen receptor and almost negligible binding to the estrogen receptor, glucocorticoid receptor and mineralcorticoid receptor.
- DNG has strong oral progestational activity but antiandrogenic activity.
- An oral DNG dose of 1 mg/day is required for inhibition of ovulation in cyclic women.
- DNG has an inhibitory effect on growth and cytokine production of endometriotic cells.
- DNG is as effective as triptorelin (gonadotropin-releasing hormone agonist) for consolidation therapy after surgery for the treatment of endometriosis.
- DNG is as effective as intranasal buserelin acetate for the relief of pain symptoms associated with endometriosis.(82)

Treatment with a GnRH-a followed by long-term dienogest therapy maintains the relief of endometriosis-associated pelvic pain achieved with GnRH-a therapy for at least 12months. This regimen reduces the amount of irregular uterine bleeding that often occurs during the early phase of dienogest therapy.(83)

Complex mechanisms involving promoter regulation may be responsible for the observed aberrations in (Estradiol Receptor a, b) ERa, ERb, and PR (progesterone Receptor) expression in endometriosis. The stromal cell component of endometriotic tissue may be the primary site of these abnormalities. In endometriotic stromal cells, ERb promoter is pathologically hypomethylated and therefore hyperactive, leading to very high ERb levels. ERb suppresses ERa expression and results in strikingly high ERb-to-ERa ratios in endometriotic cells.

It is possible that this consequence of PR-B deficiency is only the tip of the iceberg with regard to pathogenesis of endometriosis, and that numerous other molecular aberrations may also contribute to the development of resistance to hormone treatments in women with endometriosis. Selective ERb ligands that target high levels of ERb in endometriotic tissue may be clinically beneficial via disrupting this mechanism.(84) PR deficiency is likely responsible for increased levels of E2 in endometriosis because progesterone fails to induce the E2-metabolizing enzyme HSD17B2 in endometriotic tissue. Some conclusion resonates with gene expression microarray studies performed on eutopic endometrium of women with endometriosis compared with that from disease-free women.(85, 86) These studies on eutopic endometrium identified distinct molecular defects that are consistent with the progesterone resistance hypothesis.

ER b agonists act as immunomodulators, enhancing the immunologic response to the explants; a second possible explanation lies an antiangiogenic effect because ER b are present in endothelial cells of endometrial vasculature. Finally, it is possible that b receptor acts intracellularly as an ERa inhibitor, by dimerizing with the ERa molecules to form a faulty product (87).

b. Antiprogestins:
- Danazol 400-800 mg/day
- Gestrinone 1.25-2.5 Twice /week

The first medication approved for the treatment of endometriosis in the United States was the androgen danazol. The predominant mechanism of action appears to be suppression of midcycle luteinizing hormone (LH) surge, creating a chronic anovulatory state as a result, danazol creates a hypoestrogenic, hyperandrogenic state, inducing endometrial atrophy in endometriotic implants. The recommended dosage of danazol is 600 to 800 mg daily. Unfortunately, significant androgenic side effects develop at this dosage and include acne, hot flashes, hirsutism, adverse serum lipid profiles, voice deepening (possibly irreversible), elevation of liver enzymes, and mood changes. Moreover, due to possible teratogenicity, this medication should be taken in conjunction with effective contraception. Because of this adverse side-effect profile, danazol is prescribed less frequently, and when administered, its duration should be limited. Gestrinone (ethylnorgestrienone; R2323) is an antiprogestational agent prescribed in Europe for the treatment of endometriosis. Gestrinone equals the effectiveness of danazol and of GnRH agonists for relief of endometriosis-related pain. Mifepristone is a PA (Progestron Antagunist) currently approved only for use in medication abortion and, in some countries, as an emergency contraceptive, but 3 small trials have demonstrated a reduction in endometriosis symptoms with Mifepristone therapy.(88 ,89)

II. Gn-RH agents

- Lueprolide 500mg/DAY SC or 3.75 mg /month IM
- Gosereline 3.6 mg /month SC
- Buserelin IN 300 /day
- Nafarelin IN 200/day
- Triptorelin 3.75 mg /month IM

Treatment with GnRHa for 3 months is as effective as the 6-months treatment as far as pain is concerned, and when combined with estro-progestational agents ('add-back therapy') up to a maximum of 2 years, is effective for pain and safe in terms of protecting bone density.(77)

Like GnRH agonists, the GnRH antagonists share some homology with the native GnRH molecule. These drugs act by blocking the GnRH receptor directly and preventing it from activating. This result in a downregulation of the pituitary gland, a reduction of gonadotropin secretion, and a suppression of ovarian steroid production Unlike GnRH agonists, however, these drugs do not cause an initial stimulation of gonadotropin and ovarian hormone secretion. At the molecular level, GnRH antagonists interrupt the basic activation process of the GnRH receptor, blocking the receptor dimerization synthesis and secretion of luteinizing hormone (LH) and follicle stimulating hormone (FSH). Given the high binding affinity, relative abundance and long half-life of the antagonist, these molecules monopolize the GnRH receptors. As a result of the above characteristics, the

GnRH antagonists offer the theoretical advantage of working faster and more effectively than GnRH agonists, with better patient compliance because of earlier amelioration of symptoms (90).

III. COC (Combined Oral Contraceptives)

Hormone therapy obtains a good initial response, is well tolerated by patients, and can be discontinued if there are adverse effects. Combined hormone therapy with estrogens and progesterone [91] has been used for small lesions, with total or partial remission of the symptoms in a high percentage of cases. Medical treatment alone does not lead to the definitive cure of deep, severe endometriosis but only induces temporary disappearance of active lesions [92]

These drugs can be used conventionally in a cyclic regimen or may be used continuously, without a break for withdrawal menses. The continuous regimen may be preferable for its decreased frequency of menses for women who fail to achieve pain relief with cyclic COC therapy. To maintain relief from pelvic pain while minimizing hypoestrogenic side effects, several regimens are proposed. Oral contraceptives plus dienogest, a novel progestogen, or a gonadotropin-releasing hormone agonist with estrogen supplementation (add-back therapy) can be used in long-term administration. The relief from pelvic pain achieved with a gonadotropin-releasing hormone agonist can be sustained by long-term administration of a tapered dose of danazol or medium-to-low doses of oral contraceptives. Local treatment with the levonorgestrel-releasing intrauterine system is an option for long-term suppression of pelvic pain.(93) For patients with recurrent ovarian endometriosis after conservative surgery or conservative surgery plus medical therapy, LNG-IUS and COC (combined oral contraceptives) may be used to control and reduce endometriotic cysts, relieve pain and reduce the level of CA125. LNG-IUS has the advantages of a greater convenience and minor systemic side effects (94). Long-term OCP therapy can be a reliable adjuvant post-operative measure to prevent or reduce frequency/severity of recurrent dysmenorrhoea and anatomical relapse of endometriosis. Since both continuous and cyclic OCP administration regimens seem to have comparable effects, the choice of regimen can be modulated according to patient preferences. The protective effect seems to be related to the duration of treatment.(95)

IV. Aromatase inhibitor & NSAIDs and cox2- inhibitors

Large quantities of estrogen can be produced locally within ectopically located endometrium via an intracrine mechanism, via the expression of the enzyme aromatase. This enzyme, not expressed in normal endometrium, is stimulated by prostaglandin E2 (PGE2); the resulting estrogen production then stimulates PGE2, further enhancing estrogen. An obvious therapeutic target would thus be this aromatase enzyme and aromatase inhibitors were tested in the rodent endometriosis model, with good success [96].

The expression of COX-2 was recently demonstrated in ectopic endometrial cells, showing higher concentration with respect to the eutopic endometrium [97]. COX-2 selective inhibitor given at the minimal dosage is effective against the pelvic pain symptoms (dysmenorrhoea, dispareunia, and chronic pelvic pain) associated to endometriosis [98].

Aromatase inhibitors have similar hypoestrogenic side-effect profiles as GnRH agonists, but hold promise in severe, refractory cases of endometriosis.

Treatment of rats with induced endometriosis using the nonsteroidal aromatase inhibitor fadrozole hydrochloride or YMsl 1 resulted in a dose-dependent volume reduction of endometriosis transplants.(99, 100)

In a pilot study, preliminary data were generated suggesting a potential future use of this drug, but randomized controlled trials are needed to confirm these data.(101) The effect of medical treatment in terms of pain relief in women with rectovaginal endometriosis appear substantial.(102)

V. Chinese Medications (CM)

In recent years, the Chinese medicine treatment of EM has won favorable therapeutic effects with few adverse reactions. The CM treatment of EM puts stress on therapy according to syndrome differentiation, varying the treatment for different individuals and emphasizing different sides in different stages of a menstrual cycle. It is non-traumatic with less adverse effect and good long-term effectiveness. It is favorable in combination with various approaches like acupuncture and moxibustion, retention enema and Western medical treatment, and could be extensively applied in clinical practice to function effectively in improving clinical symptoms and physical signs of patients and raising their quality of life.(103) Dong, et al treated EM with Guizhi Fuling capsule combined with intervention paracentesis implemented under ultrasonographic guidance to achieve good efficacy. The patients' cystic fluid was drawn out through puncturing and then the cystic cavity was washed repeatedly with 0.5% Lidocaine, then absolute alcohol was injected into the cavity The outcome shows that the therapeutic efficacy in the two groups was the same, but adverse reaction of Guizhi Fuling Capsule was significantly less than that of Gestrinone.(104)

Xue treated 41 patients with Mifepristone (25 mg/d, starting from the 1st day of the menstruation) combined with Chinese decoction, consisting of chuanxiong, dragon's blood, peach kernel, achyranthes root, yanhusuo rhizome, typha, trogopterus dung, red peony root, Chinese angelica root, cyperus tuber, red sage root, etc., one dose a day for 6 successive months, and the total effective rate obtained was 92.7%, which was better than that of Mifepristone or Chinese herbal medicine alone.(105)

Yu used Xiaoyi Zhitong Decoction combined with Mifepristone to treat 76 patients for 3 months, which resulted in a total effective rate of 92% and a recurrent rate of 5.3%.(106)

VI. Angiogenesis inhibitors

The most prominently studied among angiogenic factors is the vascular endothelial growth factor (VEGF), which is responsible for inducing early vascular growth. In any event, one logical therapeutic step would be to attempt inhibition of these new vascular structures as a way of deterring the development of endometriosis. The only human study thus far conducted with an angiogenesis inhibitor was the treatment of endometriosis associated pain with thalidomide; pain relief was noted in these patients [107].

VII. Gene Therapy

HOX genes, encoding homeodomain transcription factors, are dynamically expressed in endometrium, where they are necessary for endometrial growth, differentiation, and implantation. In human endometrium, the expression of HOXA10 and HOXA11 is driven by sex steroids, with peak expression occurring at time of implantation in response to rising progesterone levels. However, the maximal HOXA10 and HOXA11 expression fails to occur in women with endometriosis resistance to progesterone which can explain inhospitable implantation environment and medical treatment failures in endometriosis. Alterations in progesterone receptor expression and decreased HOX gene expression secondary to hypermethylation of its promoter region are the possible mechanisms of the progesterone resistance. A gene therapy approach involving the manipulation of HOXA10 expression or by using DNA demethylation agents to restore methylation aberrations can potentially have a role in the future treatment of endometriosis.(108-110)

A new study compared women suffering chronic pelvic pain (CPP) secondary to endometriosis with women experiencing CPP due to either myofascial abdominal/pelvic pain or pelvic adhesions to determine if there are specific psychological variables uniquely associated with endometriosis .No differences were obtained across the three groups for any of the outcome measures. Effect size computation supported the absence of clinical differences across the groups for these measures. These findings fail to support the presence of a unique psychological profile or disproportionate psychological disturbance for women with CPP due to endometriosis. These data illustrate the importance of considering control groups that include chronic pain when exploring psychological contributions to specific chronic pain conditions.(111)

VIII. Modulation of Cytokines, lnhibition of Matrix Metalloproteinase

In rats with experimental endometriosis, recombinant human TNF-α-binding protein can reduce 64% of the size of endometriosis-like peritoneal lesions (112).

In nude mice, suppression of MMPs by progesterone or by a natural inhibitor slows the establishment of ectopic lesions by human endometrium. (113)

14.2 Surgical treatments

The goal of surgery is to excise all visible endometriotic lesions and associated adhesions-peritoneal lesions, ovarian cysts, deep rectovaginal endometriosis-and to restore normal anatomy.

Laparoscopy is the gold standard for diagnosis and the primary means of treatment at this time. Laparoscopy is used with different goals such as diagnosis, ablation, excision and lysis of adhesions.

Excisional removal of ovarian endometriomas seems superior to drainage and ablation for both improved spontaneous pregnancy rates and improved pain symptoms. Laparoscopic treatment of endometriosis carries a long-term substantial relief of symptoms for a significant percentage of women. (114) Laser ablation does not appear to be more effective than conventional electrosurgical ablation of endometriosis.

Radical procedures such as oophorectomy or total hysterectomy are indicated only in severe situations and can be performed either laparoscopically or by laparotomy. Laparotomy should be reserved for patients with advanced-stage disease who cannot undergo a laparoscopic procedure and for those in whom fertility conservation is not necessary.

In patients with severe endometriosis it has been recommended that surgical treatment be preceded by a 3-month course of medical treatment to reduce vascularization and nodular size (115).

Postoperative medical treatment is rarely indicated because it does not work based on randomized trials, because it prevents pregnancy, and the highest pregnancy rates occur during the first 6 to 12 months after conservative surgery (116, 117).

Presacral Neurectomy (PSN):

For some women, transection of presacral nerves lying within the interiliac triangle may provide relief of chronic pelvic pain. PSN is used in a limited manner and not recommended routinely for management of endometriosis related pain.

Laparoscopic presacral neurectomy can be offered to treat midline pelvic pain.(114, 118)

Deep Rectovaginal and Rectosigmoidal Endometriosis:

Surgical treatment of DIE (Deeply Infiltrating Endometriosis) requires a professional who is able to perform surgery in the gynaecological, urological, gastrointestinal and nervous structures of the pelvis, as the disease 'knows no boundaries'. There is no scientific validation either that a multispecialty team approach is superior for the treatment of bowel endometriosis, which could also make the multisurgeon model 'experimental' and therefore unethical. (119)

Preoperative laxatives, starch-free diet, and full bowel preparation are needed to allow perioperative bowel suturing, if needed. Ureter stents may be required before excision of peritoneal endometriosis surrounding the ureter. A multidisciplinary approach involving gynecologic and gastroenterologic surgeons and urologists is desirable.

Bladder endometriosis is rare .The common clinical manifestations of bladder endometriosis include menouria and urethral and pelvic pain syndrome occurring cyclically. Cystoscopy is the most useful diagnostic test with confirmation by histologic study. Treatment must be individualized according to the patient's age, desire for future pregnancies, the severity of the symptoms, the site affected, and whether other organs are involved. transurethral resection-endometrioma biopsy to confirm the diagnosis and hormone blockade with LH–RH analogues is the initial treatment most commonly used in recent years, despite an estimated recurrence of 25–35% .(120)

Analogues have been the medical treatment of choice because their introduction, and the estrogens, androgens, progestogens, and danazol used in previous years have fallen into disuse because they lead to more adverse effects. Analogues induce a postmenopause like anovulatory state, a hypogonadotropic hypogonadism with serum estrogen concentrations dropping to sterilization levels, which causes the endometrial tissue to regress. (121, 122)

Ureter endometriosis was related with reproductive tract endometriosis. It has insidious process resulting in difficulty for early diagnosis. It's important to treat pelvic deep infiltrating endometriosis and ovarian endometrioma to prevent ureter from further involvement. Post-operative treatment of pelvic endometriosis is the key point of preventing relapse of ureter endometriosis.(123) The laparoscopic approach for ureteral endometriosis is very well tolerated and has a reasonable incidence of complications, as well as a low rate of recurrence.

Considering the difficulty of achieving a strictly scientific approach to low disease prevalence, the surgeon dealing with ureteral endometriosis must adapt surgery to achieve a balance between conservative purposes and the risk of recurrence on the one hand, and a radical approach and risk of morbidity on the other. Ureterolysis could be used as the initial surgical step for patients with ureteral endometriosis, and may be the only treatment if the extension of ureteral involvement is limited in length and there is no residual ureteral damage or dilatation.

For patients displaying extended severe ureteral involvement, stenosis, or moderate or severe hydronephrosis with a high risk of having intrinsic ureteral disease, ureterolysis is probably insufficient and ureteroneocystostomy likely represents a wiser surgical strategy (124).

Long-term probability of pain recurrence after repeat conservative surgery for recurrent endometriosis varies between 20 and 40%. The association of presacral neurectomy to the treatment of endometriosis might be effective in reducing midline pain; however, no studies have evaluated this procedure among patients with recurrent disease. The medium-term outcome of hysterectomy for endometriosis-associated pain is quite satisfactory; nevertheless, probability of pain persistence after hysterectomy is 15% and risk of pain worsening 3–5%, with a six times higher risk of further surgery in patients with ovarian preservation as compared to ovarian removal. The conception rate among women undergoing repetitive surgery for recurrent endometriosis associated with infertility is 26%, whereas the overall crude pregnancy rate after a primary procedure is 41%.

Repeat conservative surgery for pelvic pain associated with recurrent endometriosis has the same limitations as primary surgery, with long-term cumulative recurrence rates ranging from 20 to 40%. Conversely, only one woman out of four will conceive after repeat conservative surgery for infertility, almost half the pregnancy rate after primary surgery and with no substantial advantages over IVF. (102)

Assisted Reproduction and Endometriosis:

The treatment of endometriosis-related infertility is dependent on the age of the woman, the duration of infertility, the stage of endometriosis, the involvement of ovaries, tubes, or both in the endometriosis process, previous therapy, associated pain symptoms, and the priorities of the patient, taking into account her attitude toward the disease, the cost of treatment, her financial means, and the expected results.

The success of surgery in relieving infertility is probably related to the severity of endometriosis. A recent retrospective multicenter analysis (125) reported cumulative pregnancy rates of 39%, 31%, 30%, and 25% in patients with endometriosis stages I , II, III, and IV, respectively ,12 months after surgical treatment.

Endometriosis-associated infertility can be successfully treated with intrauterine insemination, but only if it is done in combination with ovarian stimulation (126).

However, there is clear evidence that the pregnancy rate in an insemination program is lower in women with endometriosis than in women with unexplained infertility. (127, 128) More recent studies that reported a normal fertilization rate but a reduced implantation rate per embryo transferred in women obtaining oocytes from donors with endometriosis (129, 130). This reduced implantation rate could be related to increased interleukin-6 levels in follicular fluid of women with endometriosis when compared with controls (131).

15. Recurrence

Endometriosis tends to recur unless definitive surgery is performed. The recurrence rate is about 5% to 20% per year, reaching a cumulative rate of 40% after 5 years. Liu and coworkers found an approximately 15-percent rate of recurrence at 2 years following initial surgery. Pain recurs within 5 years in about one in five patients with pelvic pain treated by complete laparoscopic excision of visible endometriotic lesions (132).

16. References

[1] Baldi A, Campioni M, Signorile P G. Endometriosis: pathogenesis, diagnosis, therapy and association with cancer. Oncology Reports 2008; 19: 843–6.
[2] Shroen D. Disputatioin auguralis medica de ulceribus uteri. Jena: Krebs; 1690. p. 6–17.
[3] Sampson J A. Peritoneal endometriosis due to menstrual dissemination of endometrial tissue into the peritoneal cavity. American Journal of Obstetric and Gynecology 1927; 14:422–69.
[4] Koninckx P R, Meuleman C, Demeyere S, Lesaffre E, Cornillie F J. Suggestive evidence that pelvic endometriosis is a progressive disease, where as deeply infiltrating endometriosis is associated with pelvic pain. Fertil Steril. 1991; 55:759–765.
[5] Razzaghi M R, Rahjoo T, Golshan A. Endometriosis with Pure Urinary Symptoms. Urol J. 2009; 6:132-4.
[6] Halis G, Arici A. Endometriosis and inflammation in infertility. Ann NY Acad Sci. 2004;1034,300-315.
[7] Wu M H, Shoji Y, Chuang P C, Tsa S J. Endometriosis: disease pathophysiology and the role of prostaglandins. Mol med. 2007; 9(2):
[8] Brosens IA. Endometriosis–a disease because it is characterized by bleeding. Am J Obstet Gynecol. 1997; 176,263-267.
[9] Fauconnier A, Chapron C. Endometriosis and pelvic pain: epidemiological evidence of the relationship and implications. Hum Reprod Update. 2005; 11,595-606.
[10] Cramer D W. Epidemiology of endometriosis in adolescents. In: Wilson EA (ed) Endometriosis. Alan Liss, (1987) NewYork pp5–8
[11] Kuohung W, Jones GL, Vitonis AF etal. Characteristics of patients with endometriosis in the United States and the United Kingdom. Fertil Steril. 2002; 78:767–772.
[12] VanGorp T, Amant F, Neven P, VergoteI, Moerman P. Endometriosis and the development of malignant tumors of the pelvis: a review of literature. Best Pract Res Clin Obstet Gynaecol. 2004; 18:349–371.

[13] Kennedy S, Bergqvist A, Chapron C, et al: ESHRE guideline for the diagnosis and treatment of endometriosis. Hum Reprod. 2005; 20(10):2698.

[14] Marchino GL, Gennarelli G, Enria R, et al: Diagnosis of pelvic endometriosis with use of macroscopic versus histologic findings. Fertil Steril. 2005; 84:12.

[15] Farquhar C. Endometriosis. BMJ 2007; 334:249-53

[16] Montalto M, Santoro L, D'Onofrio F, Gallo A, Campo S, Campo V, Gasbarrini A, Gasbarrini G. Endometriosis, need for a multidisciplinary clinical setting: the internist's point of view. Intern Emerg Med. 2010; 5(6):463-7.

[17] Halme J, Hammond MG, Hulka JF, Raj SG, Talbert LM. Retrograde menstruation in healthy women and in patients with endometriosis. Obstet Gynecol. 1984; 64:151-154

[18] Troyer MR. Differential Diagnosis of Endometriosis in a Young Adult Woman With Nonspecific Low Back Pain. Physical Therapy. 2007; 87(6): 801-10

[19] Keettel WC, Stein RJ. The viability of the cast-off menstrual endometrium. Am J Obstet Gynecol. 1951 Feb;61(2):440-2.

[20] Mungyer G, Willemsen WN, Rolland R, Vemer HM, Ramaekers FC, Jap PH, Poels LG. Cell of the mucous membrane of the female genital tract in culture: a comparative study with regard to the histogenesis of endometriosis. In Vitro Cell Dev Biol. 1987 Feb;23(2):111-7.

[21] Ridley JH, Edwards IK. Experimental endometriosis in the human. Am J Obstet Gynecol. 1958 Oct;76(4):783-9

[22] Signorile PG, Baldi A. Endometriosis: new concepts in the pathogenesis. Int J Biochem Cell Biol. 2010 Jun;42(6):778-80.

[23] Nisolle M, Donnez J. Peritoneal endometriosis, ovarian endometriosis, and adenomyotic nodules of the rectovaginal septum are three different entities. Fertility and Sterility. 1997;68:585–95.

[24] Bulun SE. Endometriosis. New England Journal of Medicine.2009;360:268–79.

[25] Matsuura K, Ohtake H, Katabuchi H, et al: Coelomic metaplasia theory of endometriosis: evidence from in vivo studies and an in vitro experimental model. Gynecol Obstet Invest 47(Suppl 1):18, 1999

[26] Mitchell AO, Hoffman AP, Swartz SE, et al: An unusual occurrence of endometriosis in the right groin: a case report and review of the literature. Mil Med 156:633, 1991

[27] Pollack R, Gordon PH, Ferenczy A, et al: Perineal endometriosis. A case report. J Reprod Med 35:109, 1990

[28] Wu MH, Shoji Y, Chuang PC, Tsai SJ. Endometriosis: disease pathophysiology and the role of prostaglandins. Expert Rev Mol Med. 2007 Jan 16;9(2):1-20.

[29] Tsai SJ etal.(2001)Regulation of steroidogenic acute regulatory protein expression and progesterone production in endometriotic stromal cells. J Clin Endocrinol Metab 86, 5765-5773

[30] Noble LS. etal. (1996) Aromatase expression in endometriosis. J Clin Endocrinol Metab 81, 174-179

[31] Guo SW. Epigenetics of endometriosis. Mol Hum Reprod. 2009 Oct;15(10):587-607.

[32] Seli E, Arici A: Endometriosis: interaction of immune and endocrine systems. Semin Reprod Med 21:135, 2003

[33] Zhang RJ, Wild RA, Ojago JM. Effect of tumor necrosis factor-alpha on adhesion of human endometrial stromal cells to peritoneal mesothelia cells: an invitro system. Fertil Steril. 1993;59:1196–1201.

[34] Bullimore DW. Endometriosis is sustained by tumour necrosis factor-alpha. Med Hypotheses. 2003; 60:84–88.

[35] Eisermann J, Gast MJ, Pineda J, Odem RR, Collins JL. Tumor necrosis factor in peritoneal fluid of women undergoing laparoscopic surgery. Fertil Steril. 1988; 50:573–579.

[36] Calhaz-Jorge C, Costa AP, Barata M, Santos MC, Melo A, Palma-Carlos ML. Tumour necrosis factor alpha concentrations in the peritoneal fluid of infertile women with minimal or mild endometriosis are lower in patients with red lesions only than in patients without red lesions. Hum Reprod. 2000; 15:1256–1260.

[37] Bedaiwy MA, Falcone T, Sharma RK, et al. Prediction of endometriosis with serum and peritoneal fluid markers: a prospective controlled trial. Hum Reprod. 2002; 17:426–431.

[38] Kauppila A, Puolakka J, Ylikorkala O. Prostaglandin biosynthesis inhibitors and endometriosis. Prostaglandins. 1979; 18:655–661.

[39] Dawood MY, Khan-Dawood FS, Wilson L Jr. Peritoneal fluid prostaglandins and prostanoids in women with endometriosis, chronic pelvic inflammatory disease, and pelvic pain. Am J Obstet Gynecol. 1984; 148:391–395.

[40] Koike H, Egawa H, Ohtsuka T, Yamaguchi M, Ikenoue T, Mori N. Correlation between dysmenorrheic severity and prostaglandin production in women with endometriosis. Prostaglandins Leukot Essent Fatty Acids. 1992; 46:133–137.

[41] Matsuzaki S, Canis M, Pouly J-L, Wattiez A, Okamura K, Mage G. Cyclooxygenase-2 expression in deep endometriosis and matched eutopic endometrium. Fertil Sterill. 2004; 82:1309–15.

[42] Ota H, Igarashi S, Sasaki M, Tanaka T. Distribution of cycloozygenase-2 in eutopic endometrium in endometriosis and adenomyosis. Human Reprod. 2001; 16:561–6.

[43] Tietjen GE, Bushnell CD, Herial NA, et al. Endometriosis is associated with prevalence of comorbid conditions in migraine. Headache. 2007; 47:1069–1078.

[44] Pasoto SG, Abrao MS, Viana VS, et al. Endometriosis and systemic lupus erythematosus: a comparative evaluation of clinical manifestations and serological autoimmune phenomena. Am J Reprod Immunol. 2005; 53:85–93.

[45] Sinaii N, Cleary SD, Ballweg ML, et al. High rates of autoimmune and endocrine disorders, fibromyalgia, chronic fatigue syndrome and atopic diseases among women with endometriosis: a survey analysis. Hum Reprod. 2002; 17:2715–2724.

[46] Lamb K, Nichols TR. Endometriosis: a comparison of associated disease histories. Am J Prev Med. 1986; 2:324–329.

[47] Simpson J, Elias S, Malinak LR, et al. A Heritable aspect of endometriosis: genetic studies. Am J Obstet Gynecol. 1980; 137:327–331.

[48] Di W, Guo SW. The search for genetic variants predisposing women to endometriosis. Curr Opin Obstet Gynecol. 2007; 19:395–401.

[49] Weiss G, Maseela llP,Schott LL, Brockwell SE, Schocken M, Johnston JM. Adenomyosis a variant not a disease? Evidence from hysterectomized menopausal women in the Study of Women's Health Across the Nation (SWAN). Fertil Steril 2008
[50] Zondervan KT, Cardon LR, Kennedy SH. (2002) What makes a good case-control study? Design issues for complex traits such as endometriosis. Hum Reprod. 17,1415-1423
[51] Foster WG, Agarwal SK. (2002) Environmental contaminants and dietary factors in endometriosis. Ann NY Acad Sci. 955, 213-229
[52] Tsutsumi O. (2005) Assessment of human contamination of estrogenic endocrine-disrupting chemicals and their risk for human reproduction. J Steroid Biochem Mol Biol. 93,325-330
[53] Missmer SA. etal. (2004) Inutero exposures and the incidence of endometriosis. Fertil Steril. 82,1501-1508
[54] Arisawa K,Takeda H, Mikasa H.(2005) Background exposure to PCDDs/PCDFs/PCBs and its potential health effects: a review of epidemiologic studies. J Med Invest. 52,10-21
[55] Bock KW, Kohle C. Ah receptor: dioxin-mediated toxic responses as hints to deregulated physiologic functions. Biochem Pharmacol. 2006; 72:393–404.
[56] Puga A,Tomlinson CR, Xia Y. Ah receptor signals cross-talk with multiple developmental pathways. Biochem Pharmacol. 2005;69:199–207.
[57] Ohtake F, Takeyama K, Matsumoto T, Kitagawa H, Yamamoto Y, Nohara K, Tohyama C, Krust A, Mimura J, Chambon P. Modulation of estrogen receptor signal ling by association with the activated dioxin receptor. Nature 2003;423:545–550.
[58] Breech LL, Laufer MR: Obstructive anomalies of the female reproductive tract. J Reprod Med 44:233, 1999
[59] Schattman GL, Grifo JA, Birnbaum S: Laparoscopic resection of a non-communicating rudimentary uterine horn. A case report. J Reprod Med 40:219, 1995
[60] Schifrin BS, Erez S, Moore JG.Teen-age endometriosis. Am J Obstet Gynecol. 1973; 116:973–980.
[61] Goldstein DP, deCholnoky C, Leventhal JM, et al. New insights into the old problem of chronic pelvic pain. J Pediatr Surg. 1979; 14:675–680.
[62] Sanfilippo JS, Wakim NG, Schikler KN, et al. Endometriosis in association with uterine anomaly. Am J Obstet Gynecol. 1986;154:39–43.
[63] Dovey S, Sanfilippo J. Endometriosis and the adolescent. Clin Obstet Gynecol. 2010 Jun;53(2):420-8.
[64] Houston DE, Noller KL, Melton LJ III, et al: Incidence of pelvic endometriosis in Rochester, Minnesota, 1970–1979. Am J Epidemiol 125:959, 1987
[65] Adamson GD, Pasta DJ. Endometriosis fertility index: the new, validated endometriosis staging system. Fertil Steril. 2010 Oct;94(5):1609-15.
[66] Chapron C, Fauconnier A, Vieira M, Barakat H, Dousset B, Pansini V, Vacher-Lavenu MC, Dubuisson JB. Anatomical distribution of deeply infiltrating endometriosis: surgical implications and proposition for a classification. Hum Reprod. 2003;18(1):157-61.

[67] Koninckx PR, Meuleman C, Demeyere S, Lesaffre E, Cornillie FJ. Suggestive evidence that pelvic endometriosis is a progressive disease, whereas deeply infiltrating endometriosis is associated with pelvic pain. Fertil Steril. 1991 Apr;55(4):759-65.

[68] Arruda MS, Petta CA, Abrão MS, Benetti-Pinto CL. Time elapsed from onset of symptoms to diagnosis of endometriosis in a cohort study of Brazilian women. Hum Reprod. 2003 Apr;18(4):756-9.

[69] Hadfield R, Mardon H, Barlow D, Kennedy S. Delay in the diagnosis of endometriosis: a survey of women from the USA and the UK. Hum Reprod. 1996 Apr;11(4):878-80.

[70] Talley N, Zinsmeister AR, VanDyke C, Melton Lrd (1991) Epidemiology of colonic symptoms and the irritable bowel syndrome. Gastroenterology. 101:927–934

[71] Teke Z, Aytekin FO, Atalay AO, Demirkan NC (2008) Crohn's disease complicated by multiple stenoses and internal fistulas clinically mimicking small bowel endometriosis. World J Gastroenterol 14:146–151

[72] Onen F (2006) Familial Mediterranean fever. Rheumatol Int 26:489–496

[73] Poliness A, Lee A, Wein P, Moss S(2004) Pelvic helminthic disease masquerading as endometriosis. Aust NZ J Obstet Gynaecol 44:72–74

[74] Griffin Y, Sudigali V, Jacques A. Radiology of benign disorders of menstruation. Semin Ultrasound CT MR. 2010 Oct;31(5):414-32.

[75] Marcal L, Nothaft MA, Coelho F, Choi H. Deep pelvic endometriosis: MR imaging. Abdom Imaging. 2010 Dec;35(6):708-15. Review.

[76] Catenacci M, Sastry S, Falcone T. Laparoscopic surgery for endometriosis. Clin Obstet Gynecol. 2009 Sep;52(3):351-61.

[77] Luisi S, Lazzeri L, Ciani V, Petraglia F. Endometriosis in Italy: from cost estimates to new medical treatment. Gynecol Endocrinol. 2009 Nov;25(11):734-40.

[78] Bahamondes L, Petta CA, Fernandes A, Monteiro I. Use of the levonorgestrel-releasing intrauterine system in women with endometriosis, chronic pelvic pain and dysmenorrhea. Contraception 2007;75:S134-9.

[79] Petta CA, Ferriani RA, Abrao MS, et al. Randomized clinical trial of a levonorgestrel-releasing intrauterine system and a depot GnRH analogue for the treatment of chronic pelvic pain in women with endometriosis. Hum Reprod 2005;20:1993-8.

[80] Petta CA, Ferriani RA, Abrao MS, et al. A 3-year follow-up of women with endometriosis and pelvic pain users of the levonorgestrel-releasing intrauterine system. Eur J Obstet Gynecol Reprod Biol 2009;143:128-9.

[81] 81. Vercellini P, Frontino G, De Giorgi O, Aimi G, Zaina B, Crosignani PG. Comparison of a levonorgestrel-releasing intrauterine device versus expectant management after conservative surgery for symptomatic endometriosis: a pilot study. Fertil Steril 2003;80:305-9.

[82] Harada T, Taniguchi F. Dienogest: a new therapeutic agent for the treatment of endometriosis. Womens Health (Lond Engl). 2010 Jan;6(1):27-35. Review.

[83] Kitawaki J, Kusuki I, Yamanaka K, Suganuma I. Maintenance therapy with dienogest following gonadotropin-releasing hormone agonist treatment for endometriosis-associated pelvic pain. Eur J Obstet Gynecol Reprod Biol. 2011 Apr 5. [Epub ahead of print]

[84] Bulun SE, Cheng YH, Pavone ME, Yin P, Imir G, Utsunomiya H, Thung S, Xue Q, Marsh EE, Tokunaga H, Ishikawa H, Kurita T, Su EJ. 17Beta-hydroxysteroid dehydrogenase-2 deficiency and progesterone resistance in endometriosis. Semin Reprod Med. 2010 Jan;28(1):44-50.
[85] Kao LC, Germeyer A, Tulac S, et al. Expression profiling of endometrium from women with endometriosis reveals candidate genes for disease-based implantation failure and infertility. Endocrinology 2003;144(7):2870–2881
[86] Burney RO, Talbi S, Hamilton AE, et al. Gene expression analysis of endometrium reveals progesterone resistance and candidate susceptibility genes in women with endometriosis. Endocrinology 2007;148(8):3814–3826
[87] Pavao M, Traish AM. Estrogen receptor antibodies: specificity and utility in detection, localization and analyses of estrogen receptor a and b. Steroids 2001;66:1–16.
[88] Speroff L, Darney PF. A clinical guide for contraception. Philadelphia: Lippincott Williams & Wilkins; 2005
[89] Chabbert-Buffet N, Meduri G, Bouchard P, Spitz IM. Selective progesterone receptor modulators and progesterone antagonists: mechanisms of action and clinical applications. Hum Reprod Update 2005;11:293-307.
[90] Kupker W, Felberbaum RE, Krapp M, Schill T, Malik E, Diedrich K. Use of GnRH antagonists in the treatment of endometriosis. Reprod Biomed Online 2002;5:12–16.
[91] Westney OL, Amundsen CL, McGuire EJ (2000) Bladder endometriosis: conservative management. J Urol 163:1814–1817
[92] Vercellini P, Frontino G, Pietropaolo G, Gattei U, Daguati R, Crosignani PG (2004) Deep endometriosis: definition, pathogenesis, and clinical management. J Am Assoc Gynecol Laparosc 11:153–161
[93] Kitawaki J. Maintenance therapy for endometriosis. Nippon Rinsho. 2010 Jan;68(1):163-7.
[94] Xu XW, Wang LD, Zhu XQ, Yan LZ, Guan YT, Zhu SC, Hu Y. Levonorgestrel-releasing intrauterine system and combined oral contraceptives as conservative treatments for recurrent ovarian endometriosis: a comparative clinical study. Zhonghua Yi Xue Za Zhi. 2011 Apr 19;91(15):1047-50.
[95] Seracchioli R, Mabrouk M, Manuzzi L, Vicenzi C, Frascà C, Elmakky A, Venturoli S. Post-operative use of oral contraceptive pills for prevention of anatomical relapse or symptom-recurrence after conservative surgery for endometriosis. Hum Reprod. 2009 Nov;24(11):2729-35. Epub 2009 Jul 22.
[96] Bulun SE, Zeitoun KM, Takayama K, Sasano H. Molecular basis for treating endometriosis with aromatase inhibitors. Human Reprod Update 2000;6:413–418
[97] Ota H, Igarashi S, Sasaki M, Tanaka T. Distribution of cyclooxygenase-2 in eutopic and ectopic endometrium in endometriosis and adenomyosis. Hum Reprod 2001;16:561- 566.
[98] Cobellis L, Razzi S, De Simone S, Sartini A, Fava A, Danero S, Gioffre` W, Mazzini M, Petraglia F. The treatment with a COX-2 specific inhibitor is effective in the management of pain related to endometriosis. EJOGRB 2004;116: 100–102.

[99] Kudoh M, Susaki Y, Ideyama Y, et al. Inhibitory effects of a novel aromatase inhibitor, YM5 1 I, in rats with experimental endometriosis. J Steroid Biochem Mol Biol 19971'63:.1

[100] Takayama K, Zeitoun K, Gunby RT, et al. Treatment of severe postmenopausal endometriosis with an aromatase inhibitor. FertiI SteriI 1998: 69: '70 9-i | 3

[101] Ailawadi RK, Jobanputra S, Kataria M, et al. Treatment of endometriosis and chronic pelvic pain with letrozole and norethindrone acetate: a pilot study. Fertil Steril 2004;81(2):290-296.

[102] Vercellini P, Crosignani PG, Somigliana E, Berlanda N, Barbara G, Fedele L.Medical treatment for rectovaginal endometriosis: what is the evidence? Hum Reprod. 2009 Oct;24(10):2504-14.

[103] Jiang H, Shen Y, Wang XG. Current progress of Chinese medicinal treatment of endometriosis. Chin J Integr Med. 2010 Jun;16(3):283-8. Epub 2010 Aug 8.

[104] Dong SW, Wang SZ, Chen LY, Li GH. Effect of Guizhi Fuling Capsule combined with interventional ultrasound puncture in treatment of ovarian endometriosis cyst. Chin J Integr Tradit West Med Intens Crit Care, 2003;10:313-314.

[105] Xue XH, lian XL. Effect of 41 cases with endometriosis in treatment of integrative medicine. Shaanxi J Tradit Chin Med 2007;28:1194-1195 .

[106] Yu JS. Clinical observation on endometriosis in treatment of integrative medicine. J Pract Diagn Therapy 2005;19:383-384.

[107] Scarpellini F, Sbracia M, Lecchini S, Scarpellini L. Antiangiogenesis treatment with thalidomide in endometriosis: a pilot study. Fertil Steril 2002;78:87.

[108] Cakmak H, Taylor HS. Molecular mechanisms of treatment resistance in endometriosis: the role of progesterone-hox gene interactions. Semin Reprod Med. 2010 Jan;28(1):69-74.

[109] Jones PA, Baylin SB. The fundamental role of epigenetic events in cancer. Nat Rev Genet 2002;3(6):415–428

[110] Robertson KD. DNA methylation and human disease. Nat Rev Genet 2005;6(8):597–610

[111] Roth RS, Punch M, Bachman JE. Psychological Factors in Chronic Pelvic Pain due to Endometriosis: A Comparative Study. Gynecol Obstet Invest. 2011 May 21. [Epub ahead of print]

[112] D'Antonio M, Martelli F, Peano S, et al. Ability of recombinant human TNF binding protein-1 (r-hTBPl) to inhibit the development of experimentally induced endometriosis in rats. "/ Reprod Immunol 2000;48:81-98

[113] Bruner KL, Matrisian LM, Rodgers WH, et al. Suppression of matrix metalloproteinases inhibits establishment of ectopic lesions by human endometrium in nude mice. J Clin Invest 1997 | '99:2851-2857

[114] Catenacci M, Sastry S, Falcone T. Laparoscopic surgery for endometriosis. Clin Obstet Gynecol. 2009 Sep;52(3):351-61.

[115] Koninckx PR, Oosterlynck D, D'Hooghe TM, et al. Deeply infiltrating endometriosis is a disease where as mild endometriosis could be considered a non-disease. Ann N Y Acad Sci 1994;734:333-341

[116] Vercellini P, Crosignani PG, Fadini R, et al. A gonadotropin-releasing hormone agonist compared with expectant management after conservative surgery for symptomatic endometriosis B r J Obstet Gynecol 1999; 106:672471

[117] Parazzini F Fedele L, Busacca M, et al, Postsurgical treatment of advanced endometriosis: results of a randomized clinical trial. Am J Obstet Gynecol 1994;171:1205-1207.

[118] Porproa MG, Koninchx PR, Piazze J, et al. Correlation between endometriosis and pelvic pain. J Am Assoc Gynecol Laparosc. 1999;6:429–434.

[119] Pereira RM, Zanatta A, Serafini PC, Redwine D.The feasibility of laparoscopic bowel resection performed by a gynaecologist to treat endometriosis. Curr Opin Obstet Gynecol. 2010 Aug;22(4):344-53.

[120] Sanchez Merino JM, Guillan Maquieira C, Garcia Alonso J (2005) Tratamiento de la endometriosis vesical. Revisión de la literature española. Arch Esp Urol 58:189-194

[121] Bologna RA, Whitmore KE (2001) La endometriosis genitourinaria. In: Ball TP (ed) AUA update series, vol 1 (Spanish ed). Medical Trends, Barcelona, pp 21–29

[122] Leiva O, Ortiz Vico F (1998) Endocervicosis de la vía urinaria: sistema mülleriano secundario. In: Patologías excepcionales en Urología. Ed. Luzán, Madrid, pp 11–43

[123] Li L, Leng JH, Lang JH, Liu ZF, Sun DW, Zhu L, Fan QB, Shi JH. Diagnosis and treatment of ureter endometriosis. Zhonghua Fu Chan Ke Za Zhi. 2011 Apr;46(4):266-70.

[124] Marco Camanni, Elena M. Delpiano, Luca Bonino and Francesco Deltetto Current Opinion in Obstetrics and Gynecology 2010, 22:309–314

[125] Guzick DS,Canis M, Silliman NP, et al. Prediction of pregnancy in infertile women based on the ASRM's revised classification for endometriosis. FertiI SteriI 1997; 67 :822-83 6.

[126] Ttrmmon IS, Asher LS, Martin JRB, et al. Randomized controlled trial of superovulation and insemination for infertility associatedw ith minimal or mild endometriosis. Fertil Steril 1991;68:8-12.

[127] Nuojua HS, Tomas C, Bloigu R, et al. Intrauterine insemination treatment in subfertility: an analysis of factors affecting outcome. Hwn Reprod 1999:14:698-703

[128] Omland AK, Tanbo T, Dale PO, et al. Artificial insemination by husband in unexplained infertility compared with infertility associated with peritoneal endometriosis. Hum Reprod 1998;13:2602-2605.

[129] Simon C, Guttierez A, Vidal A, et al. Outcome of patients with endometriosis in assisted reproduction: results from in-vitro fertilization and oocyte donation. Hum Reprod 1994;9:725-729.

[130] Arici A, Oral E, Bukulmez O, et al. The effect of endometriosis on implantation: results from the Yale University in vitro fertilization and embryo transfer program. Fertil Steril 1996;65:603-6O7.

[131] Pellicer A, Valbuena D, Bauset C, et al. The follicular endocrine environment in stimulated cycles of women with endometriosis: steroid levels and embryo quality. Fertil Steril 1998;69:1135-1141

[132] Redwine DB. Conservativela paroscopice xcisiono f endometriosisb y sharpd issection:life table analysis of reoperation and persistent of recurrent disease. Fertil Steril 1991;56:628-634

2

Urinary Tract Endometriosis

Aliasghar Yarmohamadi and Nasser Mogharabian
Ghaem Hospital, Mashhad University of Medical Sciences, Mashhad, Iran

1. Introduction

Endometriosis is defined as the presence of functional endometrial tissue in an ectopic site (outside of the uterus). Although endometriosis is usually confined to the ovaries, uterosacral ligaments, and cul-de-sac, it has been documented in almost every organ system in the body.

Endometriosis was first described by Russel in 1955. Endometriosis is a common disorder of the female reproductive organs and is the leading cause of chronic pelvic pain in women.

It is one of the most complex and least understood diseases in their field and, despite many theories, we still do not have a clear understanding of its causes.

There is no relationship of endometriosis to race or socioeconomic status but it has a strong familial link. If sister or mother of a woman has the condition, then she is approximately five to six times more likely to develop it.

Because ovarian function is necessary for the development and maintenance endometrial implants, endometriosis has been reported only in the reproductive ages and so, is normally not seen before age 15 or after menopause. Endometriosis is most common in women between the ages of 25 and 35. However, after menopause, there are two factors which may promote or maintain endometriosis. One is the use of estrogen replacement therapy and the other is the presence of high endogenous estrogen in obese patients.

There have been several case reports of histological endometriosis in men , all of them in the prostate. These have occurred all in men with cancer of the prostate who were undergoing high-dose estrogen therapy.

The prevalence of endometriosis in specific categories of patients has been reported (Table.1), but the prevalence in the general population is not definitely known because a majority of patients are asymptomatic. It is estimated that affect 10% to 20% of women of reproductive age, with a peak incidence in the mid-20s. However, in women with severe menstrual cramps, the incidence of endometriosis has been reported to be between 25 and 35 percent.

Although endometriosis is a benign condition but it may have an aggressive clinical behaviour. Many women with urinary tract endometriosis have few or no symptoms. Some present with infertility. Other manifestations include urgency, frequency, pain on passing urine, pain in the flank or the back region or recurrent urinary tract infections. Some women have cyclic hematuria at times of menstruation. Some patients give a history of gynecologic surgeries such as hysterectomy many years ago.

Women of reproductive age(overall)	10 to 20 percent
Women with a history of major surgery for any gynecologic indication	1 percent
Women undergoing tubal sterilization	1 to 7 percent
Following laparoscopy to determine the cause of pelvic pain	12 to 32 percent
Women undergoing laparoscopy for infertility	9 to 50 percent
Women undergoing laparoscopy without infertility	6.7 percent
Teenagers undergoing laparoscopy for evaluation of chronic pelvic pain or dysmenorrheal	50 percent

Table 1. The prevalence of endometriosis in women groups of reproductive age.

It can be associated with many distressing and debilitating symptoms may be asymptomatic, and incidentally discovered at laparoscopy or exploratory surgery. Usually, endometriosis is confined to the pelvic and lower abdominal cavity; however, it has occasionally been reported to be in other areas. Endometriotic lesions of the urinary tract are present in 1 to 4 percent of women with endometriosis and often coexists with disease at other sites of the body.

Although ureteral and bladder endometriosis both occur in the urinary tract, they do not frequently coexist and their clinical presentation and management are different. Bladder endometriosis often mimicks recurrent cystitis, but rarely results in severe sequelae. Ureteral endometriosis is often asymptomatic, but can lead to silent loss of renal function. Renal and urethral involvements are rare and only as case reports.

Overall	unclear but may occur in 1 -4% of all cases of endometriosis
Bladder	70 – 80 percent of all urinary tract involvements
Ureter	15 – 20 percent of all urinary tract involvements
Kidney	4 percent of all urinary tract involvements
Urethra	2 percent of all urinary tract involvements

Table 2. The prevalence of endometriosis in urinary tract.

The optimal way to diagnose endometriosis is by direct visualization and biopsy of the implant(s) anywhere through the body.

2. Ethiology and pathogenesis

The classic definition of endometriosis is as the presence of endometrial glands and stroma at extrauterine sites. These ectopic endometrial implants are usually located in the pelvis, but can occur nearly anywhere in the body. It can be associated with many distressing and debilitating symptoms or may be asymptomatic, and incidentally discovered at laparoscopy or exploratory surgery.

The pathogenesis of endometriosis has not been definitively established but predominant hypotheses are as follows:

- **The implantation theory:** This theory proposes that endometrial cells are either transported during menstruation through the fallopian tubes and implanted on pelvic structures (transtubal regurgitation or retrograde menstruation) or are transplanted to surgical scars (episiotomy, laparotomy) as a result of surgery or delivery.
- **Lymphatics and blood vessels dissemination:** This theory is specially useful for explanation of endometriosis at locations outside the pelvis(extraperitoneal disease).
- **Coelomic metaplasia:** This theory proposes that the peritoneal cavity contains undifferentiated cells capable of differentiating into endometrial tissue. It is said that repeated inflammation may induce metaplasia of mesothelial cells to the endometrial epithelium.

Genetic factors probably influence an individual's susceptibility to endometriosis. The possibility of a familial tendency for endometriosis has been recognized for several decades. If a woman has endometriosis, a first-degree relative has a 7 percent likelihood of developing the disorder as compared with 1 percent in unrelated persons. Concordance in twins has also been observed.

There is evidence for altered humoral and cell-mediated immunity in the pathogenesis of endometriosis such as Deficient cellular immunity, improper Natural killer cell activity and increased concentration of leukocytes and macrophages in the peritoneal cavity and ectopic endometrium. These variations in immune system may result in an inability to recognize the presence of endometrial tissue in abnormal locations, decreased cytotoxicity to autologous ectopic endometrium and finally, secretion of cytokines and growth factors by leukocytes and macrophages into the peritoneal fluid of women with endometriosis.

One hypothesis is that secretion of various cytokines by inflammatory cells into the peritoneal cavity leads to proliferation of implants and recruitment of capillaries. Oxidative stress may be another component of the inflammatory reaction. Thus, the immune system may play a role in determining who will develop endometriosis, as well as the extent and clinical manifestation of the disease.

It is said that these women had higher rates of autoimmune inflammatory diseases, hypothyroidism, fibromyalgia, chronic fatigue syndrome, allergies and asthma, compared with the general female population so, it could provide support for the theory of altered immune system in women with endometriosis.

Vesical endometriosis is said that may be due to bladder adenomyosis or an extension of adenomyosis from the uterus into the bladder or because of imperfect closure of the uterus during a cesarean delivery.

The risk of endometriosis developing into a cancerous lesion is very low(1 - 2.5%) and the same as normal endometrium and ovaries.

Endometriosis is a common, benign, chronic, estrogen-dependent disorder with a relapsing/remitting nature. The endometrial tissue acts just like the normal ones in the uterus, responding to cyclical hormone levels, growing and bleeding at certain times of the cycle. If the tissue is in the ovaries, then bleeding of it results in accumulation of blood, named chocolate cysts. During menstruation, the ectopic tissue bleeds, causing the surrounding tissues to become inflamed. This inflammation causes fibrosis, leading to adhesions that produce pain and other complications such as infertility. Inflammation that happens at the site of the endometrial tissue results in and adhesions in the abdomen and pelvis. These can lead to a frozen pelvis and other complications such as infertility. It can be associated with many distressing and debilitating symptoms, such as pelvic pain, severe dysmenorrhea, dyspareunia and infertility, or it may be asymptomatic, and incidentally discovered at laparoscopy or exploratory surgeries.

Active endometriosis usually occurs between ages 30 and 40, but may be seen before age 20. Severe symptoms of endometriosis may have an abrupt onset or develop over many years. This disorder usually becomes progressively severe during the menstrual years but after menopause, it tends to subside.

The most common sites of endometriosis are respectively the ovaries, anterior and posterior cul-de-sac, posterior broad ligaments, uterosacral ligaments, uterus, fallopian tubes, sigmoid colon and appendix, and round ligaments. Other less commonly involved regions include the vagina, cervix, rectovaginal septum, cecum, ileum, inguinal canals, abdominal or perineal scars, urinary bladder, ureters, and umbilicus. Rarely, endometriosis has been reported in the breast, pancreas, liver, gallbladder, kidney, urethra, extremities, vertebrae, bone, peripheral nerves, lung, diaphragm, central nervous system, and even in the prostate. Endometriosis is multifocal in most patients. The disease is staged according to site and severity of involvements.

Diagnosis of urinary tract endometriosis requires a careful history and thorough physical examination. High index of suspician to all symptomatic women with a history of caesarian delivery or other gynaecological surgery gives a clue to the diagnosis.

Ultrasonography is the initial step of investigation to detect the vesical endoluminal mass or upper urinary tract dilatation. On ultrasound examination, the lesions usually appears as hypoechoic, vascular, and solid masses, although cystic changes can be present . The lesions have no definite margines and may appear to infiltrate adjacent tissues. IVU is still very much useful to detect the integrity of the upper tract and ureter. MRI is better than computed tomography for identifying hemorrhage and soft tissue planes. Fine needle aspiration will yield chocolate-colored fluid.

Cystoscopy and laparoscopy together with biopsy are fundamental to the assessment of urinary tract endometriosis specially before operation. Wide local excision is performed either for confirmation diagnosis or as treatment.

Optimal management requires a team of specialists including gynaecologists, colorectal surgeons and urologists, working together to thoroughly assess the risks and benefits of treatments and to determine the optimal care.

Treatment varies according to the severity and site of involvement of each case. Hormonal therapy with danazole does have a definite roll in regressing the lesion but in cases with urinary tract involvement, surgical treatment is a better option because the condition may lead to kidney loss up to 25%.

Aggressive surgical removal of ectopic tissues, relief of urinary obstruction and castration with or without hysterectomy is the recommended surgical treatment for urinary tract endometriosis. In the younger patients and in order to preserve fertility, endometriosis should be resected but with preservation of ovarian function and strict periodic surveillance of urinary tract.

3. Upper tract involvement

3.1 Renal endometriosis

Since renal endometriosis is rarely encountered, it is briefely mentioned in the clinical guidelines and literatures.

3.2 Ureteral endometriosis

Endometriosis of the urinary tract is predominantly found in the bladder, accounting for 70% to 80% of the cases. The ureter may be involved in 15% to 20% of the urinary tract cases. Bilateral disease has been reported in up to 23% of cases. The left side is more often affected, which may be because the sigmoid colon prevents the regurgitated endometrial cells to be cleared by the peritoneal fluid on the left side.

Ureteral involvement may be either intrinsic or extrinsic. If endometrial glands and stroma are within the lamina propria, tunica muscularis, or ureteral lumen it is said Intrinsic endometriosis and if they are localized within periureteral tissue extrinsic endometriosis ensues. Eighty percent of ureteral endometriosis is extrinsic and most commonly involves the distal ureter. Differentiation between these two forms of ureteral endometriosis has histologic and pathogenetic importance, but has little impact on clinical management since the precise location of the lesion cannot be determined preoperatively. Moreover, both intrinsic and extrinsic forms of the disease may result in ureteral stenosis.

Silent loss of renal function has been reported in 25% to 43% of patients with ureteral endometriosis, which may result in total loss of function of the affected kidney. Historically, up to one third of kidneys affected by ureteral endometriosis were lost. So, *it has been* recommended to take image of the upper urinary tract in all patients with pelvic endometriosis with ultrasonography or IVU.

Gynecologic laparoscopy for treatment of endometriosis is responsible for a large percentage of ureteral injuries. The reasons for this may be as follows: (1) endometrioma can involve the ureter either extrinsically or intrinsically; (2 adhesions from endometriosis makes ureteral visualization difficult; and (3) the disease can deviate the ureters medially resulting in abnormal anatomy.

In addition, the most commonly affected portions of the ureter are the distal third, followed by the middle third. Involvement of the proximal ureter is rare. Thus, the most frequent sites of ureteral endometriosis are below the level of tubal efflux. The lesions of the distal ureter usually coexist with posterior pouch endometriosis, as the lesions of the middle third of the ureter may be together with involvement of the ovary.

3.2.1 Clinical manifestations

Classic symptoms and signs of urinary tract endometriosis include cyclical flank pain, dysuria, urgency, urinary tract infection, and hematuria. As a rule, we can say that intrinsic endometriosis is more symptomatic than extrinsic disease. Notably, a significant portion of patients with ureteral endometriosis do not have genitourinary symptoms and as a consequence, ureteral endometriosis can lead to silent loss of renal function.

Ureteral endometriosis presents with colicky flank pain in approximately 25 percent of patients and gross hematuria in 15 percent, while up to 50 percent of patients are asymptomatic and is generally discovered at the time of laparotomy or laparoscopy for evaluation of pelvic pain or other indications.

3.2.2 Diagnosis

Ureteral endometriosis should be included in the differential diagnosis of obstructive ureteral lesions in women, particularly those involving the lower third of the left ureter. Because a large percentage of ureteral endometriosis can result in loss of renal function due to asymptomatic obstruction, all patients with pelvic endometriosis should undergo the upper urinary tract imaging. Initial imaging may be ultrasonography as a noninvasive test to look for hydroureteronephrosis.Although, IVU may be a better test in high suspicious cases. Intrinsic disease appears in IVU as ureteral filling defects, whereas extrinsic disease causes smooth strictures. The exact location and volume of the disease can be defined through retrograde ureteropyelography, CT or MRI , which can be valuable for planning treatment.

The diagnosis of ureteral endometriosis requires a high index of suspicion and is aided by clinicians' awareness of the condition. The diagnosis of ureteral endometriosis is suggested by the finding of hydronephrosis in a patient with known or suspected endometriosis, particularly if symptoms consistent with ureteral involvement are present but, definite diagnosis can be reached through direct visualization and biopsy of implants. Histologic confirmation is the gold standard for diagnosis of endometriosis .

The differential diagnosis of ureteral endometriosis includes any conditions that result in hydronephrosis such as stones and malignancies.

3.2.3 Management

Treatment has several goals including preservation of renal function, management of the original disease process, maintenance of the patient's fertility, and relief of the patient's symptoms.

Medical treatment does not treat the fibrotic component of endometriotic lesions, which is largely responsible for ureteral obstruction so, medical therapy is usually not effective at relieving ureteral obstruction and treatment of ureteral endometriosis with hydronephrosis is surgical.

Patients with mild or intermittent hydronephrosis can be treated initially with a combination of medical therapy and insertion of a ureteral stent. In such cases, close monitoring of renal function is required.

3.2.3.1 Medical treatment

While medical therapy is effective for pain relief, symptoms often recur once treatment is completed. If renal function is normal and there is minimal to mild hydronephrosis with no functional obstruction as determined by radionuclide renal scanning, hormone therapy may be prescribed.

Ureteral endometriosis is rare, and there are few studies of medical therapy. Ovarian hormonal ablation with gonadotropin-releasing hormone agonists has been utilized with success in some series. Hormonal therapy is not as effective for patients with extensive endometriosis.The aromatase inhibitors such as anastrazole and danazol was unsuccessful in relieving ureteral obstruction in few case reports.

3.2.3.2 Surgeries

The goals of surgical treatment of ureteral endometriosis are to remove the endometriotic lesion(s) and relieve ureteral stricture or kinking. Surgery is indicated if fertility is a major goal, where symptoms fail to respond to medical therapies, or where ureteric obstruction has been confirmed. Untreated ureteric obstruction may lead to irreversible kidney damage.

Surgical intervention is the treatment of choice for most patients with significant hydroureteronephrosis and periureteral disease. Ureterolysis may correct ureteral obstruction in those with extrinsic disease. If laparoscopic ureterolysis is undertaken, a transperitoneal approach is preferable in that it allows a superior assessment of endometrial implants on the peritoneum.

In the case of intrinsic disease, removal of lesions may be difficult because, endometriotic lesions infiltrate the ureteral wall and there may be no apparent margin of them to be resrcted. So, when intrinsic disease is present or in case of ureterolysis failure, distal ureterectomy with reimplantation is preferred.

As a matter of fact, all lesions adjuscent to the ureters to prevent future stenosis and renal damage, since the progression of endometriosis is unpredictable.Thus any lesion found incidentally during surgery proximal to ureters should be removed.

Ureterolysis is performed by most surgeons laparoscopically. A laparoscopic approach may be offered to patients with ureteral stricture disease. Although, ureteroneocystostomy may require laparotomy.

As the first step of the procedure ureterolysis is done. Since the ureter and peritoneum are almost never affected at the level of the pelvic brim, the peritoneum is opened upon the ureter at this site and the ureter is dissected from adjuscent tissues to the level of the cardinal ligament, sharply or bluntly.

If endometriosis invades the ureteral adventitia it may be necessary to cut the adventitial sheath without any manipulation of muscular layer. Any ureteral perforation can be repaired with two interrupted 4-0 polydioxanone sutures.

After ureterolysis is complete, the decision is made regarding whether further intervention is required, based upon visual inspection of the ureter. Then if required, ureteral stent or resection of a diseased segment of ureter must be done to prevent future stenosis and obstruction.

Since most lesions are located in the distal ureter, ureteral resection is usually combined with ureteroneocystostomy. The involved segment of ureter is excised and reimplantation into the bladder is performed. When the endometriotic lesion is in the middle or upper third of the ureter, end ureteroureterostomy should be done after resection of lesions.

Whether to proceed with resection of an endometriotic segment of the ureter or aggressive ureterolysis and stenting is a subjective decision based upon intraoperative visual with no definite criteria to predict normal postoperative ureteral function. In presence of stenosis and significant hydronephrosis, most surgeons have found that the risk of recurrence is lower after ureteral resection and ureteroneocystostomy rather than aggressive ureterolysis and stent insertion. In the case of surface ovarian endometriotic lesions or an endometrioma ipsilateral oophorectomy should be performed as needed. Bilateral oophorectomy is performed in some women to prevent recurrence of endometriosis.

In the cases incidentally discovered at time of laparoscopy or laparotomy, if ureteral adhesions are present, ureterolysis should be performed.

Complications of these surgeries include general complications the same as other abdominal laparoscopy or laparotomy and specific complications to this procedure such as ureteral fistula.

The rates of recurrence for each type of surgical procedures are included in Table.3. Complications are few and most common of them is ureteral fistula. Ureterolysis alone is associated with higher rates of both recurrence and complications compared with ureteroneocystostomy and Ureteroureteral anastomosis

Ureteroneocystostomy	3 percent
Ureterolysis alone	8 percent
Ureteroureteral anastomosis	11 percent

Table 3. The rates of recurrence for each type of surgical procedures for ureteral endometriosis.

4. Lower tract involvement

4.1 Urethral endometriosis

Since urethral endometriosis is rarely encountered the clinical guidelines and literature are briefe. Eendometriosis have been described within urethral diverticula. urethral endometriosis do not involve the urethral meatus.

4.2 Bladder endometriosis

Bladder endometriosis is defined as the presence of endometrial glands and stroma at detrusor muscle.

4.2.1 Clinical manifestations

Bladder endometriosis causes nonspecific urinary symptoms, including urinary frequency, urgency, dysuria, or urinary retention. Occurrence of these symptoms during menses is suggestive. Cyclic hematuria is uncommon but characteristic. The ureteral openings are usually not involved by the vesical lesions so, hydronephrosis is rare.

Some women with bladder endometriosis are asymptomatic and present with an incidental finding of a bladder nodule on pelvic imaging or as a result of pelvic surgery. Some patients are asymptomatic for the first few years and will only realize that they have the disease when it is already in its serious stage, manifesting more severe symptoms.

The most common complaint of women that have bladder endometriosis is pain in the abdominal or pelvic area. The degree of pain can be mild to severe or acute to subacute. Usually, this pain will be more intense during monthly period. Many women suffer from endometriosis silently because they feel that the pain is just the normal pain of premenstrual syndrome. However, if the premenstrual pain in a woman hampers her normal activities she is suspected to has endometriosis.

Women with bladder endometriosis also experience various urinary problems. It is common to feel a burning sensation during voiding. Since the cause of your urinary problems is endometrium cells in the bladder wall, antibiotics will not cure or alleviate the symptoms.

4.2.2 Diagnosis

The gold standard for diagnosis of bladder endometriosis is biopsy and histologic confirmation of visualized lesions during cystoscopy or laparoscopy.

Symptoms compatible with bladder endometriosis, specially togetherwith known endometriosis at other sites or characteristic symptoms such as pelvic pain, dysmenorrhea, dyspareunia and infertility, and finding of a bladder nodule on ultrasound suggest vesical endometriosis and further evaluation is needed.

The differential diagnosis of bladder endometriosis includes urinary tract infection, interstitial cystitis, and a bladder stone or neoplasm. So, proper tests and examinations must be done based on patient's clinical presentation to rule out these conditions. In more than 70% of cases the presenting symptoms of bladder endometriosis are identical to those of interstitial cystitis. Therefore, endometriosis should always be considered in the patient referred for frequency, urgency and pain with no documented infection.

Pelvic and renal sonography may show a bladder nodule or hydronephrosis, although, endometriosis is often not visualized on imaging studies. Endometriosis itself and its surgical treatments are capable of VVF formation. Nevertheless, endometriosis of the bladder must be differentiated from VVF because both of them may present with cyclic hematuria.

In the case of a bladder nodule, cystoscopy and biopsy is performed to rule out malignancy and confirm diagnosis. The distance of the lesion from the ureteral openings is important since, removal of the lesions adjuscent to ureteral orifices may requires ureteral surgery, as well. Magnetic resonance imaging may be useful to detect Lesions that are not visible with cystoscopy. If there is hydronephrosis , radiologic evaluation of the same ureter is required.

4.2.3 Management

Bladder endometriosis, if left unmanaged, may lead to more severe urinary problems in the future such as urinary obstruction or incontinence. However, treatment of vesical endometriosis is indicated only if there is any symptoms or resulted in hydronephrosis. First line treatment is medical therapy, since this approach avoids the risk of surgical complications. Medical therapy must be continued until menopause is not effective in all cases. Surgery must be reserved for cases in whom medical therapy have failed or is contraindicated, who wish to avoid chronic medical treatment, or who have hydronephrosis.

4.2.3.1 Medical treatment

Hormonal therapy is reasonable and effective management for bladder endometriosis and because it preserves fertility, is especially attractive to younger women. While medical therapy is effective for pain relief, symptoms often recur once treatment is completed.

Medical therapy of symptomatic bladder endometriosis is the same as for other sites of the disease. Oral contraceptives, progestins, and gonadotropin releasing hormone agonists all have been reported to improve symptoms and regress the lesions.

A tolerable and safe medication should be chosen. Oral contraceptive on the usual cyclic regimen may be efficient. Although, If perimenstrual symptoms do not resolve with a cyclic regimen, it should be substituted by a continuous regimen. Low dose progestin is also effective and safe.

4.2.3.2 Surgeries

Definitive treatment of bladder endometriosis is surgical removal of the lesions. Surgery is indicated if fertility is a major goal, where symptoms fail to respond to medical therapies, or where ureteric obstruction has been confirmed. Untreated ureteric obstruction may lead to irreversible kidney damage.

If the lesion deeply infiltrates the bladder wall then, a full thickness resection and subcequent repair of the bladder wall is needed, which can be done laparoscopically. Although, in the case of partial thickness involvements one can only resect the lesions without opening the bladder wall.

In the face of the complicated conditions there may be the need for more advanced procedures which should be performed via laparotomy and only by more experient surgeons (table.4).

1	Any possiblility for endometriosis of the ureter such as hydronephrosis.
2	The lesion is less than 2 cm away from the inter-ureteric ridge.
3	Another bladder lesion has been recently resected.

Table 4. The complicated bladder endometrioses.

If the inferior border of the endometriotic lesion is less than 2 cm away from the interureteric ridge,then ureteral catheters should be inserted at the beginning of the procedure.

Removal of endometriotic nodules at the bladder dome may not require any dissection but, in the face of nodules involving the posterior or inferior aspects, the bladder must be dissected from the uterus just enough below the inferior margin of the nodule in order to achieve complete resection. The lesions is then excised with cold scissors or electrosurgery and the bladder is closed with two layers of transverse sutures.

For lesions at the vesical base, where the bladder is apposed to the uterus, resection of a 0.5 to 1 cm deep portion of the myometrium contiguous with the endometriotic nodule may prevent recurrence.

At the end of the procedure, the bladder is filled to confirm that the closure is watertight and the bladder catheter is left in place for 7 to 10 days to prevent fistula formation.

The removal of bladder endometriosis is contraindicated in pregnant women as well during cesarean section, because high endometrial blood flow can result in massive hemorrhagia.

General complications are the same as other laparoscopic or cystoscopic procesures. Special complications include vesicovaginal hematoma and vesicovaginal fistula. Ureter–fallopian tube fistula has also been reported as a consequence of laparoscopic fulguration of endometriosis.

The overall outcome of surgical treatment for bladder endometriosis has been good and complications or need for reoperations had been low.

5. Summery

- Endometriosis is defined as the presence of functional endometrial tissue in an ectopic site (*outside of the uterus*). Endometriosis is a common, benign, chronic, *estrogen-dependent* disorder with a *relapsing/remitting* nature.
- Although endometriosis is usually confined to the ovaries, uterosacral ligaments, and cul-de-sac, it has been documented in almost every organ system in the body.
- Because ovarian function is necessary for the development and maintenance endometrial implants, endometriosis has been reported only in the *reproductive age* and so, is normally not seen before age 15 or after menopause. Endometriosis is most common in women between the ages of *25 and 35*.
- The prevalence of endometriosis in specific categories of patients has been reported (Table.1), but the prevalence in the general population is not definitely known because a majority of patients are asymptomatic. It is estimated that affect *10% to 20%* of women of reproductive age.
- Endometriosis can be associated with many distressing and debilitating symptoms *may be asymptomatic,* and incidentally discovered at laparoscopy or exploratory surgery.
- Endometriotic lesions of the urinary tract are present in *1 to 2 percent* of women with endometriosis and often *coexists with* disease at other sites of the body. Actually, endometriosis *is multifocal* in most patients.
- The pathogenesis of endometriosis has not been definitively established but predominant hypotheses are *the implantation theory, lymphatics and blood vessels dissemination, and coelomic metaplasia. Genetic* factors and altered humoral and cell-mediated *immunity* may also *play a role in endometriosis.*
- The endometrial tissue in the endometriotic lesions acts just like the normal ones in the uterus, *responding to cyclical hormone* levels, growing and bleeding at certain times of the cycle, causing the surrounding tissues to become inflamed. This *inflammation* causes *fibrosis,* leading to *adhesions* that produce pain and other complications such as infertility.
- Since renal and urethral endometriosis is rarely encountered, they are briefely mentioned in the clinical guidelines and literatures.

- Endometriosis of the urinary tract is predominantly found in the bladder, accounting for 70% to 80% of the cases. The ureter may be involved in *15% to 20%* of the urinary tract cases and *the left side* is more often affected. *Bilateral ureteral* disease has been reported in up to 23% of cases.
- Ureteral involvement may be either *intrinsic or extrinsic*. Eighty percent of ureteral endometriosis is extrinsic and most commonly involves the *distal ureter*. Differentiation between these two forms of ureteral endometriosis has histologic and pathogenetic importance, but has little impact on clinical management.
- Because a large percentage of ureteral endometriosis can result in silent loss of renal function due to asymptomatic obstruction, all patients with pelvic endometriosis should undergo the *upper urinary tract imaging*.
- Classic symptoms and signs of urinary tract endometriosis include cyclical flank pain, dysuria, urgency, urinary tract infection, and hematuria. As a rule, we can say that *intrinsic endometriosis is more symptomatic* than extrinsic disease.
- The exact location and volume of the ureteral disease can be defined through retrograde ureteropyelography, CT or MRI , which can be valuable for planning treatment.
- The diagnosis of ureteral endometriosis requires a high index of suspicion and is aided by clinicians' awareness of the condition. Definite diagnosis can be reached through direct visualization and biopsy of implants.
- Treatment of ureteral endometriosis has several goals including preservation of renal function, management of the main disease process, maintenance of the patient's fertility, and relief of the patient's symptoms. If renal function is normal and there is minimal to mild hydronephrosis with no functional obstruction as determined by radionuclide renal scanning, hormone therapy may be prescribed otherwise, surgery is indicated.
- Since most lesions are located in the distal ureter, ureteral resection is usually combined with *ureteroneocystostomy* but, when the endometriotic lesion is in the middle or upper third of the ureter, *end ureteroureterostomy* should be done after resection of lesions.
- Bladder endometriosis is defined as the presence of endometrial glands and stroma *through detrusor muscle*. The ureteral openings are usually not involved by the vesical lesions so, hydronephrosis is rare.
- Bladder endometriosis causes nonspecific urinary symptoms, including urinary frequency, urgency, dysuria, or urinary retention . Occurrence of these symptoms during menses is suggestive. *Cyclic hematuria is uncommon but characteristic.*
- Treatment of vesical endometriosis is indicated only if there is any symptoms or resulted in hydronephrosis. First line treatment is *medical therapy*. Surgery must be reserved for cases in whom medical therapy have failed or is contraindicated, who wish to avoid chronic medical treatment, or who have hydronephrosis.
- If the inferior border of the endometriotic lesion is less than 2 cm away from the interureteric ridge, then *ureteral catheters* should be inserted at the beginning of the procedure.
- Removal of endometriotic nodules at the bladder *dome* may not require any dissection but, in the face of nodules involving the *posterior or inferior* aspects, the bladder must be dissected from the uterus just enough below the inferior margin of the nodule in order to achieve complete resection.
- For lesions at the vesical base, where the bladder is apposed to the uterus, resection of a 0.5 to 1 cm deep portion of the myometrium contiguous with the endometriotic nodule may prevent recurrence.

6. References

Abbott J, Hawe J, Hunter D, et al. Laparoscopic excision of endometriosis: a randomized, placebo-controlled trial. Fertil Steril 2004; 82:878.

Abeshouse BS, Abeshouse G. Endometriosis of the urinary tract: a review of the literature and a report of four cases of vesical endometriosis. J Int Coll Surg 1960; 34:43.

Abeshouse BS, Abeshouse G. Endometriosis of the urinary tract: a review of the literature and a report of four cases of vesical endomertiosis. J Int Coll Surg 1960;34:43-63.

Abrao MS, Dias JA Jr, Bellelis P, et al. Endometriosis of the ureter and bladder are not associated diseases. Fertil Steril 2009; 91:1662.

Abrao MS, Gonçalves MO, Dias JA Jr, et al. Comparison between clinical examination, transvaginal sonography and magnetic resonance imaging for the diagnosis of deep endometriosis. Hum Reprod 2007; 22:3092.

Ahn M, Loughlin KR. Psoas hitch ureteral reimplantation in adults--analysis of a modified technique and timing of repair. Urology 2001; 58:184.

Al-Khawaja M, Tan PH, MacLennan GT, et al. Ureteral endometriosis: clinicopathological and immunohistochemical study of 7 cases. Hum Pathol 2008; 39:954.

Allen WM, Masters WH. Traumatic laceration of uterine support; the clinical syndrome and the operative treatment. Am J Obstet Gynecol 1955; 70:500.

Anaf V, Simon P, El Nakadi I, et al. Relationship between endometriotic foci and nerves in rectovaginal endometriotic nodules. Hum Reprod 2000; 15:1744.

Antonelli A, Simeone C, Frego E, et al. Surgical treatment of ureteral obstruction from endometriosis: our experience with thirteen cases. Int Urogynecol J Pelvic Floor Dysfunct 2004; 15:407.

Antonelli A, Simeone C, Zani D, et al. Clinical aspects and surgical treatment of urinary tract endometriosis: our experience with 31 cases. Eur Urol 2006; 49:1093.

Ballard K, Lane H, Hudelist G, et al. Can specific pain symptoms help in the diagnosis of endometriosis? A cohort study of women with chronic pelvic pain. Fertil Steril 2010; 94:20.

Ballard KD, Seaman HE, de Vries CS, Wright JT. Can symptomatology help in the diagnosis of endometriosis? Findings from a national case-control study--Part 1. BJOG 2008; 115:1382.

Barbieri RL, Niloff JM, Bast RC Jr, et al. Elevated serum concentrations of CA-125 in patients with advanced endometriosis. Fertil Steril 1986; 45:630.

Bazot M, Lafont C, Rouzier R, et al. Diagnostic accuracy of physical examination, transvaginal sonography, rectal endoscopic sonography, and magnetic resonance imaging to diagnose deep infiltrating endometriosis. Fertil Steril 2009; 92:1825.

Bazot M, Malzy P, Cortez A, et al. Accuracy of transvaginal sonography and rectal endoscopic sonography in the diagnosis of deep infiltrating endometriosis. Ultrasound Obstet Gynecol 2007; 30:994.

Bedaiwy MA, Falcone T, Mascha EJ, Casper RF. Genetic polymorphism in the fibrinolytic system and endometriosis. Obstet Gynecol 2006; 108:162.

Bennett GL, Slywotzky CM, Cantera M, Hecht EM. Unusual manifestations and complications of endometriosis--spectrum of imaging findings: pictorial review. AJR Am J Roentgenol 2010; 194:WS34.

Berlanda N, Vercellini P, Carmignani L, et al. Ureteral and vesical endometriosis. Two different clinical entities sharing the same pathogenesis. Obstet Gynecol Surv 2009; 64:830.

Berlanda N, Vercellini P, Carmignani L, et al. Ureteral and vesical endometriosis. Two different clinical entities sharing the same pathogenesis. Obstet Gynecol Surv 2009; 64:830.

Bese T, Simsek Y, Bese N, et al. Extensive pelvic endometriosis with malignant change in tamoxifen-treated postmenopausal women. Int J Gynecol Cancer 2003; 13:376.

Bischoff FZ, Simpson JL. Heritability and molecular genetic studies of endometriosis. Hum Reprod Update 2000; 6:37.

Blanco RG, Parithivel VS, Shah AK, et al. Abdominal wall endometriomas. Am J Surg 2003; 185:596.

Bohrer J, Chen CC, Falcone T. Persistent bilateral ureteral obstruction secondary to endometriosis despite treatment with an aromatase inhibitor. Fertil Steril 2008; 90:2004.e7.

Bordin L, Fiore C, Donà G, et al. Evaluation of erythrocyte band 3 phosphotyrosine level, glutathione content, CA-125, and human epididymal secretory protein E4 as combined parameters in endometriosis. Fertil Steril 2010; 94:1616.

Bosev D, Nicoll LM, Bhagan L, et al. Laparoscopic management of ureteral endometriosis: the Stanford University hospital experience with 96 consecutive cases. J Urol 2009; 182:2748.

Bricou A, Batt RE, Chapron C. Peritoneal fluid flow influences anatomical distribution of endometriotic lesions: why Sampson seems to be right. Eur J Obstet Gynecol Reprod Biol 2008; 138:127.

Brinton LA, Lamb EJ, Moghissi KS, et al. Ovarian cancer risk associated with varying causes of infertility. Fertil Steril 2004; 82:405.

Brosens IA, Fusi L, Brosens JJ. Endometriosis is a risk factor for spontaneous hemoperitoneum during pregnancy. Fertil Steril 2009; 92:1243.

Bulletti C, Montini A, Setti PL, et al. Vaginal parturition decreases recurrence of endometriosis. Fertil Steril 2010; 94:850.

Bulun SE. Endometriosis. N Engl J Med 2009; 360:268.

Busacca M, Chiaffarino F, Candiani M, et al. Determinants of long-term clinically detected recurrence rates of deep, ovarian, and pelvic endometriosis. Am J Obstet Gynecol 2006; 195:426.

Busard MP, Mijatovic V, van Kuijk C, et al. Magnetic resonance imaging in the evaluation of (deep infiltrating) endometriosis: the value of diffusion-weighted imaging. J Magn Reson Imaging 2010; 32:1003.

Campbell IG, Thomas EJ. Endometriosis: candidate genes. Hum Reprod Update 2001; 7:15.

Carmignani L, Ronchetti A, Amicarelli F, et al. Bladder psoas hitch in hydronephrosis due to pelvic endometriosis: outcome of urodynamic parameters. Fertil Steril 2009; 92:35.

Carmignani L, Vercellini P, Spinelli M, et al. Pelvic endometriosis and hydroureteronephrosis. Fertil Steril 2010; 93:1741.

Carmignani L, Vercellini P, Spinelli M, et al. Pelvic endometriosis and hydroureteronephrosis. Fertil Steril 2010; 93:1741.

Chapron C Dubisson JB. Laparoscopic management of bladder endometriosis. Acta Obstet Gynecol Scand 1999;78:887-90.

Chapron C, Barakat H, Fritel X, et al. Presurgical diagnosis of posterior deep infiltrating endometriosis based on a standardized questionnaire. Hum Reprod 2005; 20:507.

Chapron C, Bourret A, Chopin N, et al. Surgery for bladder endometriosis: long-term results and concomitant management of associated posterior deep lesions. Hum Reprod 2010; 25:884.

Chapron C, Chiodo I, Leconte M, et al. Severe ureteral endometriosis: the intrinsic type is not so rare after complete surgical exeresis of deep endometriotic lesions. Fertil Steril 2010; 93:2115.

Chapron C, Chopin N, Borghese B, et al. Deeply infiltrating endometriosis: pathogenetic implications of the anatomical distribution. Hum Reprod 2006; 21:1839.

Chapron C, Dubisson JB, Fauconnier A, Da-Costa VM. Laparoscopy and bladder endometriosis. Gynecol Obstet Fertil 2000;28:232-7.

Chapron C, Dubuisson JB. Laparoscopic management of bladder endometriosis. Acta Obstet Gynecol Scand 1999; 78:887.

Chapron C, Fauconnier A, Dubuisson JB, et al. Deep infiltrating endometriosis: relation between severity of dysmenorrhoea and extent of disease. Hum Reprod 2003; 18:760.

Chatman DL, Ward AB. Endometriosis in adolescents. J Reprod Med 1982; 27:156.

Chatman DL, Ward AB. Endometriosis in adolescents. J Reprod Med 1982; 27:156.

Cheng YM, Wang ST, Chou CY. Serum CA-125 in preoperative patients at high risk for endometriosis. Obstet Gynecol 2002; 99:375.

Clement PB. The pathology of endometriosis: a survey of the many faces of a common disease emphasizing diagnostic pitfalls and unusual and newly appreciated aspects. Adv Anat Pathol 2007; 14:241.

Comiter CV. Endometriosis of the urinary tract. Urol Clin North Am 2002; 29:625.

Czernobilsky B, Morris WJ. A histologic study of ovarian endometriosis with emphasis on hyperplastic and atypical changes. Obstet Gynecol 1979; 53:318.

De Cicco C, Corona R, Schonman R, et al. Bowel resection for deep endometriosis: a systematic review. BJOG 2011; 118:285.

Deligdisch L, Pénault-Llorca F, Schlosshauer P, et al. Stage I ovarian carcinoma: different clinical pathologic patterns. Fertil Steril 2007; 88:906.

D'Hooghe TM, Debrock S, Hill JA, Meuleman C. Endometriosis and subfertility: is the relationship resolved? Semin Reprod Med 2003; 21:243.

Dmowski WP, Gebel HM, Braun DP. The role of cell-mediated immunity in pathogenesis of endometriosis. Acta Obstet Gynecol Scand Suppl 1994; 159:7.

Donnez J, Nisolle M, Squifflet J. Ureteral endometriosis: a complication of rectovaginal endometriotic (adenomyotic) nodules. Fertil Steril 2002; 77:32.

Donnez J, Spada F, Squifflet J, Nisolle M. Bladder endometriosis must be considered as bladder adenomyosis. Fertil Steril 2000; 74:1175.

Dwivedi AJ, Agrawal SN, Silva YJ. Abdominal wall endometriomas. Dig Dis Sci 2002; 47:456.

Efstathiou JA, Sampson DA, Levine Z, et al. Nonsteroidal antiinflammatory drugs differentially suppress endometriosis in a murine model. Fertil Steril 2005; 83:171.

Engemise S, Gordon C, Konje JC. Endometriosis. BMJ 2010; 340:c2168.

Erzen M, Rakar S, Klancnik B, et al. Endometriosis-associated ovarian carcinoma (EAOC): an entity distinct from other ovarian carcinomas as suggested by a nested case-control study. Gynecol Oncol 2001; 83:100.

Eyster KM, Klinkova O, Kennedy V, Hansen KA. Whole genome deoxyribonucleic acid microarray analysis of gene expression in ectopic versus eutopic endometrium. Fertil Steril 2007; 88:1505.

Faccioli N, Manfredi R, Mainardi P, et al. Barium enema evaluation of colonic involvement in endometriosis. AJR Am J Roentgenol 2008; 190:1050.

Faucheron JL, Pasquier D, Voirin D. Endometriosis of the vermiform appendix as an exceptional cause of acute perforated appendicitis during pregnancy. Colorectal Dis 2008; 10:518.

Fauconnier A, Chapron C, Dubuisson JB, et al. Relation between pain symptoms and the anatomic location of deep infiltrating endometriosis. Fertil Steril 2002; 78:719.

Fedele L, Bianchi S, Montefusco S, et al. A gonadotropin-releasing hormone agonist versus a continuous oral contraceptive pill in the treatment of bladder endometriosis. Fertil Steril 2008; 90:183.

Fedele L, Bianchi S, Zanconato G, et al. Is rectovaginal endometriosis a progressive disease? Am J Obstet Gynecol 2004; 191:1539.

Fedele L, Bianchi S, Zanconato G, et al. Long-term follow-up after conservative surgery for bladder endometriosis. Fertil Steril 2005; 83:1729.

Fedele L, Piazzola E, Raffaelli R, Bianchi S. Bladder endometriosis: deep infiltrating endometriosis or adenomyosis? Fertil Steril 1998; 69:972.

Fernando S, Breheny S, Jaques AM, et al. Preterm birth, ovarian endometriomata, and assisted reproduction technologies. Fertil Steril 2009; 91:325.

Francica G, Giardiello C, Angelone G, et al. Abdominal wall endometriomas near cesarean delivery scars: sonographic and color doppler findings in a series of 12 patients. J Ultrasound Med 2003; 22:1041.

Fremont RD, Rice TW. Splenosis: a review. South Med J 2007; 100:589.

Frenna V, Santos L, Ohana E, et al. Laparoscopic management of ureteral endometriosis: our experience. J Minim Invasive Gynecol 2007; 14:169.

Fukunaga M, Nomura K, Ishikawa E, Ushigome S. Ovarian atypical endometriosis: its close association with malignant epithelial tumours. Histopathology 1997; 30:249.

Gagnon RF, Arsenault D, Pichette V, Tanguay S. Acute renal failure in a young woman with endometriosis. Nephrol Dial Transplant 2001; 16:1499.

Garcia GJ, Extramiana CJ, Esteban CJ, et al. Vesical endometriosis after caesarian section: diagnistico-tharapeutic aspects. Acta Urol Esp 1997;21:785-8.

Gardner B, Whitaker RH. The use of danazol for ureteral obstruction caused by endometriosis. J Urol 1981; 125:117.

Ghezzi F, Cromi A, Bergamini V, et al. Outcome of laparoscopic ureterolysis for ureteral endometriosis. Fertil Steril 2006; 86:418.

Goldstein DP, deCholnoky C, Leventhal JM, Emans SJ. New insights into the old problem of chronic pelvic pain. J Pediatr Surg 1979; 14:675.

Goncalves MO, Dias JA Jr, Podgaec S, et al. Transvaginal ultrasound for diagnosis of deeply infiltrating endometriosis. Int J Gynaecol Obstet 2009; 104:156.

Goncalves MO, Podgaec S, Dias JA Jr, et al. Transvaginal ultrasonography with bowel preparation is able to predict the number of lesions and rectosigmoid layers affected in cases of deep endometriosis, defining surgical strategy. Hum Reprod 2010; 25:665.

Grasso RF, Di Giacomo V, Sedati P, et al. Diagnosis of deep infiltrating endometriosis: accuracy of magnetic resonance imaging and transvaginal 3D ultrasonography. Abdom Imaging 2010; 35:716.

Gustofson RL, Kim N, Liu S, Stratton P. Endometriosis and the appendix: a case series and comprehensive review of the literature. Fertil Steril 2006; 86:298.

Hadfield RM, Lain SJ, Raynes-Greenow CH, et al. Is there an association between endometriosis and the risk of pre-eclampsia? A population based study. Hum Reprod 2009; 24:2348.

Harada T, Iwabe T, Terakawa N. Role of cytokines in endometriosis. Fertil Steril 2001; 76:1.

Hediger ML, Hartnett HJ, Louis GM. Association of endometriosis with body size and figure. Fertil Steril 2005; 84:1366.

Hensen JH, Van Breda Vriesman AC, Puylaert JB. Abdominal wall endometriosis: clinical presentation and imaging features with emphasis on sonography. AJR Am J Roentgenol 2006; 186:616.

Holland TK, Yazbek J, Cutner A, et al. Value of transvaginal ultrasound in assessing severity of pelvic endometriosis. Ultrasound Obstet Gynecol 2010; 36:241.

Hornstein MD, Thomas PP, Sober AJ, et al. Association between endometriosis, dysplastic naevi and history of melanoma in women of reproductive age. Hum Reprod 1997; 12:143.

Horton JD, Dezee KJ, Ahnfeldt EP, Wagner M. Abdominal wall endometriosis: a surgeon's perspective and review of 445 cases. Am J Surg 2008; 196:207.

Hsieh YY, Chang CC, Tsai FJ, et al. Estrogen receptor alpha dinucleotide repeat and cytochrome P450c17alpha gene polymorphisms are associated with susceptibility to endometriosis. Fertil Steril 2005; 83:567.

Hudelist G, English J, Thomas AE, et al. Diagnostic accuracy of transvaginal ultrasound for non-invasive diagnosis of bowel endometriosis: systematic review and meta-analysis. Ultrasound Obstet Gynecol 2011; 37:257.

Hudelist G, Oberwinkler KH, Singer CF, et al. Combination of transvaginal sonography and clinical examination for preoperative diagnosis of pelvic endometriosis. Hum Reprod 2009; 24:1018.

Hudelist G, Tuttlies F, Rauter G, et al. Can transvaginal sonography predict infiltration depth in patients with deep infiltrating endometriosis of the rectum? Hum Reprod 2009; 24:1012.

Huhtinen K, Suvitie P, Hiissa J, et al. Serum HE4 concentration differentiates malignant ovarian tumours from ovarian endometriotic cysts. Br J Cancer 2009; 100:1315.

Husby GK, Haugen RS, Moen MH. Diagnostic delay in women with pain and endometriosis. Acta Obstet Gynecol Scand 2003; 82:649.

Jansen RP, Russell P. Nonpigmented endometriosis: clinical, laparoscopic, and pathologic definition. Am J Obstet Gynecol 1986; 155:1154.

Jenkins S, Olive DL, Haney AF. Endometriosis: pathogenetic implications of the anatomic distribution. Obstet Gynecol 1986; 67:335.

Jepsen JM, Hansen KB. Danazol in the treatment of ureteral endometriosis. J Urol 1988; 139:1045.

Kane C, Drouin P. Obstructive uropathy associated with endometriosis. Am J Obstet Gynecol 1985; 151:207.

Kennedy S, Bergqvist A, Chapron C, et al. ESHRE guideline for the diagnosis and treatment of endometriosis. Hum Reprod 2005; 20:2698.

Kennedy S. Genetics of endometriosis: a review of the positional cloning approaches. Semin Reprod Med 2003; 21:111.

Kinkel K, Frei KA, Balleyguier C, Chapron C. Diagnosis of endometriosis with imaging: a review. Eur Radiol 2006; 16:285.

Koninckx PR, Meuleman C, Demeyere S, et al. Suggestive evidence that pelvic endometriosis is a progressive disease, whereas deeply infiltrating endometriosis is associated with pelvic pain. Fertil Steril 1991; 55:759.

Kovoor E, Nassif J, Miranda-Mendoza I, Wattiez A. Endometriosis of bladder: outcomes after laparoscopic surgery. J Minim Invasive Gynecol 2010; 17:600.

Laufer MR, Goitein L, Bush M, et al. Prevalence of endometriosis in adolescent girls with chronic pelvic pain not responding to conventional therapy. J Pediatr Adolesc Gynecol 1997; 10:199.
Lebovic DI, Mueller MD, Taylor RN. Immunobiology of endometriosis. Fertil Steril 2001; 75:1.
Lousquy R, Borghese B, Chapron C. [Deep bladder endometriosis: how do I...to perform a laparoscopic partial cystectomy?]. Gynecol Obstet Fertil 2010; 38:697.
Lucero SP, Wise HA, Kirsh G, Devoe K, Hess ML, Kandawalla N, et al. Ureteric obstruction secondary to endometriosis. Report of three cases with review of literature. Br J Urol 1988;61:201-4.
Management of endometriosis in the presence of pelvic pain. The American Fertility Society. Fertil Steril 1993; 60:952.
Marinis A, Vassiliou J, Kannas D, et al. Endometriosis mimicking soft tissue tumors: diagnosis and treatment. Eur J Gynaecol Oncol 2006; 27:168.
Matalliotakis I, Cakmak H, Dermitzaki D, et al. Increased rate of endometriosis and spontaneous abortion in an in vitro fertilization program: no correlation with epidemiological factors. Gynecol Endocrinol 2008; 24:194.
Matorras R, Rodríguez F, Gutierrez de Terán G, et al. Endometriosis and spontaneous abortion rate: a cohort study in infertile women. Eur J Obstet Gynecol Reprod Biol 1998; 77:101.
Matsuura K, Kawasaki N, Oka M, et al. Treatment with danazol of ureteral obstruction caused by endometriosis. Acta Obstet Gynecol Scand 1985; 64:339.
McArthur JW, Ulfelder H. The effect of pregnancy upon endometriosis. Obstet Gynecol Surv 1965; 20:709.
Melin A, Sparén P, Bergqvist A. The risk of cancer and the role of parity among women with endometriosis. Hum Reprod 2007; 22:3021.
Mereu L, Gagliardi ML, Clarizia R, et al. Laparoscopic management of ureteral endometriosis in case of moderate-severe hydroureteronephrosis. Fertil Steril 2010; 93:46.
Minaglia S, Mishell DR Jr, Ballard CA. Incisional endometriomas after Cesarean section: a case series. J Reprod Med 2007; 52:630.
Missmer SA, Hankinson SE, Spiegelman D, et al. Incidence of laparoscopically confirmed endometriosis by demographic, anthropometric, and lifestyle factors. Am J Epidemiol 2004; 160:784.
Missmer SA, Hankinson SE, Spiegelman D, et al. Incidence of laparoscopically confirmed endometriosis by demographic, anthropometric, and lifestyle factors. Am J Epidemiol 2004; 160:784.
Missmer SA, Hankinson SE, Spiegelman D, et al. Reproductive history and endometriosis among premenopausal women. Obstet Gynecol 2004; 104:965.
Modesitt SC, Tortolero-Luna G, Robinson JB, et al. Ovarian and extraovarian endometriosis-associated cancer. Obstet Gynecol 2002; 100:788.
Modugno F, Ness RB, Allen GO, et al. Oral contraceptive use, reproductive history, and risk of epithelial ovarian cancer in women with and without endometriosis. Am J Obstet Gynecol 2004; 191:733.
Mol BW, Bayram N, Lijmer JG, et al. The performance of CA-125 measurement in the detection of endometriosis: a meta-analysis. Fertil Steril 1998; 70:1101.
Montagnana M, Lippi G, Ruzzenente O, et al. The utility of serum human epididymis protein 4 (HE4) in patients with a pelvic mass. J Clin Lab Anal 2009; 23:331.

Moore JG, Hibbard LT, Growdon WA, Schifrin BS. Urinary tract endometriosis: Enigmas in diagnosis and management. Am J Obstet Gynaecol 1979;134:162-72.

Muzii L, Bianchi A, Bellati F, et al. Histologic analysis of endometriomas: what the surgeon needs to know. Fertil Steril 2007; 87:362.

Nazhat C, Nazhat F, Nazhat CH, Nasserbakht F, Rosati M, Seidman DS. Urinary tract endometriosis tr eated by laparoscopy. Fertil Steril 1996;66:920-4.

Nerli RB, Reddy M, Koura AC, et al. Cystoscopy-assisted laparoscopic partial cystectomy. J Endourol 2008; 22:83.

Nezhat C, Nezhat F, Nezhat CH, et al. Urinary tract endometriosis treated by laparoscopy. Fertil Steril 1996; 66:920.

Nezhat CH, Malik S, Osias J, et al. Laparoscopic management of 15 patients with infiltrating endometriosis of the bladder and a case of primary intravesical endometrioid adenosarcoma. Fertil Steril 2002; 78:872.

Nezhat F, Datta MS, Hanson V, et al. The relationship of endometriosis and ovarian malignancy: a review. Fertil Steril 2008; 90:1559.

Ogawa S, Kaku T, Amada S, et al. Ovarian endometriosis associated with ovarian carcinoma: a clinicopathological and immunohistochemical study. Gynecol Oncol 2000; 77:298.

Olive DL, Henderson DY. Endometriosis and mullerian anomalies. Obstet Gynecol 1987; 69:412.

Olive DL, Schwartz LB. Endometriosis. N Engl J Med 1993; 328:1759.

Oosterlynck DJ, Cornillie FJ, Waer M, et al. Women with endometriosis show a defect in natural killer activity resulting in a decreased cytotoxicity to autologous endometrium. Fertil Steril 1991; 56:45.

Pastor-Navarro H, Giménez-Bachs JM, Donate-Moreno MJ, et al. Update on the diagnosis and treatment of bladder endometriosis. Int Urogynecol J Pelvic Floor Dysfunct 2007; 18:949.

Pérez-Utrilla Pérez M, Aguilera Bazán A, Alonso Dorrego JM, et al. Urinary tract endometriosis: clinical, diagnostic, and therapeutic aspects. Urology 2009; 73:47.

Piketty M, Chopin N, Dousset B, et al. Preoperative work-up for patients with deeply infiltrating endometriosis: transvaginal ultrasonography must definitely be the first-line imaging examination. Hum Reprod 2009; 24:602.

Pisanu A, Deplano D, Angioni S, et al. Rectal perforation from endometriosis in pregnancy: case report and literature review. World J Gastroenterol 2010; 16:648.

Porpora MG, Koninckx PR, Piazze J, et al. Correlation between endometriosis and pelvic pain. J Am Assoc Gynecol Laparosc 1999; 6:429.

Prefumo F, Todeschini F, Fulcheri E, Venturini PL. Epithelial abnormalities in cystic ovarian endometriosis. Gynecol Oncol 2002; 84:280.

Propst AM, Laufer MR. Endometriosis in adolescents. Incidence, diagnosis and treatment. J Reprod Med 1999; 44:751.

Redwine DB. Diaphragmatic endometriosis: diagnosis, surgical management, and long-term results of treatment. Fertil Steril 2002; 77:288.

Reese KA, Reddy S, Rock JA. Endometriosis in an adolescent population: the Emory experience. J Pediatr Adolesc Gynecol 1996; 9:125.

Revised American Society for Reproductive Medicine classification of endometriosis: 1996. Fertil Steril 1997; 67:817.

Rivlin ME, Krueger RP, Wiser WL. Danazol in the management of ureteral obstruction secondary to endometriosis. Fertil Steril 1985; 44:274.

Sanchez Merino JM, Parra Muntaner L, Guillan Maquieira C, Gomez Cisner os SC, Alonso Ortiz J, Garcia Alonso J. Bladder endometriosis. Arch Esp Urol 1999;52:933-5
Sangi-Haghpeykar H, Poindexter AN 3rd. Epidemiology of endometriosis among parous women. Obstet Gynecol 1995; 85:983.
Sangi-Haghpeykar H, Poindexter AN 3rd. Epidemiology of endometriosis among parous women. Obstet Gynecol 1995; 85:983.
Savelli L, Manuzzi L, Pollastri P, et al. Diagnostic accuracy and potential limitations of transvaginal sonography for bladder endometriosis. Ultrasound Obstet Gynecol 2009; 34:595.
Savoca G, Trombetta C, Troiano L, Guaschino S, Raber M, Belgrano E. Ecographic, MRI and CT featur es in a case of bladder endometriosis. Arch Ital Urol Androl 1996;68:193-6.
Schenken RS, Williams RF, Hodgen GD. Effect of pregnancy on surgically induced endometriosis in cynomolgus monkeys. Am J Obstet Gynecol 1987; 157:1392.
Schneider A, Touloupidis S, Papatsoris AG, et al. Endometriosis of the urinary tract in women of reproductive age. Int J Urol 2006; 13:902.
Scioscia M, Molon A, Grosso G, Minelli L. Laparoscopic management of ureteral endometriosis. Curr Opin Obstet Gynecol 2009; 21:325.
Seaman HE, Ballard KD, Wright JT, de Vries CS. Endometriosis and its coexistence with irritable bowel syndrome and pelvic inflammatory disease: findings from a national case-control study--Part 2. BJOG 2008; 115:1392.
Seidman JD. Prognostic importance of hyperplasia and atypia in endometriosis. Int J Gynecol Pathol 1996; 15:1.
Sener A, Chew BH, Duvdevani M, et al. Combined transurethral and laparoscopic partial cystectomy and robot-assisted bladder repair for the treatment of bladder endometrioma. J Minim Invasive Gynecol 2006; 13:245.
Seracchioli R, Mabrouk M, Manuzzi L, et al. Importance of retroperitoneal ureteric evaluation in cases of deep infiltrating endometriosis. J Minim Invasive Gynecol 2008; 15:435.
Seracchioli R, Mannini D, Colombo FM, et al. Cystoscopy-assisted laparoscopic resection of extramucosal bladder endometriosis. J Endourol 2002; 16:663.
Simpson JL, Elias S, Malinak LR, Buttram VC Jr. Heritable aspects of endometriosis. I. Genetic studies. Am J Obstet Gynecol 1980; 137:327.
Sinaii N, Cleary SD, Ballweg ML, et al. High rates of autoimmune and endocrine disorders, fibromyalgia, chronic fatigue syndrome and atopic diseases among women with endometriosis: a survey analysis. Hum Reprod 2002; 17:2715.
Sinaii N, Plumb K, Cotton L, et al. Differences in characteristics among 1,000 women with endometriosis based on extent of disease. Fertil Steril 2008; 89:538.
Somigliana E, Vercellini P, Gattei U, et al. Bladder endometriosis: getting closer and closer to the unifying metastatic hypothesis. Fertil Steril 2007; 87:1287.
Somigliana E, Viganò P, Abbiati A, et al. 'Here comes the sun': pigmentary traits and sun habits in women with endometriosis. Hum Reprod 2010; 25:728.
Somigliana E, Vigano' P, Parazzini F, et al. Association between endometriosis and cancer: a comprehensive review and a critical analysis of clinical and epidemiological evidence. Gynecol Oncol 2006; 101:331.
Stanley Ke Jr, Utz Dc, Dockerty Mb. Clinically Significant Endometriosis Of The Urinary Tract. Surg Gynecol Obstet 1965; 120:491.
Stanley KE Jr, UTZ DC, Dockerty MB. Clinically Significant Endometriosis Of The Urinary Tract. Surg Gynecol Obstet 1965; 120:491.

Steed H, Chapman W, Laframboise S. Endometriosis-associated ovarian cancer: a clinicopathologic review. J Obstet Gynaecol Can 2004; 26:709.

Steele RW, Dmowski WP, Marmer DJ. Immunologic aspects of human endometriosis. Am J Reprod Immunol 1984; 6:33.

Stegmann BJ, Sinaii N, Liu S, et al. Using location, color, size, and depth to characterize and identify endometriosis lesions in a cohort of 133 women. Fertil Steril 2008; 89:1632.

Stephansson O, Kieler H, Granath F, Falconer H. Endometriosis, assisted reproduction technology, and risk of adverse pregnancy outcome. Hum Reprod 2009; 24:2341.

Stovall TG, Ling FW. Splenosis: report of a case and review of the literature. Obstet Gynecol Surv 1988; 43:69.

Sutton CJ, Ewen SP, Whitelaw N, Haines P. Prospective, randomized, double-blind, controlled trial of laser laparoscopy in the treatment of pelvic pain associated with minimal, mild, and moderate endometriosis. Fertil Steril 1994; 62:696.

Sutton CJ, Pooley AS, Ewen SP, Haines P. Follow-up report on a randomized controlled trial of laser laparoscopy in the treatment of pelvic pain associated with minimal to moderate endometriosis. Fertil Steril 1997; 68:1070.

Thomas EJ, Campbell IG. Molecular genetic defects in endometriosis. Gynecol Obstet Invest 2000; 50 Suppl 1:44.

Tran LV, Tokushige N, Berbic M, et al. Macrophages and nerve fibres in peritoneal endometriosis. Hum Reprod 2009; 24:835.

Treloar SA, Bell TA, Nagle CM, et al. Early menstrual characteristics associated with subsequent diagnosis of endometriosis. Am J Obstet Gynecol 2010; 202:534.e1.

Van Gorp T, Amant F, Neven P, et al. Endometriosis and the development of malignant tumours of the pelvis. A review of literature. Best Pract Res Clin Obstet Gynaecol 2004; 18:349.

Van Langendonckt A, Casanas-Roux F, Donnez J. Oxidative stress and peritoneal endometriosis. Fertil Steril 2002; 77:861.

Vercammen EE, D'Hooghe TM. Endometriosis and recurrent pregnancy loss. Semin Reprod Med 2000; 18:363.

Vercellini P, Aimi G, De Giorgi O, et al. Is cystic ovarian endometriosis an asymmetric disease? Br J Obstet Gynaecol 1998; 105:1018.

Vercellini P, Busacca M, Aimi G, et al. Lateral distribution of recurrent ovarian endometriotic cysts. Fertil Steril 2002; 77:848.

Vercellini P, Frontino G, Pietropaolo G, et al. Deep endometriosis: definition, pathogenesis, and clinical management. J Am Assoc Gynecol Laparosc 2004; 11:153.

Vercellini P, Frontino G, Pisacreta A, et al. The pathogenesis of bladder detrusor endometriosis. Am J Obstet Gynecol 2002; 187:538.

Vercellini P, Pisacreta A, Pesole A, et al. Is ureteral endometriosis an asymmetric disease? BJOG 2000; 107:559.

Vercellini P, Trespidi L, De Giorgi O, et al. Endometriosis and pelvic pain: relation to disease stage and localization. Fertil Steril 1996; 65:299.

Victory R, Diamond MP, Johns DA. Villar's nodule: a case report and systematic literature review of endometriosis externa of the umbilicus. J Minim Invasive Gynecol 2007; 14:23.

Viganò P, Somigliana E, Parazzini F, Vercellini P. Bias versus causality: interpreting recent evidence of association between endometriosis and ovarian cancer. Fertil Steril 2007; 88:588.

Wang G, Tokushige N, Markham R, Fraser IS. Rich innervation of deep infiltrating endometriosis. Hum Reprod 2009; 24:827.

Watson WJ, Sundwall DA, Benson WL. Splenosis mimicking endometriosis. Obstet Gynecol 1982; 59:51S.
Westney OL, Amundsen CL, McGuire EJ. Bladder endometriosis: conservative management. J Urol 2000; 163:1814.
Wiegand KC, Shah SP, Al-Agha OM, et al. ARID1A mutations in endometriosis-associated ovarian carcinomas. N Engl J Med 2010; 363:1532.
Winkel CA. Evaluation and management of women with endometriosis. Obstet Gynecol 2003; 102:397.
Witz CA. Interleukin-6: another piece of the endometriosis-cytokine puzzle. Fertil Steril 2000; 73:212.
Wykes CB, Clark TJ, Khan KS. Accuracy of laparoscopy in the diagnosis of endometriosis: a systematic quantitative review. BJOG 2004; 111:1204.
Yamamoto K, Mitsuhashi Y, Takaike T, et al. Tubal endometriosis diagnosed within one month after menarche: a case report. Tohoku J Exp Med 1997; 181:385.
Yates-Bell AJ, Molland MB, Pryor JP. Endometriosis of the ur eter. Br J Urol 1972;44:58-67.
Yohannes P. Ureteral endometriosis. J Urol 2003; 170:20.
Zanetta G, Webb MJ, Segura JW. Ureteral endometriosis diagnosed at ureteroscopy. Obstet Gynecol 1998; 91:857.
Zhao X, Lang J, Leng J, et al. Abdominal wall endometriomas. Int J Gynaecol Obstet 2005; 90:218.

3

Diagnosis and Treatment of Perineal Endometriosis

Lan Zhu, Na Chen and Jinghe Lang
Dept. of O/G of Peking Union Medical College Hospital, Chinese Academy of Medical Science, Beijing, P. R. China

1. Introduction

1.1 Introduction and epidemiology

Endometriosis is the extrauterine occurrence of endometrial glands and stroma, most often involving the ovaries or dependent visceral peritoneal surfaces. This tissue responds to the hormone variations in the cycle similar to eutopic endometrium.

Endometriosis is most commonly a disease of women in the second half of their reproductive life, between 30 and 45 years, and tends to regress at the menopause or even before. As a significant gynecological problem, endometriosis occurs in 7%-10% of the general population and up to 50% of premenopausal women (Wheeler, 1989). It is found in 20%-50% (mean 38%) of infertile women (Rawson, 1991; Strathy, 1982; Verkauf, 1987), and in 71%-87% of those with chronic pelvic pain (Carter, 1994; Koninckx et al., 1991; Ling, 1999). Endometriosis is responsible for 20% of all gynecologic operations and is the single leading nonobstetric cause (.5%) of hospitalization for women age 15-44 years. Although benign, endometriosis is progressive, tends to recur, may be locally invasive, may have widespread disseminated foci (rare), and may exist in pelvic lymph nodes (30%) (Martin & Pernoll, 2001).

Endometriosis is commonest in the pelvis. It is very occasionally found in bizarre sites such as the pleura, umbilicus, Caesarean section scars, perineam or vagina, diaphragm, arm, leg or kidney, but these cases are rare. The following statistical data shows the order of frequency: ovaries (30%), uterosacral and large ligaments (18-24%), fallopian tubes (20%), pelvic peritoneum, pouch of Douglas and gastrointestinal tract. Extraperitoneal locations include cervix (0.5%), vagina and rectovaginal septum, round ligament and inguinal hernia sac (0.3-0.6%), navel (1%), abdominal scars after gynecological surgery (1.5%) and cesarean section (0.5%). Endometriosis rarely affects extra-abdominal organs such as the lungs, urinary system, skin and central nervous system (Bergqvist, 1993; Lin et al., 2006).

Perineal endometriosis (PEM) is the presence of endometrial tissues in the perineal sites. It has been published in obstetric and gynecologic literature since 1949. A retrospective study in Peking Union Medical College Hospital shows 17263 women received surgical treatment for endometriosis between Jan 1992 and Apr 2011. Of them, 64 women (3.7‰) were with PEM. Of these 64 women, cases of PEM with anal sphincter involvement were 31 (1.8‰). That is, in nearly half of women with PEM, the lesions erode into anal sphincter.

2. Pathogenesis

The etiology and pathogenesis of endometriosis are complex and still incompletely understood. So many theories have been developed:

1. Implantation theory. Theory of implantation was described by Sampson in 1921 (Sampson JA, 1921). Retrograde menstruation (Sampson's theory) occurs possibly as a result of a hypotonic uterotubal junction in women with endometriosis, allowing increased menstrual regurgitation. Endometrial cells shed from the uterus at menstruation spread in a retrograde manner passing along the fallopian tube to the peritoneal cavity. This theory would account for by far the highest incidence of endometriosis occurring in the pelvis.
2. Coelomic metaplasia. Under the influence of certain unspecified stimuli, mesothelial cells might undergo a metaplastic change to endometrium.
3. Transplantation of exfoliated endometrium. Lymphatic, vascular and iatrogenic routes may disseminate endometriosis. Transtubal regurgitation is the most common route.
4. Altered immunological recognition of endometrial tissues allowing acceptance of emboli of endometrium in these sites. Probably a combination of the first and last theories is most likely to be responsible for endometriotic lesions in different sites of the body.

Transplantation theory actually is divided from the first theory (implantation theory). During vaginal delivery, viable endometrial cells become implanted in the perineum, including the site of episiotomy and result in endometriotic lesions. Perineal lesion often occurs during vaginal delivery, but the incidence of PEM is rare. The reasons for rare incidence may include: (1) Bacteria existing in the perineal wound which can cause infection or even necrosis of the local tissues. The infection and necrosis is not appropriate for transplanted endometrial cells to live. (2) After delivery, the level of estrogen decreases, which also makes the growth of transplanted endometrial cells difficult.

We reported one case of PEM with no history of surgical manipulation or trauma of her perineal area. Perineal endometriosis without history of delivery can not be explained by transplantation theory. We tried lymphatic dissemination theory on this patient (Zhu et al., 2003). As there are rich lymphatic communications between uterus, cervix, vaginal and perineum, endometrial tissues can be transported by lymphatic routes and result in perineal endometriosis.

Nicola Cinardi et al., reported a special case of perineal scar endometriosis ten years after Miles' procedure for rectal cancer. The patient was a 35-year-old-female who was treated 10 years earlier at the same institution for a low rectal cancer. She presented with two discrete subcutaneous bulges within her perineal wound. Since the patient was asymptomatic and the complete work up for recurrent disease showed no evidence of malignancy, first line therapy was conservative. After two pregnancies and a caesarean section, the patient presented at our observation with enlarged and tender perineal nodules. The patient was treated with a wide excision of the perineal scar en-bloc with the nodules. Final pathology report was consistent with perineal scar endometriosis. In the report, the author suggests that direct implantation of endometrial tissue cannot explain all the cases. There are a variety of cases of primary cutaneous endometriosis without previous abdominal surgery at different sites such as umbilicus, vulva, perineum, groin, and extremities (Healy et al., 1995;

Ideyi et al., 2003). From an etiologic perspective, the present case can be explained with postoperative menstrual implantation within the open perineal wound resulting from the procedure. Another mechanism of transplantation would see silent foci of unknown, asymptomatic pelvic endometriosis that could have been present at the time of surgery and have been disseminated within the wound edges. These foci developed into overt disease several years after surgery (Nicola et al., 2011).

3. Malignant transformation

There is a growing awareness of risk of possible transformation of endometriosis into an invasive malignancy. This is rare but well documented, and theoretically, it can occur in any gonadal or extragonadal site of endometriosis. Since 1925, more than 200 cases of malignant transformation of endometrioma have been reported in the literature (English). Heaps et al. found that 79% of such cases occurred in the ovary, the reminder occurring in extragonadal sites, usually in rectovaginal septum, pelvic peritoneum, colon, rectum, and vagina. The 5-year survival rate in patients with localized disease treated with surgery and postoperative radiation is about 80% (Heaps et al., 1990). Malignant transformation of extraovarian endometriosis is uncommon and only 60 cases have been reported world widely until 1990; of them, ninety percent are endometroid carcinomas (Johana et al., 2007).

Johana Castillo Bustamante et al. reported a 41 year-old female patient with an episiotomy in her delivery and a myomectomy performed at 31 year-old. She had symptoms for a year like progressive pain and tumour at the perineum and glutei area and cyclic bleeding. The core biopsy reported endometrioid carcinoma of perineum. She was diagnosed of "1. Pelvic tumour: Hematometra or ovarian tumour; 2. Solid tumour of right isquiorrectal area: endometroid carcinoma". When laparotomy was performed, the uterus was absent, a left ovarian endometrioma cyst and a right follicular cyst were detected, and appendix had endometrial tissues. Six months after the surgery the patient had liver metastases and she died 2 months later (Johana et al., 2007).

4. Clinical findings and diagnosis

4.1 Clinical features

Almost all patients with PEM are of reproductive ages and has a history of vaginal delivery. The perineal mass is often found in the episiotomy site or laceration site after vaginal delivery. Most patients have perineal cyclic pain corresponding to menstrual periods. Usually there is a mass between left labium majora and labium minora close to the clitoris. Perineal mass can be big and tender. Mostly the color of mass is normal. Sometimes the color of perineum is blue. Some patients have cyclic bleeding in perineal mass.

We analyzed 36 patients with perineal endometriosis who were operated on between 1983 and 2007 at Peking Union Medical College Hospital (PUMCH) retrospectively. The mean age of the 36 patients was 30.7 years (range, 23-44 years). Mean gravidity was 2.05 (range, 1-6) and mean parity was 1.03 (range 1-2). The median latent period (time from delivery to the women having perineal pain or nodule) of these 36 cases was between 4 months and 13 years after delivery. All cases had cyclical perineal pain, which was progressive and correlated with their menstrual cycles (Zhu et al, 2009).

4.2 Physical examination

A thorough physical examination, which included a bimanual gynecologic examination, a trimanual gynecologic examination and a digital rectal examination (DRE), was performed on each case. The exam revealed a hard perineal nodule corresponded to the episiotomy scar or perineal laceration scar. In a patient with PEM and anal sphincter involvement, the nodule was also associated with part of the anal sphincter. In nearly half of all patients with PEM at PUMCH, the endometrioma eroded into the anal sphincter. Thus, it is imperative that further examination (including DRE and endoanal ultrasonography) should be used to confirm whether the anal sphincter is involved in a patient with PEM. Physical examination (including DRE) could provide extremely important additional clues. The mass is generally hard, frequently adjacent to an existing episiotomy scar or previous site of tearing or injury. For some patients, the skin color over the perineal lesions may be brownish on examination. Some may have cyclic ulceration or bleeding from the perineal mass.

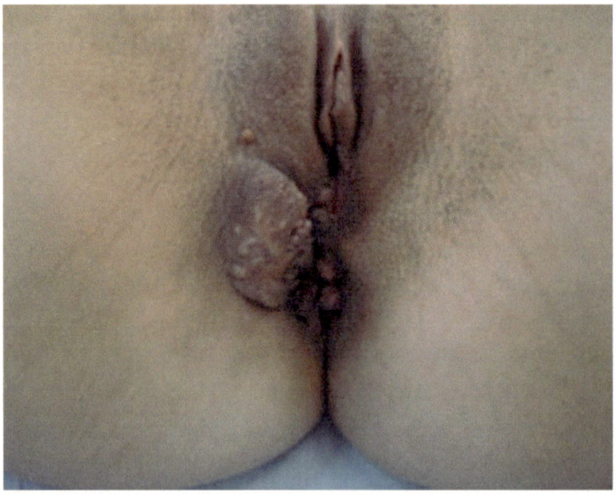

Fig. 1. Preoperative status with firm nodule in the episiotomy scar (Odobasic et al., 2010)

4.3 Lab examination

Our study of 36 patients with Perineal Endometriosis (PEM) between 1983 and 2007 in PUMCH revealed serum CA_{125} was elevated in 2 (6.7%) of 30 patients (CA_{125} levels were measured in 30 patients of these 36 patients) (Zhu et al., 2009). In 31 cases of perineal endometriosis with anal sphincter involvement, level of serum CA_{125} was elevated (>35U/ml) in 2 (6.5%) cases because of simple PEM with anal sphincter involvement. An analysis Of 101 patients with abdominal wall endometriosis (AWE) between 1992 and 2005 in PUMCH showed level of serum CA_{125} was abnormal (>35U/ml) in 20.5% of them (Cheng et al., 2007). These studies indicate the preoperative level of serum CA_{125} is insensitive for the diagnosis of AWE, PEM or PEM with anal sphincter involvement.

Ultrasound is an easy and non-invasive examination that could be prescribed in general practice. Perineal ultrasonography shows irregular hypoechoic mass in the perineal region with rounded or oval anechoic areas in it. With some patients of PEM, the examination shows a heterogeneous mass containing cystic anechoic and hyperechoic areas. Perineal ultrasonography can help in the diagnosis of the lesion, but it fails in revealing the involvement of anal sphincter. Preoperative endoanal ultrasonography, on the contrary, is a reliable technique for visualizing perianal endometriosis and for diagnosing anal sphincter involvement. The ultrasonographic features of the lesion are similar to those mentioned above. Its advantage over perineal ultrasonography is that it can reveal the involvement of anal sphincter clearly. Besides, endoanal ultrasonography can also help in the differential diagnosis of perianal lesions: ultrasonography of perianal abscess shows homogeneous hypoechoic lesions; ultrasonography of perianal fistula shows hypoechoic fistula passes through the longitudinal muscle tissues; ultrasonography of anal carcinoma and melanoma show solid lesions. As 16.7% of patients with PEM are concomitant with pelvic endometriosis, pelvic examination and pelvic ultrasonography should be taken to exclude pelvic endometriosis (Bacher et al., 1999; Toyonaga, 2006; Watanabe et al., 2003).

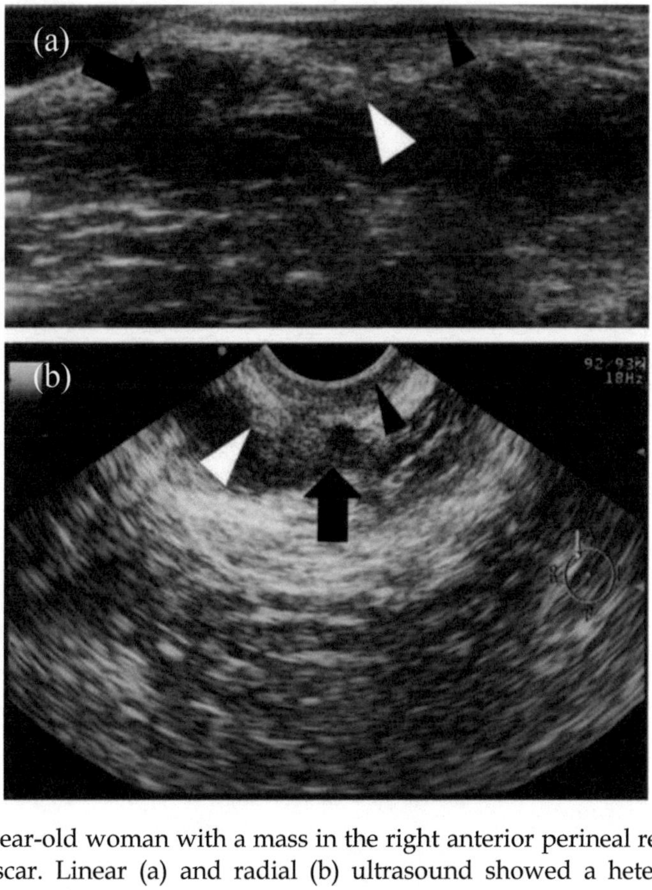

Fig. 2a,b. A 30-year-old woman with a mass in the right anterior perineal region adjacent to an episiotomy scar. Linear (a) and radial (b) ultrasound showed a heterogeneous mass containing cystic anechoic areas (black arrow) in the right anterior perianal region;the mass seemed to involve the external anal sphincter (white arrowhead) and not to involve the internal anal sphincter (black arrowhead). (Toyonaga, 2006)

Computer tomography (CT) also can be used in the diagnosis of perineal endometriosis by some authors. The value of CT however remains to be determined as it is both expensive and uses ionizing radiation. (Amato& Levitt, 1984). Fine needle aspiration cytology of the lesion to demonstrate histological evidence of endometriosis is recommended for an accurate diagnosis (Griffin & Betsill, 1985).

4.4 Diagnosis

Perineal endometriosis can be diagnosed on the basis of clinical features. According to our retrospective study of the 36 cases of PEM, 26 were PEM with anal sphincter involvement (Zhu et al., 2009). The early diagnosis and treatment of PEM is important for the prevention of progressive involvement of surrounding tissue (especially the anal sphincter), thus decreasing the risk of postoperative fecal incontinence. A detailed medical history is of great significance for the diagnosis. Three typical characteristics of perineal endometriosis for women of reproductive ages should be considered when taking a history: (1) past perineal tearing of episiotomy during vaginal delivery; (2) a tender nodule or mass at the perineal lesion; and (3) progressive and cyclic perineal pain. If these 3 criteria were met, the predictive value of perineal endometriosis was 100% (Zhu et al., 2009).

All cases of PEM (including 31 cases of PEM with anal sphincter involvement) at PUMCH met the abovementioned criteria on history and physical examination. Preoperative endoanal ultrasonography is a reliable technique for visualizing perianal endometriosis and for diagnosing anal sphincter involvement. Preoperative endoanal ultrasonography enables the surgeon to determine the operative approach and to explain the possible complications of sphincteroplasty to the patient (Bacher et al., 1999; Toyonaga, 2006; Watanabe et al., 2003).

Serum CA_{125} levels are of great clinical importance in the diagnosis of pelvic endometriosis. In other types of EM, the serum level of CA_{125} is of little significance. However, pelvic examination and ultrasonography should be performed when serum CA_{125} levels are elevated in a patient with PEM to exclude pelvic endometriosis.

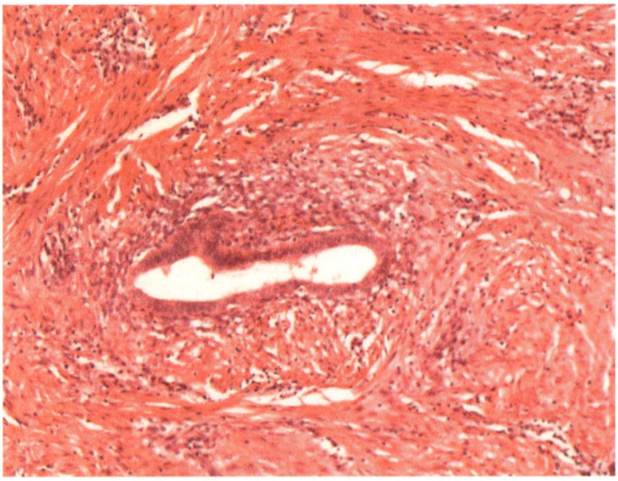

Fig. 3. Histopathology: an endometrial gland in the sphincteric muscular tissue (H & E, ×100)

The pathology result of the excised lesions (endometrial glands and stroma in hyperplastic connective tissues) confirmed the diagnosis.

5. Management

Management of perineal endometriosis can be classified into surgical management and medical management.

5.1 Surgical management

Surgical excision of endometrioma is recommended in all perineal endometriotic cases, in spite of a case of spontaneous regression of endometrioma after subsequent pregnancy reported in the literature. Wide excision of the endometrial tissues with a good healthy margin is important even if this necessitates primary sphincteroplasty when the anal sphincter is involved. It has the best chance of cure and is recommended in all cases where such an excision does not compromise function of adjacent structures and organs (Barisic et al., 2006).

In our analysis of 36 cases of perineal endometriosis in 2007, 10 patients with no anal sphincter involvement had complete excision of the endometrial tissue and did not receive hormonal treatment before or after surgery. None of these 10 patients had recurrence or fecal incontinence at the follow-up between 4 and 11 years. There were no postoperative complications after surgical excision. Surgical intervention with complete excision of the mass included a resection margin of 0.5–1 cm of surrounding healthy tissue (Zhu et al., 2009).

Of the 26 patients with perineal endometriosis and anal sphincter involvement, 18 cases received complete excision and had no recurrence or fecal incontinence during follow-up between 4 and 11 year. Of these 18 patients, 7 patients had no hormonal treatment and remaining patients had hormonal treatment after surgery. Of the remaining 8 patients with anal sphincter involvement, disease recurred after incomplete excision in 7 of them and complete excision in 1 of them. After a second complete wide surgical excision of perineal endometriomas, there were no recurrence during follow-up between 6 months to 5 years (Zhu et al., 2009).

Based on this analysis, Lan Zhu et al. suggest surgical excision is the first choice of treatment for perineal endometriosis. The relevance between the recurrence rate of perineal endometriosis and anal sphincter involvement makes preoperative evaluation of anal sphincter important (Zhu et al., 2009).

Anal sphincter invasion of the endometrioma provides an interesting dilemma. The goal is to excise the endometrioma completely, which may compromise the anal sphincter. This may necessitate primary sphincteroplasty to lesson the risk of fecal incontinence. A PubMed search showed only 13 cases of perineal endometriosis with anal sphincter involvement in eleven different case reports since 1957 (Bacher et al., 1999; Barisic et al., 2006; Beischer et al., 1966; Dougherty & Hull, 2000; Gordon et al., 1976; Hambrick et al., 1979; Kanellos et al., 2001; Martı´nez et al., 2002; Prince & Abrams, 1957; Sayfan et al., 1991; Toyonaga, 2006). In the 13 cases of PEM with anal sphincter involvement, the wide excision (WE) and primary sphincteroplasty (PSp) were performed in 6 cases, narrow excision (NE) and PSp in 5 cases, and incomplete excision (IE) in 1 case, and spontaneous regression after a subsequent delivery was registered in 1 case. In cases where NE was performed, there were no complications associated with this procedure, but, in two cases, recurrence developed requiring subsequent hormonotherapy (Prince & Abrams, 1957; Gordon et al., 1976). In the group where WE was performed, there were no complications, no incontinence or recurrence during variable follow-up (minimal 3 months, maximal 36 months). Based on these studies, WE and PSp is recommended as the best treatment for PEM with anal sphincter involvement (Barisic et al., 2006; Dougherty & Hull, 2000; Kanellos et al., 2001; Martı´nez et al., 2002; Sayfan et al., 1991; Toyonaga, 2006).

Some authors suggest in younger patients, wide excision with PSp may be optimal to obviate the need for additional therapy. In older patients closer to menopause, narrow or incomplete excision with subsequent hormonal therapy could (when endometriosis tends to regress) lessen the risk of incontinence with sphincter resection (Dougherty & Hull, 2000).

In another analysis of 31 cases of perineal endometriosis with anal sphincter involvement in our hospital, NE and PSp was carried out in 30(96.8%) patients. IE was applied in the remaining 1 (3.2%) patient because her endometrioma was too large to excise completely. Of these 31 cases, hormonotherapy was applied to 21 (67.7%) cases preoperatively. For patients who received hormonotherapy preoperatively, pathological examination of the resected lesions showed gland atrophy and interstitial hyperplasia. These provided evidence for the effectiveness of hormonotherapy. As an adjuvant treatment, hormonotherapy in PUMCH (GnRH-agonist as the first choice) should be administered preoperatively for 2-4 months when physical examinations of patients revealed lesions involved with the anal sphincter. The aim was to reduce the size of endometrioma and make boundaries of these lesions clearer, thus to make the complete excision of lesions easier and reduce damage to surrounding tissues. With no recurrence in the NE and Psp group, we suggest preoperative hormonotherapy for every PEM with anal sphincter involvement patinet. For patients (≥40 years) whose perineal lesions are too large to excise clearly, to avoid postoperative fecal incontinence and recurrence, hysterectomy and bilateral salpingo oophorectomy could be considered instead after discussing with the patient.

No recurrence or fecal incontinence was found in the NE group and 1 recurrence occurred with the IE patient during a variable follow-up period from 6 to 78 months. This may be relevant to the use of preoperative hormonotherapy in the NE group. We recommend NE and PSp with preoperative hormonotherapy as an appropriate treatment for PEM with anal sphincter involvement. Hormonotherapy immediately after surgery could be omitted, provided the lesion was resected completely.

5.2 Medical management

Medical management (including oral contraceptives, danazol, progestogens, gonadotrophin-releasing hormone agonists (GnRH- agonists and gestrinone) could produce temporary relief of symptoms. No drug eradicates endometriosis or produces long-term cure.

Beischer et al. reported that 1 patient had spontaneous regression of perineal endometriosis after a subsequent pregnancy, suggesting that the endometriosis was related to the change in hormone levels (Beischer et al., 1966). In our analysis of 36 cases with perineal endometriosis, one patient underwent hysterectomy and bilateral salpingo-oophorectomy for a recurrence of perineal endometrioma seven years after complete excision of perineal endometriosis. The patient was then followed up for 2 years; the perineal endometrioma decreased gradually and then could not be detected (Zhu et al., 2009). This also supports the theory that endometriosis was related to the change in hormone levels.

In all the masses resected from our patients who had hormone treatment before surgery, the pathologic examination of the excised specimens showed gland atrophy and interstitial hyperplasia. These cases confirmed the effectiveness of hormone treatment. However, hormone treatment provided only short-term success in alleviation of symptoms and recurrence was common after the hormone therapy was stopped, so the hormone could be used only as an adjuvant therapy. In our hospital, GnRH agonists are the first choice. We also use oral contraceptive pills, progestogens either preoperatively or postoperatively (Zhu et al., 2009).

In our analysis of 31 cases of perineal endometriosis with anal sphincter involvement in our hospital, hormonal treatment was applied to 21 (67.7%) cases preoperatively and 14 (45.2%) cases postoperatively. For patients received hormonal therapy preoperatively, pathological examination of the resected lesions revealed responsive tissues after medical treatment. These provided evidence for the effectiveness of hormonal therapy preoperatively. As an adjuvant treatment, GnRH- agonists are the first choice in our hospital nowadays.

GnRH- agonists could effectively deplete the pituitary of endogenous gonadotropins and inhibit further synthesis, thus interrupting the menstrual cycle and resulting in a hypoestrogenic state, endometrial atrophy, and amenorrhea. In our hospital, the aim of GnRH- agonists used preoperatively for 3-4 months was to reduce the size of endometrioma, make boundaries of these lesions clearer thus to reduce intraoperative damage to the surrounding tissues and make the complete resection of lesions easier.

6. Conclusion

Three typical characteristics of perineal endometriosis for women of reproductive ages include: (1) past perineal tearing of episiotomy during vaginal delivery; (2) a tender nodule or mass at the perineal lesion; and (3) progressive and cyclic perineal pain. If these 3 criteria were met, the predictive value of perineal endometriosis was 100% (Zhu et al., 2009). Based on these two studies of patients of perineal endometriosis in our hospital, Lan Zhu et al. suggests complete excision of the endometrioma is the first choice of treatment for perineal endometriosis (Zhu et al., 2009). When the perineal endometrioma invades into anal sphincter, we recommend NE and PSp with preoperative hormonal therapy as an appropriate treatment.

7. References

Amato M, Levitt R. (1984). Abdominal wall endometrioma: CT findings. *J Comput Assisted Tomography*, Vol.8, (1984), pp. 1213-1214, ISSN 0363-8715

Bacher H, Schweiger W, Cerwenka H & Mischinger HJ. (1999). Use of anal endosonography in diagnosis of endometriosis of the external anal sphincter: report of a case. *Dis Colon Rectum*, Vol.42, No.5, (May, 1999), pp. 680-682, ISSN 0012-3706

Barisic G, Krivokapic Z & Jovanovic D. (2006). Perineal endometriosis in episiotomy scar with anal sphincter involvement: report of two cases and review of the literature. *Int Urogynecol J*, Vol.17, (2006), pp. 646-649, ISSN 0937-3462

Beischer NO. (1966). Endometriosis of an episiotomy scar cured by pregnancy. *Obstet Gynecol*, Vol.28, (1966), pp. 15-21, ISSN 0029-7844

Bergqvist A. (1993). Different types of extragenital endometriosis: a review. *Gynecol Endocrinol*, Vol.7, (1993), pp. 207-221, ISSN 1473-0766

Carter JE. (1994). Combined hysteroscopic and laparoscopic findings in patients with chronic pelvic pain. *J Am Assoc Gynecol Laparosc*, Vol.2, (1994), pp. 43-47, ISSN 1074-3804

Cheng Ninghai , Zhu Lan et al. (2007). Clinical analysis of 101 cases of abdominal wall endometriosis. *J Reprod Med*, Vol.16, No.2, (2007), pp. 82-85, ISSN 0024-7758

Dougherty LS & Hull T. (2000). Perineal endometriosis with anal sphincter involvement: report of a case. *Dis Colon Rectum*, Vol.43, (2000), pp. 1157–1160, ISSN 0012-3706

Gordon PH, Schottler JL, Balcos EG & Goldberg SM. (1976). Perianal endometrioma: report of five cases. *Dis Colon Rectum*, Vol.19, (1976), pp.260-265, ISSN 0012-3706

Griffin JB & Betsill WL. (1985). Subcutaneous endometriosis diagnosed by fine needle aspiration cytology. *Acta Cytol*, Vol.29, (1985), pp. 584-588, ISSN 0001-5547.

Hambrick E, Abcarian H & Smith D. (1979). Perineal endometrioma in episiotomy incisions: clinical features and management. *Dis Colon Rectum*, Vol.22, (1979), pp. 550-552, ISSN 0012-3706

Healy JT, Wilkinson NW & Sawyer M. (1995). Abdominal wall endometrioma in a laparoscopic trocar tract: a case report. *Am Surg*, Vol.61, (1995), pp. 962-963, ISSN 0002-9610

Heaps JM, Nieberg RK & Berek JS. (1990). Malignant neoplasms arising in endometriosis. *Obstet Gynecol*, Vol.75, (1990), pp. 1023-1028, ISSN 0029-7844

Ideyi SC, Schein M, Niazi M & Gerst PH. (2003). Spontaneous endometriosis of the abdominal wall. *Dig Surg*, Vol.20, (2003), pp. 246-248, ISSN 0253-4886

Johana Castillo Bustamante, Francisco Loreto & Doris Digianmarco, et al. (2007). Endometriosis Perineal Malignizada. *Rev venez Oncol*, Vol.19, No.4, (2007), pp. 337-343, ISSN 0798-0582

Kanellos I, Kelpis T, Zaraboukas T & Betsis D. (2001). Perineal endometriosis in episiotomy scar with anal sphincter involvement. *Tech Coloproctol*, Vol.5, (2001), pp. 107-108, ISSN 1123-6337

Koninckx PR, Meuleman C, Demeyere S, Lesaffre E & Cornillie FJ. (1991) .Suggestive evidence that pelvic endometriosis is a progressive disease, whereas deeply infiltrating endometriosis is associated with pelvic pain. *Fertil Steril*, Vol.55, (1991), pp. 759-765, ISSN 0015-0282

Lin YH, Kuo LJ & Chuang AY. (2006). Extrapelvic endometriosis complicated with colonic obstruction. *J Chin Med Assoc*, Vol.69, (2006), pp. 47-50, ISSN 1726-4901

Ling FW. MD.& The Pelvic Pain Study Group. (1999). Randomized controlled trial of depot leuprolide in patients with chronic pelvic pain and clinically suspected endometriosis. *Obstet Gynecol*, Vol.93, (1999), pp. 51-58, ISSN 0029-7844

Martin L, Pernoll, M.D. (2001). Endometriosis and Adenomyosis, In: Benson & Pernoll's handbook of Obstetrics & Gynecology 10th ed, 0071383522, McGraw-Hill Companies, United States of America

Martı´nez P, Villanueva E & Alvarez F, et al. (2002). Endoanal sonography in the assessment of perianal endometriosis with external anal sphincter involvement. *J Clin Ultrasound*, Vol.30, (2002), pp. 245-8, ISSN 0091-2751

Nicola Cinardi, Salvatore Franco & Danilo Centonze, et al. (2011). Perineal scar endometriosis ten years after Miles' procedure for rectal cancer: Case report and review of the literature. *International Journal of Surgery Case Reports*, Vol.2, (2011), pp. 150-153, ISSN 2210-2612

Odobasic, A., A. Pasic & Iljazovic-Latifagic, et al. (2010). Perineal endometriosis: a case report and review of the literature. *Tech Coloproctol*, Vol.14, No. Suppl 1, (Nov 2010), pp. S25-27, ISSN 1123-6337

Prince LN, Abrams J. (1957). Endometriosis of the perineum: review of the literature and case report. *Am J Obstet Gynecol*, Vol.73, (1957), pp. 890-893, ISSN 0002-9378

Rawson JM. (1991). Prevalence of endometriosis in asymptomatic women. *J Reprod Med*, Vol.36, (1991), pp. 513-515, ISSN 0024-7758

Sampson JA. (1921). Perforateing hemorrhagic cysts of the ovary: their importance and especially their relation to pelvic adenomas of emdometrial type ('adenoma' of the uterus, rectovaginal septum, sigmoid etc.). *Arch Surg*, Vol.3, (1921), pp. 245, ISSN 0004-0010

Sayfan J, Benosh L, Segal M & Orda R. (1991). Endometriosis in episiotomy scar with anal sphincter involvement. Report of a case. *Dis Colon Rectum*, Vol.34, No.8, (Aug 1991), pp. 713-716, ISSN 0012-3706

Strathy JH, Molgaard CA, Coulam CB & Melton LJ 3d. (1982).Endometriosis and infertility: a laparoscopic study of endometriosis among fertile and infertile women. *Fertil Steril*, Vol.38, (1982), pp. 667-672, ISSN 0015-0282

T. Toyonaga, M. Matsushima & Y.Tanaka, et al. (2006). Endoanal ultrasonography in the diagnosis and operative management of perianal endometriosis: report of two cases. *Tech Coloproctol*, Vol.10, (2006), pp. 357-360, ISSN 1123-6337

Watanabe M, Kamiyama G & Yamazaki K, et al. (2003). Anal endosonography in the diagnosis and management of perianal endometriosis: report of a case. *Surg Today*, Vol.33 , (2003), pp. 630-632, ISSN 0941-1291

Wheeler JM. (1989). Epidemiology of endometriosis-associated infertility. *J Reprod Med*, Vol.34, (1989), pp. 41-46, ISSN 0024- 7758

Zhu L, Lang JH, Wong F & Guo L. (2003). Perineal endometriosis without perineal trauma: a case report. *Chin Med J*, Vol.116, No.4, (2003), pp. 639-640, ISSN 0366-6999

Zhu Lan, Lang Jinghe & Wang Hanbi, et al. (2009). Presentation and management of perineal endometriosis. *Int J Gynaecol Obstet*, Vol.105, No.3, (Jun 2009), pp. 230-232, ISSN 0020-7292

4

Abdominopelvic Complications of Endometriosis

Arturo del Rey-Moreno
Department of General Surgery, Hospital de Antequera, Málaga, Spain

1. Introduction

Endometriosis is a painful chronic disease occurring in 4 to 17% of menstruating women. Its aetiology is unknown, although there is a high incidence in sterile females (10-25%) (Pritts *et al.*, 2003), 60-70% in women with chronic pelvis pain as well as in those who have a family history (Bianchi *et al.*, 2007). It is characterized by the presence of functional endometrial tissue consisting of glands and/or stroma located outside the uterus.

Endometriosis can be divided into intra and extraperitoneal sites. The intraperitoneal locations are ovaries (30%), uterosacral and large ligaments (18-24%), fallopian tubes (20%), pelvic peritoneum, pouch of Douglas and gastrointestinal tract. Extraperitoneal locations include cervical portio (0.5%), vagina and rectovaginal septum, round ligament, inguinal hernia sac, abdominal scars after gynaecological surgery (1.5%) and caesarean section (0.5%). This disease rarely affects extra-abdominal organs such as the lungs, urinary system, skin and the central nervous system (Chapron *et al.*, 2003; Veeraswamy *et al.*, 2010).

Clinical manifestations of endometriosis fall into three general categories: pelvic pain, infertility and pelvis mass. The goal of therapy is to relieve these symptoms. There is no high quality evidence that one medical therapy is superior to another for managing pelvic pain due to endometriosis, or that any type of medical treatment will affect future fertility. Therefore, treatment decisions are individualized, taking into account the severity of symptoms, the extent and location of disease, desire for pregnancy, the age of the patient, medication side effects, surgical complication rates, and cost (Berlanda *et al.*, 2010; Shakiba *et al.*, 2008).

2. General indications for surgery of endometriosis

Indications for surgical management of endometriosis include:

- Symptoms that are severe, incapacitating, or acute.
- Symptoms that have failed to resolve or have worsened under medical management.
- Advanced disease: anatomic distortion of the pelvic organs, endometriotic cysts, obstruction of the bowel or urinary tract, etc.
- Patient reluctance to use hormonal/non-surgical treatments.
- Adnexal mass suspicious for malignancy.

3. Pre and postoperative medical therapy

3.1 Preoperative medical therapy

Hormonal suppression has been used prior to surgery to decrease the size of endometriotic implants (Yap *et al.*, 2004). However, there is no evidence that preoperative hormonal intervention decreases the extent of surgical dissection and recurrence rates, prolongs the duration of pain relief, or increases future pregnancy rates.

3.2 Postoperative medical therapy

The hypothetical advantages of short-term postoperative medical treatment, including resorption of residual visible foci and sterilisation of microscopic implants, should result in a reduction of postoperative lesions and symptoms recurrence rates (Vercellini *et al.*, 2003).

Progestins, danazol, estrogen-progestin pills, and GnRH agonists have been used in conjunction with laparotomy or laparoscopic conservative or definitive surgical treatment. Several trials have reported that these agents increase the duration of pain relief and delayed recurrence of symptoms (Kennedy *et al.*, 2005). However, a meta-analysis of eight trials, considered that postoperative hormonal suppression of endometriosis decreased recurrence rates, but there was no significant benefit for the outcomes of pain or pregnancy rates (Yap *et al.*, 2004). The main problem in interpreting the above data is the short-instead of long-term use of medications. In fact, the rationale for suggesting adjuvant therapy for a few months is far from clear. When this treatment is deemed opportune, oestrogen-progestogen combinations should be considered because of their tolerable side effects, limited costs, and antalgic efficacy similar to GnRH agonists and danazol (Kennedy *et al.*, 2005).

The lowest effective dose of hormone replacement should be used shortly after definitive surgery or as soon as menopausal symptoms arise. Avoidance of oestrogen-only treatment and the use of combined preparations or tibolone are suggested (Vercellini *et al.*, 2009). Oestrogen-only therapy has been associated with an increased risk of malignant transformation of ectopic foci (Modesitt *et al.*, 2002).

4. Treatment of pelvic pain and recurrent symptomatic endometriosis

Several physiopathological mechanisms might explain the relation between endometriosis and pelvic pain: (i) recurrent cyclic micro-bleeding in the endometriotic lesions responsible for hyperpressure; (ii) production of inflammatory mediators by endometriotic lesions, which can stimulate the nerves; (iii) adhesions responsible for fixed position of pelvic structures; (iv) compression and/or infiltration of the sub-peritoneal nerve fibres by deep implants (Fauconnier & Chapron, 2005).

Women with pelvic pain and suspected endometriosis may be managed with empiric medical therapy prior to establishing a definitive diagnosis by laparoscopy. It is suggested analgesics and/or combined oral estrogen-progestin contraceptives for women with no more than mild pelvic pain and a GnRH agonist for those with moderate to severe pelvic pain. Although 80 to 90% of patients will have some improvement in symptoms with medical therapy, medical interventions neither enhance fertility nor diminish endometriomas or adhesions, and they are more appropriately managed surgically (Kennedy *et al.*, 2005). The growing popularity and widespread diffusion of operative laparoscopy has fostered a spread of surgical procedures in women with endometriosis (Vercellini *et al.*, 2009). However, due to the relapsing tendency of the disease, postoperative recurrences are very common (20-40%), and a further surgical procedure is performed in 15-20% of cases (Busacca *et al.*, 1998; Fedele *et al.*, 2006).

4.1 Repetitive conservative surgery

Conservative surgery preserves the uterus and as much ovarian tissue as possible. Very limited information is available on the effect of repetitive conservative surgery for recurrent symptomatic endometriosis in terms of postoperative pain relief (Vercellini *et al.*, 2009). Pain relief is achieved in most patients who undergo laparoscopic ablation of endometriosis and adhesiolisis. However, the long-term outcome appears suboptimal, with a cumulative probability of pain recurrence between 20% and 40% and a further surgical procedure between 15% and 20% (Fedele *et al.*, 2006; Vercellini *et al.*, 2009).

Busacca *et al.* (1998) compared surgical outcomes in patients reoperated either at laparatomy or at laparoscopy. The crude recurrence rates of moderate to severe dysmenorrhea, deep dyspareunia, and pelvic pain were, respectively, 22%, 30%, and 35% in the laparotomy group and 29%, 25%, and 32% in the laparoscopy group. The 24-month cumulative probability of recurrence of dysmenorrhea (34% and 43%, respectively) and non-cyclical pelvic pain was not significantly different in the two groups. However, in the patients operated by laparotomy, the rate of recurrence of deep dyspareunia and the number of patients requiring a third intervention was higher.

The effect of repetitive laparoscopic surgery on pain is similar to that observed after first-line surgery, with a 5-year cumulative pain recurrence rate of 20% after the first surgical procedure and 17% after the second one and cumulative rates of retreatment of 19% and 17%, respectively. This fact confirm the effectiveness of repeat conservative surgery in the treatment of recurrent pain, which is more likely to be associated with severe disease, adhesions and deep intraovarian or multilocular cysts (Fedele *et al.*, 2006).

High recurrence rate is the demonstration that surgery alone is a suboptimal treatment for a chronic disease such endometriosis. In order to possibly reduce recurrences of endometriosis, it is important that all surgical procedures including primary surgery are performed by experienced surgeons and that prolonged ovarian suppression is established postoperatively (Vercellini *et al.*, 2009).

4.2 Pelvic denervating procedures

In these conditions, one of the clinical dilemmas regards the indication for and the potential benefit of reoperation. In women wishing for conception, uterine denervation may be performed in addition to repetitive ablation of endometriotic lesion to improve long-term antalgic results. Laparotomy or laparoscopy plus presacral neurectomy has better results than surgery only in regard to: recurrence of dysmenorrhea at 1-year follow-up (17% and 25%, respectively), dysmenorrhea relief at 6 and 12 month follow-up (87% vs 60%, and 86% vs 57%, respectively), severity of dysmenorrhea, dyspareunia, non-menstrual pelvic pain and health-related quality of life at 24-month follow-up (Zullo *et al.*, 2004). However, this technique presents limitations that must be taken into account: first, it is effective in reducing midline pain only, whereas lateral, adnexal pain is not influenced; second, denervation of bowel and bladder cause *de-novo* constipation (15%) and urinary urgency (5%) (Latthe *et al.*, 2007; Zullo *et al.*, 2004); third, great care must be taken to avoid damaging the right ureter and major and midsacral vessels (Berlanda *et al.*, 2010). Systematic performance of presacral neurectomy cannot be recommended, only in patients with central, hipo-gastric pain (Latthe *et al.*, 2007; Vercellini *et al.*, 2009).

The addition of uterosacral ligament resection (i.e., laparoscopic uterosacral nerve ablation) to laparoscopic surgical treatment of endometriosis was not associated with a significant difference in any pain outcomes (Latthe *et al.*, 2007).

4.3 Definitive surgery

Definitive surgery in women with chronic pain is a controversial procedure, especially in young women. However, this factor should be carefully evaluated in order to offer a reliable prognosis to women affected by an oestrogen-responsive disease (Vercellini *et al.*, 2009). The surgical solution in women with recurrent symptoms after previous conservative procedures for endometriosis should be based on the desire for conception, and the pre-operative patient assessment must be complete, including testing for bowel dysmotility, urologic disorders, musculoskeletal lesions, and psycho-socio-environmental factors (Berlanda *et al.*, 2010). The risk of depressive symptoms after definitive procedures must be taken into account, particularly in young patients (Vercellini *et al.*, 2009). The definitive therapy for endometriosis is represented by total hysterectomy, bilateral salpingo-oophorectomy and removal of all endometriotic lesions, in particular deep lesions involving the pouch of Douglas, the anterior pouch or the ureter. The operation mimic radical hysterectomy (Berlanda *et al.*, 2010).

When pregnancy is no longer an issue and the woman reveals good psychological stability, hysterectomy with or without bilateral salpingo-oophorectomy may be considered and offers the best outcome. The presence of multiple pelvic symptoms, previous use of a GnRH agonist, and absence of pain resolution predict the likelihood of subsecuent hysterectomy (Learman *et al.*, 2007). Few studies address the advantages of hysterectomy for severe pelvic pain associated with endometriosis. Standard extrafascial hysterectomy is associated with increased recurrence of pain than radical hysterectomy with removal of deep endometriotic lesions (31% vs 0%) (Fedele *et al.*, 2005a).

The decision to preserve or remove the ovaries should be based on patient's age and intraoperative gonadal conditions. Bilateral oophorectomy substantially reduces the risk of recurrent symptoms and reoperation due to pelvic pain over the ovarian-preserving surgery (10% vs 62%, and 3.7-8% vs 19.2-31%, respectively). Preservation of both ovaries at hysterectomy for symptomatic endometriosis increased the risk of reoperation by 2.4 to 8.1 (Shakiba *et al.*, 2008). Nonetheless, whenever possible at least one gonad should be preserved in young women, especially in those with objections to the use of oestrogen-progestogens (Shakiba *et al.*, 2008). The effect of postoperative medical treatment on the probability of pain relapse should be taken into account after both conservative and definitive procedures.

5. Deep infiltrating endometriosis

The term deep infiltrating endometriosis (DIE) is used to describe infiltrative forms of the disease that involve the uterosacral ligaments, rectovaginal septum, bowel, bladder, or ureters, but is histologically defined in arbitrary manner when endometriotic lesions extending more than 5 mm beneath the peritoneal surface (Chapron *et al.*, 2009) suggest, regardless of location (bladder, intestine, ureter, etc.) that endometriosis is only considered to be DIE when the muscularis is involved (Yantiss *et al.*, 2001). This entity is responsible for refractory pelvic pain, of which the intensity is correlated with the depth of infiltration, and occurs in 30%-40% of the patients with endometriosis (Chapron *et al.*, 2003).

DIE is thought to arise from several possible mechanisms: (i) The Sampson's retrograde menstruation theory: during menstruation, endometrial tissue refluxes trough the fallopian tubes, implanting and growing on the serosal surface of abdominal and pelvic organs, influenced by local hormones and immune, genetic and environmental factors. This results in peritoneal and ovarian endometrial deposits. (ii) The coelomic metaplasia theory proposes that endometriosis develops from metaplasia of the cells that line the pelvic peritoneum. These cells share a common embryological origin with the germinal endometrium of the ovary and the müllerian ducts. Infectious, hormonal or inflammatory stimuli could result in metaplasia of these cells and endometriosis. This theory is supported by the rare occurrence of endometriosis in men and in prepubertal girls. (iii) The embryonic rest theory proposes that metaplasia of müllerian duct remnants in the rectovaginal septum could result in the rectovaginal nodules. (iv) Another theory implies the migration of cells through the lymphatic system or vía hematogenous spread. (v) The neurologic hypothesis is a new concept in the pathogenesis of endometriosis: the lesions seem to infiltrate the large bowel wall along the nerves, at a distance from the primary lesion (Anaf *et al.*, 2004). It is thought that the growth and invasion of endometrial tissue at ectopic sites is due to a process of neovascularizacion mediated by pro-angiogenic factors such as vascular endothelial growth factor (VEGF) (Taylor *et al.*, 2009). Histologically, endometrial nodules are composed of hypertrophic smooth muscle and endometrial glands, similar in appearance to adenomyosis in the uterus (Brouwer & Woods, 2007).

The multifocal distribution of DIE lesions indeed prompted us to cease considering this disease as a single organ pathology but rather, to see it as an "abdomino-pelvic multifocal pathology" (Chapron *et al.*, 2010). The pre-operative work-up (questioning, clinical examination and imaging information) aims to clarify the exact location and likely extension of DIE lesions. This is essential in order to: (i) Specify the surgical procedures required to achieve complete excision of symptomatic DIE lesions, the only way to prevent the recurrence. (ii) Thoroughly describe the surgical risks to the patient. (iii) Obtain the patient's full informed consent, as necessary prior to surgery for a benign pathology responsible for painful symptoms (Chapron *et al.*, 2010). It must take into account that the discovery of a DIE nodule during clinical and/or imaging investigations is not always followed by surgery. Only lesions that give rise to symptoms should be operated on.

Although medical treatment may be effective in some DIE patients, the treatment of choice is surgical excision. The multifocal nature of DIE lesions must be taken into account when defining the surgical strategy (Chapron *et al.*, 2003). Generally, DIE is presented as a pathology with a high risk of recurrence, estimated at around 30%. Often, however, recurrence corresponds to persistence of DIE lesions that were left in place as the result of an incomplete initial surgical removal (Vignali *et al.*, 2005).

6. Bowel endometriosis

Endometriosis affects the gastrointestinal tract of 5-12% of women with this condition (Wills *et al.*, 2009). The rectum and the rectosigmoid junction are the most common sites of bowel endometriosis (70-93% of all bowel lesions). The rectovaginal septum, appendix, caecum and distal ileum may also be affected, with a lower incidences (12%, 3-18%, 2-5% and 2-20%, respectively). (Chapron *et al.*, 2003; De Cicco *et al.*, 2011). In most cases, intestinal endometriosis is associated to genital endometriosis. Rectal involvement is associated with DIE and adnexal endometriosis in 70% and 80% of the patients, respectively (Chapron *et al.*, 2003).

Bowel endometriosis is considered an infiltration or invasion phenomenom, found that there is a histological continuity between the superficial and underlying deep lesions originating from the serosa progressively invade the muscularis propria (Anaf *et al.*, 2004). Endometriosis infiltrating the muscularis propria may lead to localized fibrosis, strictures, and small or large bowel obstruction (Yantiss et al, 2001).

Bowel endometriosis is difficult to diagnose because of the lack of characteristic symptoms. The patients present with relapsing bouts of abdominal pain, abdominal distention, tenesmus, constipation, diarrhoea, rectal bleeding and pain during defecation (Brouwer & Woods, 2007). Colicky abdominal pain is the most common symptom. Rectal bleeding may be caused by mucosal injury during the passage of stools through a stenosed colon with the intramural endometriotic tissue increased at the time of menses if it occurs. Bowel endometriosis can mimic other abdominal pathologies such as malignancy, inflammatory bowel disease, ischaemic colitis, infectious diseases and irritable bowel syndrome (Bianchi *et al.*, 2007). Hematochezia is an uncommon symptom due to low incidence of mucosal involvement. Endometriosis of the small bowel should be suspected in young, nulliparous patients with abdominal pain, in conjunction with signs of obstruction (Del Rey-Moreno *et al.*, 2008).

Clinical examination has been shown to have a low sensitivity and moderate specificity for uterosacral, high rectovaginal and rectal involvement. The presence of a large, palpable rectovaginal nodule identifies the patient at risk of rectal involvement. The low percentage of rectal endometriosis extending to the mucosa means colonoscopy has too low a sensitivity to be a reliable test for rectal involvement. Preoperative colonoscopy should be performed on an individualised basis to exclude other pathology and suspicious mucosal lesions should be biopsied to exclude malignancy (Wills *et al.*, 2009). Endorectal ultrasound has shown a sensitivity of more than 90% for rectovaginal septum endometriosis and a lower specifity for rectal wall invasion. Transvaginal ultrasound may be as effective as endorectal ultrasound (Chapron *et al.*, 2004). Magnetic resonance imaging of cul-de-sac obliteration, deep pelvic nodules and rectal involvement have an accuracy of 72-90% in predicting disease when measured against findings at surgery (Kataoka *et al.*, 2005). Currently, MRI is the best imaging modality for enteric endometriosis with a sensitivity of between 77-93% (Bianchi *et al.*, 2007). When endoscopic and radiologic examinations (computed tomography, endorectal ultrasound, magnetic resonance imaging) are performed, an extrinsic process is revealed and nearly all patients undergo a diagnostic laparoscopy as part of their investigations their symptoms (De Cicco *et al.*, 2011). This is often the first test that identifies rectal involvement. Brouwer & Woods (2007) have proposed a preoperative approach that minimizes the use of endorectal ultrasound and magnectic resonance imaging and focuses on assessing the possibility of rectal involvement on laparoscopy and clinical examination under anaesthetic. A significant number of patients have more than one laparoscopy and the number of laparoscopies has been shown to correlate to extent of rectal involvement.

Treatment consists of surgical excision, or segmental resection. Excision should be complete in order to achieve maximal pain relief and minimal recurrences (De Cicco *et al.*, 2011). When the rectum is involved there are several approaches to be considered. The choice of technique depends on the size, location, degree and depth of involvement of the endometriotic implant. As a general rule, less is better when it comes to removal of rectal endometriosis as long as the implant can be completely excised. The nodule can be shaved off the rectal wall leaving it intact if superficial serosal deposits are present, alternatively if there is a solitary penetrating nodule there may be the opportunity to perform a full-thickness disc resection of the rectal wall, or it may be necessary to consider a segmental resection of the rectum and/or sigmoid colon (Brouwer & Woods, 2007; Wills *et al.*, 2009). All these procedures can be carried out by either a laparoscopic, combined or open approach (Brouwer & Woods, 2007; Dousset *et al.*, 2010; Wills *et al.*, 2009). Robotic assistance may allow more bowel resections to be carried out by laparoscopy (Veeraswamy *et al.*, 2010). An initial laparoscopy is carried out unless the preoperative assessment mandate a laparotomy. It appears that most authors decide to perform a bowel resection before surgery, based on preoperative examinations. This approach seems to result in a very high incidence of bowel resection. The indication reported is based on dimensions of the nodule >2 cm or 3 cm, and/or on muscularis involvement and/or occupation of more than one-third of the rectal circumference (Brouwer & Woods, 2007). The other approach is to decide during surgery based on findings such as the size, localisation and extension of the disease. Laparoscopic conversion rates is from 0% to 13%, due to extent of disease, dense adhesions, bowel perforation, difficulty stapling a bowel anastomosis, bleeding and poor visualisation (Wills *et al.*, 2009).

Surgery is only indicated in enteric endometriosis in acute or subacute small bowel obstruction that fails to resolve, in endometriotic tumours or when it is impossible to exclude malignancy. In an emergency setting, the main aim of surgery should be to relieve the obstruction, and if the disease is suspected intra-operatively, then as many ectopic deposits as possible should be excised (Bianchi *et al.*, 2007; Del Rey-Moreno *et al.*, 2008). It can be difficult to exclude a malignancy intra-operatively, in such case is appropriate to carry out an oncological resection.

Appendiceal endometriosis may present as an incidental finding with or without pelvic disease. Acute symptoms are similar to those of appendicitis. The appendix should be inspected in all patients undergoing surgery for endometriosis and appendectomy is recommended if it seems abnormal (Veeraswamy *et al.*, 2010).

The overall complication rate after surgery is 22.2%. Major complications occur in 7%-12.6% of women: colorectal anastomotic leakage (3.7%-11%), recto-vaginal fistula (4%-8.5%), severe obstruction (2.7%), haemorrhage (2.5%), pelvic abscess (1-4.2%), delayed ureteral ischemic necrosis (2%). Minor complications occur in 14.7% of women: temporary bowel dysfunction (4%), bladder dysfunction (8%-17%) (De Cicco *et al.*, 2011; Dousset *et al.*, 2010). The combination of systematic diverting ileostomy, interposition of omentoplasty and nonjuxtaposed vaginal and colorectal sutures are major factors in preventing and facilitating the conservative treatment of anastomotic leaks, and the increased use of preoperative endoscopic ureteral double pig-tail stenting may help to prevent delayed ureteral ischemic necrosis related to extensive ureterolysis. The most frequent specific complication of compete surgery for low rectal endometriosis is transient peripheral neurogenic bladder. The inferior hypogastric nerves are recognized and preserved during surgery but may require resection in cases with lateral pelvic wall invasion (Dousset *et al.*, 2010).

The recurrence of symptoms for follow-up periods of 2-5 years varies between 4% and 54%. The recurrence of pain requiring surgery is 0% to 34%. Proven bowel endometriosis recurrence is 0-25% (De Cicco *et al.*, 2011; Dousset *et al.*, 2010), and is higher for dissection off the rectal wall (22.2%) that anterior rectal wall excision (5.2%) and segmental rectal resection (0-4.7%) (Brouwer & Woods, 2007; Dousset *et al.*, 2010). Recurrence of endometriosis can be explained by the significant proportion of rectal lesions that extend into the submucosa (36%) (Brouwer & Woods, 2007). The overall improvement in pain-related symptoms is of 87%-94% and in quality of life assessment of 90% (Dousset *et al.*, 2010). Dousset y cols (2010) believe that the very low recurrence in rectal endometriosis is related to a "carcinologic" surgical approach: (i) all additional extrarectal sites of endometriosis were removed, (ii) total mesorectal excision and en-bloc resection of the rectal nodule together with posterior vaginal fornix and uterosacral to ensure free anterior and circumferential resection margins, (iii) rectal section at least 2-cm below the endometriotic nodule, and (iv) all additional intestinal and urologic endometriotic deposits were resected with 2-cm-free surgical margins.

The results of several series show that with a multidisciplinary approach (gynaecologic, gastrointestinal and urologist surgeons, radiologist) to the management of endometriosis involving the rectum and radical surgery to excise the disease as completely as possible at one operation, excellent results can be achieved with low morbidity and recurrence (Brouwer & Woods, 2007; De Cicco *et al.*, 2011; Dousset *et al.*, 2010).

7. Abdominal wall endometriosis

Abdominal wall endometriosis is defined as endometrial tissue within the abdominal wall, superficial to the peritoneum. This entity occurs in 0.03 to 1.08% of women with previous history of obstetric or gynaecologic procedures, particularly after histerotomy The time from surgery to the onset of symptoms ranges from months to 17.5 years, with an average of 30 months. The association between abdominal wall endometriosis and pelvic endometriosis is found in 2.5% - 25% of the cases (Bektas *et al.*, 2010; Horton *et al.*, 2008).

The pathogenesis of abdominal wall endometriosis is explained by a combination of theories: (i) Iatrogrenic direct implantation during the surgical procedure, endometrial tissue is seeded into the wound; this theory alone is not enough to completely explain the physiopathology, given the low incidence of this disease and the reports of endometriosis without previous surgery, (ii) endometrial cells may reach a caesarean section via lymphatic or hematogenous routes, (iii) coelomic metaplasia and, (iv) cell immunity change theory (Bektas *et al.*, 2010). Malignant transformation of abdominal wall endometriosis is a rare complication (1%).

It should always be considered when a mass appears in or near a caesarean section scar or other gynaecologic operative procedure sites, in the umbilicus or in the inguinal region, more so when pain accompanying the patient's menstrual cycle. The diagnosis may become difficult if cyclical pain is not present (43%). Also be diagnosed in patients without previous surgery. Moreover, abdominal wall endometriosis patients are often referred to the general surgeons and were diagnosed after surgical techniques such as appendectomy, inguinal hernia repair, or laparoscopic procedures. Accurate preoperative diagnosis varies between 20% and 50% (Bektas *et al.*, 2010; Horton *et al.*, 2008).

Additional studies such as ultrasound, CT scan, MRI, or fine-needle aspiration may be obtained if the lesion is very large, there is concern for fascial involvement, or if the diagnosis is in doubt. This information may assist with surgical planning especially when an abdominal wall reconstruction is anticipated (Veeraswamy *et al.*, 2010). Ultrasonography is the most commonly used investigational procedure for abdominal masses; the mass may appear hypoechoic and heterogeneous with scattered internal echoes, solid, or with cystic changes. The findings on computed tomography scan depend on the phase of the menstrual cycle, the proportions of stromal and glandular elements, the amount of bleeding, and the degree of surrounding and fibrotic response, without pathognomonic findings. Owing to the relatively vascular nature of these lesions, enhancement often occurs when intravenous contrast material is used. Magnetic resonance imaging enables very small lesions to be detected and can distinguish the hemorrhagic signal of endometriotic lesions. Fine needle aspiration cytology can confirm the diagnosis and eliminate the possibility of malignancy. This is justified only in cases of large masses, doubtful diagnosis and atypical clinical manifestations. However, its use is still controversial of the risk of causing new implants at the puncture site (Bektas *et al.*, 2010; Horton *et al.*, 2008).

The treatment of choice is surgical excision with at least 1 cm margin, even for recurrent cases and, if necessary, placement of mesh for fascia defects. A combination of surgical re-excision with hormonal therapy is also recommended (Bektas *et al.*, 2010; Horton *et al.*, 2008).

During violation of endometrial cavity, inoculum of endometrial tissue spill and implant on the abdominal wound. Thus, it is strongly recommended that the abdominal wound be cleaned at the conclusion of the cesarean section. Other recommendations are delivering the uterus outside the abdomen to repair, not using the same suture material to close the abdomen as used for uterine closure, not swabbing out the uterine cavity following the delivery of the placenta or discarding the swab used to clean the endometrial cavity after delivery of placenta, or using wound edge protector to separate the edges of the incision from contact with the patient's abdominal contents, instruments, and gloves during the procedure (Bektas *et al.*, 2010; Horton *et al.*, 2008).

8. Urinary tract endometriosis

Endometriosis expanding and invading the urinary tract is a rare occurrence found in 0.3%-5% of all endometriotic patients (Chapron *et al.*, 2003; Mereu *et al.*, 2010). The bladder is the most frequently involved organ, followed by the ureters and the kidneys with a proportion of 40:5:1. The endometriosis that comprises the urinary tract cannot be considered to be primary lesions from these organs (Abrao *et al.*, 2009).

8.1 Bladder endometriosis

Bladder is the most frequent location in cases of urinary endometriosis. Amongst women suffering from DIE, 11% present lesions that affect the bladder. According to the three major etiopathogenic theories proposed, vesical endometriosis may develop from mulleriam remnants in the vesicouterine septum, or as an extension of an adenomyotic nodule of the anterior uterine wall, or from implantation of regurgitated endometrium (Chapron *et al.*, 2003).

Patients may present with variable urinary symptoms (cystalgia 43%-58.3%, dysuria 21%-25%, urinary frequency 16.6%-71%, macroscopic hematuria 12.5%-19%) (Le Tohic *et al.*, 2009) and/or symptoms related to endometriosis (dysmenorrhea 70.8%, dyspareunia 21%-50%, chronic pelvic pain 43%-75%); these symptoms may be cyclic (34.6%-100%) (Abrao *et al.*, 2009; Le Tohic *et al.*, 2009). This entity should also be considered in postmenopausal patients receiving hormonal replacement therapy who report voiding symptoms and who are unsuccessfully treated for interstitial cystitis. During pelvic examination an anterior nodule is palpated in 41.7% to 97.5% of the patients. When a bladder nodule is diagnosed, it has to be differentiated from bladder carcinoma, varices, papillomas or angiomas (Chapron *et al.*, 2010; Le Tohic *et al.*, 2009).

The diagnosis of bladder endometriosis is often difficult to make and it is based on ultrasound, MRI, and cystoscopy. Generally, pelvic ultrasound is the first imaging test performed and allows the bladder nodule DIE in the 38%-100% of patients (Le Tohic *et al.*, 2009). Transvaginal ultrasound is capable of diagnosing bladder nodules in 58.3% of patients. Cystoscopy may reveal typical red and/or bluish lesions (30%-38.4%), extrinsic compression (38.4%), or may be normal (Chapron *et al.*, 2010; Le Tohic *et al.*, 2009); and also helps to rule out vesical epithelial malignancy, to ascertain the precise location of bladder DIE nodule (distance with the ureteral meata and the lower endometriotic margin) and to define the ureteral status (Chapron *et al.*, 2010). The presentation of endometriosis varies over the menstrual cycle; the lesions are more obvious and congestive during menstruation (Pang *et al.*, 2008). MRI shows the presence of a nodule in 77.2%-100% of patients. Generally, the bladder DIE nodule is unifocal in the bladder wall (posterior wall 62.5%-74.7%, vesical dome 25.3%-37.5%). The mean size of the bladder nodule at pathological examination is 23.6 mm (range 8-50 mm). Bladder DIE is isolated in 36% of the cases, and 64% of the patients is associated with posterior DIE lesions (intestinal 32%, ureteral 9.3%, unilateral or bilateral ovarian endometriomas 24%, uterosacral ligament 33.3%, vagina 26.7%); therefore, should not be considered as an independent form of the disease (Chapron *et al.*, 2010; Fedele *et al.*, 2005b, Le Tohic *et al.*, 2009).

Treatment of bladder endometriosis can be medical therapy with antiestrogenic agents or surgical excision. Medical therapy often results in temporary improvement of the symptoms, but relapse may occur. Most clinicians agree that surgery is the best option and resection should be complete. This can be carried out by laparotomy or laparoscopy depending on the lesion, skill, and experience of the surgeon (Chapron *et al.*, 2010; Fedele *et al.*, 2005b; Le Tohic *et al.*, 2009). Cystoscopic transillumination was used to better define the edges of the lesion and to maximize sparing of unaffected mucosa (Fedele *et al.*, 2005b). During the surgical procedure complete excision of all associated symptomatic posterior DIE lesions are performed (uterosacral resection, colpectomy, intestinal resection).

Transurethral resection is not an optimal treatment because it does not permit complete excision of the disease –the disease originates outside (from the peritoneum) the bladder- (Chapron *et al.*, 2010; Le Tohic *et al.*, 2009), radicality would imply bladder perforation, and the patients have a high recurrence (11.5 %) (Le Tohic *et al.*, 2009). Pang *et al.* (2008) have reported a case treated with combined transurethral and laparoscopic excision followed by laparoscopic bladder reconstruction, taking advantage of both approaches.

Major complications can occur in 2.7% of patients, such as vesico-uterine or vesico-digestive fistula, intravesical or pelvic hematoma (Chapron *et al.*, 2010; Le Tohic *et al.*, 2009). The painful symptoms improved in 100% of the patients (Chapron *et al.*, 2010). The recurrence rate of clinical-instrumental evidence can range between 0% (Chapron *et al.*, 2010) and 10.9% (Fedele *et al.*, 2005b).The factors influencing rate of recurrence is the extent of surgical excision and the vesical base involvement. When the resection include both the vesical lesion and a 0.5-1 cm deep portion of the adjacent myometrium, recurrence is significantly less frequent compared to the removal of the bladder lesion only (0% vs 26%, respectively) (Fedele *et al.*, 2005b).

8.2 Ureteral endometriosis

Ureteral endometriosis is a rare but serious localization of the disease (<0.3%) (Li *et al.*, 2008) because it may cause silent loss for renal function (Abrao *et al.*, 2009; Li *et al.*, 2008; Mereu *et al.*, 2010). Disease is predominantly unilateral, with the left ureter affected more commonly than the right, although bilateral disease does occur (Li *et al.*, 2008). The lesions are localized in the lower third of the ureter (Abrao *et al.*, 2009), and associated with endometriosis elsewhere in the pelvis (Li *et al.*, 2008; Mereu *et al.*, 2010). There are two major pathologic types of ureteral endometriosis: intrinsic and extrinsic, occurring, respectively with a 1:4 ratio. In the intrinsic disease, ectopic endometrial tissue infiltrates the muscularis mucosa and the uroepithelium. In the extrinsic disease, the endometrial tissue invades only the ureteral adventitia or surrounding connective tissue. These pathologic types can coexist. Indeed, both entities can lead to ureteral obstruction with subsequent hydroureter and dilatation of the renal pelvis that can be also asymptomatic (Li *et al.*, 2008). Generally, bladder is not affected for endometriosis in the patients with ureteral endometriosis. This observations confirms that, although ureter and bladder are both part of the urinary tract, endometriotic lesions affecting these sites have a different behavior (Abrao *et al.*, 2009).

The patients have symptoms predominantly related to pelvic endometriosis (dysmenorrhea, dyspareunia, chronic pelvic pain [75%-100%]) and lower frequency patients have urologic symptoms such as renal colic or urinary frecuency (3.6%-50%). Because of the absence urologic symptoms (56.5%) and the risk for subsequent loss of renal function (20%), checking the integrity of the urinary tract of patients with endometriosis not only before surgery and after surgery but also during medical therapy is recommended (Li *et al.*, 2008; Mereu *et al.*, 2010). Rectal or vaginal infiltration by the posterior DIE is present in 74% of these patients, and extensiveness of adnexal adhesion are factors related to dysmenorrhea severity (Abrao *et al.*, 2009). The presence of retrocervical and rectum-sigmoid involvement in most patients with ureteral endometriosis suggest that the origin of ureteral endometriosis is extrinsic (Abrao *et al.*, 2009; Mereu *et al.*, 2010).

The diagnostic exams include ureteroscopy with intraluminal ultrasound, computerized tomography, abdominal ultrasound, intravenous pyelography and laparoscopy. Ultrasound as a screening tool to rule out urinary tract obstruction in patients with pelvic endometriosis is routinely used, whereas intravenous pyelography and cystoscopy are used only for patients with urologic symptoms or positive ultrasound for ureteral or bladder involvement. When ureteral involvement and cortical atrophy are revealed, renal function should be checked by kidney scintigraphy (Camanni *et al.*, 2010). Patients with renal compromise may benefit from percutaneous nephrostomy for urinary diversion before definitive surgery. The pelvic spread of the disease and its involvement of the other pelvic organs are evaluated by CT and/or MRI (Li *et al.*, 2008).

The treatment of ureteral endometriosis should be tailored to relieve urinary tract obstruction, eliminate symptoms, preserve renal function, and to avoid disease recurrence and any morbidity associated with radical surgery (Li *et al.*, 2008). Hormonal therapy has been proposed by some authors for the treatment, but others have noted that drugs are unlikely to relieve ureteral obstruction once dense fibrosis has occurred. Hormonal therapy is an appropriate option for patients with normal renal function or minimal obstructions. Surgical treatment remains the gold standard in severe forms of endometriosis: ureterolysis, segmental resection and anastomosis, or ureteroneocystostomy; taking into account that ureteral endometriosis and pelvic disease should be treated at the same time when they coexist (Li *et al.*, 2008). Minimally access procedures are equally effective as the open techniques (Camanni *et al.*, 2010; Mereu *et al.*, 2010). Ureterolysis could be used as the initial surgical step for patients if the extension of ureteral involvement is limited in length and there is no residual ureteral damage or dilatation (Camanni *et al.*, 2010; Mereu *et al.*, 2010). Preoperative endoscopic ureteral double pig-tail stenting may help to prevent delayed ureteral ischemic necrosis related to extensive ureterolysis. In cases of intrinsic ureteral endometriosis, it is necessary to perform a ureteral dissection. When the localization of the stricture is far from the bladder, an uretero-ureterostomy has to be considered. When the ureteral stenosis is reasonably close to the vesicoureteral junction the best choice is the ureteroneocystostomy. In some cases, when the localization of the stricture is halfway or in which resection of a long segment of the ureter is required, ureteroneocystostomy with a psoas bladder hitch must be carried out (Mereu *et al.*, 2010).

Ureterolysis has demonstrated to be effective as the first-line surgical approach in patients with deep endometriosis despite the rate of recurrence reported (0-15.8%) (Camanni *et al.*, 2010; Li *et al.*, 2008; Mereu *et al.*, 2010). Reintervention during hospitalization and follow-up is more frequent in patients undergoing ureterolysis than in those treated with ureteroureterostomy (33% vs 11.7%) (Mereu *et al.*, 2010).

8.3 Renal endometriosis

Renal endometriosis is a rare condition. Presenting symptoms and signs include flank or back pain, hematuria, hydronephrosis, or a renal mass (Dirim *et al.*, 2009). Additional studies are necessary to help determine its etiology (intravenous pyelography, computerized tomography scan or MRI). Unfortunately, in the absence of a biopsy there is no accurate preoperative method to exclude malignancy, so a majority of patients are treated with nephrectomy (Veeraswamy *et al.*, 2010).

9. Other sites of intra-abdominal endometriosis

9.1 Liver endometriosis

Hepatic endometriosis is rarely seen. Malignancy must be excluded when endometriosis is discovered in unusual sites like the liver. The majority of patients are symptomatic, generally with epigastric or right upper quadrant abdominal pain. Catamenial epigastric pain is characteristic, although rarely seen. Other possible presentations are malaise, nausea, vomiting, obstructive jaundice, portal vein thrombosis, hepatomegaly (Nezhat *et al.*, 2005; Schuld *et al.*, 2011) and bilioptysis, which is intermittent bile-stained sputum (Schuld *et al.*, 2011). Generally, liver involvement is superficial. The lesion size ranged from 3 to 20 cm. The principal diagnostic method is CT scan or MRI, showing a heterogeneous mass containing septated, thick-walled cystic lesions, implying complex pathophysiology (Veeraswamy *et al.*, 2010). Because of the wide range of possible morphologic features of endometriosis, there are no characteristic imaging findings that can distinguish either pelvic or extrapelvic endometriosis from other processes. Final diagnosis can only be made by pathologic evaluation. The treatment is surgical resection with adequate margins (Nezhat *et al.*, 2005).

9.2 Pancreatic endometriosis

Endometriosis involving the pancreas is an extremely rare condition. The patients have pain abdominal in the left upper quadrant and/or abdominal mass. In a woman of childbearing age with intermittent abdominal pain and a cystic lesion in the pancreas on imaging studies, endometriosis must be considered in the differential diagnosis. Partial pancreatectomy and resection of the adjacent viscera affected is the treatment of choice (Tunuguntla *et al.*, 2004).

9.3 Omentum endometriosis

Involvement of the omentum by endometriosis is not rare. Probably occur by transmission through peritoneal fluid or lymphatics. The commonest clinical features are abdominal distension, dymenorrhoea and brown or bloody ascites. Laparoscopy and biopsy may still be necessary to exclude malignancy. Treatment is by excision of endometriotic nodule and/or ovarian suppression (Naraynsingh *et al.*, 1985).

9.4 Nervous system endometriosis

The most common site of endometriosis involving the nervous system has been within nerves in or near the pelvis. Sciatic nerve endometriosis presents as sciatic pain, muscle weakness, sensory deficits, and pelvic pain. Cyclic sciatica related to menses should be considered suggestive of endometriosis. Similarly, endometriosis involving obturator nerve, produces pain and proximal muscle weakness. Theses patients are treated by excision of endometriosis and associated fibrosis surrounding the nerve. Although the direct spread of pelvic endometriosis to and along nerves coursing through the pelvis seems logical, not all patients have been found to have pelvic disease (Veeraswamy *et al.*, 2010).

10. Massive ascites and endometriosis

The association of endometriosis with massive bloody ascites is extremely rare and represent a diagnostic dilemma for gynecologists, owing to their rarity and to the fact that theses cases mimic malignant ovarian neoplasms. In these cases the endometriosis involves mainly the peritoneum, with multiple adhesions and ovarian endometriomas. Ascites is detected in large volumes (4254 mL on average) and is bloody or brown (Sait, 2008).

Ectopic endometrial tissue is influenced by hormonal levels of the uterine cycle, so it flakes off with the drop of the hormonal peak as normal endometrium. This mechanism causes an inflammatory reaction in the site of interest and possible ascites in the case of peritoneal endometriosis. The rapid production of fluid by inflamed tissue and the obstruction of subdiaphragmatic lymph vessels, which impair its reabsorption, may be responsible for the large volumes detected (Zeppa *et al.*, 2004).

Fine-needle cytology has been successfully used to diagnose endometriosis by demonstrating the presence of epithelial and stromal cells in the smears, but usually their cytological features are not specific enough to allow a definite cytological diagnosis of endometriosis, nor to exclude even a neoplastic process (Zeppa *et al.*, 2004). Endometriosis-associated ascites is commonly mistaken for ascites caused by ovarian neoplasms, especially when associated with an elevated CA-125 level (Sait, 2008), and laparoscopy and microscopic examination of tissue are generally required for diagnosis. Nonetheless, the cytological diagnosis of endometriosis in effusions, avoid more invasive diagnostic procedures (Zeppa *et al.*, 2004).

Although there is no established treatment is usually performed conservative surgical resection and suppression of ovulation with a GnRH agonist (Sait, 2008).

11. Spontaneous hemoperitoneum in pregnancy and endometriosis

Spontaneous hemoperitoneum in pregnancy is an uncommon yet dramatic cause of hemoperitoneum, associated with high perinatal mortality (31%) and 44% of these deaths attributable to maternal shock. No maternal deaths have been reported in the last 20 years. The condition is most common during the third trimester of pregnancy. Endometriosis is considered a major risk factor (Brosens *et al.*, 2009).

The cause of this condition is not fully clarified. Inoue *et al.* (1992) have suggested two possible explanations for the involvement of endometriosis: (i) chronic inflammation due to endometriosis may make utero-ovarian vessels more friable; (ii) the resultants adhesions may give further tension to these vessels when the uterus is enlarged during pregnancy. Invasiveness of severe endometriosis has been suggested as a reason for this entity, but Brosens *et al.* (2009) found no apparent correlation between spontaneous hemoperitoneum in pregnancy and stage of endometriosis.

The typical presentation of spontaneous utero-ovarian vessel rupture consists of a sudden onset of abdominal pain without vaginal bleeding, associated with signs of acute abdomen and hypovolemia. Fetal distress is an uncommon finding unless there is severe hemodynamic instability. Abdominal ultrasound examination does not reveal signs of placental abruption and fail to diagnose intraperitoneal bleeding as cause of acute pain. Transvaginal ultrasound and computerized tomography scans sometimes indicate the presence of intraperitoneal free fluid, but in most cases the diagnosis is only established at laparotomy (Brosens *et al.*, 2009). Preoperatively other potential diagnoses are placental abruption, uterine rupture, HELLP syndrome, abdominal pregnancy or rupture of the liver or spleen (Grunewald & Jördens, 2010).

At laparotomy, a substantial amount of hemoperitoneum is found (range: 500 to 4000 mL). The bleeding is not arterial but arise from superficial veins or varicosities on the posterior surface of the uterus or parametria. Treatment of bleeding is variable: thermal coagulation, hemostatic sutures or clips, or hysterectomy after caesarean section (Brossens 2009).

Since endometriosis may cause infertility, and assisted reproduction technology is increasingly used to enable patients to conceive, it is likely that there will be more cases with unprovoked hemoperitoneum in the near future (Grunewald & Jördens, 2010).

12. Malignancy

Malignant transformation is an infrequent complication of endometriosis and has been reported in 0.7-1% of patients and 62%-78.7% of the cases occur in the ovary, whereas extragonadal sites represent 21.3%-38% of tumors. The rectovaginal septum, rectosigmoid colon, vagina, and pelvic peritoneum represented the majority of extragonadal sites. Other locations include: bowel, umbilicus, lymph node, urinary tract, pleura, diaphragm, lung, etc (Slavin *et al.*, 2000; Van Gorp *et al.*, 2004; Yantiss *et al.*, 2001). Two possible explanations for the relation-ship between endometriosis and intraperitoneal cancer have been proposed: (i) endometriotic implants undergo malignant transformation secondary to genetic defects (p53 mutations) (Akahane *et al.*, 2007) that also serve to enable the endometriosis to thrive, or (ii) women with endometriosis have a defect in their immune system that enables the endometriosis to flourish, and this baseline defect leaves them more susceptible to subsequent malignant transformation (Modesitt *et al.*, 2002). It has been seen a direct transition from clearly benign epithelium through atypical endometriosis to carcinoma. This association suggest that atypical endometriosis can act as a precancerous lesion, as seen in atypical hyperplasia of the endometrium (Van Gorp *et al.*, 2004).

Among malignancies arising from endometriosis of the ovaries, endometrioid adenocarcinoma is the most common histologic type (23%-69.1%), followed by clear-cell carcinomas (13.5%-23%), sarcomas (11.6%), and rare cell types (6%) (Modesitt *et al.*, 2002). Extragonadal lesions are mostly endometrioid tumors (66%) and sarcomas (25%); clear cell histology is seen in only 4.5% of extragonadal malignancies. Tumors arising in endometriosis are predominantly low grade and confined to the site of origin (Slavin *et al.*, 2000; Van Gorp *et al.*, 2004). The histopathological criteria to classify a malignancy as arising from endometriosis include the demonstration of cancer arising in the tissue and not invading it from another source, and the presence of tissue resembling endometrial stroma surrounding the epithelial glands (Slavin *et al.*, 2000).

The risk factors for malignant transformation in endometriosis are poorly defined. An association has been noted between unopposed estrogen therapy and the development of endometrioid or clear cell epithelial ovarian tumors (Modesitt *et al.*, 2002). Increasing parity, and hormonal contraceptive use for $\geq$ 5 years, decreases the risks of both subtypes. Breast feeding and tubal ligation are inversely associated, but significantly so only for the endometrioid tumor (Nagle *et al.*, 2008; Van Gorp *et al.*, 2004). Obesity is associated only with clear cell cancers, with a two-fold increased risk. Also a significant trend of decreasing risk with increasing intensity (not duration) of smoking and education beyond high school is associated with decreased development of clear cell cancers only (Nagle *et al.*, 2008). The decreased risk of clear cell ovarian cancer amongst users of combined oestrogen and progestin hormone replacement therapy is interesting given the role of progestin as a potential chemopreventive agent in ovarian cancer (Nagle *et al.*, 2008). 86% of the patients with an extraovarian cancer had undergone a prior hysterectomy and bilateral salpingo-oophorectomy (Modessit *et al.*, 2002).

Pelvic pain or pelvic mass in a postmenopausal woman with a previous history of endometriosis should raise suspicions of reactivation or malignant transformation of endometriosis. Vaginal bleeding may signify the presence of a vaginal or rectovaginal septum lesion. Malignant transformation of colorrectal endometriosis may produce gastrointestinal dysfunction and/or bleeding. Urinary symptoms may herald urinary tract involvement with this disease (Slavin *et al.*, 2000; Van Gorp *et al.*, 2004).

The differential histological diagnosis of endometrioid and colonic adenocarcinoma is difficult because colonic adenocarcinoma has a significant mucosal component, while endometrioid adenocarcinoma usually involves the outer layers of the colon (30% are intramural) and endoscopic biopsies usually yield insufficient tissue for a definitive pathologic diagnosis (Slavin *et al.*, 2000; Yantiss *et al.*, 2001). Immunohistochemical staining seems to be useful in differentiating colonic endometrioid adenocarcinoma. The endometrioid tumor expresses cytokeratin 7 and CA-125, whereas cytokeratin 20 and carcinoembryonic antigen decorate colonic adenocarcinoma (Slavin *et al.*, 2000).

Primary surgical treatment with complete resection of pelvic tumors should be performed when feasible. Appropriate staging biopsies of lymph nodes and tissues in the upper abdomen should be performed when macroscopic disease is confined to pelvis. After surgical resection, is recommended the progestin therapy. Although postoperative treatment has not been clearly defined, 70% of these patients have been reported to receive chemotherapy or radiotherapy (Modesitt *et al.*, 2002).

Malignant transformation within endometriomas or within extragonadal endometriosis confined to the genital tract carries a much better prognosis, with a 67% 5-year survival for those with disease confined to the ovary and 100% 5-year survival for those with extragonadal disease confined to the site of the origin. Disseminated intraperitoneal disease had a poor prognosis, with a 12% 5-year survival (Van Gorp *et al.*, 2004).

13. Conclusion

The specialist approach to deep endometriosis has now evolved into a collaborative one, much like the multidisciplinary management of colorectal cancer. Preoperative assessment involves radiologist, gynaecologist, colorectal surgeon and in cases where bladder or ureteric involvement are suspected, a urologist. This approach results in the ability to achieve complete excision of all the endometriosis at the one operation.

14. Acknowledgment

This chapter has been financed by the funds of the "Asociación Jornadas Quirúrgicas de Antequera" (Málaga). Spain.

15. References

Abrao MS, Dias JA, Bellelis P, Podgaec S, Bautzer CR, Gromatsky C. (2009). Endometriosis of the ureter and bladder are not associated diseases. *Fertil Steril;* 91: 1662-1667.

Akahane T, Sekizawa A, Purwosunu Y, Nagatsuka M, Okai T. (2007). The role of p53 mutation in the carcinomas arising from endometriosis. *Int J Gynecol Pathol;* 26: 345-351.

Anaf V, El Nakadi I, Simon P, Van de Stadt J, Fayt I, Simonart T, Noel JC. (2004). Preferential infiltration of large bowel endometriosisalong the nerves of the colon. *Hum Reprod;* 19: 996-1002.

Bektas H, Bilsel Y, Sari YS, Ersöz F, Koç O, Deniz M, Boran B, Huq GE. (2010). Abdominal wall endometrioma: A 10-year experience and brief review of the literature. *J Surg Res;* 164: 77-81.

Berlanda N, Vercelllini P, Fedele L. (2010). The outcomes of repeat surgery for recurrent symptomatic endometriosis. *Curr Opin Obstet Gynecol;* 22: 320-325.

Bianchi A, Pulido L, Espin F, Hidalgo LA, Heredia A, Fantova MJ, Muns R, Suñol J. (2007). Intestinal endometriosis. Current status. *Cir Esp;* 81: 170-176.

Brosens IA, Fusi L, Brosens JJ. (2009). Endometriosis is a risk factor for spontaneous hemoperitoneum during pregnancy. *Fertil Steril;* 92: 1243-1245.

Brouwer R, Woods RJ. (2007). Rectal endometriosis: results of radical escisión and review of published work. *Aust N Z J Surg;* 77: 562-571.

Busacca M, Fedele L, Bianchi S, Candiani M, Agnoli B, Raffaelli R, Vignali M. (1998). Surgical treatment of recurrent endometriosis: Laparotomy versus laparoscopy. *Hum Reprod;* 13: 2271-2274.

Camanni M, Delpiano EM, Bonino L, Deltetto F. (2010). Laparoscopic conservative management of ureteral endometriosis. *Curr Opin Obstet Gynecol;* 22: 309-314.

Chapron C, Fauconnier A, Vieira M, Barakat H, Dousset B, Pansini V, Vacher-Lavenu MC, Dubuisson JB. (2003). Anatomical distribution of deeply infiltrating endometriosis: surgical implications and proposition for a classification. *Hum Reprod;* 18: 760-766.

Chapron C, Vieira M, Chopin N, Balleyguier C, Barakat H, Dumontier I, Roseau G, Fauconier A, Foulot H, Dousset B. (2004). Accuracy of rectal endoscopic ultrasonography and magnetic resonance imaging in the diagnosis of rectal involvement for patients presenting with deeply infiltrating endometriosis. *Ultrasound Obstet Gynecol;* 24: 175-179.

Chapron C, Pietin-Vialle C, Borghese B, Davy C, Foulot H, Chopin N. (2009). Associated ovarian endometriomas is a marker for greater severity of deeply infiltrating endometriosis. *Fertil Steril;* 92: 453-457.

Chapron C, Bourret A, Chopin N, Bousset B, Leconte M, Amsellem-Ouazana D, de Ziegler D, Borghese B. (2010). Surgery for bladder endometriosis: long-term results and concomitant management of associated posterior deep lesions. *Hum Reprod;* 25: 884-889.

De Cicco C, Corona R, Schonman R, Mailova K, Ussia A, Koninckx PR. (2011). Bowel resection for deep endometriosis: a systematic review. *BJOG;* 118: 285-291.

Del Rey Moreno A, Jiménez Martín JJ, Moreno Ruiz FJ, Hierro Martín I. (2008). Asociación de enteritis quística profunda, ileocolitis de Crohn y endometriosis como causa de obstrucción intestinal. *Cir Esp;* 83: 271.

Dirim A, Celikkaya S, Aygun C, Caylak B. (2009). Renal endometriosis presenting with a giant subcapsular hematoma: case report. *Fertil Steril;* 92: 391.e5-e7.

Dousset B, Leconte M, Borghese B, Millischer AE, Roseau G, Arkwright S, Chapron C. (2010). Complete surgery for low rectal endometriosis. Long-term of a 100-case prospective study. *Ann Surg;* 251: 887-895.

Fauconnier A, Chapron C. (2005). Endometriosis and pelvis pain: epidemiological evidence of the relationship and implications. *Hum Reprod Update;* 11: 595-606.

Fedele L, Bianchi S, Zanconato G, Berlanda N, Borrato F, Frontino G. (2005a). Tailoring radicality in demolitive surgery for deeply infiltrating endometriosis. *Am J Obstet Gynecol ;* 193: 114-117.

Fedele L, Bianchi S, Zanconato G, Bergamini V, Berlanda N, Carmignani L. (2005b). Long-term follow-up after conservative surgery for bladder endometriosis. *Fertil Steril;* 83: 1729-1733.

Fedele L, Bianchi S, Zanconato G, Berlanda N, Raffaelli R, Fontana N. (2006). Laparoscopic excision of recurrent endometriomas: long-term outcome and comparison with primary surgery. *Fertil Steril;* 85: 694-699.

Grunewald C, Jördens A. (2010). Intra-abdominal hemorrhage due to previously unknown endometriosis in the third trimester of pregnancy with uneventful neonatal outcome: A case report. *Eur J Obstet Gynecol Reprod Biol;* 148: 204-205.

Horton JD, Dezee KJ, Ahnfeldt EP, Wagner M. (2008). Abdominal wall endometriosis: a surgeon's perspective and review of 445 cases. *Am J Surg;* 196: 207-212.

Inoue T, Moriwaki T, Niki I. (1992). Endometriosis and spontaneous rupture of the uterine vessels in a pregnancy complicated by endometriosis. *Lancet;* 340: 240-241.

Kataoka ML, Togashi K, Yamaoka T, Koyama T, Ueda H, Kobayashi H, Rahman M, Higuchi T, Fujii S. (2005). Posterior cul-de-sac obliteration associated with endometriosis: MR imaging evaluation. *Radiology;* 234: 815-823.

Kennedy S, Bergqvist A, Chapron C, D'Hooghe T, Dunselman G, Greb R, Hummelshoj L, Prentice A, Saridogan E. (2005). ESHRE Special Interest Group for Endometriosis and Endometrioum Guideline Development Group. ESHRE guideline for the diagnosis and treatment of endometriosis. *Hum Reprod;* 20: 2698-2704.

Latthe PM, Proctor MI, Farquhar CM, Johnson N, Khan KS. (2007). Surgical interruption of pelvic nerve pathways in dysmenorrhoea: a systematic review of effectiveness. *Acta Obstet Gynecol;* 86: 4-15.

Learman LA, Kuppermann M, Gates E, Gregorich SE, Lewis J, Washington AE. (2007). Predictors of hysterectomy in women with common pelvic problems: a uterine survival analysis. *J Am Coll Surg;* 204: 633-641.

Le Tohic A, Chis C, Yazbeck C, Koskas M, Madelenat P, Panel P. (2009). Endométriose vésicale: diagnostic et traitment. À propos d'une série de 24 patientes. *Gynecol Obstet Fertil;* 37: 216-221.

Li CY, Wang HQ, Liu HY, Lang JH. (2008). Management of ureteral endometriosis: a report of ten cases. *Chin Med Sci J;* 23: 218-223.

Mereu L, Gagliardi JL, Clarizia R, Mainardi P, Landi S, Minelli L. (2010). Laparoscopic management of ureteral endometriosis in case of moderate-severe hydroureteronephrosis. *Fertil Steril;* 93: 46-51.

Modesitt SC, Tortolero-Luna G, Robinson JB, Gershenson DM, Wolf JK. (2002). Ovarian and extraovarian endometriosis-associated cancer. *Obstet Gynecol;* 100: 788-795.

Nagle CM, Olsen CM, Webb PM, Jordan SJ, Whiteman DC, Green AC. (2008). Endometrioid and clear cell ovarian cancers - A comparative analysis of risk factors. *Eur J Cancer*; 44: 2477-2484.

Naraynsingh V, Raju GC, Ratan P, Wong J. (1985). Massive ascites due to omental endometriosis. *Postgrad Med J*; 61: 539-540.

Nezhat C, Kazerooni T, Berker B, Lashay N, Fernandez S, Marziali M. (2005). Laparoscopic management of hepatic endometriosis: report of two cases and review of the literature. *J Minim Invasive Gynecol*; 12: 196-200.

Pang ST, Chao A, Wang CJ, Lin G, Lee CL. (2008) Transurethral partial cystectomy and laparoscopic reconstruction for the management of bladder endometriosis. *Fertil Steril*; 90: 2014.e1-e3.

Pritts EA, Taylon RN. (2003). An evidence-based evaluation of endometriosis-associated infertility. *Endocrinol Metab Clin North Am*; 32: 653-667.

Sait KH. (2008). Massive ascites as a presentation in a young woman with endometriosis: a case report. *Fertil Steril*; 90: 2015.e17-e19

Schuld J, Justinger C, Wagner M, Bohle RM, Kollmar O, Schilling MK, Richter S. (2011). Bronchobiliary fistula: a rare complication of hepatic endometriosis. *Fertil Steril*; 804.e15-e18.

Shakiba K, Bena JF, McGill KM, Minger J, Falcone T. (2008). Surgical treatment of endometriosis: a 7-year follow-up on the requirement for further surgery. *Obstet Gynecol*; 1285-1292.

Slavin RE, Krum R, Van Dinh T. (2000). Endometriosis-associated intestinal tumours: A clinical an pathological study of 6 cases with a review of the literature. *Hum Pathol*; 31: 456-463.

Taylor RN, Yu J, Torres PB, Schickedanz AC, Park JK, Mueller MD, Sidell N. (2009). Mechanistic and therapeutic implications of angiogenesis in endometriosis. *Reprod Sci* ; 16: 140-146.

Tunuguntla A, Van Buren N, Mathews MR, Ehrenfried JA. Endometriosis of the pancreas presenting as a cystic pancreatic neoplasm with possible metastasis.

Van Gorp T, Amant F, Neven P, Vergote I. (2004). Endometriosis and the development of malignant tumours of the pelvis. A review of literature. *Best Pract Res Clin Obstet Gynaecol*; 18: 349-371.

Veeraswamy A, Lewis M, Mphil AM, Kotikela S, Hajhosseini B, Nezhat C. (2010). Extragenital Endometriosis. *Clin Obstet Gynecol*; 53; 449-466.

Vercellini P, Frontino G, De Giorgi O, Pietropaolo G, Pasin R, Crosignani PG. (2003). Endometriosis preoperative and postoperative medical treatment. *Obstet Gynecol N Am*; 30: 163-180.

Vercellini P, Barbara G, Abbiati A, Somigliana E, Viganò P, Fedele L. (2009). Repetitive surgery for recurrent symptomatic endometriosis: What to do? *Eur J Obstet Gynecol Reprod Biol*; 146: 15-21.

Vignali M, Bianchi S, Candiani M, Spadaccini G, Oggioni G, Busacca M. (2005). Surgical treatment of deep endometriosis and risk of recurrence. *J Minim Invasive Ginecol*: 12: 508-513.

Wills HJ, Reid GD, Cooper MJ, Tsaltas J, Morgan M. Woods RJ. (2009). Bowel resection for severe endometriosis: An Australian series of 177 cases. *Aust N Z J Obstet Gynaecol*; 49: 415-418.

Yantiss RK, Clement PB, Young RH. (2001). Endometriosis of the intestinal tract: a study of 44 cases of a disease that may cause diverse challenges in clinical and pathologic evaluation. *Am J Surg Pathol*; 25: 445-454.

Yap C, Furness S, Farquar C. (2004). Pre and postoperative medical therapy for endometriosis surgery. *Cochrane Databese Sys Rev*; 3.CD003678.

Zeppa P, Vetrani A, Cozzolino I, Palombini L. (2004). Endometrial glands in ascites secondary to endometriosis. *Diagn Cytopathol*; 30: 131-132.

Zullo F, Palomba S, Zupi E, Russo T, Morelli M, Sena T, Pellicano M, Mastrantonio P. (2004). Long-term effectiveness of presacral neurectomy for the treatment of severe dysmenorrhea due to endometriosis. *J Am Assoc Gynecol Laparosc*; 11: 23-28.

5

Endometrial Tumors in Postoperative Scars - Pathogenesis, Diagnostics and Treatment

Stanisław Horák and Anita Olejek
Chair and Clinical Department of Gynecology, Obstetrics and Gynecological Oncology, Silesian Medical University Poland

1. Introduction

Endometriosis is defined as the presence of endometrial glands and stroma in another places of the female body than the uterine cavity. Despite of being a relatively common disease it still remains a diagnostic and therapeutic enigma, mainly thanks to its variable presentations. When endometriosis is localized intraperitoneally, the major problem in young women is involuntary sterility, whereas by extraperitoneal localization they suffer predominantly of bothersome pain.

In 1903 Robert Mayer was the first, who described the presence of endometriosis in the postoperative scar, as mentioned in Bytom study (43), and from this time the number of publications in this field is slowly rising, but still a lot of problems ought to be satisfactory elucidated. An investigation of this disease and making firm conclusions is not easy because of inconsistent and small series of patients, often casuistic (2, 5, 6, 8, 11, 12, 13, 16, 19, 22, 30, 36, 39, 42, 46, 48, 52). Up to now only one large systemic review (29) was published and two biggest single retrospective studies (57, 41) included 81 and 72 patients appropriately.

2. Pathogenesis

Endometriosis is doubtless a multifactorial disease.

The most widely accepted theory of arising of the endometriosis is an implantation of endometrial fragments brought by retrograde menstrual flow in a peritoneal surface (50). This should be typical for intraperitoneal lesions.

Meyer's theory explains the origin of endometriosis by celomic metaplasia mainly in the ovaries, peritoneum and urinary bladder due to their common development from the celomic epithelium. Mesenchymal cells with retained multi-potential under the properties circumstances undergo metaplasia into endometriotic cells. This theory may explain the incidence of endometriosis in women with uterine agenesis or in males treated by estrogens (3).

Vascular dissemination theory (27), in turn, with endometrial cells spread into blood or lymphatic circulation may explain distal locations of endometriosis. Very interesting was one of cases described by Agarwal and Fong (1). This Chinese woman suffering from sterility and a lump in right inguinal region had twice laparoscopy and ablation of endometriotic intraperitoneal lesions without managing of the lump. Third laparoscopy revealed endometriotic deposits along the right round ligament contiguous with this lump which was afer excision diagnosed as an endometrioma. It may be speculated, that in some conditions endometriotic cells can infiltrate per continuitatem like a malignant tumour.

The etiopathogenetic mechanism of endometriosis localized in surgical scars would be related to iatrogenic transplantation of endometrium during delivery or surgery, mostly gynecological.

All the mentioned above theories could only elucidate mainly the way on which endometrial cells or fragments could be transported to their improper localizations. But still remains unclear why in these places the endometrial cells survive and proliferate.

Endometriosis is defined as a steroid-dependent condition with a particular genetic background (37). It is well known, that estrogens promote the development of endometriotic lesions and anti-estrogen or gestagen therapy can diminish the symptoms.

There is substantial evidence that not only hormonal but first of all immunologic factors play a role in the pathogenesis of endometriosis (3, 54, 56). Immune alterations include increased number and activation of macrophages, decreased T cells reactivity and NK cells cytotoxicity, increased circulating antibodies and changes in the cytokine system. These alterations are responsive for implantation and survival of the ectopic endometrial cells and concomitant inflammatory reaction and pain. Increased oxidative stress appears to be a common contributory factor in the pathogenesis of endometriosis (3). Wicherek et al. (56) in discussion consider that endometral cells are implanted in ectopic places usually during the maintenance of higher immunotolerance, including pregnancy. The ectopic endometrium preserves the ability to undergo reversible decidualization. Once implanted develops further when estrogens level raise with a concomitant lack of adequate progesterone level.

The next factor, playing a potent role are endometrial stromal cells themselves. When stimulated by estrogens the endometriotic cells may proliferate until they become symptomatic. Moreover, endometriotic lesions can thanks to aromatase activity produce estrogens locally themselves (9).

It is known, that in patients suffering from endometriosis higher activity of integrins and cadherin E on surface of endometrial and mesothelial cells is expressed (24). This may explain the better ability of adhesion of these cells in another places than uterine cavity. The invasion of them is enhanced by metalloproteinases. It was shown, that in patients with endometriotic lesions even eutopic endometrium expresses higher activity of matrix metalloproteinase -2 (MMP-2) whereas lower of tissue matrix metalloproteinase inhibitor – 2 (TIMP-2) (14). The ability of endometrial cells to regulate the cytotoxic immune activity by expression of factors such as RCAS 1 or metallothionein enables their survival in ectopic localizations (56). After invasion the endometrial cells are producing growth factors and cytokinins, such as vascular endothelial growth factor (VEGF), macrophage colony stimulating factor (MCSF) and a lot of others, what stimulates neovascularization of the lesions and further development (25).

The role of genetics (32) and exogenous environmental pollutants (47) as contributing factors is also considered.

3. Occurrence and diagnostics

The disease is uncommon but not so rare. The extraperitoneal localizacion of the lesion is mainly the abdominal wall scar, but should be also in episotomy scar, bowel, bladder, lung, kidneys, brain, umbilicus, groin (29) and even in male urinary tract (51). Leite et al. (38) mentioning except those liver, extremities and pericardium, confirm the opinion that extrapelvic endometrioma occurs mainly as a complication of cesarean section, hysterectomy and episiotomy. Akagi et al. (2) reported an asymptomatic case of endometriosis of the appendix. Endometriosis in the inguinal channel usually occurs on the right side (90%) and in 32% may be associated with an hernia (15, 20). This feature seems to be due to the clockwise circulation of the peritoneal fluid and to the presence of sigmoid colon that shields the left inguinal ring (20). Vulvar involvement of endometriosis is extremely rare. Buda et al. (8) described a case of endometriosis in a scar after excicion of the Bartholin gland.

According to Chaterjee (11) endometriosis of the abdominal wall occurs in 0,03 - 1,08% of women with previous history of obstetric or gynecologic procedures. Leite et al. (38) reviewing bibliography estimates the incidence of abdominal wall endometrioma on 0,03 - 3,5%. Nominato et al. (41) in their large series report the incidence of scar endometrioma in 0,2% women submitted former to cesarean section but only in 0,06% when episiotomy was made. Singh et al. (52) reported three cases, considering that the true incidence of this disease (0,8%) is underestimated because a lot of cases remains undetected. Agarwal and Fong (1) reporting 10 cases (among them six in Pfannenstiel scar) estimate the frequency of cutaneous localization of disease 1,1%. Unusually high percent (5,2%) of cutaneous localization of endometriosis was reported from Glasgow (18).

Concerning the coincidence of peritoneal and abdominal wall endometriosis das Chagas Medeiros et al. (10) basing on literature data estimates the frequency of abdominal wall endometriosis on about 0,5 - 1% in women with pelvic endometriosis. According to another data in 13% both of the forms of disease are present (29), more often by spontaneous abdominal wall endometriosis without any previous surgery (1).

The diagnosis of endometriosis in the postoperative scars is usually established basing on characteristic clinical symptoms as the presence of slowly developing immobile lump, which seems to be attached to the anterior fascia, in the scar or near of them, often swelling during menstruation and painful, especially in this period in most of cases. Sometimes occurs periodical bleeding from the superficial lesions and lower abdominal pain (1, 4, 29). The boundary of the mass is not clear usually. Incision of it looks grey or slightly yellowish (59). Leite et al. (38) in turn, describe it as whitish fibrous tumor with thick chocolate-like colored liquid areas.

Horton et al. (29) summarized their review of 445 cases from 29 reports till 2006 as follows (table 1):

Data	Result	95% CI
Mean age (years)	31,4	29,1 - 33,8
Mean interval to symptoms (years)	3,6	2,5 - 4,8
Presenting with mass	96%	93 - 99,7%
Presenting with pain	87%	80 - 93%
Cyclic symptoms	57%	44 - 70%
Concurrent pelvic endometriosis	13%	5,6 - 20%
Mean size of mass (cm)*	2,7	2,1 - 3,2
Recurrence rate	4,3%	1,2 - 7,4%
Associated with a cesarean section scar	57%	NC
Associated with a hysterectomy scar	11%	NC
Associated with other surgeries	13%	NC
Spontaneous abdominal wall endometriosis	20%	NC

* largest single dimension

NC = not calculated

Table 1. Summary of review data of cases of abdominal wall endometriosis

No other diagnostic tools are necessary if the anamnesis and physical examination are classical. In another cases, especially if the lesion is large, further investigation should be very useful (29).

The preoperative diagnosis should be confirmed by ultrasound scan of the lesion (21, 52, 59). Francica et al. (21) described extensionally ultrasonographic picture of small (0,7 - 2,6 cm) and large (3 - 6 cm) lesions. The most typical ultrasound pattern was that of a solid nonhomogenous hypoechoic nodule with infiltrating margins, echogenic rim and increased vascularity in the musculocutaneous planes of the abdominal wall near the cesarean section incision. In large lesion there was significantly higher grey-scale, higher incidence of cystic areas and fistulous tracts, loss of round or oval shape, multiple vascular pedicles and central vascularity comparing to small lesions.

Very useful should be a computerized tomography or magnetic resonace imaging. The data from these diagnostic procedures may be helpful even during planning a reconstructional operation of the abdominal wall (29, 39), though Francica et al. (21) consider that they often are nonspecific.

Sometimes, if the lesion is very superficial, epiluminescence microscopy should be used (23) to exclude melanoma.

Fine-needle aspiration cytology (10, 26) in suspicious cases is very good and cheap diagnostic tool if an incisional hernia is ruled out, of course. Epithelial endometrial-like cells, stromal cells or hemosiderin-laden macrophages are essential to confirm endometriosis on cytology. Some authors (12) consider, that needle biopsy may be dangerous, because of dissemination of endometrial or even neoplasmatic cells.

The diagnostic pitfalls are more common among general surgeons, who are very often first contact physicians (5, 13, 34), especially when no palpable masses are present. Sometimes are misleading the age of the patient (4) or enormously long time between the cesarean section and occurrence of the first symptoms. The disease most often occurs in adult young women in their twenties till forties but Attia et al. (4) also reported a case of 15 years old girl.

Abdominal wall endometriosis is often misdiagnosed as a hernia, hematoma, lyphadenopathy, lymphoma, lipoma, abscess, subcutaneous cyst, suture granuloma, neuroma, soft tissue sarcoma, desmoid tumours and metastatic cancer, particularly as many endometrial tumours of the abdominal wall are not related to prior surgical procedures (29). Even cellulites is mentioned as a possible misdiagnostic condition (1). Gajjar et al. (22) and Khoo (33) described a case of cesarean scar endometriosis presenting as an acute abdomen. Umbilical endometriosis can pose a next diagnostic dilemma (1, 48) simulating malignant melanoma or the "sister Mary Joseph nodule" - a manifestation of intraabdominal malignancy. Endometriosis should mimick hernia recurrence in tne inguinal region, especially if it is painless (19). On the other hand not only endometrial tissue can implant into postoperative scars. Neumann et al. (40) reported a rare case of implantation of adenosquamous cervical carcinoma in an episiotomy scar mentioning 13 another cases reported to date.

The occurrence of the endometriosis in an postoperative scar is usually the result of a previous caesarean section or abdominal hysterectomy but any other surgery might be a cause of this disease. Harry et al. (28) presented a case of the scar endometriosis converting in a clear cell adenocarcinoma more than 30 years after an open tubal sterilization. Zhu et al. (59) basing on another reports, are of opinion, that tubal mucosa after simply tubal ligation brought into the incision is able to transform to the endometrial tissue. Kaunitz and Di Saint'Agnese reported about endometriosis as a complication of amniocentesis (30). One of the cases presented by Agarwal and Fong (1) had an endometriotic lesion after appendectomy. Kurotsuchi et al. (36) described a case of abdominal scar endometriosis as a complication of laparotomy performed because of uterine perforation during dilatation and curettage. Aydin (4) mentioned about rising incidence of endometriomas in port sites after laparoscopy.

4. Surgical treatment

A surgical resection with complete and wide negative margins is the treatment of choice of endometriotic lesions in the abdominal wall, taking into account the risk of recurrence and the potential for their malignant transformation (1, 8, 12, 13, 28, 29, 43, 59). If the endometriosis is incorporated into the musculature, en bloc resection of all the myofascial elements is recommended and often mesh repair of the abdominal wall is necessary (1, 29, 43, 59). Figures 1 - 6 illustrate the procedure in such a case of 15 cm endometrioma in Bytom clinical centre.

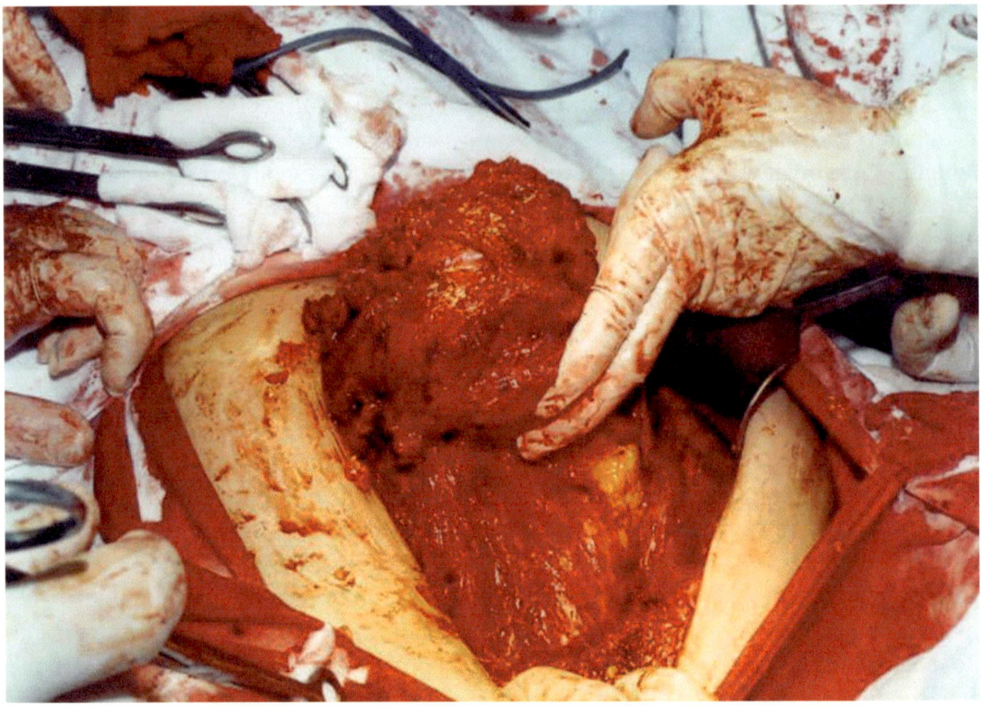

Fig. 1. Large endometrioma penetrating abdominal wall.

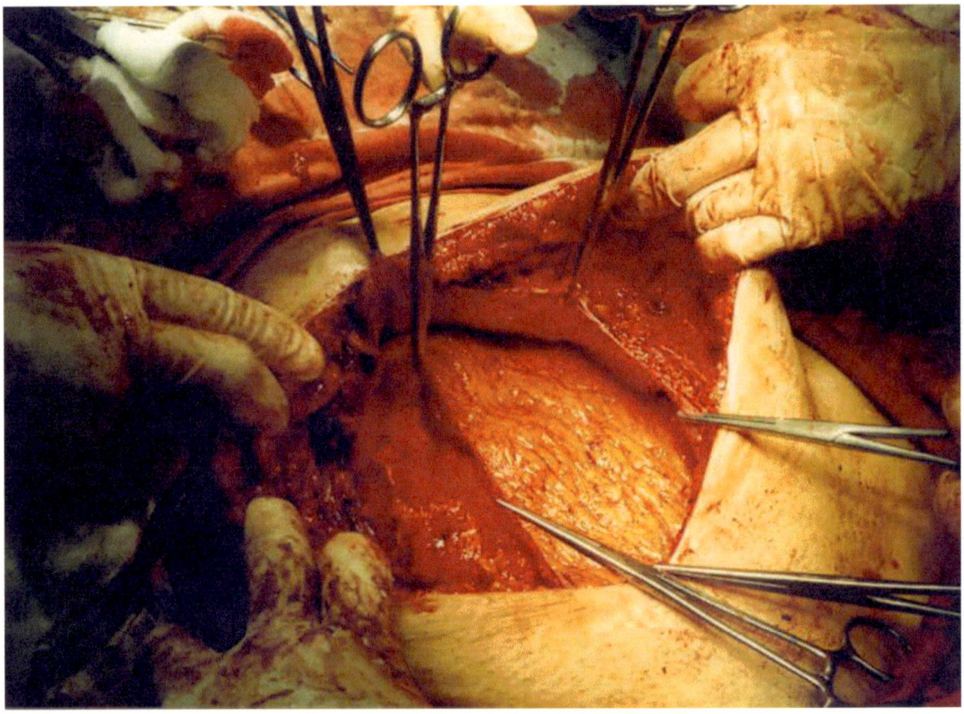

Fig. 2. Endometrioma is totally excised with wide margins including peritoneum

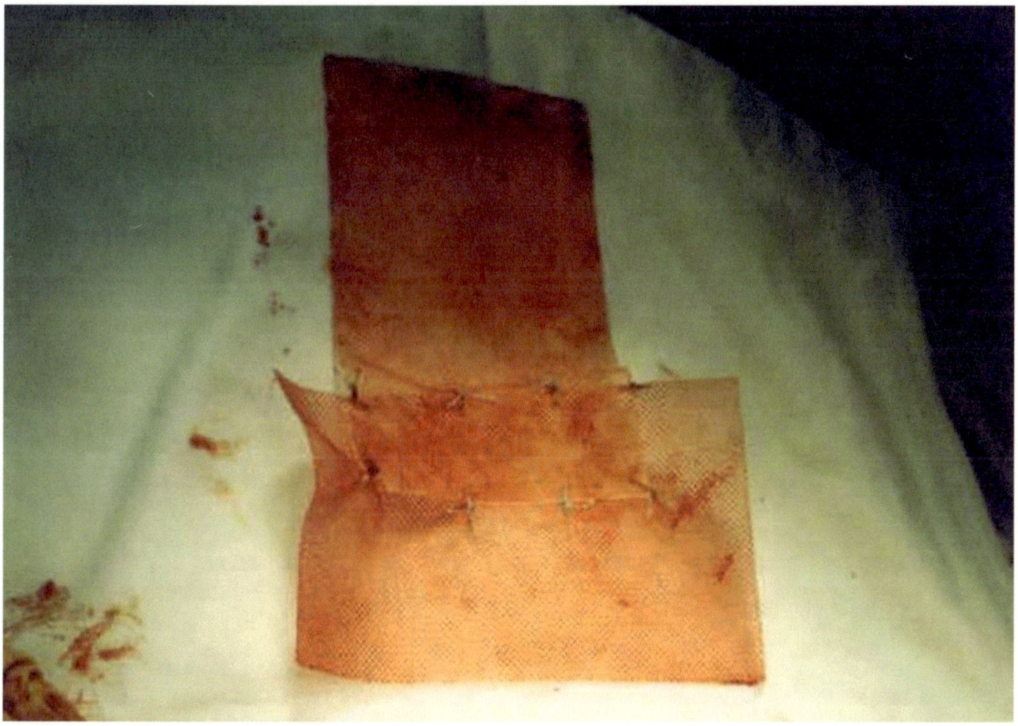

Fig. 3. The polypropylene mesh ready to use

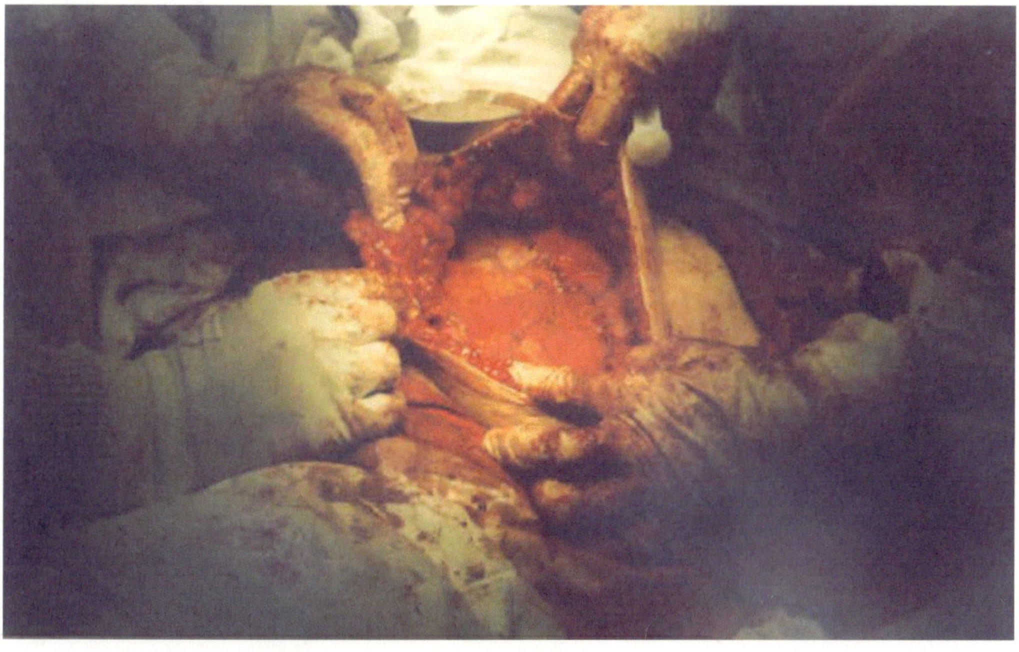

Fig. 4. Abdominal wall thoroughly repaired by mesh

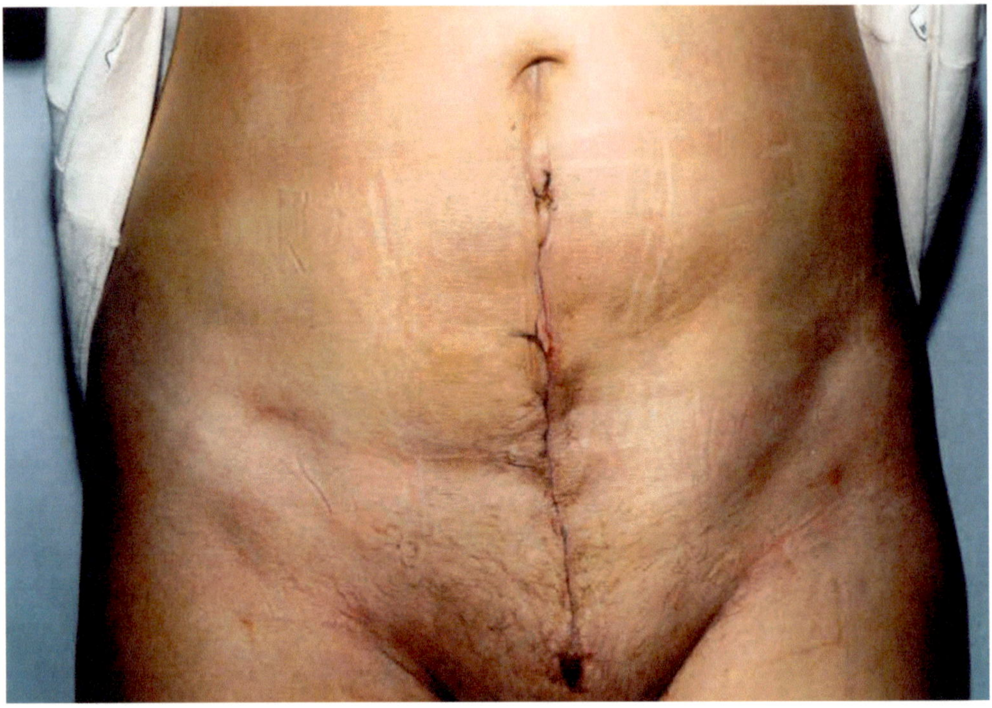

Fig. 5. The skin is sutured.

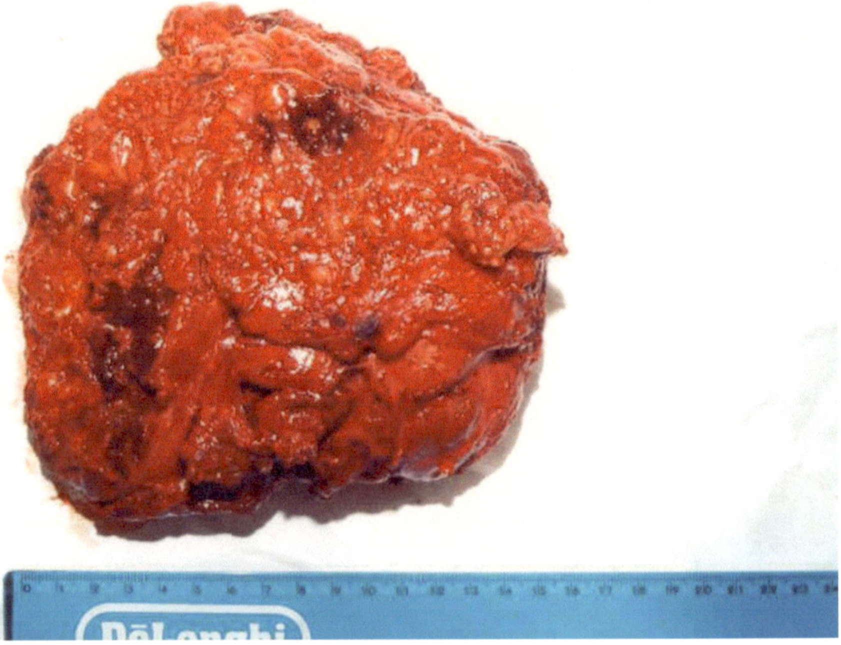

Fig. 6. The excised endometrioma of size 15 cm.

A large use of coagulation is advised to diminish bleeding and a risk of recurrences (35).

A wide surgical resection is also the therapy of choice when the endometrioma is localized in perineal scars (8, 11, 41, 51). If necessary, even anal sphincter reconstruction ought to be performed (6). Dougherty and Hull (11) clearly demonstrated in their series of patients that narrow excision only gives a very high rate of recurrences whereas wide excision does not.

Fedele et al. (20) advise in cases of inguinal endometriosis also the removal of the extraperitoneal portion of the round ligament to avoid recurrences.

5. Histopathology

All the excised specimen must be examined histopathologically because of mentioned above reasons (12, 38, 43). The frozen section is advisable (59). Histopatological examination reveals usually ectopic endometrial glands with surrounding cellular stroma, occasionally associated with extravasation of erythrocytes and some inflammatory infiltrates around the glands (5, 33, 38).

Recently, the largest and exhausting study on histopatology of cutaneous endometriosis basing on 73 patients presented Kazakov et al. (31). The excised nodules looked out macroscopically as a gray-white scar-like tissue with or without an evidence of hemorrhage containing tiny cysts when viewed under a magnifying glass. Two cases were excluded from study because of fibrotic granulation tissue in the first and cutaneous endosalpingiosis in the second one with a complete lack of endometriotic tissue in both. The resting cases showed typical endometriotic glands with a characteristic stroma. The müllerian epithelium is apt to show a broad spectrum of metaplastic changes. The authors discovered in glandular component in most of cases tubal metaplasia (61%), less often reactive atypia (23%), oxyphilic metaplasia (15%), hobnail metaplasia (10%), atypical mitoses in glands (6%), mucinous metaplasia (4%), papillary syncytial metaplasia in two cases and hyperplasia in one. The stromal component revealed mostly myxoid changes (69%), less often smooth muscle metaplasia (31%) and in single cases decidual changes, stromal endometriosis, micronodular stromal endometriosis and elastosis. In ¾ of specimens were observed large granular CD56 positive lymphocytes. Quite frequently occurred lipoblast like cells (15%), intranuclear inclusions in adipocytes (10%), atypically appearing myocytes (10%) and spiral arteries (4%). Perineural invasion was present in one case. The authors also advertised, that endometrioid or clear cell cancer can occur in the skin lesions.

Zhang et al. (58) evidenced that bothersome pain caused usually by endometriotic lesion is caused by sensory nerve fibres which are present mainly in deeply infiltrating endometriosis.

6. Pharmacological treatment

Medical management of the endometriosis by drugs as danazol, GnRH-analogues, progestagens or oral contraceptives, results usually in the temporary relief of pain (53). Opinions concerning combined therapy are different. According to Horton et al. (29) there are no data to support postoperative hormonal therapy. Sometimes might be useful preoperative treatment by GnRH-analogues for three months to diminish the tumour size

(1). On the other hand Zhu et al. (59) in a part of their patients administered postoperative analogues of GnRH. Ding and Hsu (16) prescribed danazol for six months postoperatively. Korczyński and Sobkiewicz (35) are of opinion, that pharmacological treatment can be applied in some cases as a complementary therapy. Kurotsuchi et al. (36) suggest that GnRH-agonist therapy might be an alternative to surgical treatment.

The presence of aromatase activity in endometriotic lesions might be a new target of therapeutical actions. Oner et al. (45) in an animal model showed significant regression of endometriotic implants by letrozol and metformin. Moreover, in the metformin group thanks to its antiproliferative and anti-inflammatory properties the authors observed less adhesions.

Basing on the results from animal studies it seems be effective in future to treat and prevent endometriosis by vaccination using immunomodulators like RESAN, DETOX or BCG (54).

New therapeutical options mentioned by Skrzypczak (53) may represent statins and selective progesterone receptor modulators.

Antioxidants and nonsteroidal antiinflammatory drugs are considered as a possible additive therapeutical options (3).

7. Risk factors

The most evident risk factor for the scar endometriosis are obstetrical surgical procedures, especially cesarean section (38,41). It is believed that the opening of uterine cavity mainly during cesarean section causes the risk of decidualized endometrium implantation (10,29,53,57). The risk of scar endometriosis is significantly higher, when the cesarean section is performed before the term (44,56,57), though Nominato et al. (41) does not confirm this suggestion. There is no correlation between the parity, number of cesarean sections and the disease prevalence (38) but de Oliveira et al. (44) are of opinion that low parity may increase the risk.

The risk of scar endometrioma is augmented when not proper operative techniques are used (not closing the visceral and parietal peritoneum, using of the same surgical material during opening and closing uterus and abdominal wall, failure to shielding the wound during lack of placenta extraction with subsequent curettage and thorough washing before definitive closure) (38,55).

On the other hand, as it is mentioned by Zhu et al. (59) endometriosis in the postoperative scar may occur not only after operations that need not open the uterus (for example tubal operations).

Pelvic endometriosis seems to be the risk factor of arising scar endometriosis when treated by laparoscopy (10,29). The laparoscopic procedure may cause transportation of endometrial cells in the abdominal wall in women with a predisposition to endometriosis. Agarval and Fong (1) found that spontaneous cutaneous endometriosis was associated with more severe pelvic disease.

Non-surgical risk factors of scar endometrioma are also alcohol consumption and increased menstrual flow (44).

Hyperestrogenismus, even relative, seems to be also a risk factor of endometriosis, though there is a lack of valuable literature data confirming it in relation to scar endometriomas.

The important risk factor is the genetic one. Lattuada et al. (37) reported that the frequency of the PROGINS allele T2 in affected women was 17,2% compared with 11% in controls. They are of opinion that the progesterone receptor mutation increases the risk of endometriosis morbidity two fold. Teng et al. (56) discussing their results mentioned that the antiapoptotic function of the survivin gene may play an important role in endometriotic implant survival and invasion.

8. Prophylaxis

First of all one should avoid unnecessary cesarean sections (41, 59). To prevent the iatrogenic inoculation of the endometrium into the surgical wound during the cesarean section it is strongly recommended to protect the abdominal wall by a quadrangular bandage during curettage of an uterine cavity after removal of the placenta, discard immediately after cleaning the uterine cavity swabs or sponges, not to reuse the suture material used to suturing of the uterus during the closure of the abdominal wall. The surgical wound should be thoroughly cleaned and irrigated by saline before final closure, especially at the operators side in Pfannenstiel incision (16, 55). Zhu et al. (59) recommend during suturing the myometrium to avoid penetration of endometrium.

Performing another surgical procedures lifting the uterus outside of the pelvis before making uterine incision and removing a functional corpus luteum during hysterectomy may reduce the likelihood of arising the scar endometriosis (11,29). Before endometrial cystectomy all the cystic content should be sucked out, the incision of the abdominal wall covered by swabs and before closure abdominal cavity and incision thoroughly flushed by saline (59).

Wicherek et al. (57) clearly demonstrated, that cesarean section performed before spontaneous onset of labor significantly increases the risk of abdominal wall scar endometriosis thanks to higher immunotolerance. This might also explain higher rate of endometriomas in scars after cesarean section comparing to episiotomy.scars. Thus, if it is possible, the decision on cesarean section should be delayed till the natural onset of the labour.

It should be avoided estrogen monotherapy in obese patients, becuse such treatment augments the risk of rising and malignant degeneration of endometriotic lesions (7).

A prolonged breast feeding is well known protecting factor because of causing hypoestrogenic status that does not support endometriosis development.

Administering of antioxidant agents and proper diet (3) seem to be to some extent helpful, so as endometriosis coexists with local inflammatory reaction.

9. Complications

The typical complications of scar endometriosis are relatively high recurrence rate, malignancy and anatomical defects. Olejek et al. (43) reported a very high recurrence rate – 8 from 33 (over 24%) operated patients during on an average 19 months. It might be caused by larger size of endometriomas and no medical therapy after their excision. Leite et al. (38) described only two cases (6,0%).

Sampson (49) was the first to document the possibility of malignant changes in ectopic endometrial tissue. Chene et al. (12) consider that 0,3 - 1% of scar endometriosis undergo malignant degeneration reporting a case of serous papillary cystadenocarcinoma. In our clinical material (43) also in one patient after two surgical removals of the cesarean scar endometriosis preformed in other centers (where endometrioma was diagnosed) papillary adenocarcinoma was recognized. Matsuo et al. (39) described primary clear cell carcinoma developed in previous abdominal scar post endometriosis surgery. Authors mentioned that endometrioid adenocarcinoma, clear cell adenocarcinoma and adenosarcoma are also common enough in extragenital localization. Razzouk et al. (46) reported a case of mixed clear cell and endometrioid carcinoma arising in a recurrent cesarean section scar endometrioma.

10. Closing remarks

All the menstruating women or postmenopausal, especially using hormone replacement therapy, in whose cases any lesion in any postoperative scar or nearby them appear, should be suspected of endometriosis. It should be kept in mind that lesions of an abdominal wall or another regions of the body even without operation in past might be of endometriotic origin. In unclear cases additional proper diagnostic examinations are advised preoperatively.

The wide excision of the lesion with possible fascial or muscular repair should be offered in these cases and histopatological examination ought to be performed by an experienced histopathologist because of a possibility of malignancy. One should remember that diagnostic pitfalls, particularly among general surgeons often occur.

Medical treatment being less invasive than the surgical one, may be developed and seems to be promising in the future.

Unnecessary operations, especially cesarean sections, should be avoided and if performed, one should be aware of the transmission of endometrial cells in the wound.

Further systematic investigations in the field of scar endometriosis are still needed.

11. References

[1] Agarwal A. & Fong Y.F.: *Cutaneous endometriosis.* Singapore Med J 2008, 49, 704-9.

[2] Akagi T., Yamamoto S., Kobayashi Y., Fujita S., Akadu T., Moria Y. & Kato T.: *A case of endometriosis of the appendix with adhesion to right ovarian cyst presenting as intususpection of a mucocele of the appendix.* Surg Laparosc Endosc Percutan Tech 2008, 18, 622-5.

[3] Alpay Z., Saed G.M. & Diamond M.P.: *Female infertility and free radicals: potential role in adhesions and endometriosis.* J Soc Gynecol Investig 2006, 13, 390-8.

[4] Attia L., Ben Temime R., Sidhom J., Sahli A., Makhlouf T., Chachia A., Koubaa A. & Zermani R.: *A case of cutaneous endometriosis developed on an abdominal scar.* Tunis Med 2010, 88, 841-3.

[5] Aydin Ö.: *Scar endometriosis – a gynecologic pathology often presented to the general surgeon rather than the gynaecologist: report of two cases.* Langenbecks Arch Surg 2007, 392, 105-9.

[6] Barisić G., Krivokapić Z. & Jovanović D.: *Perineal endometriosis in episiotomy scar with anal sphincter involvement: report of two cases and review of the literature.* Int Urogynecol J 2006, 17, 646-9.

[7] Benoit L., Arnould L., Cheynel N., Diane B., Causeret A., Machado A., Collin F., Fraisse J. & Cuisenier J.: *Malignant extraovarian endometriosis: a review.* Eur J Surg Oncol 2006, 32, 6-11.

[8] Buda A., Ferrari L., Marra C., Passoni P., Perego P. & Milani R.: *Vulvar endometriosis in surgical scar after excision of the Bartholin gland: report of a case.* Arch Gynecol Obstet 2008, 277, 255-6.

[9] Bulun S.E., Imir G., Utsunomyia H., Thung S., Gurates B., Tamura M. & Lin Z.: *Aromatase in endometriosis and uterine leiomyomata.* J Steroid Biochem Mol Biol 2005, 95, 57-62.

[10] das Chagas Medeiros F., Magno Cavalcante D.I., da Silva Medeiros M.A. & Eleutério J.: *Fine-needle aspiration cytology of scar endometriosis: study of seven cases and literature review.* Diagn Cytopathol 2011, 39, 18-21.

[11] Chatterjee S.K.: *Scar endometriosis: a clinicopathologic study of 17 cases.* Obstet Gynecol 1980, 56, 81-4.

[12] Chene G., Darcha C., Dechelotte P., Mage G. & Canis M.: *Malignant degeneration of perineal endometriosis in episiotomy scar, case report and review of the literature.* Int J Gynecol Cancer 2007, 17, 709-14.

[13] Chiang D.T. & The W.T.: *Cutaneous endometriosis – surgical presentations of a gyanecological condition..* Aust Fam Physician 2006, 35, 887-8.

[14] Chung H.W., Lee J.Y., Moon H.S., Hur S.E., Park M.H., Wen Y. & Polan M.L.: *Matrix metalloproteinase-2, membranous type 1 matrix metalloproteinase, and tissue inhibitor of metalloproteinase-2 expression in ectopic and eutopic endometrium.* .Fertil Steril 2002, 78, 787-95.

[15] Clausen I. & Nielsen KT.: *Endometriosis in the groin.* Int J Gynaecol Obst 1987, 25, 469-71.

[16] Ding D.C. & Hsu S.: *Scar endometriosis at the site of cesarean section.* Taiwan J Obstet Gynecol 2006, 45 247-9.

[17] Dougherty L.S. & Hull T.: *Perineal endometriosis with anal sphincter involvement.* Dis Colon Rectum 2000, 43, 1157-60.

[18] Douglas C. & Rotimi O.: *Extragenital endometriosis – a clinicopathological review of a Glasgow hospital experience with case illustrations.* J Obstet Gynaecol 2004, 24, 804-8.

[19] Ducarme G., Uzan M. & Poncelet C. : *Endometriosis mimicking hernia recurrence.* Hernia 2007, 11, 175-7.

[20] Fedele L., Bianchi S., Frontino G., Zanconato G. & Rubino T.: *Radical excision of inguinal endometriosis.* Obstet Gynecol 2007, 110, 530-3.

[21] Francica G., Scarano F., Scotti L., Angelone G. & Giardiello C.: *Endometriomas in the region of a scar from cesarean section: sonographic appearance and clinical presentation vary with the size of the lesion.* J Clin Ultrasound 2009, 37, 215-20.

[22] Gajjar K.B., Mahendru A.A. & Khaled M.A.: *Caesarean scar endometriosis presenting as an acute abdomen: a case report and review of literature.* Arch Gynecol Obstet 2008, 277, 167-9.

[23] de Giorgi V., Massi D., Mannone F., Stante M. & Carli P.: *Cutaneous endometriosis: non invasive analysis by epiluminescence microscopy.* Clin Exp Dermatol 2003, 28, 315-7.

[24] Groothuis P.G., Koks C.A. & de Goeij A.F.: *Adhesion of human endometrial fragments to peritoneum in vitro.* Fertil Steril 1999, 71, 1119-23.

[25] Grümmer R., Schwarzer F., Bainczyk K., Hess-Stumpp H., Regidor P.A., Schindler A.E. & Winterhager E.: *Peritoneal endometriosis: validation of an in-vivo model.* Hum Reprod 2001, 16, 1736-43.

[26] Gupta R.K.: *Fine-needle aspiration cytodiagnosis of endometriosis in cesarean section scar and rectus sheath mass lesions – a study of seven cases.* Diagn Cytopathol 2008, 36, 224-6.

[27] Halban J.: *Metastatic hysteroadenosis.* Wien Klin Wochenschr 1924, 37, 1205-6.

[28] Harry V.N., Shanbhag S., Lyall M., Narayansingh G.V. & Parkin D.E.: *Isolated clear cell adenocarcinoma in scar endometriosis mimicking an incisional hernia.* Obstet Gynecol 2007, 110, 469-71.

[29] Horton J.D., DeZee K.J., Ahnfeldt E.P. & Wagner M.: *Abdominal wall endometriosis: a surgeon's perspective and review of 445 cases.* Am J Surg 2008, 196, 207-12.

[30] Kaunitz A. & Di Saint'Agnese P.A.: *Needle tract endometriosis: an unusual complication of amniocentesis.* Obstet Gynecol 1979, 54, 753-5.

[31] Kazakov D.V., Ondič O., Zámečník M., Shelekhova K.V., Mukenšnábl P., Hes O., Dvořák V. & Michal M.: *Morphological variations of scar-related and spontaneous endometriosis of the skin and superficial soft tissue: a study of 71 cases with emphasis on atypical features and types of müllerian differentiations.* J Am Acad Dermatol 2007, 57, 134-46.

[32] Kennedy S.: *The genetics of endometriosis.* J Reprod Med 1998, 43, 263-8.

[33] Khoo J.J.: *Scar endometriosis presenting as an acute abdomen.* Aust N Z J Obstet Gynaecol 2003, 43, 164-5.

[34] Kocakusak A., Arpinar E., Arikan S., Demirbag N., Tarlaci A. & Kabaca C.: *Abdominal wall endometriosis: a diagnostic dilemma for surgeons.* Med Princ Pract 2005, 14, 434-7.

[35] Korczyński J. & Sobkiewicz S.: *Diagnostyka i postępowanie lecznicze w przypadkach endometriozy powłok brzusznych.* Ginekol Pol 2001, 73, 358-72.

[36] Kurotsuchi S., Iwase A., Goto M., Hariyama Y. & Kikkawa F.: *Scar endometriosis after a laparotomy for uterine perforation as a complication of dilatation and curettage.* Arch. Gynecol Obstet 2009, 279, 941-3.

[37] Lattuada D.,Somigliana E., Viganò P., Candiani M., Pardi G., Di Blasio A.M.: *Genetics of endometriosis: a role for the progesterone receptor gene polymorphism PROGINS?* Clinical Endocrinology 2004, 61, 190-4.

[38] Leite G.K.C., de Carvalho L.F.P., Koreks H., Guazzelli T.F., Kenj G. & de Toledo V.: *Scar endometrioma following obstetric surgical incisions: retrospective study on 33 cases and review of the literature.* Sao Paulo Med J 2009, 127, 270-7.

[39] Matsuo K., Alonsozana E.L.C., Eno M.L., Rosenhein N.B. & Im D.D.: *Primary peritoneal clear cell adenocarcinoma arising in previous abdominal scar for endometriosis surgery.* Arch Gynecol Obstet 2009, 280, 637-41.

[40] Neumann G., Rasmussen K.L. & Petersen L.K.: *Cervical adenosquamous carcinoma. Tumor implantation in an episiotomy scar.* Obstet Gynecol 2007, 110, 467-9.

[41] Nominato N.S., Prates L.F.V.S., Lauar I., Morais J., Maia L. & Geber S.: *Caesarean section greatly increases risk of scar endometriosis.* Eur J Obstet Gynecol Reprod Biol 2010, 152, 83-5.

[42] Odobasić A., Pasić A,. Iljazović-Latifagić E., Arnautalić L., Odobasić Ad., Idrizović E., Dervisefendić M. & Dedić L.: *Perineal endometriosis: A case report and review of the literature.* Tech Coloproctol 2010, 14 (Suppl), S25-7.

[43] Olejek A., Zamłyński J., Podwińska E., Horák S., Paliga-Żytniewska M. & Kellas-Ślęczka S.: *Guzy endometrialne w bliznach po cięciu cesarskim. [Abdominal Wall endometrioma in the cesarean section scar].* Ginekol Pol 2008, 79, 612-5.

[44] de Oliveira M.A., de Leon A.C., Freire E.C., de Oliveira H.C. & Study S.O.: *Risk factors for abdominal scar endometriosis atfer obstetrics hysterotomies: a case control study.* Acta Obstet Gynecol Scand 2007, 86, 73-80.

[45] Oner G., Oczelik B., Ozgun M.T., Serin I.S., Ozturk F. & Basbug M.: *The effects of metformin and letrozole on endometriosis and comparison of the two treatment agents in a rat model.* Hum Reprod 2010, 25, 932-7.

[46] Razzouk K., Roman H., Chanavaz-Lacheray I., Scotté M., Verspyck E. & Marpeau L.: *Mixed clear cell and endometrioid carcinoma arising in parietal endometriosis.* Gynecol Obstet Invest 2007, 63, 140-2.

[47] Rier S.E., Martin D.C., Bowman R.E., Dmowski W.P. & Becker J.L.: *Endometriosis in rhesus monkeys (Macaca mulatta) following chronic exposure to 2,3,7,8-tetrachlorodibenzo-p-dioxin.* Fundam Appl Toxicol 1993, 21, 433-41.

[48] Rosina P., Pugliarello S., Colato C. & Girolomoni G.: *Endometriosis of umbilical cicatrix: Case report and review of the literature.* Acta Dermatovenerol Croat 2008, 16, 218-21.

[49] Sampson J.A.: *Endometrial carcinoma of the ovary arising in endometrial tissue in that organ.* Arch Surg 1925, 10, 1-72.

[50] Sampson J.A.: *The development of the implantation theory for the origin of peritoneal endometriosis.* Am J Obstet Gynecol 1940, 40, 549

[51] Schrodt G.R., Alcorn M.O. & Ibanez J.: *Endometriosis in the male urinary system: a case report.* J Urol 1980, 124, 722-3.

[52] Singh M., Sivanesan K., Ghani R. & Granger K.: *Caesarean scar endometriosis.* Arch Gynecol Obstet 2009, 279, 217-9.

[53] Skrzypczak J.: *Farmakologiczne leczenie endometriozy.* In: *Endometrioza.* (red. Wielgoś M.), Ed: *Via Medica,* Gdańsk, 2010, 24-38.

[54] Szymanowski K., Chmaj-Wierzchowska K., Yatczenko A., Niepsuj-Biniaś J., Florek E., Opala T. & Murawski M.: *Endometriosis prophylaxis and treatment with the newly developed xenogenic immunomodulator RESAN in an animal model.* Eur J Obstet Gynecol Reprod Biol 2009, 142, 145-8.

[55] Teng C.C., Yang H.M., Chen K.F., Yang C.J., Chen L.S. & Kuo C.L.: *Abdominal wall endometriosis: an overlooked but possibly preventable complication.* Taiwan J Obstet Gynecol 2008, 47, 42-8.

[56] Wicherek Ł., Dutsch-Wicherek M., Gałązka K., Banaś T., Popiela T., Lazar A. & Kleinrok-Podsiadło B.: *Comparison of RCAS 1 and metallothionein expression and the*

presence and activity of immune cells in human ovarian and abdominal wall endometriomas. Reprod Biol Endocrinol 2006, 4, 41-9.

[57] Wicherek Ł., Klimek M., Skręt-Magierło J., Czekierdowski A., Banaś T., Popiela T.J., Kraczkowski J., Sikora J., Opławski M., Nowak A., Skręt A. & Basta A.: *The obstetrical history in patients with Pfannenstiel scar endometriomas – an analysis of 81 patients.* Gynecol Obstet Invest 2007, 63, 107-13.

[58] Zhang X., Yao H,. Huang X., Lu B., Xu H. & Zhou C.: *Nerve fibres in ovarian endometriotic lesions in women with ovarian endometriosis.* Hum Reprod 2010, 25, 392-7.

[59] Zhu Z., Al.-Beiti M.A.M., Tang L., Liu X. & Lu X.: *Clinical characteristic analysis of 32 patients with abdominal incision endometriosis.* J Obstet Gynaecol 2008, 28, 742-5.

6

Pathological Aspects of Endometriosis

Agatha Kondi-Pafitis
Aretaieion University Hospital Athens Medical School, Greece

1. Introduction

Endometriosis is one of the most enigmatic diseases of the female because its cause and pathophysiology remain poorly understood. Although the histological diagnosis of endometriosis is usually easy to make, there are diagnostic problems in relation to certain aspects such as the atypias and neoplastic alterations of the endometriotic glandular and stromal components and in cases of endometriosis in unusual places the small size of specimens available for histological examination does not aid the correct diagnosis. An effort will be made in this chapter to address the various problems and the most commonly asked questions about endometriosis.

2. Definition of endometriosis

Endometriosis is the presence of tissue resembling endometrial components outside the uterus. Usually both, glands and stroma are observed but occasionally the diagnosis can be made when only one component is present. Endometriosis is distinct from adenomyosis or endometriosis interna which is defined by the presence of endometrial components in the myometrium. These two entities were linked in the past by common terminology but present different clinical presentation, epidemiologic and etiologic patterns.

3. Clinical features of endometriosis

Endometriosis is a condition described in European Medical history for over 300 years (Knapp , 1999) and afflicts women in their reproductive years. It is the third leading cause of gynecologic hospitalization in the USA and although the true incidence is unknown, it is estimated that it afflicts about 4-13% of all women in reproductive age,25-50% of women with infertility problems, 5-25%of those that are hospitalized because of pelvic pain,50% of young girls with severe dysmenorrhea and up to 7% of women hospitalized with the diagnosis of pelvic masses(Cramer & Missmer, 2002, Allaire, 2006, Anaf et al, 2000).There is a shift of the time of diagnosis from the late thirties and early forties to the twenties and the cause of this my be extensive use of laparoscopy and delayed childbearing. The use of hormones in menopausal women and obesity may be responsible for the occurrence of endometriosis in postmenopausal age. Most women with endometriosis present some or all of four major problems: infertility, secondary dysmenorrhea, dyspareunia and pelvic pain, but many women are asymptomatic. The intensity of the pain is poorly correlated with the actual extend of the disease and the various local biochemical factors and the local action of activated mast cells may be responsible for this symptom. In rare cases with ovarian endometriosis, acute abdomen because of rupture of ovarian cystic masses and ascites raise the suspicion of malignancy (Henkel et al, 1999).

4. Serum markers in endometriosis

Levels of CA-125 may be elevated in the serum and peritoneal fluid of women with endometriosis and the concentration of serum CA-125 usually correlate with the severity and the clinical course of the disease. The sensitivity of the serum test is low for the screening of general population, but sensitive in the monitoring the response to hormonal treatment of women with endometriosis. Antiendometrial antibodies are found in 83% of women with confirmed endometriosis and the titers low after hormonal treatment and a good response.

5. Etiologic factors of endometriosis

Genetic, hormonal, immunological, and environmental and angiogenetic factors are implicated in the pathogenesis of endometriosis. Heritable factors are important and there is strong evidence that a large proportion of female relatives are affected by the disease by a severe form of the disease. The relative risk of endometriosis in a first-degree relative is 7.2 and there are high concordance rates for the presence of endometriosis in monozygotic but not dizygotic twins (Kennedy, 1997, Kennedy, 1999). The finding of endometriosis in reproductive years and the hormone dependent response of endometrium implicates hormonal factors in the pathogenesis of endometriosis. The ovarian function is considered an important factor. The concentrations of microenvironmental steroid hormone are high, measuring 1000-fold higher in the ovarian follicles than the plasma .The peritoneal fluid is derived mainly by peri-follicular and corpus luteum exudates and presents high steroid hormone levels. It is estimated that the concentration of peritoneal estradiol during follicular phase increases progressively and reaches after the ovulation levels 100-fold higher that the plasma concentrations while the progesterone peritoneal levels are low in the follicular and increase rapidly after ovulation. There is evidence that the peritoneal fluid in women with endometriosis contain multiple types of free floating cells such as macrophages, leucocytes, lymphocytes, eosinophils and mast cells in greater numbers than in healthy women (Arid, 1997). Macrophages secret a high number of growth factors such as epidermal and transforming growth factor, fibroblast growth factor, interleukins 1,6 and 8, tumor necrosis factor-a. These factors play a role in the growth and regulation of the endometriotic foci. There is also reported a reduced T-mediated cytotoxicity to autologous endometrial cells and a decreased lymphocyte stimulation response to autologous endometrial antigens in patients with endometriosis. This findings support the theory that certain cell-mediated immune mechanisms limiting the growth of endometriotic implants may be impaired. Cyclo-0xygenase-2, involved in the synthesis of prostaglandins E2 may also play a role in the development of endometriosis. In the peritoneal fluid of women with endometriosis, potent angiogenetic growth factors were observed produced from peritoneal fluid macrophages, which probably are important in the development of endometriosis (Haney, 1991).

6. Theories about the histogenesis of endometriosis

The many theories proffered to explain the histogenesis of endometriosis may be divided in

a. theories that propose the transplantation on endometrium in extra-uterine site,
b. theories that favor the induction of mesenchyme to produce endometriotic tissues under the influence of various factors and
c. theories proposing that endometriosis arise on sites of metaplastic change of the coelomic peritoneum.

The theory of transplantation is the most widely accepted. According to this theory the menstrual flow products flow in a retrograde fashion through the fallopian tubes into the peritoneal cavity. The endometrial products implant, grow and produce tissues with morphology of endometrial glands and stroma. Laparoscopic studies show that during menstruation there is blood in the peritoneal cavity of most women and the retrograde menstrual flow is indeed a usual phenomenon which explains the endometriotic implantation in the ovary and the uterosacral ligaments. Sigmoid colon partly forms a shield and entraps the retrograde menstrual flow products and this fact explains the finding that endometriosis is observed mainly in the left ovary. Also the uterine position is important for the development of endometriosis which is observed anteriorly in patients with anterior uteri. Experimental findings support the transplantation theory and suggest that endometriosis develop in two distinct phases. In the first phase the uterine products are invasive and ovarian hormone -dependent and in the second phase express endogenous estrogen biosynthesis. By the first month after inoculation of primate models with menstrual endometrial tissues these elements attach, grow and invade through the peritoneal mesothelial covering and express estrogen receptor-beta, although aromatase activity is expressed later (Fazleabas et al, 2002). Other routes of implantation such as vascular and/or lymphatic spread and direct implantation are reported and explain the development of endometriosis in distant and unusual places such as lung or lymph nodes.

The metaplastic theory proposes that the peritoneum adjacent to ovaries is a multipontential tissue which may obtain characteristics of endometrial tissue (Lauchlan 1972, Lauchlan, 1994). This theory is supported by the observation that endometriosis may develop in cases where no retrograde menstrual flow is possible such as in Rokitansky-Kuster-Hauser syndrome (Acien et al, 1988), in young girls and in men. Finally, according to the induction theory which adds information to transplantation theory, the endometriotic glands and stroma develop de novo from the host tissues, stimulated by the transplanted endometrium.

Most pathologists favor a combination of the metastatic and metaplastic theories and support the theory that endometriosis represents a polygenetic disorder, with alterations in multiple biological pathways (Donnez et al, 2002, Sasson & Taylor, 2008) leading to a metaplastic process under the irritating effect of endometrial tissue shed during retrograde menstrual flow.

7. The theory of the secondary Mullerian system

Lauchlan (1972) first used this term to describe the propensity of the peritoneum which covers the ovary and the lower peritoneal cavity to Mullerian differentiation. The mesothelial covering and the sub-mesothelial stroma of peritoneum exhibit a full spectrum of Mullerian differentiation from benign to malignant .Many lesions of secondary Mullerian system are described, which are benign, such as endosapingiosis, endocervicosis, of low grade of malignancy, serous and mucinous and malignant ,described as extraovarian peritoneal serous and mucinous carcinomas. The sub-mesothelial stroma gives rise to peritoneal leiomyomatosis and may undergo decidual reaction .Amongst the lesions of secondary Mullerian system are also classed lesions of the retroperitoneal lymph node such as Mullerian inclusions, leiomyomatosis and decidual reaction. Endometriosis is considered as the main lesion of the secondary Mullerian system (Clement & Young, 2008) It has been postulated that the peritoneum of the lower abdominal cavity retains the ability to differentiate to Mullerian tissues due to the proximity to the coelomic epithelium from which the primary Mullerian system is derived. Lauchlan (1994) proposes that the development of peritoneal Mullerian lesions may be secondary to the proximity of pelvic peritoneum to tubal fibria, and the exposure of the peritoneal surfaces to external agents , such as talk, that stimulate the peritoneal Mullerian differentiation.

8. Histological features of the secondary Mullerian system

The secondary Mullerian system consists of the covering mesothelial layer and the sub-mesothelial mesenchyme, on and adjacent to the ovaries, the pelvic peritoneum, the omentum and the retroperitoneal lymph nodes. The most common type of epithelial differentiation is a tubal-like epithelium, with ciliated cells. In the omentum and the ovaries cystic inclusions of tubal type epithelium are often observed intermingled with endometrial-type epithelium. Differentiations to mucinous, transitional and squamous type epithelial lesions, benign and malignant are also described. The sub-mesothelial stroma retains the ability to differentiate towards endometrial stroma and smooth muscle tissue and to undergo decidual reaction.

9. Elevated serum CA- 125 levels may be expressed in endometriosis

CA 125 is an antigenic determinant recognized by the monoclonal antibody OC125 against an ovarian cancer cell line. The serum CA125 levels are increased in women with benign conditions such as endometriosis, pelvic inflammatory disease and pregnancy. Ca125 is detected by immunohistochemical methods in fetal coelomic epithelium, fetal Mullerian ducts and Mullerian-derived epithelia in the adult. In the fetus, CA125 is detected in the peritoneum, ovaries and Mullerian ducts after 15 weeks gestation and after the 23rd week it is strongly expressed in endometrium, tubes and cervical tissues.CA125 is considered a differentiation antigen associated with fetal coelomic tissues, derived from embryonic mesoderm Lesions derived from embryonic coelomic tissues either the primary or the secondary Mullerian systems, such as endometriosis, retain the ability to express CA 125.

10. Common locations of endometriosis

Most patients with endometriosis have multiple sites of involvement. Endometriosis is located in uterosacral ligaments (63%), ovaries (56%), ovarian fossae (33%) anterior vesicle pouch (22%) pouch of Douglas (19%), intestines, fallopian tube and uterus (5%) There is variation of the distribution among the various series, depending on the diagnostic criteria used, histological or clinical. When histological criteria are used, the ovaries are the most common site (36%) the fallopian tubes, uterus and cul-de-sac account for 6-14% of biopsies, and the uterosacral ligaments account only for 2% of specimens examined. On a clinical basis, 5-12% of women present extrapelvic endometriosis and in descending order in the sigmoid, the appendix, and omentum, on operative scars and in inguinal region. Rarely endometriosis is observed in distant sites such as lungs, brain, bones and skin (Jenkins et al, 1986).

11. The effect of pregnancy on endometriosis

Endometriosis during pregnancy presents a variable behavior among different patients and a variable behavior in the same patient during different pregnancies. The endometriotic lesions usually shrink and an amelioration of the symptoms is observed. In early pregnancy the lesions may enlarge and bleed. The endometriotic stromal decidual transformation during pregnancy may cause softening and rupture of the lesion causing acute abdomen and hemoperitoneum.

12. Eendometriosis may cause a Meigs-like syndrome

In patients with extensive abdominal endometriosis, a sero-sanguinous ascites may occur and in one third of these patients a right pleural effusion may be observed. In these cases, there is also present an ovarian lesion caused by endometriosis, and the whole clinical picture is consistent with malignancy. The exact mechanism of the development of ascites and the pleural effusion is not clear, and as the most probable cause is considered the stimulation of the mesothelial layer by the endometriosis to produce ascites.

13. Gross features of endometriosis

The location and the age of the endometriotic lesion and the patients' age affect the morphological appearance of endometriosis and may lead to diagnostic difficulties. Gross appearance of endometriotic lesions is affected by their age and this is reflected by the various colors they present. Red color characterizes early lesions and yellow-red color reflect the breakdown of blood products. These lesions eventually progress into old or advanced lesions presenting black color. Hemosiderin is indicated by a yellowish color and occasionally white lesions may be observed indicating the presence of fibrosis. It is possible that the same patient presents endometriotic foci in various stages of development. The size of the lesions varies as well. In early stages blister-like blebs are observed measuring 0.2-0.3 cms in diameter, corresponding to the early red lesion observed mainly in adolescents .As the lesions age, they may enlarge up to 1 cms in diameter and are pigmented , bluish-red, black and eventually white and puckered because of fibrosis. Endometriotic foci are frequently associated with adhesions. The older the patient the more fibrotic the endometriotic lesion is and eventually it atrophies with obliteration of its components Endometriotic lesions become grossly cystic only in the ovaries reaching a diameter up to 15 cms. Ovarian endometriotic cysts present a fibrous wall of various thickness and are filled by chocolate-like contend. The interior surface may be smooth or shaggy. Rarely, endometriosis obtains the form of polypoid masses projecting from serosal surfaces and is referred as polypoid endometriosis.

14. Microscopic features of endometriosis

Typically endometriosis in women of reproductive age presents histologically as one or more endometrioid glands surrounded by stromal cells, resembling the endometrial stromal cells of the proliferative phase. The glandular epithelium is one layer thick with cuboidal or tall cells and eosinophilic cytoplasm. Nuclei are ovoid with vertical orientation and very rare mitoses. The whole picture is usually consistent with inactive or irregular proliferative endometrium, although typical proliferative or secretory changes may be observed. Cilia may be observed as well. Stromal cells are supported by a delicate reticulin network in which hyperemic small vessels may be observed. In the case of exogenous administration of progestins, cyclically functionic endometriosis or pregnancy, a stromal decidual reaction may be observed. A diffuse infiltration of histiocytes is usually observed. The histiocytes convert the red blood cells into glucolipid and brown pigment (pseudoxanthoma cells) .The pigment is usual a ceroid such as lipofuscin and to a lesser extend hemosiderin .The amount of the pigment increases with the age of the lesion. Inflammatory cells may be present and a small component of smooth muscle cells especially in the wall of endometrioid cysts may be observed. Not all the above described elements are easily identified in endometriosis. Especially in the cases of ovarian endometrioid cysts the lesion appears to be composed of stroma, with fibrosis, lined by hemosiderin-laden macrophages. Many histological sections may be necessary to identify the glandular component of endometriosis. One must keep in mind that macrophages may be connected with hemorrhagic follicles or corpora lutea and only the presence of glandular epithelium or luteinized cells is diagnostic. The degree of cyclic changes of the glandular component depend on the amount of fibrous tissue, the amount of stroma round the glands, the degree of vascularity and the steroid receptor content Endometriosis in places with native smooth muscle component may induce marked hypertrophy identical to that observed in cases of adenomyosis that leads to creation of adenomyomata or adenomyomatous nodules (Anaf et al, 2000).

15. Common problems in the differential diagnosis of endometriosis

In the ovary, the presence of hemorrhagic follicle cysts or cystic corpora lutea may cause diagnostic problems, although the presence of granular layer cells or luteinized cells aid to the diagnosis. Serosal inclusion cysts lined by serous cells are diagnosed as such because of the absence of a stromal component and associated alterations. Rete ovarii present a characteristic ramifying pattern and absence of stromal cells and hemorrhage. Mesonephric and paramesonephric remnants are surrounded by smooth muscle and are lined with low cuboidal epithelium. Dermoid cysts may be lined by macrophages and granulation tissue but in multiple sections squamous cells and hair fragments will be observed. It must be noted that there are cases that the laparoscopic picture is diagnostic but the typical picture of endometriosis cannot be established and only stromal cells and other changes such as hemorrhage and macrophages are observed. In these cases the most appropriate diagnosis is that the lesion is "compatible with endometriosis".

16. Metaplastic and hyperplastic glandular changes observed in endometriosis

The glandular cells of endometriosis may present metaplastic changes such as ciliated, eosinophilic, clear cell and rarely squamous, transitional and rarely mucinous metaplasia usually of endocervical type. It is reported that in cases with extensive metaplastic changes in endometriosis an association with an ovarian epithelial tumor is observed. Glandular epithelium may present hyperplastic changes due to endogenous or exogenous hormonal action resembling hyperplastic endometrial changes from simple cystic to complex atypical hyperplasia. In cases of ovarian endometrioid adenocarcinoma remnants of endometriosis with hyperplastic changes are observed. Metaplastic changes are observed in the endometriotic stroma as well, of smooth muscle type. Concomitant hyperplastic changes may create endomyometriotic nodules or uterus-like masses, in the ovary, broad ligament, the bowel and lymph nodes.

17. Histological characteristics of stromal endometriosis

The presence of stromal elements in the absence of glandular epithelium in foci of endometriosis constitutes the stromal endometriosis. This is encountered in the ovary, in the cervix and the peritoneum and usually is associated with a focus of typical endometriosis.

18. Hormonal receptor status in endometriosis

In endometriotic glands and stroma, estrogen and progesterone receptors are present in lower concentrations and without the cyclical variation observed in the normal endometrium. There is not correlation between the hormonal receptor status of endometriosis and the severity of symptoms.

19. Classification of endometriosis

The American Society for Reproductive Medicine proposed a classification of endometriosis with the aim to predict the chance of conception based on the severity of the disease. This system proposes a point score that assesses: the extend of endometriosis among organs and within an organ, scoring the superficial versus the invasive disease, the size of endometriomas, the development of endometriosis uni-or bilaterally in ovaries ,and the type of adhesions. The cumulative score results in a stage designation of the disease, from minimal (stage 1) to extensive (stage 4). The reproducibility of the classification system is limited, according the operative method used and the surgeon's experience (Hoeger & Guzick, 1997).

20. Morphology and histogenesis of Liesegang rings

These rings are acellular eosinophilic structures composed from colloidal solutions, encountered in endometrioid cysts, in areas of inflammation and necrosis. On histological examination, these structures look like parasites and foreign material and may be recognized by their association to endometriosis and lack of staining by specific histochemical methods.

21. Histological features of pseudoxanthomatous salpingitis

This is a form of tubal inflammation characterized histologically by the presence of histiocytes filled with lipofuscin and hemosiderin. In multiple sections there is always a typical focus of endometriosis of the fallopian tube and / or the ovary.

22. Histological features of necrotic pseudoxanthomatous nodules

These lesions occur to postmenopausal women and are multiple nodules usually attached to peritoneum or floating free in the peritoneal cavity. They consist of a central fibrotic or hyalinized core with central necrosis surrounded by lipid laden histiocytes. Occasionally multiple sections will reveal remnants of endometriotic foci, and typical ovarian endometriosis co-exists.

23. Histological features of superficial and deep cervical endometriosis

Superficial cervical endometriosis is observed in the lamina propria of ectocervix as a solitary or multiple hemorrhagic nodules (endovervix is rarely involved by endometriosis). The predisposing factor is cervical trauma and implantation of endometrioid tissue after surgery. Deep cervical endometriosis is created by the extension of a cul-de-sac lesion and is observed in widespread pelvic endometriosis. Similar mechanisms underlie superficial and deep vaginal endometriosis as well.

24. Histology of the three types of tubal endometriosis

Tubal endometriosis may occur as: a direct extension of endometrial tissue with replacement of tubal mucosa, as a growth of endometrial tissue into the lumen with total occlusion causing infertility and associated with tubal pregnancy and, as post-salpingectomy endometriosis, following tubal ligation.

25. Histological features of spontaneous umbilical endometriosis

Endometriosis of the umbilicus in the absence of previous caesarian section or hysterectomy is described as spontaneous endometriosis and it is caused by lymphatic dissemination of endometrial tissue, through lymphatic vessels extending between pelvis and umbilicus. Umbilical endometriosis may recur after surgical resection (Chen, 1998).

26. Histological features of pleuropulmonary endometriosis

There are 21 cases of documented pleural endometriosis involving exclusively the right side of thorax and 17 cases of pulmonary endometriosis. These cases were associated with abdominal endometriosis in one third of the cases and with uterine operations in half of the cases. The development of pulmonary endometriosis suggests an embolic origin of the endometrial implants, while the pleural involvement is explained by the passage of endometrial implants through diaphragmatic lymphatics or defects.

27. Histological features of endometriosis of the nervous system

There are about 30 cases reported of endometriosis of the sciatic nerve, one case of endometriosis of the lumbar spinal cord and one case of cerebral endometriomas. These cases developed probably by "metastatic" implantation of endometrial tissue, through the perineural lymphatics (Abrao et al, 1999, Ichida et al, 1993).

28. Endometriosis in male patients

There are a few reports of endometriosis that develops in male patients under hormonal therapy for prostatic carcinoma. The usual sites that endometriosis develops are: the urinary bladder, the prostate, the para-testicular region and the abdominal wall.

29. Histological features of the peritoneal decidual reaction and the peritoneal leiomyomatosis

Peritoneal decidual reaction is an incidental finding, usually discovered during a caesarian section or postpartum tubal ligation, as small whitish or yellow peritoneal nodules, mimicking metastatic disease. Histological examination shows an extensive decidual reaction of the sub-mesothelial mesenchymal cells. This reaction may also be observed at the omentum, appendix and uterine ligaments. Due to the presence of hyperemic vessels in these lesions, the development of hemoperitoneum during labor may be a rare complication Peritoneal leiomyomatosis presents as multiple small white nodules in the peritoneum and arise from smooth muscle-cell metaplasia of the sub-mesothelial mesenchymal cells. This is a self-limiting disease successfully treated with GHRH antagonists. There is no evidence that these two conditions are related to endometriosis, but they probably represent lesions of the secondary Mullerian system (Clement, 1995).

30. Neoplasms related to endometriosis

The exact rate of neoplastic transformation of endometriosis is not known because of the fact that the neoplasm obliterates the endometriotic features of the underlying lesion. Neoplastic transformation of both the glandular and the stroma component of endometriosis may occur. There are benign and malignant lesions that may develop in endometriotic foci. Tumor-like benign lesions in the form of nodules or even larger, uterus-like masses are reported. Histological examination showed hyperplastic chances of the glandular component of endometriosis and extensive leiomyomatous metaplasia of the stromal component. These lesions may be described as endometrioid adenomas or endometrioid cystadenomas. Malignant transformation of the glandular component presents the pathological features of an endometrioid adenocarcinoma. In 75% of cases the malignant transformation of the glandular component arises in the ovaries. Ovarian endometrioid and clear cell adenocarcinomas are strongly related to ovarian endometriosis and atypical endometriotic lesions were observed in 60% of those carcinomas. Endometriosis -associated ovarian adenocarcinomas are well differentiated tumors in stage I and have a better prognosis that the other ovarian epithelial carcinomas. There are strict criteria for establishing the origin of an adenocarcinoma from endometriosis: Both elements must co-exist, atypical hyperplastic and dysplastic changes of endometriosis must be observed and t no extension of carcinoma from another source is established. Extra ovarian sites where malignant transformation of endometriosis is reported are the rectovaginal septum and the colon (Benoit et al, 2006). Malignant transformation of the stromal component of the endometriosis gives rise to stromal sarcomas similar to uterine stromal tumors (Dogan et al, 2006, Han, 1998). In the table below, tumor-like conditions and tumors, benign and malignant, associated with endometriosis are presented. This classification is based on the WHO classification of Ovarian Tumors (IARC Press, Lyon 2003) modified to contain the tumor-like conditions and premalignant changes.

Tumor-like Conditions
Polypoid endometriosis
Benign Tumors
Adenoma endometrioid
Adenofibroma endometrioid
Cystadenofibroma endometrioid
Cystadenoma endometrioid
Premalignant changes
Atypical endometriosis
Bordeline tumors
Endometrioid cystic Adenofibroma
Endometrioid Cystadenofibroma
Malignant tumors
Endometrioid adenocarcinoma
With squamous elements
With clear cell elements
Stromal sarcoma
Low grade
High grade
Malignant tumors with mixed components
Adenosarcoma
Carcinosarcoma

Table 1. Tumor-like conditions and tumors associated with endometriosis

31. Pathogenesis of malignant transformation of endometriosis

The molecular pathology studies of both atypical and malignant glandular epithelium of endometriosis have shown aneuploid DNA, in contrast to adjacent benign epithelium which is diploid, and a loss of heterozygosity on the arm of chromosome 12 or X-chromosome inactivation, consistent with a common lineage. Aneuploidy of chromosome 17, implicated in the genesis of ovarian cancer, was discovered in about 65% of the endometrioid cells (Jiang et al, 1998). There is evidence that malignant transformation of endometriosis is a multistep pathway involving somatic genetic changes and changes in hormone receptor status (Hompes & Mijatovitc, 2007).

In conclusion, endometriosis is a chronic gynecological disease that results in severe morbidity, including chronic pain and infertility. The pathogenesis of the condition is multifactorial and various factors, genetic, immunological, environmental are implicated Recent data provide evidence that there is an endometrial stem/progenitor cell capable of establishing endometriotic implants .The functions of this stem cell may represent the primary defect in the endometriosis pathway. Current research uses the endometrial stem-cell system as a model to study the molecular biology regulating endometriosis (Sasson & Taylor, 2007).

32. References

Abrao MS, Podgaec S, Carvalho FM, Pinotti JA (1999). Endometriosis in the presacral nerve. *Int J Gynecol Obstet* 64:173-175.

Acien P, Lloret M, Chehab H (1988). Endometriosis in a patient with Rokitansky- Kuster-Hauser syndrome. *Gynecol Obstet Invest* 25:70-72.

Allaire C. Endometriosis and infertility - a review (2006). *J Reprod Med* 51:164-8.

Anaf V, Chapron C, El Nakadi I, De Moor V, Simonart T, Noel JC (2006). Pain, mast cells, and nerves in peritoneal, ovarian, and deep infiltrating endometriosis. *Fertil Steril* 86:1336-43.

Anaf V, Simon P, Fayt I, Noel J (2000). Smooth muscles are frequent components of endometriotic lesions. *Hum Reprod* 15:767-71.

Arid A, Oral E (1997). The peritoneal environment in endometriosis. In: Diamond MP, Osteen KG, eds. *Endometrium and Endometriosis*. Oxford: Blackwell Science; 161-73.

Benoit L, Arnould L, Cheynel N, et al (2006). Malignant extraovarian endometriosis: a review. *EJSO* 32:6-11.

Chen TH(1998). Umbilical endometriosis. *Eur J Plast Surg* 21:51-2.

Clement PB (1995). Reactive tumor-like lesions of the peritoneum. *Am J Clin Pathol* 103:673-6.

Clement PB and Young RH (2008). *Atlas of Gynecologic Surgical Pathology*, 2nd Ed. Saunders-Elsevier ISBN 978-1-4160-2972-4, China.

Cramer DW, Missmer SA (2002). The epidemiology of endometriosis. In: Yoshinaga, Parrott EC, eds. *Endometriosis: Emerging Research and Intervention Strategies.* New York: New York Academy of Sciences, 11-22.

Dogan S. Agic A, Eilers W, Finas D, Diedrich K, Hornung D (2006). Endometriosis and risk of malignancy. *Geburt Frauenheil* 66:739-44.

Donnez J, Van Langendonckt A, Casanas-Roux F, et al (2002). Current thinking on the pathogenesis of endometriosis. *Gynecol Obstet Invest* 54(Suppl):52-62.

Fazleabas AT, Brudney A, Gurates B, Chai D, Bulun S (2002). A modified baboon model for endometriosis. In: Yoshinaga K, Parrott EC, eds. *Endometriosis: Emerging Research and Intervention Strategies.* New York: New York Academy of Sciences, 308-17.

Han AC, Hovenden S. Rosenblum NG, Salazar H (1998). Adenocarcinoma arising in extragonadal endometriosis: an immunohistochemical study. *Cancer* 83:1 163-9.

Haney AF. The pathogenesis and etiology of endometriosis (1991). In: Thomas EJ, Rock JA, eds. *Modern Approaches to Endometriosis.* Dordrecht: Kluwer Academic, 113-28.

Henkel A, Christensen B, Schindler AE (1999). Endometriosis: a clinically malignant disease. *Eur J Obstet Gynecol Reprod Biol* 82:209-11.

Hoeger KM, Guzick DS (1997). Classification of endometriosis. *Obstet Gynecol Clin North Am* 24:347-59.

Hompes PGA, Mijatovic V (2007). Endometriosis: the way forward. *Gynecol Endocrinol* 23:5-12.

Ichida M, Gomi A, Hiranouchi N, et al (1993). A case of cerebral endometriosis causing catamenial epilepsy. *Neurology* 43:2708-9.

Jenkins S, Olive DL, Haney AF (1986). Endometriosis: pathogenetic implications of the anatomic distribution. *Obstet Gynecol* 67:335-8.

Jiang XX, Morland SJ, Hitchcock A, Thomas EJ, Campbell IG (1998). Allelotypi of endometriosis with adjacent ovarian carcinoma reveals evidence of a common lineage. *Cancer Research* 58:1707-12.

Kennedy S (1997). Is there a genetic basis to endometriosis? *Semin Reprod Endocrinol* 15:309-18.

Kennedy S (1999). The genetics of endometriosis. *Eur J Obstet Gynecol Reprod Biol* 82:129-33.

Knapp VJ (1999). How old is endometriosis? Late 17th- and 18th-century European descriptions of the disease. *Fertil Steril* Jul;72(1):10-4.
Lauchlan SC (1972). The secondary Mullerian system. *Obstet Gynecol Surv* 27(3):133-46
Lauchlan SC (1994). The secondary Mullerian system revisited. *Int J Gynecol Pathol* 13(1):73-9
Sasson IE,Taylor HS (2008). Stem cells and the pathogenesis of endometriosis. Ann. NY Acad. Sci. 1127:106-115

Section 2

Pathogenesis

7

Involvement of Prostaglandins in the Pathophysiology of Endometriosis

Gabriela F. Meresman and Carla N. Olivares
Instituto de Biología y Medicina Experimental (IBYME-CONICET) Buenos Aires, Argentina

1. Introduction

Prostaglandins (PGs), thromboxanes (TXs) and leukotrienes (LTs) collectively called eicosanoids, are cyclooxygenase (COX) and lipoxygenase (LOX) products. Prostanoids, PGs and TXs, are known effectors of a wide range of actions in most cells and tissues. They have been described to be involved in muscle contraction and relaxation, neurotransmitter release/unrelease, fever, sleep induction, apoptosis, cell proliferation and oncogenesis; but respecting endometriosis, what matters us mostly, is that they are central molecules involved in the reproductive system (Jabbour & Sales, 2004; Narumiya et al., 1999).

1.1 Prostaglandin synthesis and function

Arachidonic acid (AA) is the precursor of all eicosanoids. Phospholipase A_2 splits AA from plasma membrane phospholipids; once free in the cytosol it is cyclized, oxygenated and reduced to the intermediary PGH_2 by the COX enzymes; or to hydroperoxyeicosatetraenoic acid (HPETE) by LOX enzymes, when the LT pathway is followed.

Two *COX* genes are known to be highly conserved throughout the species. *COX-1* gene has several splice variants: the most widely known COX-1 enzyme, the less known counterparts COX-3 and other smaller variants of the COX-1 (Chandrasekharan et al., 2002; Chandrasekharan & Simmons, 2004). *COX-2* gene has, up to now, only one known protein. COX-1 is ubiquitously and constitutively expressed. It was long thought of COX-1 as the enzyme that was involved only in physiological conditions, but was proven to be upregulated in various carcinomas and to be involved in tumorigenesis (Hwang et al., 1998; Kitamura et al., 2002; Sales et al., 2002). COX-2 enzyme is physiologically induced by growth factors and cytokines; it functions when the concentrations of AA are very low (Fortier et al., 2008). Furthermore COX-2 was seen to be overexpressed in several pathological circumstances as different types of cancers, where its high expression correlates with a negative prognosis, and other inflammation related diseases, as endometriosis (Matsuzaki et al., 2004; Ota et al., 2001).

PGH_2 synthesized by the COXs, is used as a substrate to produce the terminal prostanoids by the PG synthases; each of them is named by their product: PGD_2, PGE_2, $PGF_{2\alpha}$, prostacyclin (PGI_2) and thromboxane (TX) A_2 are produced by PGD synthase (PGDS), PGE synthase (PGES), PGF synthase (PGFS), PGI synthase (PGIS) and TX synthase (TXS), respectively. Once synthesized prostanoids are rapidly exported by a PG transporter out of the cell and they function very close to their liberation site, in an autocrine or paracrine fashion. They exert their biological actions through G protein coupled receptors (GPCRs) and, as it happens with the synthases, each prostanoid has a distinctive receptor to which to bind to. DP, EP, FP, IP and TP are the receptors for PGD_2, PGE_2, $PGF_{2\alpha}$, PGI_2 and TXA_2, respectively (Figure 1). The EP receptor has four known subtypes (EP1-EP4), each encoded by a different gene; furthermore, EP3 has eight splice variants; TP and FP have also been described to have two splice variants each (Fortier et al., 2008).

Sequence homology analysis revealed that receptors sharing a common signaling pathway are more closely related than do receptors binding the same ligand. After binding to the corresponding GPCR there is generation of soluble second messengers. Coupled to Gq, DP receptor increases cyclic adenosine monophosphate (cAMP) concentration, whereas IP receptor is coupled to Gs and increases not only cAMP but also mediates responses by phosphatidylinositol increasing free Ca^{2+} concentration (Narumiya et al., 1999). Both isoforms of TP activate phopspholipase C (PLC), but TPα activates adenylate cyclase while TPβ inhibits it (Narumiya et al., 1999). FP receptors also act through Gq, PLC and Ca^{2+} release; while EP receptors have distinctive signaling pathways depending on the subtype binding PGE_2: EP1 is coupled to Gi and Ca^{2+} channels, EP2 and EP4 share the pathway coupling to Gs and increasing cAMP intracellular concentration, whereas the EP3 has specific responses depending on the splice variant, but is usually assumed as an inhibitory receptor coupled to Gi (Fortier et al., 2008) (Figure 1).

2. Role of endometrial prostaglandins in reproduction

The uterus plays a crucial role in the implantation process of the fertilized egg. Humans and old-world primates have the particularity that they shed part of their endometrium if fertilization or implantation does not take place. Consequently, endometrium is a dynamic tissue that undergoes regulated phases of proliferation, differentiation and degradation, cyclically. PGs are known to be important actors of this process; different reports have implicated COX enzymes and PGs in several stages of reproduction (Jabbour et al., 2006).

COX-2 is physiologically expressed at different levels along the menstrual cycle. It has been shown to be expressed at its lowest level during ovulation and slightly start augmenting during the secretory phase, peaking at the late secretory and menstrual phases after which it starts decreasing again (Jones et al., 1997).

The importance of COX and PGs in reproduction has been revealed from studies of knockout mice. Even if COX-1 deficient mice were fertile, their gestation period was prolonged while parturition and viable offspring were reduced. These findings demonstrated that COX-1 is essential for normal labor in the mouse (Gross et al., 1998; Jabbour et al., 2006). On the other side, selective COX-2 ablation impairs ovulation, fertilization and implantation; and a combined approach showed that COX-2 inhibition in COX-1(-/-) mice induced complete reproductive failure, suggesting a lack of alternative sources of PG synthesis (Reese et al., 2001).

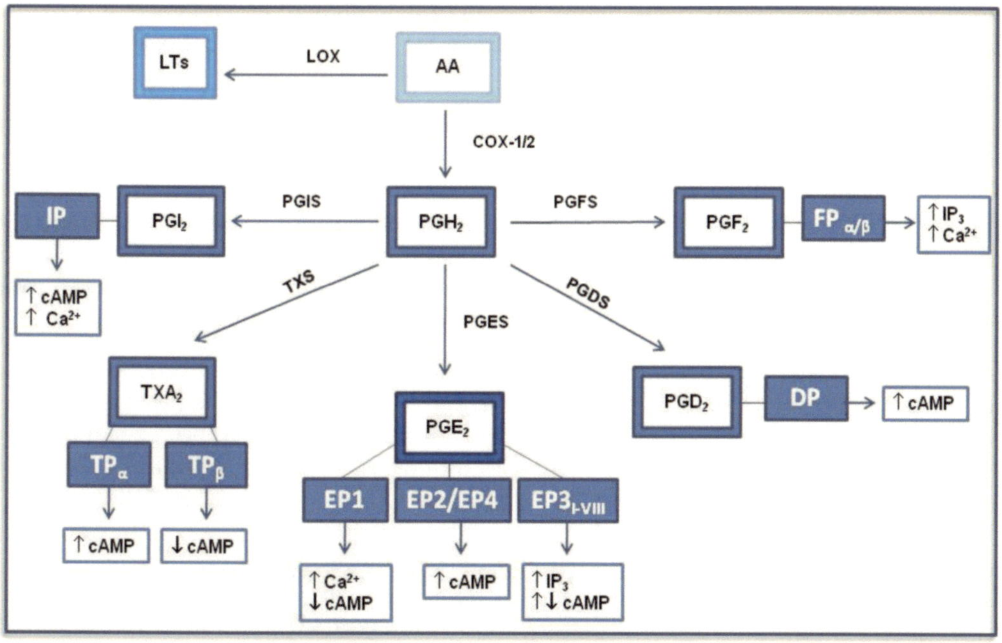

Arachidonic acid is the precursor for leukotrienes and prostaglandins. Each prostaglandin has a specific seven transmembrane G protein coupled receptor; after binding with its receptor, prostaglandins produce the up (↓) or downregulation (↑) of second messengers.

AA: arachidonic acid; **LTs**: leukotrienes; **LOX**: lipooxygenase; **COX-1/2**: cyclooxygenase-1 or 2; **PGH$_2$:** prostaglandin H_2; **PGIS**: prostacyclin synthase; **PGI$_2$**: prostacyclin; **TXS**: thromboxane synthase; **TXA$_2$**: thromboxane; **PGE$_2$:** prostaglandin E_2; **PGD$_2$:** prostaglandin D_2; **PGF$_2$:** prostaglandin F_2; **PGES**: PGE_2 synthase; **PGDS**: PGD_2 synthase; **PGFS**: $PGF_{2\alpha}$ synthase; **IP, TP$_{\alpha/\beta}$, EP1-4, DP, FP$_{\alpha/\beta}$**: specific PG receptors; **cAMP**: cyclic adenosine monophosphate; **IP$_3$**: inositol triphosphate; **Ca^{2+}**: calcium.

Fig. 1. Prostaglandin synthesis and signal transduction

In addition, studies using EP and FP knockout mice have demonstrated the specific roles of PGE_2 and $PGF_{2\alpha}$ in reproduction. It has been shown that EP2 receptors are essential for ovulation and fertilization (Kennedy et al., 1999; Ushikubi et al., 2000) and FP are indispensible for parturition (Sugimoto et al., 1998). These studies indicate not only the essential role of PGE_2 in the fertilization process, but also the importance of $PGF_{2\alpha}$ in natural parturition.

As well, it has been described that PGs serve as endogenous ligands for nuclear receptors. In this respect, other prostanoids were identified as good peroxisome proliferator-activated receptors (PPAR) agonists with varying specificity. 15-deoxy-Δ 12,14 prostaglandin J2 (15dPGJ2), a natural PPARγ ligand, has high affinity for PPARγ and has been proposed as a regulator of the inflammatory response (Nosjean & Boutin, 2002; Scher & Pillinger, 2009). Another PPAR ligand is PGI_2 that was found to play an important role via PPAR-δ nuclear receptor in implantation and decidualization (Pakrasi & Jain, 2008).

The process of implantation is considered to be analogous to pro-inflammatory responses, hence the speculation that PGs play a role in this event (Kennedy, 1979; Maybin et al., 2011; Tranguch et al., 2005). As well, several nonsteroidal anti-inflammatory drugs (NSAIDs) and selective COX-2 inhibitors were implicated in the inhibition of endometrial vascular permeability and implantation in a variety of species (Diao et al., 2007; Sookvanichsilp & Pulbutr, 2002).

In particular in the endometrium, COXs and PGs are known to be involved in the initiation of implantation and decidualization (Kennedy et al., 2007; Tranguch et al., 2005). It is well known that endometrial vascular permeability and proliferation and differentiation of endometrial stromal cells to decidual cells are mediated by PGs (Kennedy, 1979; Kennedy & Doktorcik, 1988). The initial studies of Chakraborty and coworkers suggest an important role for PGs in the implantation process; specifically this report demonstrated that COX-2 expression during the blastocyst attachment is critical to implantation (Chakraborty et al., 1996).

In an effort to identify which PGs are involved in the implantation process, different researchers have confirmed the presence of PGE and PGF receptors in the peri-implantation endometrium (Kennedy et al., 2007). However, no single type of PG has been unequivocally associated to this event. There may be species differences and also different PGs may be involved in the implantation or decidualization processes (Kennedy et al., 2007).

3. PGE_2 and its role in the aetiopathogenesis of endometriosis

COX-2, the crucial enzyme for the production of PGs, has been described to be upregulated in different pathological inflammatory conditions. Endometriosis is characterized by the high proliferation rate of endometrial cells in an ectopic site, inflammation and pain. COX-2 is highly expressed in eutopic endometrium, both in the proliferative and secretory phases, and in ectopic lesions from endometriosis patients compared to disease free women (Ota et al., 2001). Wu and coworkers also described that COX-2 is expressed in stromal and epithelial cells derived from endometriosis patients, and is in agreement with the work from Ota and coworkers, in that this expression is higher in patients (Ota et al., 2001; Wu et al., 2002).

3.1 Sources of prostaglandins

It is well known that the elevated levels of PGs found in the peritoneal fluid from patients with endometriosis are mainly produced by peritoneal macrophages and endometriotic tissues (Raiter-Tenenbaum et al., 1998; Wu et al., 2002; Wu et al., 2010). COX-2 is overexpressed in peritoneal macrophages and in ectopic and eutopic endometrial tissue derived from patients with endometriosis (Banu et al., 2008; Ota et al., 2001; Wu et al., 2002; Wu et al., 2005b). Peritoneal macrophages from endometriosis-free women express no or minimal amounts of COX-2, while the overexpression of COX-2 found in endometriosis has been associated with the elevated concentrations of PGs and the severity of the disease (Wu et al., 2002). Explicitly, induction of COX-2 expression correlated with the evidence that peritoneal macrophages from patients with endometriosis release significantly more PGE_2 and $PGF_{2\alpha}$ compared with peritoneal macrophages from control women (Karck et al., 1996; Raiter-Tenenbaum et al., 1998). Many pro-inflammatory and pro-angiogenic factors contribute to increase PGs levels: interleukin (IL)-1β, tumor necrosis factor (TNF)-α, vascular endothelial growth factor (VEGF), macrophage migration inhibition factor (MIF) and even PGE_2 have been shown to induce COX-2 expression in peritoneal macrophages from women with endometriosis (Wu et al., 2002) and in endometrial and endometriotic stromal cells (Carli et al., 2009; Tamura et al., 2002; Wu et al., 2005b) (Figure 2).

The mitogenic effects of estrogens are mediated by the upregulation of several growth factors and also by PGs. Specifically, aromatase and steroidogenic acute regulatory protein (StAR) are known to be regulated by PGE_2 in endometriotic stromal cells (Bulun et al., 2004; Noble et al., 1997; Sun et al., 2003; Tsai et al., 2001). PGE_2 alone via the EP2/EP4 receptor is sufficient to induce de novo synthesis of estrogen from cholesterol (Attar et al., 2009). As well, estrogen further stimulates the synthesis of PGE_2 in ectopic endometrial tissue (Bulun et al., 2000; Noble et al., 1997). In conclusion, estrogens, pro-inflammatory and pro-angiogenic peptides contribute to elevate the expression of COX-2 and consequently the levels of PGE_2 in endometriotic tissue and in peritoneal macrophages from patients with endometriosis (Figure 2).

3.2 Regulation of aromatase activation and estrogen production by PGE_2

Aromatase is the key enzyme in the conversion of the androgens, androstenedione and testosterone, to estrone and estradiol (E_2) respectively (Bulun et al., 2001). This protein was seen to be overexpressed in the eutopic endometrium of patients with endometriosis compared to controls (Noble et al., 1996) and it has been described to be expressed in the ectopic endometriotic lesion. PGE_2 induces not only aromatase expression but also its activity, as seen in studies conducted in endometriotic stromal cells *in vitro* (Noble et al., 1997); and its product, E_2, induces COX-2 expression with the consequent synthesis of PGE_2 (Tamura et al., 2004). It is clear that given the way these molecules interact, a positive feedback loop is established favoring the activity of aromatase, provoking high levels of E_2 locally in the vicinity of the lesion (Figure 2). These high levels of E_2 also give the endometriotic cells a high capability of proliferating; as it has been demonstrated that, through its estrogen receptor (ER)β, E_2 enhances stromal cell proliferation (Trukhacheva et al., 2009).

Another mitogenic factor is fibroblast growth factor (FGF)-9. This molecule was found to be regulated by estrogen in endometriotic stromal cells in culture and, if added exogenously, cell proliferation was enhanced in a dose dependent manner. On the contrast, when cells were incubated with an aromatase or an ER inhibitor, the rate of cell proliferation diminished significantly compared to the untreated control (Wing et al., 2003). In the same study by Wing and coworkers, it was observed that not only FGF-9 is regulated by E_2, but also, FGF receptors 2IIIc and 3IIIc. More recently, a study revealed that PGE_2, acting through its receptor EP3 induces the expression of FGF-9 in a dose dependent manner in endometriotic cells *in vitro* (Chuang et al., 2006) (Figure 2).

3.3 PGE_2 and angiogenesis

Endometrial cells at the ectopic site are urged to establish their own irrigation network, this is essential for the further maintenance and growth of the endometriotic lesion. It is widely known that VEGF is crucial for the process of angiogenesis; this is the process by which new blood vessels can be developed from preexisting ones. It has been shown that patients with endometriosis have a higher VEGF concentration in peritoneal fluid than endometriosis free women (Mahnke et al., 2000). Moreover, it was seen that VEGF stimulates COX-2 expression (Tamura et al., 2006) and that PGE_2 increases VEGF production (Gately & Li, 2004; Liu et al.,

2002); as it happens with aromatase, a positive feedback loop is established in which COX-2 activity and PGE_2 production are favored, giving the characteristic inflammation site of endometriosis (Figure 2).

3.4 Prostaglandins as immune and inflammatory mediators in endometriosis

Immune dysfunction has been proposed to play an important role in endometriosis (Dmowski W.P. & Braun, 2004; Vinatier et al., 1996). Peritoneal macrophages may play a key role in this respect, and may control the function of other immune cells. One of the altered mechanisms involved in the implantation and propagation of endometrial tissues ectopically is the decrease of the phagocytic ability of peritoneal macrophages (Chuang et al., 2009).

In their earlier studies, Braun and coworkers reported that the decrease in peritoneal macrophages cytotoxic function is controlled by PG synthesis (Braun et al., 1992) (Figure 2). To elucidate the molecular mechanism implicated in the reduced phagocytic ability of peritoneal macrophages in endometriosis, recent *in vitro* and *in vivo* studies demonstrated that PGE_2, via the EP2 receptor-dependent signaling pathway, inhibits the expression of the scavenger receptor CD36 in peritoneal macrophages. Reduced expression of any one of the scavenger receptors may result in loss of phagocytic ability of macrophages (Chuang et al., 2010). Another work suggests that the expression and the enzymatic activity of MMP-9, a metalloproteinase that plays important roles in the scavenger activity of macrophages, is reduced by PGE_2 in peritoneal macrophages derived from endometriosis patients compared to controls (Wu et al., 2005a). Wu and coworkers also reported that this inhibitory effect of PGE_2 may be mediated via the EP2/EP4-dependent PKA pathway (Wu et al., 2005a). These data allow us to explain some of the disruptions observed in the endometriotic macrophage functions and provide a functional link between COX-2 overexpression and endometriosis development (Ota et al., 2001; Tamura et al., 2002; Wu et al., 2005b).

There is abundant evidence demonstrating that endometriosis is accompanied by inflammatory reactions in the peritoneum, resulting in abnormal levels of a variety of cytokines, chemokines and pro-inflammatory factors in the peritoneal fluid (Gazvani & Templeton, 2002; Lousse et al., 2010). It is also well known, that the number of macrophages is increased in the peritoneal fluid of endometriosis patients and that they are in a hyperactive state (Halme & Surrey, 1990; Raiter-Tenenbaum et al., 1998). Production of inflammatory cytokines by these macrophages such as monocyte chemoattractant protein (MCP)-1, IL-1β, TNF-α and IL-6 is also increased in peritoneal fluid (Wu et al., 2007). As well, we found that the release of PGE_2 by peritoneal macrophages was 100-fold higher in advanced endometriosis patients than in controls (Raiter-Tenenbaum et al., 1998).

It has also been demonstrated that the overexpression of COX-2 is markedly induced by IL-1β, TNF-α and MIF and that these pro-inflammatory agents strongly stimulate the production of PGE_2 (Carli et al., 2009; Wu et al., 2002) (Figure 2). However, not only the overexpression of COX-2 increases the production of PGE_2, but also a decrease in the deactivating enzyme 15-PGDH was found, showing an imbalance between eicosanoid biosynthesis and degradation in endometriosis patients compared with controls (Lousse et al., 2010). As a result, the concentration of PGE_2 in the peritoneal fluid is elevated in patients with endometriosis, which leads to a more severe pathological process.

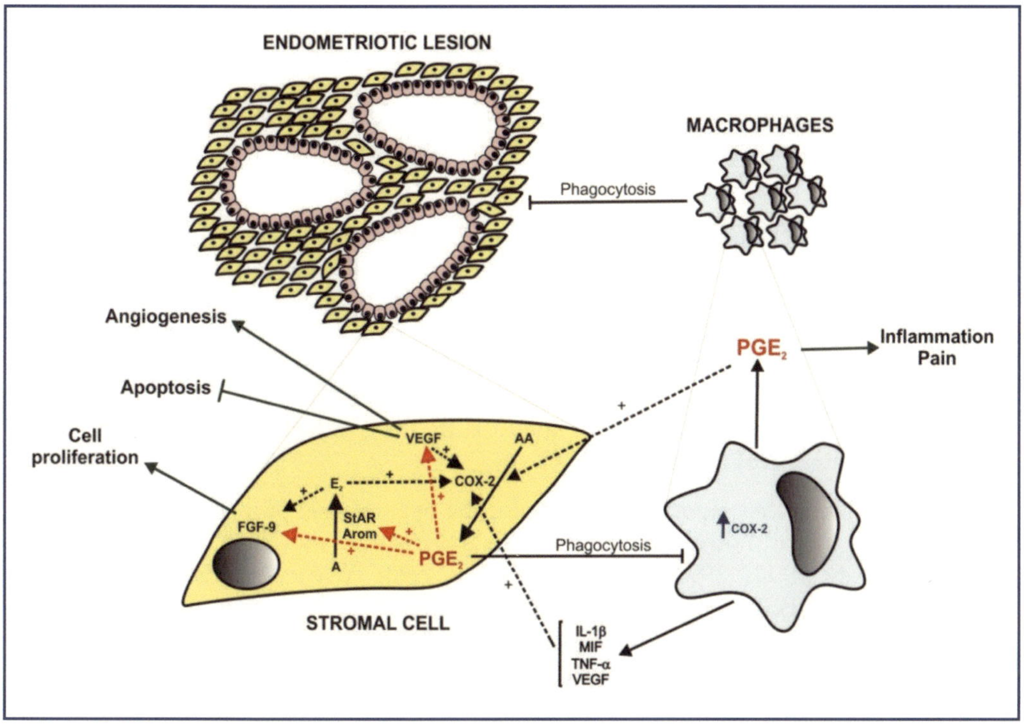

Macrophages synthesize and liberate PGE_2, VEGF, MIF, IL-1β, TNF-α; all of these factors stimulate the expression and/or activity of COX-2 producing higher concentrations of PGE_2. The high levels of PGE_2 stimulate the expression of the angiogenic factor VEGF and the steroidogenic capacity of endometriotic cells by the upregulation of StAR and aromatase, which augments the byosinthesis of estrogen. E_2 and PGE_2 further induce FGF-9 expresion to stimulate endometriotic cell proliferation. As a result, angiogenesis and cell proliferation are augmented while apoptosis is inhibited. Moreover, PGE_2 suppresses the phagocytic ability of macrophages, which fail to phagocytase the retrograde endometrial tissue and allow the implantation and proliferation of endometriotic lesion.

A: androstenedione; **AA**: arachidonic acid; **Arom:** aromatase P450; **COX-2**: cyclooxygenase-2; **E_2**: estradiol; **IL-1β**: interleukin 1β; **MIF**: macrophage migration inhibitory factor; **PGE_2**: prostaglandin E_2; **StAR**: steroidogenic acute regulatory protein; **TNF-α**: tumor necrosis factor α; **VEGF**: vascular endothelial growth factor; **FGF-9**: fibroblast growth factor-9.

Fig. 2. Peritoneal environment in endometriosis

4. Prostaglandins and pelvic pain

Endometriosis has been traditionally included among the most important causes of pelvic pain in women of reproductive age. A recent case-control study described that 73% of women with endometriosis reported experiencing abdominopelvic pain, dysmenorrhea, or menorrhagia compared with only a 20% of the controls (Ballard et al., 2008).

The role of PGs has been examined in women suffering from heavy menstrual bleeding and dysmenorrhea (Maybin et al., 2011). Dysmenorrhea is defined as the excessive pain during menstruation; and menorraghia or heavy menstrual bleeding is the excessive menstrual blood loss during the menstrual periods. These may be primary disorders or secondary to endometrial pathology such as endometriosis (Maybin et al., 2011; Tietjen et al., 2006).

The pelvic pain of dysmenorrhea has been demonstrated to be mediated through the action of PGE_2 and a direct relationship between the severity of dysmenorrhea and the production of PGs has been observed in endometriosis (Coco, 1999; Koike et al., 1992; Nasir & Bope, 2004). As well, analysis of menstrual fluid from women suffering from dysmenorrhea revealed augmented levels of PGE_2 and $PGF_{2\alpha}$ (Dawood & Khan-Dawood, 2007a, 2007b; Lumsden et al., 1983).

Increased synthesis of PGE_2 and $PGF_{2\alpha}$ in the endometrium has important implications for menstruation (Baird et al., 1996). PGE_2 is a potent vasodilator leading to increased oedema and contributing to pain at time of menstruation. Increased COX-2 and enhanced PGE_2–EP-induced cAMP production has been found by Smith and coworkers in the endometrium of women with objective heavy menstrual bleeding. These authors suggest that the increased expression of the rate-limiting COX enzymes in the endometrium of women with heavy menstrual blood loss will lead to an increase in PG production and to a magnified inflammation (Smith et al., 2007).

In addition, there is well reported evidence for the hyperalgesic properties of PGs; and EP receptors have been shown elevated in sensory neurons that lead to increased pain perception (Bley et al., 1998; Levine & Taiwo, 1990). Wienecke and coworkers also demonstrated that PGE_2 induces headache in healthy subjects by sensitization of cranial perivascular sensory afferents (Wienecke et al., 2009). Therefore, PG inhibition usually resolves the pain and many studies have demonstrated the efficacy of NSAIDs and specific COX-2 inhibitors in relieving dysmenorrheic pain (Coco, 1999; Hayes & Rock, 2002). Suprofen, ibuprofen and acetaminophen were shown to be efficient not only for pain relief but for menstrual fluid PGs suppression as well (Dawood & Khan-Dawood, 2007a, 2007b).

A recent study suggests that the major modality to substantially alleviate pain in endometriosis is suppression of ovarian function and induction of a steady hormonal condition, anovulation and, eventually, amenorrhea (Vercellini et al., 2011). Hormonal manipulation and surgery have been found to be efficient in the management of pelvic pain associated to endometriosis (Vercellini et al., 2011). Oral contraceptives, GnRH agonists, danazol and progestins have been shown to reduce the production of PGs, which are responsible in large part for pelvic pain (Crosignani et al., 2006; Venturini et al., 1997).

Given that, further investigations should focus on how to inhibit the production of PGs in endometriosis to control the pain and the development of the pathology.

5. Endometriosis and its therapies

As an estrogen-dependent disease, endometriosis treatment has aimed at reducing estrogen concentrations with reversible therapies, using oral contraceptives in a cyclical or continuous fashion as well as with GnRH analogues as first line medical treatments. Progestins, aromatase inhibitors (AIs) and, less frequently, androgens are also used. Removing lesions in a conservative surgery, or even having a radical intervention when the extent of the disease is major, is the surgical approach nowadays available. The most ordinary way of treating endometriosis is attacking from both flanks, with the surgical intervention and dealing with the symptoms with the drug therapy. In any case, the disease is likely to reappear after cessation of therapy; in fact, recurrence rate for endometriosis is between 4-25% (Meuleman et al., 2011).

5.1 PGE_2 synthesis inhibition and pain treatment

One of the most inhabilitating symptoms of endometriosis for carrying a normal life is the elevated pelvic pain patients experience. It includes pain before and during periods, during sexual intercourse, while urinating or defecating and during menstruation. It has been of great importance to provide the patient with a better quality of life ameliorating pain symptoms. Elevated concentrations of PGE_2 in peritoneal fluid from endometriosis patients is the major cause thought to be involved in pain and inflammation processes (Wu et al., 2002).

There have been done a large number of studies focusing on the inhibition of COXs activity. Whether it is blocking simultaneously COX-1 and COX-2 or with selective COX-2 inhibitors, the ultimate goal is to lower the concentrations of PGE_2.

NSAIDs, among them: ibuprofen, naproxen, diclofenac or aspirin; are used primarily for pain treatment, from a headache to menstrual cramps, from a backache to treating an inflammation due to a sprain. These NSAIDs are non-selective COX inhibitors; this means that they prevent the synthesis of PGs from both COXs. Of course, as a constitutively and ubiquitously expressed enzyme, COX-1 inhibition has side effects that should be avoided. Gastrointestinal ulcer is not a rare effect after long term inhibition of COX-1 (Wadman, 2007); this is why COX-2 selective inhibitors have been developed.

Celecoxib belongs to the family of NSAIDs with high selectivity for COX-2 inhibition. Other coxibs have been developed too (rofecoxib, valdecoxib) but were withdrawn from the market in the mid 2000s by the Federal Drug and Food Administration (FDA) of the United States of America because they were proven to have serious cardiovascular adverse events. Coxibs were and are mostly used in arthritis; the one still available for purchase, celecoxib, is prescribed in familial adenomatous polyposis and as an adjuvant in breast cancer (Basu et al., 2006; Falandry et al., 2009; Iwama, 2009; Jankowski & Hunt, 2008; Lynch et al., 2010). Celecoxib has not been approved yet for the treatment of endometriosis. There is one study that evaluated the effectiveness of a COX-2 specific inhibitor on relieving pain symptoms associated to endometriosis after a conservative surgery. Cobellis and coworkers demonstrated in their study that rofecoxib was effective for the management of pain and no recurrence occurred during the six months of treatment (Cobellis et al., 2004).

Ferrero and coworkers, recently published a review where they compilated information on the use of AIs and how they contributed to diminish endometriosis related pain. This systematic study shows that the AIs, letrozole and anastrozole, are effective in treating pain symptoms; when withdrawn symptoms reappear, but they cannot be used for a long term therapy because of the adverse effects these compounds have on bone density (Ferrero et al., 2011). Endometriosis patients need chronic treatment, and this could be achieved combining AIs with a hormonal therapy to reduce the loss of bone density (Ferrero et al., 2011).

5.2 PGE_2 synthesis inhibition and the control over endometriosis development

There have been conducted several studies in which AIs were used and the progression of endometriosis was evaluated. When letrozole or anastrozole were added to endometrial epithelial cells from endometriosis patients in culture, cell proliferation was inhibited and apoptosis augmented (Meresman et al., 2005). When the same two compounds were used for the treatment of surgically induced endometriosis in mice, not only cell proliferation was diminished and apoptosis increased within the endometriotic like lesion, but PGE was also decreased in the peritoneal fluid of mice treated with letrozole but not with anastrozole (Bilotas et al., 2010).

Much research has been done evaluating the effects of inhibiting COXs activity regarding the development of endometriosis with *in vivo* and *in vitro* approaches. Celecoxib has been shown to have anti-proliferative and pro-apoptotic effects over endometrial epithelial cells in culture obtained from biopsies of women with and without endometriosis; it was also effective in diminishing COX-2 expression, reducing the synthesis of VEGF and PGE_2 (Olivares et al., 2008). Similar results had previously been achieved in various cancer models (Basu et al., 2005; Chun & Surh, 2004). Given that the endometrial cells at the ectopic site have a very similar behaviour to neoplasic cells; it is not surprising that treatments aim at the same targets.

There is one very complete work from Efstathiou and coworkers where they compared seven different selective (rofecoxib and celecoxib) and non-selective (aspirin, ibuprofen, indomethacin, naproxen and sulindac) NSAIDs on the establishment and development of endometriosis in a mouse model (Efstathiou et al., 2005). In this work, celecoxib given orally twice daily and indomethacin administered subcutaneously daily for four weeks, were both effective in significantly diminishing the percentage of established lesions compared to the control group. All the NSAIDs evaluated in the same study, except for aspirin, significantly inhibited the growth of the established lesions compared to the control group (Efstathiou et al., 2005). A study in a rat model of endometriosis, evaluated the effect of parecoxib, another selective COX-2 inhibitor, and showed not only a significant reduction in lesion size, but also, a significant inhibition on the expression of VEGF, its receptor Flk-1 and COX-2 compared to the untreated group with endometriosis (Machado et al., 2010). Machado and coworkers also observed a significant reduction of the levels of PGE_2 in endometriotic homogeneized tissue treated with parecoxib compared to the untreated group (Machado et al., 2010).

More recently a new approach targeting more than one molecule to prevent the development of the disease has gained importance. Promising results were achieved firstly in cancer models, which targeted COX-2 and PPARγ. This combinational therapy resulted in the inhibition of cell proliferation and apoptosis enhancement *in vitro* and increased overall survival rate *in vivo* (Mustafa & Kruger, 2008; Sun et al., 2009). When celecoxib was combined with rosiglitazone, a PPARγ agonist, for the treatment of surgically induced endometriosis in a mouse model, a reduced number of established lesions was observed as well as the volume of established ones; also induction of apoptosis and reduction of the cell proliferation rate and vascularization was achieved (Olivares et al., 2011).

Reducing PGE_2 concentration in the peritoneal environment would not only be relieving the pain caused by the disease but would also be affecting its development. This is one of the main goals of endometriosis treatments; now it is time to decide whether the drugs used to achieve these results are the appropriate ones to manage with this disease.

6. Conclusion

In conclusion, PGs play a substantial role in the physiological and pathological processes in the reproductive system. PGs are known to be involved in the initiation of the phsysiological implantation and decidualization. Also, COX-2 and PGE_2 were seen to be overexpressed in several pathological circumstances as different types of cancers and other inflammation related diseases.

There is no doubt that PGE_2 is implicated in the aetiopathogenesis of endometriosis and contributes to the development and maintenance of the disease. The elevated levels of PGs found in the peritoneal fluid from patients with endometriosis are mainly produced by peritoneal macrophages and endometriotic tissues. As well, the peritoneal estrogens, pro-inflammatory and pro-angiogenic molecules contribute to elevate the expression of COX-2 and consequently the levels of PGE_2 in endometriosis patients. The pelvic pain associated to endometriosis has also been demonstrated to be mediated through the action of PGE_2 and inhibition of PG production usually resolves the pain.

Given these data, further investigations should focus on how to inhibit the production of PGs in endometriosis, to control the pain and the development of the pathology.

7. Acknowledgement

We thank Dr. Gustavo Leirós for providing technical assistance in designing figures.

8. References

Attar, E., Tokunaga, H., Imir, G., Yilmaz, M.B., Redwine, D., Putman, M., Gurates, B., Attar, R., Yaegashi, N., Hales, D.B., & Bulun, S.E. Prostaglandin E2 via steroidogenic factor-1 coordinately regulates transcription of steroidogenic genes necessary for estrogen synthesis in endometriosis. *Journal of Clinical Endocrinology and Metabolism*, Vol.94, No.2, (February 2009), pp. (623-631), 0021-972X

Baird, D.T., Cameron, S.T., Critchley, H.O., Drudy, T.A., Howe, A., Jones, R.L., Lea, R.G., & Kelly, R.W. Prostaglandins and menstruation. *European Journal of Obstetrics & Gynecology and Reproductive Biology.*, Vol.70, No.1, (December 1996), pp. (15-17), 0301-2115

Ballard, K.D., Seaman, H.E., de Vries, C.S., & Wright, J.T. Can symptomatology help in the diagnosis of endometriosis? Findings from a national case-control study--Part 1. *BJOG: An International Journal of Obstetrics and Gynaecology*, Vol.115, No.11, (October 2008), pp. (1382-1391), 1470-032

Banu, S.K., Lee, J., Speights, V.O., Jr., Starzinski-Powitz, A., & Arosh, J.A. Cyclooxygenase-2 regulates survival, migration, and invasion of human endometriotic cells through multiple mechanisms. *Endocrinology*, Vol.149, No.3, (March 2008), pp. (1180-1189), 0013-7227

Basu, G.D., Pathangey, L.B., Tinder, T.L., Gendler, S.J., & Mukherjee, P. Mechanisms underlying the growth inhibitory effects of the cyclo-oxygenase-2 inhibitor celecoxib in human breast cancer cells. *Breast Cancer Research*, Vol.7, No.4, (April 2005), pp. (R422-R435), 1465-5411

Basu, G.D., Tinder, T.L., Bradley, J.M., Tu, T., Hattrup, C.L., Pockaj, B.A., & Mukherjee, P. Cyclooxygenase-2 inhibitor enhances the efficacy of a breast cancer vaccine: role of IDO. *Journal of Immunology*, Vol.177, No.4, (August 2006), pp. (2391-2402), 0022-1767

Bilotas, M., Meresman, G., Stella, I., Sueldo, C., & Baranao, R.I. Effect of aromatase inhibitors on ectopic endometrial growth and peritoneal environment in a mouse model of endometriosis. *Fertility and Sterility*, Vol.93, No.8, (May 2010), pp. (2513-2518), 0015-0282

Bley, K.R., Hunter, J.C., Eglen, R.M., & Smith, J.A. The role of IP prostanoid receptors in inflammatory pain. *Trends in Pharmacological Sciences*, Vol.19, No.4, (April 1998), pp. (141-147), 0165-6147

Braun, D.P., Gebel, H., Rotman, C., Rana, N., & Dmowski, W.P. The development of cytotoxicity in peritoneal macrophages from women with endometriosis. *Fertility and Sterility*, Vol.57, No.6, (June 1992), pp. (1203-1210), 0015-0282

Bulun, S.E., Fang, Z., Imir, G., Gurates, B., Tamura, M., Yilmaz, B., Langoi, D., Amin, S., Yang, S., & Deb, S. Aromatase and endometriosis. *Seminars in Repoductive Medicine*, Vol.22, No.1, (February 2004), pp. (45-50), 1526-8004

Bulun, S.E., Yang, S., Fang, Z., Gurates, B., Tamura, M., Zhou, J., & Sebastian, S. Role of aromatase in endometrial disease. *Journal of Steroid Biochemestry and Molecular Biology*, Vol.79, No.1-5, (December 2001), pp. (19-25), 0960-0760

Bulun, S.E., Zeitoun, K.M., Takayama, K., & Sasano, H. Estrogen biosynthesis in endometriosis: molecular basis and clinical relevance. *Journal of Molecular Endocrinology*, Vol.25, No.1, (August 2000), pp. (35-42), 0952-5041

Carli, C., Metz, C.N., Al Abed, Y., Naccache, P.H., & Akoum, A. Up-regulation of cyclooxygenase-2 expression and prostaglandin E2 production in human endometriotic cells by macrophage migration inhibitory factor: involvement of novel kinase signaling pathways. *Endocrinology*, Vol.150, No.7, (July 2009), pp. (3128-3137), 0013-7227

Chakraborty, I., Das, S.K., Wang, J., & Dey, S.K. Developmental expression of the cyclo-oxygenase-1 and cyclo-oxygenase-2 genes in the peri-implantation mouse uterus and their differential regulation by the blastocyst and ovarian steroids. *Journal of Molecular Endocrinology*, Vol.16, No.2, (April 1996), pp. (107-122), 0952-5041

Chandrasekharan, N.V., Dai, H., Roos, K.L., Evanson, N.K., Tomsik, J., Elton, T.S., & Simmons, D.L. COX-3, a cyclooxygenase-1 variant inhibited by acetaminophen and other analgesic/antipyretic drugs: cloning, structure, and expression. *Proceedings of the National Academy of Sciences of U.S.A*, Vol.99, No.21, (October 2002), pp. (13926-13931), 0027-8424

Chandrasekharan, N.V. & Simmons, D.L. The cyclooxygenases. *Genome Biology*, Vol.5, No.9, (August 2004), pp. (241-247), 1465-6906

Chuang, P.C., Lin, Y.J., Wu, M.H., Wing, L.Y., Shoji, Y., & Tsai, S.J. Inhibition of CD36-dependent phagocytosis by prostaglandin E2 contributes to the development of endometriosis. *American Journal of Pathology*, Vol.176, No.2, (February 2010), pp. (850-860), 0002-9440

Chuang, P.C., Sun, H.S., Chen, T.M., & Tsai, S.J. Prostaglandin E2 induces fibroblast growth factor 9 via EP3-dependent protein kinase Cdelta and Elk-1 signaling. *Molecular and Cellular Biology*, Vol.26, No.22, (November 2006), pp. (8281-8292), 0270-7306

Chuang, P.C., Wu, M.H., Shoji, Y., & Tsai, S.J. Downregulation of CD36 results in reduced phagocytic ability of peritoneal macrophages of women with endometriosis. *Journal of Pathology*, Vol.219, No.2, (October 2009), pp. (232-241), 0022-3417

Chun, K.S. & Surh, Y.J. Signal transduction pathways regulating cyclooxygenase-2 expression: potential molecular targets for chemoprevention. *Biochemical Pharmacology*, Vol.68, No.6, (September 2004), pp. (1089-1100), 0006-2952

Cobellis, L., Razzi, S., De Simone, S., Sartini, A., Fava, A., Danero, S., Gioffre, W., Mazzini, M., & Petraglia, F. The treatment with a COX-2 specific inhibitor is effective in the management of pain related to endometriosis. *European Journal of Obstetrics & Gynecology and Reproductive Biology*, Vol.116, No.1, (September 2004), pp. (100-102), 0301-2115

Coco, A.S. Primary dysmenorrhea. *American Family Physician*, Vol.60, No.2, (August 1999), pp. (489-496), 0002-838X

Crosignani, P., Olive, D., Bergqvist, A., & Luciano, A. Advances in the management of endometriosis: an update for clinicians. *Human Reproduction Update*, Vol.12, No.2, (March 2006), pp. (179-189), 1355-4786

Dawood, M.Y. & Khan-Dawood, F.S. Clinical efficacy and differential inhibition of menstrual fluid prostaglandin F2alpha in a randomized, double-blind, crossover treatment with placebo, acetaminophen, and ibuprofen in primary dysmenorrhea. *American Journal of Obstetrics & Gynecology*, Vol.196, No.1, (January 2007a), pp. (35-35), 0002-9378

Dawood, M.Y. & Khan-Dawood, F.S. Differential suppression of menstrual fluid prostaglandin F2a, prostaglandin E2, 6-keto prostaglandin F1a and thromboxane B2 by suprofen in women with primary dysmenorrhea. *Prostaglandins & Other Lipid Mediators*, Vol.83, No.1-2, (February 2007b), pp. (146-153), 1098-8823

Diao, H.L., Zhu, H., Ma, H., Tan, H.N., Cong, J., Su, R.W., & Yang, Z.M. Rat ovulation, implantation and decidualization are severely compromised by COX-2 inhibitors. *Frontiers in Bioscience*, Vol.12 (May 2007), pp. (3333-3342), 1093-4715

Dmowski W.P. & Braun, D.P. Immunology of endometriosis. *Best Practice & Research in Clinical Obstetrics & Gynaecology*, Vol.18, No.2, (April 2004), pp. (245-263), 1521-6934

Efstathiou, J.A., Sampson, D.A., Levine, Z., Rohan, R.M., Zurakowski, D., Folkman, J., D'Amato, R.J., & Rupnick, M.A. Nonsteroidal antiinflammatory drugs differentially suppress endometriosis in a murine model. *Fertility and Sterility*, Vol.83, No.1, (January 2005), pp. (171-181), 0015-0282

Falandry, C., Canney, P.A., Freyer, G., & Dirix, L.Y. Role of combination therapy with aromatase and cyclooxygenase-2 inhibitors in patients with metastatic breast cancer. *Annals of Oncology*, Vol.20, No.4, (April 2009), pp. (615-620), 0923-7534

Ferrero, S., Gillott, D.J., Venturini, P.L., & Remorgida, V. Use of aromatase inhibitors to treat endometriosis-related pain symptoms: a systematic review. *Reproductive Biology and Endocrinology*, Vol.9 (June 2011), pp. (89-112), 1477-7827

Fortier, M.A., Krishnaswamy, K., Danyod, G., Boucher-Kovalik, S., & Chapdalaine, P. A postgenomic integrated view of prostaglandins in reproduction: implications for other body systems. *Journal of Physiology and Pharmacology*, Vol.59 Suppl 1 (August 2008), pp. (65-89), 0867-5910

Gately, S. & Li, W.W. Multiple roles of COX-2 in tumor angiogenesis: a target for antiangiogenic therapy. *Seminars in Oncology*, Vol.31, No.2 Suppl 7, (April 2004), pp. (2-11), 0093-7754

Gazvani, R. & Templeton, A. Peritoneal environment, cytokines and angiogenesis in the pathophysiology of endometriosis. *Reproduction*, Vol.123, No.2, (February 2002), pp. (217-226), 1470-1626

Gross, G.A., Imamura, T., Luedke, C., Vogt, S.K., Olson, L.M., Nelson, D.M., Sadovsky, Y., & Muglia, L.J. Opposing actions of prostaglandins and oxytocin determine the onset of murine labor. *Proceedings of the National Academy of Sciences of U.S.A*, Vol.95, No.20, (September 1998), pp. (11875-11879), 0027-8424

Halme, J. & Surrey, E.S. Endometriosis and infertility: the mechanisms involved. *Progress in Clinical Biological Research*, Vol.323 (1990), pp. (157-178), 0361-7742

Hayes, E.C. & Rock, J.A. COX-2 inhibitors and their role in gynecology. *Obstetrical and Gynecological Survey*, Vol.57, No.11, (November 2002), pp. (768-780), 0029-7828

Hwang, D., Scollard, D., Byrne, J., & Levine, E. Expression of cyclooxygenase-1 and cyclooxygenase-2 in human breast cancer. *Journal of the National Cancer Institute*, Vol.90, No.6, (March 1998), pp. (455-460), 0027-8874

Iwama, T. NSAIDs and colorectal cancer prevention. *Journal of Gastroenterology*, Vol.44 Suppl 19 (2009), pp. (72-76), 0944-1174

Jabbour, H.N. & Sales, K.J. Prostaglandin receptor signalling and function in human endometrial pathology. *Trends in Endocrinology & Metabolism*, Vol.15, No.8, (October 2004), pp. (398-404), 1043-2760

Jabbour, H.N., Sales, K.J., Smith, O.P., Battersby, S., & Boddy, S.C. Prostaglandin receptors are mediators of vascular function in endometrial pathologies. *Molecular and Cellular Endocrinology*, Vol.252, No.1-2, (June 2006), pp. (191-200), 0303-7207

Jankowski, J. & Hunt, R. Cyclooxygenase-2 inhibitors in colorectal cancer prevention: counterpoint. *Cancer Epidemiology, Biomarkers & Prevention*, Vol.17, No.8, (August 2008), pp. (1858-1861), 1055-9965

Jones, R.L., Kelly, R.W., & Critchley, H.O. Chemokine and cyclooxygenase-2 expression in human endometrium coincides with leukocyte accumulation. *Human Reproduction*, Vol.12, No.6, (June 1997), pp. (1300-1306), 0268-1161

Karck, U., Reister, F., Schafer, W., Zahradnik, H.P., & Breckwoldt, M. PGE2 and PGF2 alpha release by human peritoneal macrophages in endometriosis. *Prostaglandins*, Vol.51, No.1, (January 1996), pp. (49-60), 0090-6980

Kennedy, C.R., Zhang, Y., Brandon, S., Guan, Y., Coffee, K., Funk, C.D., Magnuson, M.A., Oates, J.A., Breyer, M.D., & Breyer, R.M. Salt-sensitive hypertension and reduced fertility in mice lacking the prostaglandin EP2 receptor. *Nature Medicine*, Vol.5, No.2, (February 1999), pp. (217-220), 1078-8956

Kennedy, T.G. Prostaglandins and increased endometrial vascular permeabiltiy resulting from the application of artificial stimulus to the uterus of the rat sensitized for the decidual cell reaction. *Biology of Reproduction*, Vol.20, No.3, (April 1979), pp. (560-566), 0006-3363

Kennedy, T.G. & Doktorcik, P.E. Effects of analogues of prostaglandin E2 and F2 alpha on the decidual cell reaction in the rat. *Prostaglandins*, Vol.35, No.2, (February 1988), pp. (207-219), 0090-6980

Kennedy, T.G., Gillio-Meina, C., & Phang, S.H. Prostaglandins and the initiation of blastocyst implantation and decidualization. *Reproduction*, Vol.134, No.5, (November 2007), pp. (635-643), 1470-1626

Kitamura, T., Kawamori, T., Uchiya, N., Itoh, M., Noda, T., Matsuura, M., Sugimura, T., & Wakabayashi, K. Inhibitory effects of mofezolac, a cyclooxygenase-1 selective inhibitor, on intestinal carcinogenesis. *Carcinogenesis*, Vol.23, No.9, (September 2002), pp. (1463-1466), 0143-3334

Koike, H., Egawa, H., Ohtsuka, T., Yamaguchi, M., Ikenoue, T., & Mori, N. Correlation between dysmenorrheic severity and prostaglandin production in women with endometriosis. *Prostaglandins, Leukotrienes and Essential Fatty Acids*, Vol.46, No.2, (June 1992), pp. (133-137), 0952-3278

Levine, J.D. & Taiwo, Y.O. Hyperalgesic pain: a review. *Anesthesia Progress*, Vol.37, No.2-3, (March 1990), pp. (133-135), 0003-3006

Liu, X.H., Kirschenbaum, A., Lu, M., Yao, S., Dosoretz, A., Holland, J.F., & Levine, A.C. Prostaglandin E2 induces hypoxia-inducible factor-1alpha stabilization and nuclear localization in a human prostate cancer cell line. *Joournal of Biological Chemistry*, Vol.277, No.51, (December 2002), pp. (50081-50086), 0021-9258

Lousse, J.C., Defrere, S., Colette, S., Van Langendonckt, A., & Donnez, J. Expression of eicosanoid biosynthetic and catabolic enzymes in peritoneal endometriosis. *Human Reproduction*, Vol.25, No.3, (March 2010), pp. (734-741), 0268-1161

Lumsden, M.A., Kelly, R.W., & Baird, D.T. Primary dysmenorrhoea: the importance of both prostaglandins E2 and F2 alpha. *British Journal of Obstetrics and Gynaecology*, Vol.90, No.12, (December 1983), pp. (1135-1140), 0306-5456

Lynch, P.M., Ayers, G.D., Hawk, E., Richmond, E., Eagle, C., Woloj, M., Church, J., Hasson, H., Patterson, S., Half, E., & Burke, C.A. The safety and efficacy of celecoxib in children with familial adenomatous polyposis. *American Journal of Gastroenterology*, Vol.105, No.6, (June 2010), pp. (1437-1443), 0002-9270

Machado, D.E., Berardo, P.T., Landgraf, R.G., Fernandes, P.D., Palmero, C., Alves, L.M., Abrao, M.S., & Nasciutti, L.E. A selective cyclooxygenase-2 inhibitor suppresses the growth of endometriosis with an antiangiogenic effect in a rat model. *Fertility and Sterility*, Vol.93, No.8, (May 2010), pp. (2674-2679), 0015-0282

Mahnke, J.L., Dawood, M.Y., & Huang, J.C. Vascular endothelial growth factor and interleukin-6 in peritoneal fluid of women with endometriosis. *Fertility and Sterility*, Vol.73, No.1, (January 2000), pp. (166-170), 0015-0282

Matsuzaki, S., Canis, M., Pouly, J.L., Wattiez, A., Okamura, K., & Mage, G. Cyclooxygenase-2 expression in deep endometriosis and matched eutopic endometrium. *Fertility and Sterility*, Vol.82, No.5, (November 2004), pp. (1309-1315), 0015-0282

Maybin, J.A., Critchley, H.O., & Jabbour, H.N. Inflammatory pathways in endometrial disorders. *Molecular and Cellular Endocrinology*, Vol.335, No.1, (March 2011), pp. (42-51), 0303-7207

Meresman, G.F., Bilotas, M., Abello, V., Buquet, R., Tesone, M., & Sueldo, C. Effects of aromatase inhibitors on proliferation and apoptosis in eutopic endometrial cell cultures from patients with endometriosis. *Fertility and Sterility*, Vol.84, No.2, (August 2005), pp. (459-463), 0015-0282

Meuleman, C., Tomassetti, C., D'Hoore, A., Van Cleynenbreugel, B., Penninckx, F., Vergote, I., & D'Hooghe, T. Surgical treatment of deeply infiltrating endometriosis with colorectal involvement. *Human Reproduction Update*, Vol.17, No.3, (May 2011), pp. (311-326), 1355-4786

Mustafa, A. & Kruger, W.D. Suppression of tumor formation by a cyclooxygenase-2 inhibitor and a peroxisome proliferator-activated receptor gamma agonist in an in vivo mouse model of spontaneous breast cancer. *Clinical Cancer Research*, Vol.14, No.15, (August 2008), pp. (4935-4942), 1078-0432

Narumiya, S., Sugimoto, Y., & Ushikubi, F. Prostanoid receptors: structures, properties, and functions. *Physiological Reviews*, Vol.79, No.4, (October 1999), pp. (1193-1226), 0031-9333

Nasir, L. & Bope, E.T. Management of pelvic pain from dysmenorrhea or endometriosis. *Journal of the American Board of Family Practice*, Vol.17 Suppl (November 2004), pp. (S43-S47), 0893-8652

Noble, L.S., Simpson, E.R., Johns, A., & Bulun, S.E. Aromatase expression in endometriosis. *Journal of Clinical Endocrinology and Metabolism*, Vol.81, No.1, (January 1996), pp. (174-179), 0021-972X

Noble, L.S., Takayama, K., Zeitoun, K.M., Putman, J.M., Johns, D.A., Hinshelwood, M.M., Agarwal, V.R., Zhao, Y., Carr, B.R., & Bulun, S.E. Prostaglandin E2 stimulates aromatase expression in endometriosis-derived stromal cells. *Journal of Clinical Endocrinology and Metabolism*, Vol.82, No.2, (February 1997), pp. (600-606), 0021-972X

Nosjean, O. & Boutin, J.A. Natural ligands of PPARgamma: are prostaglandin J(2) derivatives really playing the part? *Cellular Signaling*, Vol.14, No.7, (July 2002), pp. (573-583), 0898-6568

Olivares, C., Bilotas, M., Buquet, R., Borghi, M., Sueldo, C., Tesone, M., & Meresman, G. Effects of a selective cyclooxygenase-2 inhibitor on endometrial epithelial cells from patients with endometriosis. *Human Reproduction*, Vol.23, No.12 (December 2008), pp. (2701-2708), 0268-1161

Olivares, C., Ricci, A., Bilotas, M., Baranao, R.I., & Meresman, G. The inhibitory effect of celecoxib and rosiglitazone on experimental endometriosis. *Fertility and Sterility*, Vol.96, No.2, (August 2011), pp. (428-433), 0015-0282

Ota, H., Igarashi, S., Sasaki, M., & Tanaka, T. Distribution of cyclooxygenase-2 in eutopic and ectopic endometrium in endometriosis and adenomyosis. *Human Reproduction*, Vol.16, No.3, (March 2001), pp. (561-566), 0268-1161

Pakrasi, P.L. & Jain, A.K. Cyclooxygenase-2 derived PGE2 and PGI2 play an important role via EP2 and PPARdelta receptors in early steps of oil induced decidualization in mice. *Placenta*, Vol.29, No.6, (June 2008), pp. (523-530), 0143-4004

Raiter-Tenenbaum, A., Baranao, R.I., Etchepareborda, J.J., Meresman, G.F., & Rumi, L.S. Functional and phenotypic alterations in peritoneal macrophages from patients with early and advanced endometriosis. *Archives of Gynecology and Obstetrics*, Vol.261, No.3, (1998), pp. (147-157), 0932-0067

Reese, J., Zhao, X., Ma, W.G., Brown, N., Maziasz, T.J., & Dey, S.K. Comparative analysis of pharmacologic and/or genetic disruption of cyclooxygenase-1 and cyclooxygenase-2 function in female reproduction in mice. *Endocrinology*, Vol.142, No.7, (July 2001), pp. (3198-3206), 0013-7227

Sales, K.J., Katz, A.A., Howard, B., Soeters, R.P., Millar, R.P., & Jabbour, H.N. Cyclooxygenase-1 is up-regulated in cervical carcinomas: autocrine/paracrine regulation of cyclooxygenase-2, prostaglandin e receptors, and angiogenic factors by cyclooxygenase-1. *Cancer Research*, Vol.62, No.2, (January 2002), pp. (424-432), 0008-5472

Scher, J.U. & Pillinger, M.H. The anti-inflammatory effects of prostaglandins. *Journal of Investigative Medicine*, Vol.57, No.6, (August 2009), pp. (703-708), 1081-5589

Smith, O.P., Jabbour, H.N., & Critchley, H.O. Cyclooxygenase enzyme expression and E series prostaglandin receptor signalling are enhanced in heavy menstruation. *Human Reproduction*, Vol.22, No.5, (May 2007), pp. (1450-1456), 0268-1161

Sookvanichsilp, N. & Pulbutr, P. Anti-implantation effects of indomethacin and celecoxib in rats. *Contraception*, Vol.65, No.5, (May 2002), pp. (373-378), 0010-7824

Sugimoto, Y., Segi, E., Tsuboi, K., Ichikawa, A., & Narumiya, S. Female reproduction in mice lacking the prostaglandin F receptor. Roles of prostaglandin and oxytocin receptors in parturition. *Advances in Experimental Medicine and Biology*, Vol.449 (1998), pp. (317-321), 0065-2598

Sun, H.S., Hsiao, K.Y., Hsu, C.C., Wu, M.H., & Tsai, S.J. Transactivation of steroidogenic acute regulatory protein in human endometriotic stromalcells is mediated by the prostaglandin EP2 receptor. *Endocrinology*, Vol.144, No.9, (September 2003), pp. (3934-3942), 0013-7227

Sun, W.H., Chen, G.S., Ou, X.L., Yang, Y., Luo, C., Zhang, Y., Shao, Y., Xu, H.C., Xiao, B., Xue, Y.P., Zhou, S.M., Zhao, Q.S., & Ding, G.X. Inhibition of COX-2 and activation of peroxisome proliferator-activated receptor gamma synergistically inhibits proliferation and induces apoptosis of human pancreatic carcinoma cells. *Cancer Letters*, Vol.275, No.2, (March 2009), pp. (247-255), 0304-3835

Tamura, K., Sakurai, T., & Kogo, H. Relationship between prostaglandin E2 and vascular endothelial growth factor (VEGF) in angiogenesis in human vascular endothelial cells. *Vascular Pharmacology*, Vol.44, No.6, (June 2006), pp. (411-416), 1537-1891

Tamura, M., Deb, S., Sebastian, S., Okamura, K., & Bulun, S.E. Estrogen up-regulates cyclooxygenase-2 via estrogen receptor in human uterine microvascular endothelial cells. *Fertility and Sterility*, Vol.81, No.5, (May 2004), pp. (1351-1356), 0015-0282

Tamura, M., Sebastian, S., Yang, S., Gurates, B., Fang, Z., & Bulun, S.E. Interleukin-1beta elevates cyclooxygenase-2 protein level and enzyme activity via increasing its mRNA stability in human endometrial stromal cells: an effect mediated by extracellularly regulated kinases 1 and 2. *Journal of Clinical Endocrinology and Metabolism*, Vol.87, No.7, (July 2002), pp. (3263-3273), 0021-972X

Tietjen, G.E., Conway, A., Utley, C., Gunning, W.T., & Herial, N.A. Migraine is associated with menorrhagia and endometriosis. *Headache*, Vol.46, No.3, (March 2006), pp. (422-428), 0017-8748

Tranguch, S., Daikoku, T., Guo, Y., Wang, H., & Dey, S.K. Molecular complexity in establishing uterine receptivity and implantation. *Cellular and Molecular Life Sciences*, Vol.62, No.17, (September 2005), pp. (1964-1973), 1420-682X

Trukhacheva, E., Lin, Z., Reierstad, S., Cheng, Y.H., Milad, M., & Bulun, S.E. Estrogen receptor (ER) beta regulates ERalpha expression in stromal cells derived from ovarian endometriosis. *Journal of Clinical Endocrinology and Metabolism*, Vol.94, No.2, (February 2009), pp. (615-622), 0021-972X

Tsai, S.J., Wu, M.H., Lin, C.C., Sun, H.S., & Chen, H.M. Regulation of steroidogenic acute regulatory protein expression and progesterone production in endometriotic stromal cells. *Journal of Clinical Endocrinology and Metabolism*, Vol.86, No.12, (December 2001), pp. (5765-5773), 0021-972X

Ushikubi, F., Sugimoto, Y., Ichikawa, A., & Narumiya, S. Roles of prostanoids revealed from studies using mice lacking specific prostanoid receptors. *Japanese Journal of Pharmacology*, Vol.83, No.4, (August 2000), pp. (279-285), 0021-5198

Venturini, P.L., Fasce, V., Gorlero, F., & Ginocchio, G. Chronic pelvic pain: oral contraceptives and non-steroidal anti-inflammatory compounds. *Cephalalgia*, Vol.17 Suppl 20 (December 1997), pp. (29-31), 0333-1024

Vercellini, P., Crosignani, P., Somigliana, E., Vigano, P., Frattaruolo, M.P., & Fedele, L. 'Waiting for Godot': a commonsense approach to the medical treatment of endometriosis. *Human Reproduction*, Vol.26, No.1, (January 2011), pp. (3-13), 0268-1161

Vinatier, D., Dufour, P., & Oosterlynck, D. Immunological aspects of endometriosis. *Human Reproduction Update*, Vol.2, No.5, (September 1996), pp. (371-384), 1355-4786

Wadman, M. The pain game. *Nature*, Vol.448, No.7152, (July 2007), pp. (400-401), 0028-0836

Wienecke, T., Olesen, J., Oturai, P.S., & Ashina, M. Prostaglandin E2(PGE2) induces headache in healthy subjects. *Cephalalgia*, Vol.29, No.5, (May 2009), pp. (509-519), 0333-1024

Wing, L.Y., Chuang, P.C., Wu, M.H., Chen, H.M., & Tsai, S.J. Expression and mitogenic effect of fibroblast growth factor-9 in human endometriotic implant is regulated by aberrant production of estrogen. *Journal of Clinical Endocrinology and Metabolism*, Vol.88, No.11, (November 2003), pp. (5547-5554), 0021-972X

Wu, M.H., Lu, C.W., Chuang, P.C., & Tsai, S.J. Prostaglandin E2: the master of endometriosis? *Experimental Biology and Medicine*, Vol.235, No.6, (June 2010), pp. (668-677), 1535-3702

Wu, M.H., Shoji, Y., Chuang, P.C., & Tsai, S.J. Endometriosis: disease pathophysiology and the role of prostaglandins. *Expert Reviews in Molecular Medicine*, Vol.9, No.2, (January 2007), pp. (1-20), 1462-3994

Wu, M.H., Shoji, Y., Wu, M.C., Chuang, P.C., Lin, C.C., Huang, M.F., & Tsai, S.J. Suppression of matrix metalloproteinase-9 by prostaglandin E(2) in peritoneal macrophage is associated with severity of endometriosis. *American Journal of Pathology*, Vol.167, No.4, (October 2005a), pp. (1061-1069), 0002-9440

Wu, M.H., Sun, H.S., Lin, C.C., Hsiao, K.Y., Chuang, P.C., Pan, H.A., & Tsai, S.J. Distinct mechanisms regulate cyclooxygenase-1 and -2 in peritoneal macrophages of women with and without endometriosis. *Molecular Human Reproduction*, Vol.8, No.12, (December 2002), pp. (1103-1110), 1360-9947

Wu, M.H., Wang, C.A., Lin, C.C., Chen, L.C., Chang, W.C., & Tsai, S.J. Distinct regulation of cyclooxygenase-2 by interleukin-1beta in normal and endometriotic stromal cells. *Journal of Clinical Endocrinology and Metabolism*, Vol.90, No.1, (January 2005b), pp. (286-295), 0021-972X

8

Genetic Polymorphisms and Molecular Pathogenesis of Endometriosis

Vijayalakshmi Kodati and Q. Hasan
Vasavi Medical & Research Centre,
India

1. Introduction

Endometriosis occupies a unique position in medicine. The natural history of the disease is uncertain, its precise etiology is unknown, the clinical presentation is inconsistent, diagnosis is difficult and can be confirmed only by invasive procedures, and the treatment is poorly standardized.

It is one of the commonest benign gynaecological conditions affecting 15 - 25% of women in the reproductive age group. Yet, it displays features similar to malignancy, ranging from neo-vascularisation to local invasion and aggressive spread to distant organs (metastasis).

The most widely accepted theory to explain endometriosis is that viable endometrial cells reach the peritoneal cavity through retrograde menstruation along the fallopian tubes. Some of the cells then adhere to the peritoneal surface and proliferate in response to the ovarian hormones. However, it is well established that menstrual debris is present in the peritoneal cavity of 90% of menstruating women, suggesting that endometrial cells from only 'some women' are capable of establishing ectopic endometrial implants. Why does this happen in only 'some (10-15%) women'? There are several possible explanations for disease susceptibility, including differences in genetic predisposition (Bischoff FZ et al, 2000), increased exposure to menstrual debris, abnormal eutopic endometrium, altered peritoneal environment, reduced immune-surveillance (Sinaii N et al, 2002), and increased angiogenic capacity (Absenger Y et al, 2004).

Endometriosis, the name by itself implies an endometrial pathology but this concept has long been disputed by Thomas and Prentice in 1992. The acceptance of an endometrial origin poses the question of whether endometrium that is able to proliferate and implant at ectopic sites is in some way abnormal. The commonest site for endometriosis is the pelvis. Endometrium reaches the pelvis most commonly by retrograde menstruation which is now accepted to be an almost ubiquitous event. Endometriosis is more common in women whose normal menstrual egress is occluded by genital tract anomalies, women with an early menarche, short menstrual cycles and prolonged menses. All these factors suggest that peritoneal soiling is important but if retrograde menstruation is ubiquitous then why do not all women have endometriosis? The truth is that the presence of ectopic endometrium within the peritoneal cavity is probably universal but the association of ectopic endometrium with either symptoms or anatomic distortion is not. It is these latter two groups of women that present with pathological endometriosis as the presence of ectopic endometrium alone is not pathological; this can clearly be seen in the case of infertility associated with minimal and mild endometriosis.

The endometrium shed at menstruation contains numerous cytokines and angiogenenic growth factors. These factors undoubtedly could promote proliferation of and angiogenesis around ectopic endometrial implants, allowing survival of the shed endometrium at ectopic sites. If they are of importance in the pathogenesis of endometriosis then it would be expected that differences would exist between those women with and those without endometriosis. However, no qualitative differences exist between either eutopic and ectopic endometrium nor between endometrium from women with and those without endometriosis. This observation is true for all growth factors and cytokines studied to date, and strongly suggests that endometriosis is not an endometrial disease.

If endometriosis is not primarily an endometrial disease, then it is uncertain what permits and facilitates the survival of endometrium at ectopic sites. It is becoming increasingly clear that the peritoneal fluid and its cellular constituents are important in the pathogenesis of endometriosis.

In many ways endometriosis can be considered to be a chronic inflammatory condition of the pelvis. The endometriotic implants have many different appearances but in early stages in particular, they are surrounded by new blood vessel formation which resembles an inflammatory response. The peritoneal fluid in endometriosis contains an increased size and number of macrophages that have an increased activation status. They secrete large number of cytokines and produce growth factors that support the establishment of the ectopic implants. Peritoneal macrophages are regulated by ovarian steroids and in their activated state produce increased levels of VEGF (vascular endothelial growth factor) that supports angiogenesis around the endometriotic implants. These macrophages are less susceptible to apoptosis which is the normal consequence of activation.

However, there is convincing evidence that the disease is inherited as a complex genetic trait (Kennedy S, 1997). Genetic factors accounted for 52% of the variation in liability to endometriosis in an Australian twin study (Treloar et al, 2000). The genetic relative - recurrence risk for sibs was estimated to be 2.34 in a cohort of Australian twins and their families. This risk indicates that polygenic and multifactorial etiology is far more likely to be the cause than Mendelian inheritance. Familial aggregation has been reported in humans and non-human primates (Kennedy S et al, 1995; Zondervan et al, 2004). A genome-wide Linkage study in 1,176 affected sister pair families identified a significant susceptibility locus for endometriosis on chromosome 10q26 (Treloar SA, Kennedy SH, et al, 2005).

Initially *cytogenetic studies* of chromosomal rearrangements in affected endometriotic tissue were conducted to uncover candidate chromosomal loci. Dangel et al, (1994), found no evidence of abnormalities in any of the 42 implants studied. However, with the application of chromosome-specific probes using multicolor fluoroscent in situ hybridization (FISH) technique, a significantly greater frequency of chromosome 17 aneuploidy in the endometriotic specimens was observed. It was proposed that acquired chromosome-specific alterations may be involved in endometriosis through a multistep pathway suggesting clonal expansion of chromosomally abnormal cells. Cytogenetic R-banding studies on human endometriosis-derived permanent cell line (FbEM-1) showed numerous chromosomal aberrations, including monosomy X, $4q^+$, $5q^+$, trisomy 7,8,10 and tetrasomy of chromosomes 17, 18, 19 and 20 (Bouquet DJ et al, 1997). A caveat for these studies is that cultured cell-lines may be unstable, which reflects growth of selectively advantaged cells and is no longer representative of the original tissue. Comparative genomic hybridization (CGH) has also been used which revealed overrepresentation of chromosomes 1, 2, 3, 5, 6p, 7, 16, 17q, 20, 21q, and 22q, whereas chromosomes 6q, 9, 11p, 12, 13q, 18 and X were underrepresented. Subsequent FISH analysis confirmed gain at 6p and 17q and loss of 1p, 22q, and chromosomeX (Gogusev J et al 2000).

Subsequent studies were conducted using the method of *quantitative genetic analysis.* To find the genes of endometriosis from nearly 30,000 total human genes, the technique of sibling-pair quantitative linkage analysis was used. Sibling-pair analysis obligatorily requires that informative DNA polymorphic markers exist every few centimorgans (10cM). The polymorphisms usually used are DNA variants, such as di-nucleotide, tri-nucleotide, or tetra-nucleotide repeats.

It has been argued that findings have been inconsistent because most studies have used inappropriate controls. However, confusion is also created by underpowered studies and/or studies investigating genes without sufficient evidence to support their biological plausibility. *Two examples are given here.*

First, significant association of GALT gene with endometriosis was reported with at least one allele with the N314D mutation, whereas *GALT* gene had been previously associated with Mullerian anomalies. The polymorphism causes reduced activity of the enzyme galactose-1-phosphate uridyl transferase, which is involved in galactose metabolism. Three subsequent studies involving more patients have failed to replicate the association (Stefansson H et al, 2001).

Second, genes that encode enzymes involved in detoxification, such as the glutathione S-transferase (GST) family, have been investigated based on the finding that the environmental pollutant 2,3,7,8-tetrachlorodibenzo-p-dioxin (dioxin) induces endometriosis in the rhesus monkey. Homozygotes for a null mutation in one of the GST family genes, *GSTM1,* were more common in endometriosis cases than in controls. Subsequently, studies in UK (Hadfield RM et al, 2001), Japanese (Morizane M et al, 2004), Chinese (Ding Y et al, 2004) and Indian (Babu KA et al, 2005) populations have failed to replicate the association. No association has been found for a mutation in a similar gene, *GSTT1.* Moreover, in a critical appraisal of all the human and nonhuman primate evidence implicating dioxin exposure as a risk factor for endometriosis, Guo SW (2004) concluded that there was insufficient evidence to support the theory, about 10 years after it was first proposed! It is possible, therefore, that research groups around the world have investigated genes involved in detoxification as functional candidates based on an entirely false premise.

Although endometriosis is a benign disorder, it has also been viewed as a neoplastic process. Evidence to support this hypothesis includes molecular similarities between endometriosis and cancer; and the increased susceptibility to develop ovarian clear-cell cancer and endometrioid cancer in the presence of endometriosis. Molecular genetic alterations in endometrioid cancers of the ovary were analyzed (Catasus L et al, 2004). Frequent alterations are seen in beta-catenin and PTEN genes, as well as MSI in low-stage ovarian carcinomas of endometrioid type. However, allelic loss studies do not provide evidence for the 'endometriosis as tumor' theory (Prowse AH et al, 2005). Ovarian endometriosis with cytological atypia has potential for malignant transformation. Endometriotic cysts seem to be monoclonal and demonstrate aggressive growth and localized invasion of the myometrium. Malignant transformation has been documented. The proposed pathway is through loss of chromosome material by causing allelic imbalance or loss of heterozygosity (LOH).Genomic instability in any form can transform a normal cell to an abnormal or malignant cell. DNA damage can cause genetic alterations and can manifest as gross DNA damage, chromosomal instability or by a more subtle genetic change like microsatellite instability.

DNA studies examining the role of LOH in endometriotic lesions have identified candidate suppressor gene loci, including 9q, 11q and 22q (Jiang X et al 1996). Alterations in chromosome arms 5q, 6q, 11q and 22q were observed in 25-30% of women with endometriosis and associated carcinoma of the ovary (Jiang X et al 1998).

Gene expression analysis by oligo-nucleotide micro-arrays indicated inflammatory immuno-reactions due to up-regulation of FCER1G and PGDS mast cell specific genes which play an important role in producing fibrosis and adhesions in endometriotic lesions (Konno R et al, 2003). Downregulated elements included the tumor suppressor Tp53, genes related to apoptosis, and the gene encoding OVGP1, a protein involved in maintenance of early pregnancy (Arimoto et al, 2003).

Eyster KM et al (2002) illustrated the use of cDNA micro-array technology by studying eutopic endometrium and endometriotic implants from three patients and reported eight genes that were over-expressed in endometriotic implants as compared to eutopic endometrium, that had roles in the cytoskeleton.

The revolutionary evolution of genetics and molecular technologies has given a new perspective to the understanding of the etiology of the perplexing disease of endometriosis. Meyer's (1919) hypothesis of coelomic metaplasia in the totipotential peritoneal cells subjected to repeated irritation by a variety of factors, as a cause of endometriosis, would explain those cases of endometriosis in primary amenorrhoea and in men on prolonged estrogen treatment. There are some unknown factors produced within the uterus which stimulate undifferentiated mesenchyme to undergo metaplastic transformation. These *unknown factors* that allow endometrial fragments to implant in the peritoneal cavity of some women and lymphatic spread to allow ectopic endometrium to develop at distant sites are presently being hypothesized to be due to genetic factors. It has been suggested that endometriosis has a genetic basis by Kennedy et al two decades back.

1.1 Definition of endometriosis

Endometriosis is defined as a disease characterized by the presence of functional endometrial cells, comprising of glands and stroma in ectopic sites outside the uterine cavity in addition to their normal presence in the innermost lining of the uterus. The ectopic endometrial tissue responds to hormones and drugs in a similar manner to eutopic endometrium.

Ectopic endometrium shares many morphological aspects with eutopic endometrium, but differs in its biological behaviour due to the fact that the cells are present in a different environment. Ectopic and eutopic endometrium are not synchronized in their histological changes; ectopic tissue implants present a maturation disorder with different degrees of maturation and organization in the same implant. Complete secretory modification is rarely found in endometriosis and this could be due to an impact on the production of progesterone dependent factors like prostaglandins.

2. Factors affecting endometriosis

There are numerous suggested etiological factors in the pathogenesis of endometriotic implants. However, only the genetic factors will be discussed here.

2.1 Genetic factors

Epidemiological data show a familial tendency of endometriosis. Patients with an affected first-degree relative have nearly a ten-fold increased risk of developing endometriosis. Concordance of twins has also been demonstrated (Bischoff FZ et al 2000). There is evidence in both, human and non-human primates that supports the theory of a genetic basis to endometriosis (Zondervan KT et al, 2001).

Attempts to explore the role of genetic and molecular factors in the etiology of endometriosis have begun in the last decade. Genetic studies also detected an association between endometriosis and polymorphic mutations of several genes, including the N-acetyltransferase 2 gene(NAT2), the glutathione S-transferase M gene (GSTM) and Estrogen Receptor alpha gene (ER-a).

2.1.1 DNA- polymorphism

Polymorphism literally means many forms and it is seen that on an average, every 1 in 500 base pairs of DNA varies between individuals. Variations in coding regions are rare because of the need to preserve function. Changes in non-coding regions of the genome are subject to very little selection pressure and generate allelic variations at a very high frequency. This variation can be an alteration in a single base, deletion or addition of bases and expansion or contraction of repeats.

DNA polymorphisms are the basis of all current *genetic markers*. A marker is any *polymorphic Mendelian* character that can be used to follow a chromosomal segment through a pedigree. Allelic human gene *expression variation* may be caused by changes in regulatory DNA, including sequences which regulate transcription and splicing. This type of sequence variation may often underlie the susceptibility to common diseases but quantitative methods to explore allelic variation in human gene expression have been developed only very recently (Yan H et al, 2002).

2.1.2 Single Nucleotide Polymorphism (SNP)

This involves a single nucleotide which is substituted by a different nucleotide. Typically, SNPs have only two alleles. Since coding DNA accounts for only about 1.5% of the human genome, most SNPs are found in the non-coding DNA, such as within introns and intergenic sequences.

3. Endometriosis and genetic polymorphism

A number of polymorphisms in candidate genes have been studied to identify the genes responsible for the etiology of endomeriosis. It was only since 2000, that reports were published establishing an association of genetic polymorphism with endometriosis.

Transforming growth factor beta (TGF-β) family members are multi-functional cytokines that play a key role in cellular growth, proliferation, and differentiation (Hsieh YY et al, 2005). It has been shown that an association of endometriosis with TGF-β 1-509 gene polymorphism exists. T homozygote and T allele for TGF-β1 are associated with higher susceptibility to endometriosis. Arg448Gly, a common polymorphism located within nuclear receptor interacting protein 1 (NRIP1) gene, is associated with endometriosis. NRIP1 gene variants, separately or in combinations, might act as predisposing factors for human endometriosis (CaballeroV, et al., 2005).

A significant linkage on chromosome 10q26 and another region of suggestive linkage on chromosome 20p13 as susceptibility loci, has been associated with endometriosis (Treloar SA et al, 2005).

It has been hypothesized that dysregulation of the normal apoptotic process takes place in the endometrium. One of the apoptotic pathways playing a crucial role in the programmed cell death within the endometrium is the Fas-FasL system. Three polymorphisms within FAS (-1377G>A and -670A>G) and FASL (-843C>T) genes, as susceptibility factors for endometriosis have been analysed. However, the differences in the distribution of the polymorphic variants were not statistically significant (Fernandez,R.M.et.al,2005). The angiotensin I-converting enzyme (ACE) A2350G and A-240T gene polymorphism has been suggested as markers of susceptibility in endometriosis as the genotypes and alleles are associated with higher susceptibility to endometriosis and might be associated with endometriosis development (HseihYY etal, 2005).

3.1 Environmental toxin genes

Endometriosis shows significantly elevated frequency in industrial areas and there is a possible genetic pre-disposition (Kennedy S et al. 2001). The glutathione-S-transferases (GSTs) constitute a family of xenobiotic-detoxifying phase-II enzymes catalyzing the conjugation of glutathione to a variety of electrophilic compounds including polycyclic aromatic hydrocarbons (PAH), which are widely present in the human environment and known to be carcinogenic.

Several GSTs are polymorphic and some allelic variants causing enzyme activity impairment are suspected to increase susceptibility to malignancies associated with environmental PAH, particularly colorectal cancer (Strange RC & Fryer AA, 1999). A very small portion of endometriosis develops into cancer later, but endometriosis itself is not a malignant disease. It has many characteristics similar to cancer, for example progressive growth, invasive growth, estrogen-dependent growth, recurrence and a tendency to metastasis (van Gorp T et al. 2004).

Environmental toxic compounds like *dioxin* may increase the risk of endometriosis. Previous association studies implicated GALT gene (a gene involved in galactose metabolism, located on chromosome 9), glutathione S transferases (GSTM 1), (GSTT1), cytochrome p 450 (CYP1A1) and N- acetyltransferase 2 (NAT2) genes, which encode for detoxification enzymes, as possible disease susceptibility genes (Zondervan KT et al, 2001; Hadfield RM et al, OXEGENE collaborative group, 2001; Deguchi M et al, 2005). The diversity of biological effects resulting from exposure to dioxin may reflect the ability of this environmental pollutant to alter gene expression by binding to the Aryl hydrocarbon receptor (AHR) gene and related genes (Watanabe T et al, 2001).

One of the genes previously implicated in endometriosis is CYP17; this encodes the enzyme P450c17alpha, which plays a vital role in steroid biosynthesis in the ovary. However, the CYP17 MspA1 polymorphism has not been associated with endometriosis in either the UK or the Japanese population(Asghar,T.et.al,2005).

A study of the association between endometriosis and polymorphisms in the N-acetyltransferase 1 (NAT1) and N-acetyltransferase 2 (NAT2) genes has previously demonstrated a positive association with NAT2 polymorphisms in a UK population. However, polymorphisms in NAT1 and NAT2 were not associated with an increased risk of endometriosis in the Japanese population (Deguchi M et al, 2005).A case control study suggested no association between endometriosis and NAT2 in South Indian-women(Arvind-Babu,K.et.al.2005).

Glutathione S-transferases (GSTs) are enzymes involved in the metabolism of many disease-causing carcinogens and mutagens that are present in human environments. An association between the incidence of endometriosis and the GST genotypes of patients has been suggested. The study inferred that GSTM1, GSTT1 and GSTP1 genetic polymorphisms are not associated with the development of endometriosis in Korean women (Hur.S.E.et.al, 2005).

3.2 Angiogenic genes

Vascular endothelial growth factor (VEGF), a major mediator of angiogenesis and vascular permeability, is known to play a key role in the pathophysiology of endometriosis.The single nucleotide polymorphisms, -460C>T and +405G>C, in the 5'-untranslated region of the VEGF gene were associated with lower promoter activity, which was significantly less common in women with endometriosis suggesting that the +405G allele may influence the likelihood of a woman developing the disease(Bhanoori M et al, 2005).

A relationship between the *alpha 2-Heremans Schmidt glycoprotein (AHSG)* gene polymorphism and endometriosis has been studied. Women not carrying the AHSG 2 allele were found to have twice the risk of endometriosis there by suggesting an association of endometriosis with the AHSG gene polymorphism in Korean women. (Kim JG et al, 2004).

3.3 Hormonal genes

3.3.1 Estrogen Receptor (ER) gene

The risk and severity of endometriosis has been associated with polymorphisms in genes coding for estradiol-synthesizing enzyme like the Ser312Gly polymorphism in 17-beta-hydroxysteroid dehydrogenase type 1 (HSD17B1). Evidence for association between the Ser312Gly polymorphism in HSD17B1 and endometriosis was found in a Japanese population. The A-allele of HSD17B1 appears to confer higher risk for endometriosis (Tsuchia M et al, 2005).

The *Alu*I polymorphism in the ERβ gene is associated with an increased risk of stage IV endometriosis in a Japanese population (Wang Z et al, 2004). The *Pvu*II polymorphism of the ERα gene is associated with the risk for endometriosis, adenomyosis and leiomyomata in Japanese women (Kitawaki J et al, 2001). The ERα dinucleotide repeat and cytochrome P450c17α gene polymorphisms are associated with susceptibility to endometriosis in Taiwanese women (Hsieh.Y Y et al, 2005).

3.3.2 Androgen Receptor (AR)

Androgen receptor gene is present in the endometrial tissue and the pelvic organs, which are the targets for endometriotic implants. The AR was detected in endometriosis, adenomyosis and endometrial carcinoma (Horie K et al 1992). Endometrial cysts are monoclonal in origin and are related to the reaction with AR. The endometrioma might be formed from an independent monoclonal ovarian endometrial cell after inactivation of AR allele in the X chromosome (Fujimoto J et al, 1999). The proliferation and differentiation of the endometrium are mediated mainly by the Estrogen and Progesterone receptors. However, Androgen receptor also plays a role in modulating the cyclic change of the endometrium.

Androgen Receptor (AR) gene trinucleotide polymorphism has been associated with endometriosis (Yao-Yuan-Hsieh et al, 2001). The AR gene has a polymorphic cytosine, adenine and guanine (CAG) microsatellite in exon 1 that codes for variable length glutamine repeats in the amino-terminal domain of the AR protein (Hsieh.Y Y et al, 2004). The 21-CAG repeats may be associated with some determinants for endometriosis formation as indicated in a study by Lattuada et al, (2004) in Italian women.

3.3.3 Progesterone Receptor (PR)

Estrogen and progesterone receptors are present in the ectopic endometrium but in lower concentrations than in eutopic endometrium. Cyclical variation in the receptor population has not been observed and also there seems to be a difference in the way that estrogen is handled by the endometrium at the two sites (Vierikko P et al, 1985).

The expression of the variants of the Progesterone Receptor (PR-A and PR-B) was shown to be aberrant in endometriotic tissues, which may indicate a role of the progesterone receptor in the pathogenesis of endometriosis (Nisolle M et al, 1994; Attia GR et al 2000).

The progesterone receptor gene is located in chromosome region 11q22-23.PROGINS polymorphism has been studied in association with breast cancer (Wang-Gohrke S et al, 2000) and ovarian cancer (Vigano P et al, 2006). The data indicate that a mutated progesterone receptor gene contributes to the development of disease in hormone-sensitive tissues

Progesterone Receptor (PR) gene PROGINS polymorphism has been shown to be associated with endometriosis in Caucasian women (Weiser F et al, 2002). The secretory phase of the menstrual cycle is controlled largely by progesterone, and this sex steroid hormone is absolutely required for normal implantation and pregnancy. PROGINS polymorphism of the progesterone receptor may be associated with an increased risk of endometriosis in Italian women (Lattuada et al, 2004).

4. Microsatellite Instability (MSI)

Microsatellites are short sequence elements that consist of mononucleotide to hexanucleotide motifs reiterated several times. This form of genomic instability is caused by defects in the DNA mismatch repair system. Genomic instability is an almost universal feature of cancer cells. Microsatellite instability is a DNA level instability seen in a number of tumors, including colon cancers. Instability is probably necessary to enable a cell to amass enough mutations and is not a chance feature, but is the result of selection. High frequency of MSI is defined as >29% of all markers and are defined as a class of MSI positive tumors (Strachanan & Read 2004).

4.1 Microsatellite (MS) markers

Genetic alterations in microsatellite marker sites among eight tumor suppressor genes in endometriosis were examined and reported that MSI is not ubiquitous in endometriosis and may be uncommon (Nakayama K et al, 2001). MSI assays reveal an allelic imbalance and loss of heterozygosity (LOH) on p16(Ink4), GALT, p53, APOA2 loci in endometriosis. The 9p21 locus may be a prognostic marker of the disease (Goumenou AG et al, 2001).

5. Gene expression

Gene expression profiles in endometriosis have been studied by two groups. In one study differentially expressed genes were investigated in epithelial and stromal cells from deep endometriosis and matched eutopic endometrium using cDNA microarrays and laser capture microdissection (Matsuzaki S et al, 2004) while Smith SK , (2003) undertook a genome-wide analysis of transcript abundance and changes in transcript level between normal endometrium in the proliferative and secretory phases of the menstrual cycle, between normal and ectopic endometrium of endometriosis and between normal and RU-486 exposed endometrium.

Gene expression profiling to identify genes involved in endometriosis has shown that Cyr61 gene, which codes for cystein-rich heparin-binding protein that promotes cell adhesion, migration and neo-vascularisation was deregulated (Absenger Y et al, 2004). Overexpression of p53 in atypical endometriosis and cancer associated with endometriosis has been reported (Sainz de la Cuesta R et al, 2004). Thymosin beta 4 (Tb4) gene expression, an actin sequestering protein, was up-regulated in uterine adenomyosis(endometriosis of myometrium) in mice (Kawahara R et al, 2003). Dysregulation of 14 genes was found to be overtly associated with endometriosis by Real- Time RT-PCR expression profiling of endometriosis (Wei Ping Hu et al, 2006).

6. Research by our group

The research work aimed to identify polymorphisms of candidate genes which increase susceptibility to endometriosis by genetic and molecular methods in 106 women who were confirmed with the diagnosis of endometriosis and with age matched 140 normal women as controls from South India. Progesterone and Androgen Hormone Receptor *gene polymorphisms;* genomic instability at ectopic and eutopic endometrial tissues resulting in *Micro Satellite Instability* (MSI); *gene expression* in ectopic endometrial tissue by Differential Display Reverse Transcriptase Polymerase Chain Reaction (DD-RT-PCR) to identify novel genes were studied. DNA was isolated from peripheral blood and from fresh tissue samples of both ectopic and eutopic endometrium. We subsequently assessed the polymorphisms of Estrogen Receptor, TNF-alpha and TLR 4 genes. The ongoing research work involves ICAM, IL-6, NOD-2, MMP-2,and MMP-9 genes polymorphism studies.

6.1 Microsatellite instability analysis by multiplex PCR

Allelic imbalance in selected loci was reported by microsatellite assays in endometriosis (Goumenou et al, 2001). Three different microsatellite markers were selected based on reports from previous studies (Luokola et al, 2001; Xing et al, 1999). These three microsatellite markers are as follows:

The mononucleotide adenine $(A)_n$ repeats-(BAT-RII) and dinucleotide $(CA)_n$ repeats-(D3S1313, D9S171).

Multiplex PCR was carried out using specific primers for the microsatellite markers selected. PCR was performed to amplify the three target sequences using specific primers. Multiplex PCR was performed on blood and tissue DNA from 12 cases and a matching number of controls. Thus 60 multiplex PCR reactions were set up using specific primers for each of the selected microsatellite markers.

6.1.1 Single strand conformation polymorphism (SSCP)

Each of the samples was analysed for all the three markers in the tissue using blood as control. MSI positivity was indicated by *mobility* difference between blood, ectopic and eutopic tissue; presence of additional band or absence of bands.

MSI is defined as a difference in length due to insertion or deletion of the amplified microsatellite markers between the normal and ectopic tissue of the same individual. MSI in the ectopic tissues is assessed by the detection of alleles of novel size that are not present in the normal tissues of the same individuals. All microsatellite markers showing instability were analyzed. Samples lacking MSI were defined as Microsatellite stable (MSS).

6.1.2 Differential display- reverse transcriptase-PCR (DD-RT-PCR)

RNA isolation and RT-PCR analysis: Biopsy material obtained from the ectopic and eutopic endometrial tissue at the time of surgery was collected in sterile normal saline and transported to the lab for storage at minus 70°C. mRNA was isolated using mRNA direct isolation kit (Qiagen, Oligotex direct mRNA micro kit, Catalogue No. 72012) according to the manufacturer's instructions. mRNA was converted to cDNA by Reverse Transcriptase (RT) step which was followed by 45 cycles of 3-stage PCR with a specific annealing temperature for each primer set. DD RT-PCR allows identification of differentially expressed genes in various cell types and under defined physiologic conditions. DD was performed by the modified method of Hasan et al (2000). PCR was performed using selected primers to study the differential expression of the selected genes in the ectopic and eutopic endometrial tissues.

cDNA DD PCR: 5 sets of random exonic primers were used. DD-PCR was repeated with a different set of seven primers, which were selected arbitrarily.

7. Results and statistical analysis

A non-parametric statistic is opted because (1) there is no *'a priori reason'* to assume a particular disease model and (2) the assignment of the status *'unaffected'* is problematic because a surgical procedure is required to exclude endometriosis.

Allele and genotype frequencies were compared in the patient and control groups. The odds ratio (OR) was used to measure the strength of the association between the frequencies of allele and genotype and endometriosis. The software MedCalc (version 7.4.3.0) was used for statistical analyses. All 'p' values two-tailed and 95% Confidence Intervals (CI) were calculated.

7.1 PROGINS analysis

* MW T1T1 T1T2

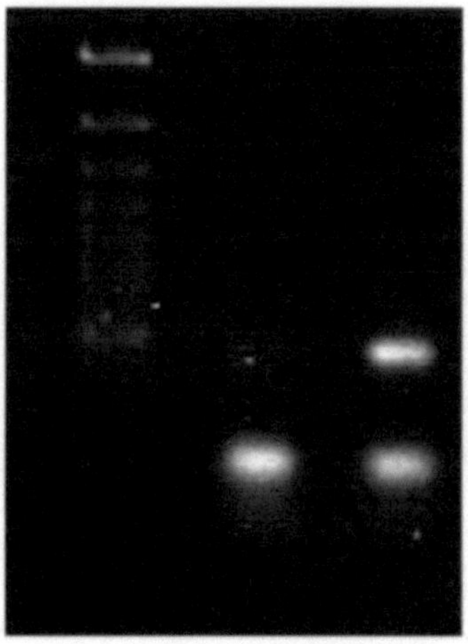

455 bp p

149 bp

*MW- Molecular Weight ladder

Fig. 1. Photograph of a 2% agarose gel stained with ethidium bromide to resolve the 306-base pair intron G insertion polymorphism of the progesterone receptor gene. The 149-base pair band represents the wild type allele (allele T1) and the 455-base pair band represents the mutant allele (allele T2). Lane 1 indicates the molecular weight markers; lanes 2 and 3 show the homozygous wild type T1T1 and the heterozygous T1T2 patterns. There is no homozygous mutant T2T2 pattern.

7.2 Androgen receptor analysis

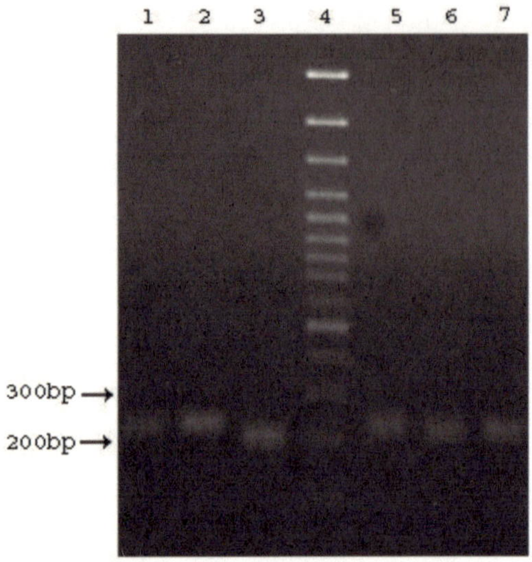

Fig. 2. Photograph of a 2% Agarose gel stained with ethidium bromide to resolve the trinucleotide CAG repeats in AR gene encompassing Exon 1.The bands appeared between 200bp - 300bp. The Lane 4 indicates the molecular weight marker.

The small repeat changes occurring between 200bp - 300bp and heterozygotic alleles could not be identified on agarose gels. Hence, analysis was done using 12% PAGE for further analysis.

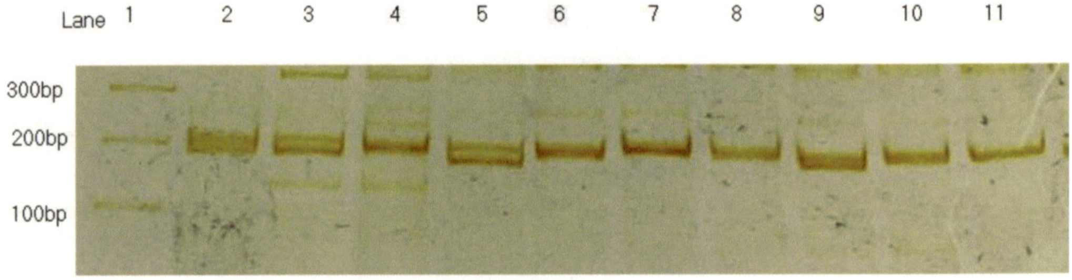

Fig. 3. Native PAGE showing heterozygous and homozygous alleles of AR gene: 200 samples processed with 12% polyacrylamide gel and silver staining showed band sizes ranging from 156 bp - 238 bp which fall within the CAG repeats range of 4-34.

7.3 MSI analysis

Multiplex PCR for 12 cases and 12 controls was carried out using blood as control. Each case had three sets of samples, viz. blood, eutopic tissue and ectopic tissue. Hence 36 multiplex PCR reactions were set up for cases. For the controls two sets of samples were set up, viz. blood and eutopic tissue. Hence 24 multiplex PCR reactions were set up for controls.

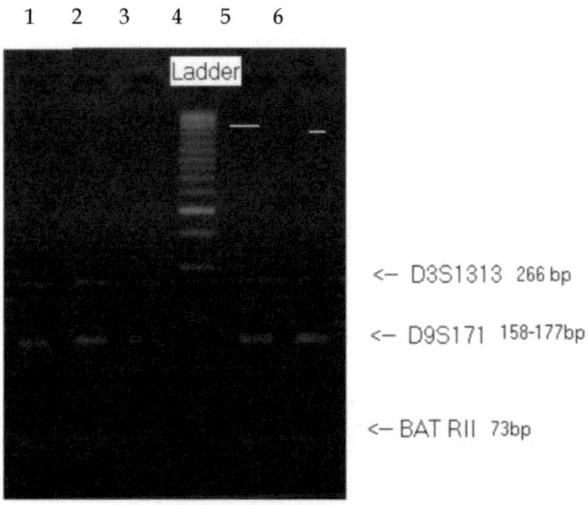

Fig. 4. 2% Agarose gel showing results of multiplex PCR both from endometriotic cases and controls with the specific MSI markers and their band sizes. Lanes 1,2,3 are of a case; Lane 4 is the DNA ladder; Lanes 5,6 are of a control

7.4 SSCP (Single Stranded Conformation Polymorphism) analysis

SSCP was carried out on 15% polyacrylamide gel to identify mobility shift, and/or additional bands at the three selected markers. SSCP PAGE gel showing mobility shift at BAT R II locus in ectopic tissue from a case of endometriosis. 2 cases of endometriosis showed mobility shift in the BAT R II locus associated with TGF beta R II receptor gene. One control showed additional band in D3 locus associated with FHIT gene.

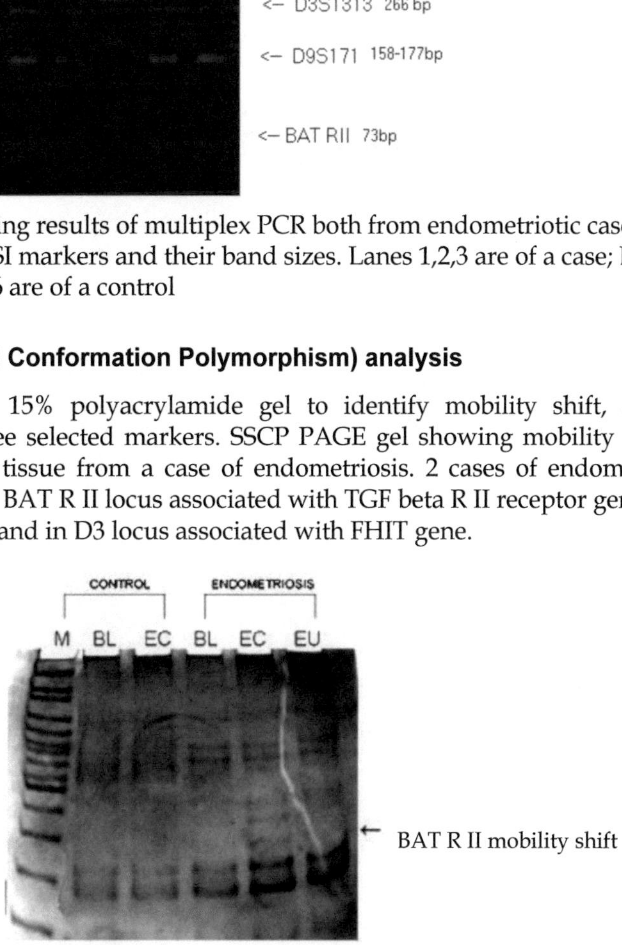

Fig. 5. Lane 1 is the DNA ladder; Lanes 2 and 3 are blood and eutopic tissue of control;

Lanes 4, 5 and 6 are blood, ectopic and eutopic tissue of a case ; Additional bands are seen in all the samples of the case but not in the control, whereas mobility shift of the band is seen in the ectopic tissue only and not in the eutopic tissue of the case.

7.5 DD – RT – PCR analysis

Differential display RTPCR helps in identifying novel genes which are expressed or suppressed in tissues with an altered pathophysiology compared to controls using two sets of five and seven arbitrary primers. A number of common bands were seen between eutopic and ectopic samples from the same patient. However, in three cases studied differential bands of 45bp in the first set, and 350bp region in the second set were observed in the ectopic tissue of patient suffering from severe endometriosis, stage IV. DD-RTPCR using first set of 5 primers. Fig. 6.

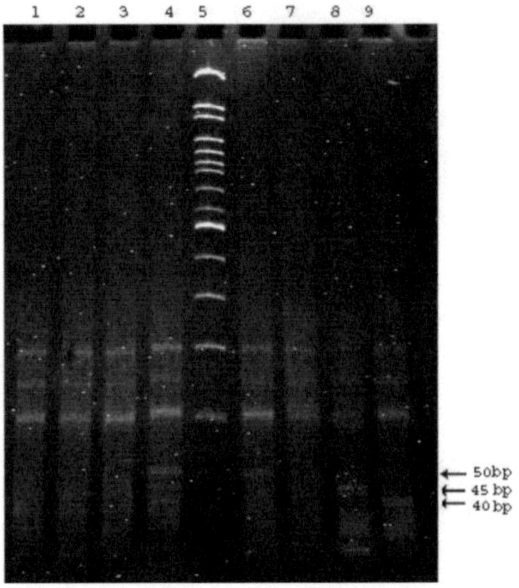

Fig. 6. DD-RT-PCR using second set of seven primers

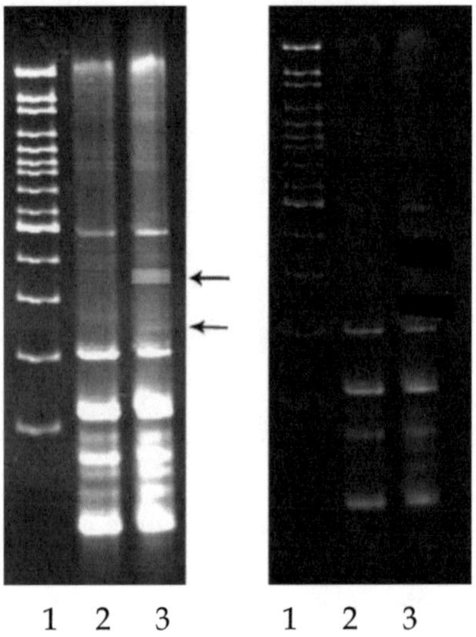

Upper arrow: differential band of 350 bp
Lower arrow: faint differential band of 250 bp

Fig. 7. Lane 1: 100 bp ladder; Lane 2: Eutopic tissue; Lane 3: Ectopic tissue.
Differentially expressed bands are seen in ectopic tissue in lane 3, as shown by the arrows (before eluting), and in lane 3 on the right side (after eluting).

The eluted bands were automatically sequenced using MWG-AG, BIOTECH, Bangalore. The sequences obtained are shown below.

Sequencing of differentially expressed bands:

I. 350bp band showing 60/65 gene sequence showing homology with Shigella species which included S. dysenteriae, S. boydii, S. sonnei.

II. 250 bp showing (a) 20/20 gene sequence showing homology with Hepatocellular carcinoma- associated antigen HCA557b, (b) 24/25 gene sequence showing homology with S. dysenteriae

8. Discussion

One hundred and six (106) cases of endometriosis, diagnosed at laparoscopy and/or laparotomy were staged according to the Revised American Fertility Society (rAFS) classification and were enrolled in the study. One hundred and forty (140) controls were also included in the study who comprised of women who either had no symptoms, or no endometriosis at the time of laparoscopy/laparotomy which was performed for other indications. Mild endometriosis (stages I & II) was diagnosed in 72% of cases and advanced endometriosis (stages III & IV) was diagnosed in 28% of cases in the cohort studied.

The aim of the present study was to identify individuals clinically suffering from endometriosis and establish genetic and molecular markers for understanding the cellular and molecular pathogenesis of this condition.

Few well-designed epidemiologic studies of risk factors for endometriosis exist. Eskanazi B et al, (1997) conducted a review of more than 100 published studies and found that only 6 (1 cohort and 5 case-control studies) included a surgically case confirmed group, provided clear criteria for control selection, and considered potential confounding factors in the analysis. Hence, the importance of the present study is that all the cases of endometriosis included were confirmed by laparoscopy/laparotomy and the controls were age matched women who were surgically proven to have no endometriosis or had no symptoms suspicious of endometriosis throughout their reproductive life.

Endometriosis plaques have been shown to have estrogen, progesterone and androgen receptors, and they grow in the presence of estrogen but atrophy when exposed to androgens. Since endometriosis is a hormone-sensitive disease, in the present study the role of hormonal genes polymorphism was analyzed in women with surgically confirmed diagnosis of endometriosis. This is the first Indian study to evaluate the hormonal genetic factors in the etiology of endometriosis.

The PROGINS polymorphism has been shown to be associated with endometriosis in Caucasian women (Weiser et al, 2002) including Italian women (Lattuada D et al, 2004). *Our study established 5% prevalence of PROGINS polymorphism in Indian population and showed no susceptibility to endometriosis.(Govindan et al 2006).* Estrogen receptor-α gene (T/C) Pvu II polymorphism in Endometriosis and Uterine Fibroids has been studued by our group. It was observed to be significantly associated with endometriosis in Asian Indian population. (Govindan et al. 2009)

The highly polymorphic trinucleotide repeat (CAG) in AR varies in length and methylation pattern which affects both AR expression and function.The AR gene CAG polymorphism has been associated with a number of benign and malignant conditions, eg. polycystic ovarian syndrome in women, and male infertility and prostate cancer in men. Its association with endometriosis in Italian women did not constitute an important factor of genetic predisposition (Lattuada D et al, 2004). The range of CAG repeats varies from 9-31 in Japanese population (Hsieh Y et al, 2001) and 14-32 in Italian population. However, there are no studies reported for the AR polymorphism in Indian women with endometriosis.

Our study proposes that the 19 CAG repeats may be associated with increased risk of endometriosis in our population. AR gene CAG repeat polymorphism may become a useful marker to predict the future development of endometriosis and to permit early therapeutic intervention in women at high risk of developing endometriosis (Shaik et al.2009)

Since endometriosis clinically mimics cancer with proliferation, angiogenesis and metastasis, three markers associated with carcinogenesis were selected for MSI analysis. TGF-beta II receptor gene is a putative tumor suppressor. It has been found that the TGFBRII gene was inactivated in a subset of colon cancer cell lines exhibiting MSI. Once generated, the proliferative advantage of cells with inactivated type II receptor would drive colon tumor progression **(Markowitz et al 1995)**. This pathway may also be operative in other human pathologies like endometriosis. Human FHIT (fragile histidine triad) protein is encoded by the FHIT putative tumor suppressor gene (Barnes et al 1996). Aberrant transcripts of the FHIT locus were found in approximately 50% of esophageal, stomach, and colon carcinomas (Ohta et al 1996). The results from several studies showed aberrant regulation of several cell cycle proteins, including CDKN (Kim et al 2005).

In endometriotic lesions the differentiation of glands and stroma is absent as the lining is attenuated, lost or replaced with granulation tissue and dense fibrous tissue. Hence it is difficult to get suitable ectopic endometrial tissue from cases for DNA isolation. Therefore MSI could be assessed in 12 cases only and tissue samples were obtained from 12 controls. Out of the 12 cases 2 (16.66%) showed microsatellite instability in the TGFbetaRII gene. *This is the first study reporting an association of TGF-beta receptor II gene with endometriosis in Indian women.* None of the samples studied showed any instability with regards to the other two markers. This suggests that D3S1313 and D9S171 may not be important markers for endometriosis.

In the present study mRNA was isolated from ectopic and eutopic tissues and DD-RT-PCR was carried out twice using 7 different sets of arbitrary primers. **Ectopic endometriotic tissue of one case showed unique band of 45bp after DD-RT-PCR using the first set, while a band in the region of 350bp was obtained using the second set of primers.** Both the 45bp and 350bp bands were cut out, eluted and automatically sequenced. The 45bp band gave multiple errors during sequencing, whereas the 350bp band could be sequenced successfully. Sequencing was carried out twice from the latter band. Both the sequences were analyzed using the BLAST search (National Centre for Biotechnology Information-NCBI; Google Search). It revealed a 60/65bp, 96% homology with Shigella dysenteriae, boydii and sonnei species. This sequence also matched a smaller 20/20bp stretch of 100% homology with human Hepatocellular carcinoma associated antigen (HCAA). Hence, a simple cost-effective technique like DD-RT-PCR has enabled the identification of novel gene sequences in ectopic tissue of endometriosis which was hither-to not associated with endometriosis.

A world-wide literature search through Medline, PubMed and Google, showed no reported work associating either the Shigella species nor the HCAA gene with endometriosis. These results open up new possibilities for the etiology of endometriosis.

The HCAA gene is a likely candidate for causing endometriosis, which needs to be further investigated.

Shigella are gram-negative, non-motile, aerobic and facultatively anaerobic bacilli from the family Enterobacteriaciae.1 *S. dysenteriae, flexneri, boydii,* and *sonnei* are highly infectious strains that can cause dysentery in humans with an ID**50** of only 100-200 bacteria. Bacterial diarrhoea in humans caused by Shigella species due to the shiga toxin is called shigellosis.

It causes inflammation in the small and large bowel, which may extend to the pelvic peritoneum. Although this organism has not been earlier associated with endometriosis, it can be hypothesized that a bacteria related to shigella which induces pelvic peritoneal inflammation, may be playing a role in the etiology of endometriosis. This may not be far-fetched after the Nobel Prize winning discovery of Warren and Marshall (Julie Parsonnet 2005), who found that inflammation caused by Helicobacter pylori is responsible for esophageal/gastric cancer (Forbes et al, 1994).

Studies on the pathogenesis of *Shigella* have revealed unique methods of mucosal invasion that result in the lesions seen with infection. Because most lesions are often centered on gut-associated lymphoid tissue (GALT) and spread outward, it is suspected that the bacteria make their initial entry into the body through the normally *phagocytic macrophage cells* overlying the lymphoid tissue (Salyers AA et al.1994) Additional studies have revealed that through a complex process involving multiple genes found on both a large plasmid and on the *Shigella* chromosome, attachment of the bacteria to mucosal epithelial cells stimulates a structural alteration of the normally nonphagocytic epithelial cell cytoskeleton and actin filaments to cause uptake of the organism in a manner similar to phagocytosis. Once within the intracellular vacuole of the invaded cell, a hemolysin produced by *Shigella* causes release of the organism into the cytoplasm. The *Shigella* then rapidly multiply and migrate along polymerized actin filaments to reach the plasma membrane so that adjacent cells can be invaded (Keusch GT et al, 1993). Early in the course of disease, low numbers of *Shigella* organisms can be found by electron microscopy within mucosal epithelial cell vacuoles. As the disease progresses, fibrinous exudate replaces the dead epithelial cells (Brady AG et al, 1998). Death of epithelial cells and sloughing of mucosa creates the ulceration, pseudomembrane formation, hemorrhage, and inflammatory response that typifies shigellosis.

An additional aspect of virulence involves the production of an exotoxin, shiga toxin, by *S. dysenteriae*. Shiga toxin also enhances the lipopolysaccharide-mediated release of cytokines, such as interleukin-1 and tumor necrosis factor-alpha (Kodati V et.al, 2009), which likely contributes to the vascular damage leading to renal failure seen in a complication of shigellosis, hemolytic uremic syndrome. Subsequent to the identification by sequencing of shigella bacterial association with peritoneal inflammation, a hypothesis was proposed by our group to explain the molecular pathogenesis of endometriosis.

9. Hypothesis

The identification of genetic sequences homologous to shigella bacteria (Kodati V et al, 2007) in the ectopic endometriotic tissue in this study unravels an understanding of the etio-pathogenesis of endometriosis, which has not yet been reported. An important element in the initiation of inflammatory responses is the activation of macrophages, resulting in the

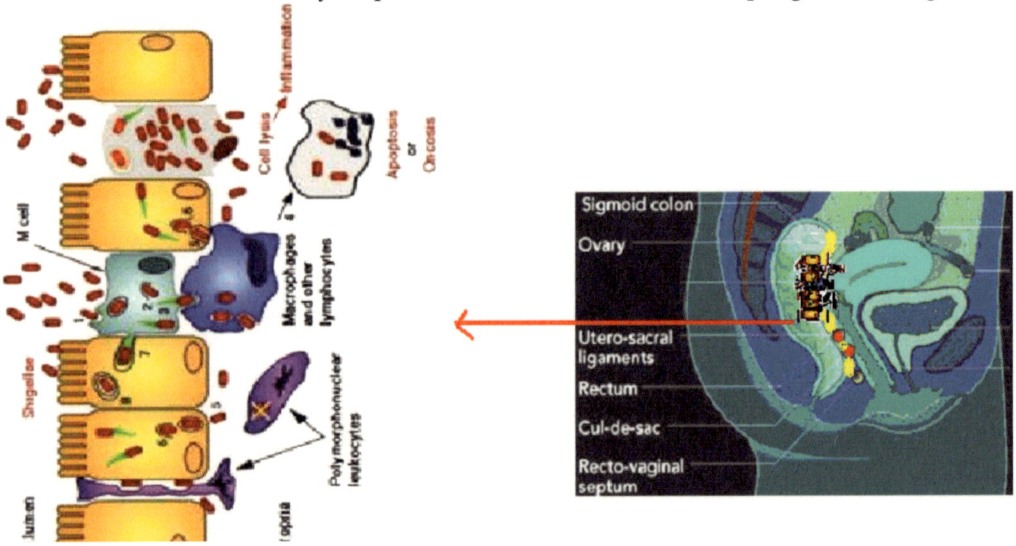

Fig. 8. Right side of the figure shows the saggittal section of the pelvis showing the route of shigella invasion from the colon to the Pouch of Douglas. Note the close proximity of the colon and Cul-de-sac/ posterior surface of uterus. Left side of the figure is the microscopic appearance of the mucous cells of the colon showing migration of the non-motile bacteria from cell to cell upto the lamina propria.

production of pro-inflammatory cytokines such as interleukins-12 (IL-12). Toll-Like Receptors (TLRs) which are expressed on macrophages, recognize microbial molecules and transmit signals that initiate transcription of cytokine genes. TLR4 recognizes the gram-negative bacterial product lipopolysaccharide (LPS). TLRs use several signaling pathways to initiate gene transcription. With the environmental toxins theory of endometriosis being now disproved, and with inconsistent results from genetic polymorphism studies amongst different ethnic groups, it could be postulated that the "infection theory" caused by Shigella or a similar bacteria may be the trigger that sets into action the immunological changes in the pelvic peritoneum resulting in the phenotype of endometriosis. While this can explain the pelvic and abdominal endometriosis, the occurrence of distant metastasis is yet unclear. Further work in this area should enhance the understanding of TLR signaling and the regulatory mechanisms controlling the inflammatory response by bacteria like shigella and their role in endometriosis.

9.1 Probable mechanism of Shigellosis to endometriosis

Commonly, shigella bacteria are known to invade the mucosa of the colon through the feco-oral route causing Shigellosis. The non-motile bacteria travel from cell to cell of the colonic epithelium through the cytoplasm by a unique mechanism called F-actin polymerization.

Thereby the bacteria reach the lamina propria of the colonic mucosa (Fig. 8). It is hypothesized that by the same mechanism the bacteria can enter the blood stream and/or travel across the colon wall to reach the outer peritoneal surface of the colon which is in close proximity to the posterior uterine surface, the site which incidentally happens to be the commonest site of early endometriosis (Cul-de-sac or Pouch of Douglas) as shown in Fig. 8. We propose that the peritoneal reaction to this bacterial invasion may be similar to any antigenic response by the host immune system resulting in the activation of macrophages and production of cytokines characteristic of acute inflammatory response. The endometrial cells that are shed during the retrograde menstruation into the cul-de-sac adhere to the inflamed peritoneal and ovarian surfaces and come under the influence of circulating ovarian hormones. The thus implanted endometrial cells in the peritoneum progress to endometriosis through angiogenesis. Our postulated bacterial hypothesis proposes that shigella or shigella-like organisms may be the trigger for the immunological changes in the pelvic peritoneum which initiate the etiopathogenesis of endometriosis. The inflammatory hypothesis is further reinforced by our subsequent research on TNF-alpha -C850T polymorphism, which showed significant association with endometriosis. (Lakshmi KV et al 2009) The bacterial hypothesis is supported by our recent research work on TLR-4 (A896G) polymorphism. Toll- Like Receptor 4 is specific for recognition of the molecular pattern of gram-negative bacteria. TLR-4 is present on the surface of endometrial cells. TLR-4 A896G is a functional polymorphism resulting in hypo-responsiveness of the receptor, causing peritoneal inflammation in the female pelvis. The molecular micro-environment of the cul-de-sac becomes favourable for initiation of endometriosis.(Latha M et al 2011)

10. Conclusion

Endometriosis remains a difficult clinical problem today and warrants more extensive research to understand the disease pathology. The future is to confirm early diagnosis by non-invasive test using a panel of potential genetic and molecular bio- markers. A long term goal is to be able to identify genetic determinants that contribute to the expression of the different phenotypes seen in endometriosis.

11. References

Absenger. Y, Hess-Stumpp. H, Kreft. B, Kratzschmar. J, Haendler. B, Schutze. N, Regidor. PA, & Winterhager E. (2004). Cyr61, a deregulated gene in endometriosis. *Mol Hum Reprod,* 10 (6): 399-407.

Alluri. RV, Mohan. V, Komandur. S, et al., (2005). MTHFR C677T gene mutation a risk factor for arterial stroke: A hospital based study. *Eur J Neurology,* 12(1): 40-4

Arimoto.T, Katagiri.T, Oda.K, et al., (2003). Genome-wide cDNA microarray analysis of gene-expression profiles involved in ovarian endometriosis. *Int. J. Oncol,* 22:551–60.

Asghar.T, Yoshida.S, Nakago. S, et al., (2005). Lack of association between endometriosis and the CYP17 MspA1 polymorphism in UK and Japanese populations. *Gynecol Endocrinol,* Feb;20(2):59-63.

Attia GR, Zeitoun K, Edwards D, et al.,(2000). Progesterone receptor Isoform A but not B is expressed in endometriosis. *J Clin. Endocrinol. Metab,* 85:2897-902.

Babu KA, Reddy NG, Deendayal M, et al., (2005). GSTM1, GSTT1 and CYP1A1 detoxification gene polymorphisms and their relationship with advanced stages of endometriosis in South Indian women. *Pharmacogenet genomics*, 15(3):167-72.

Barnes LD, Garrison PN, Siprashvili Z, et al., (1996). *Biochemistry*., 10;35(36):11529-35

Bhanoori M, Babu K, Reddy NG, et al.,(2005).The vascular endothelial growth factor (VEGF) +405G>C 5'-untranslated region polymorphism and increased risk of endometriosis in South Indian women: a case control study. *Hum Reprod*. Jul;20(7):1844-9.

Bischoff FZ & Simpson JL. (2000). Heritability and molecular genetic studies of endometriosis. *Hum Reprod Update*, 6: 37-44. .

Bouquet DJ, Validire P, Canis M, et al., (1997). Human endometriosis-derived permanent cell- line (FbEM-1): establishment and characterization. *Hum Reprod Update*, 3: 117-23

Brady AG & Morton DG. (1998). Digestive system: small and large intestine in non-human primates. *Biomedical Research Diseases*. 392-393.

Caballero V, Ruiz R, Sainz JA, et al., (2005). Preliminary molecular genetic analysis of the Receptor Interacting Protein 140 (RIP140) in women affected by endometriosis. *J Exp Clin Assist Reprod*, Aug. 30, 2(1): 11.

Catasus L, Bussaglia E, Rodrguez I, et al., (2004). Molecular genetic alterations in endometrioid carcinomas of the ovary: similar frequency of beta-catenin abnormalities but lower rate of microsatellite instability and PTEN alterations than in uterine endometrioid carcinomas. *Hum Pathol*, 35(11): 1360-8.

Cramer DW, Wilson E, Stillman RJ, et al., (1986). The relation of endometriosis to menstrual characteristics, smoking and exercise. *JAMA*, 25: 1904-9.

Dangel A, Medchill MT, Davis G, Meloni AM, & Sandberg AA. (1994). Cytogenetic studies in endometriosis tissue. *Cancer Genet Cytogenet*, 78: 172-4.

Deguchi M, Yoshida S, Kennedy S, et al., (2005). Lack of association between endometriosis and N-acetyl transferase 1 (NAT1) and 2 (NAT2) polymorphisms in a Japanese population: J Soc Gynecol Investig, Apr,12(3):208-13.

Ding Y, Chen ZF, Lin RY, et al., (2004). Relationship between endometriosis and glutathione S-transferase M1, T1 genes of the Uygurs and Hans in Xinjiang. *Zhonghua Fu Chan Ke Za Zhi*, 39(2):101-4.

Eskanazi B & Warner ML. (1997). Epidemiology of endometriosis. *Obstet Gynecol Clin North Am*, 24: 235-58.

Eyster KM, Boles AM, Brannian JD & Hansen KA. (2002). DNA microarray analysis of gene expression markers of endometriosis. *Fertil Steril*, 77:38-42.

Fernandez RM, Noval JA, Garcia-Lozano JC, et al., (2005). Polymorphisms in the promoter regions of FAS and FASL genes as candidate genetic factors conferring susceptibility to endometriosis. *Int J Mol Med*, May;15(5):865- 9.

Forbes GM, Glaser M, Cullen D, Warren JR, Marshall BJ, et al.,(1994). Seven year follow-up of duodenal ulcer treated with H. Pylori eradication therapy. *Lancet*, 343(8892) : 258-260.

Fujimoto J, Hirose R , Sakaguchi H & Tamaya T. (1999). Expression of oestrogen receptor-α and -β in ovarian endometriomata. *Mol. Hum. Reprod*. 5 (8): 742-747.

Gogusev J, Bouquet dJ, Telvi L, et al., (2000). Genetic abnormalities detected by comparative genomic hybridization in a human endometriosis derived cell line. *Mol Hum Reprod,* 6: 821-7.

Guo SW. (2004). The link between exposure to dioxin and endometriosis: a critical reappraisal of primate data. *Gynecol Obstet Invest.* 57:157-73.

Goumenou AG, Arvanitis DA, Matalliotakis IM, et al.,(2001). Microsatellite DNA assays reveal an allelic imbalance in p16(Ink4), GALT, p53, and APOA2 loci in patients with endomtriosis. *Fertil. Steril,* 75(1): 160-5.

Govindan S, Ahmad SN, Vedicherla B, Kodati V, et al., (2006). Association of progesterone receptor gene polymorphism (PROGINS) with endometriosis, uterine fibroids and breast cancer. *Cancer Biomarkers,* 22, 1-6

Govindan. S, Ahmad SN, Vedicharla B, Kodati V, et al., (2009). Estrogen receptor-α gene (T/C) Pvu II polymorphism in Endometriosis and Uterine Fibroids. *Disease Markers,* 26: 1-6

Hadfield RM, Manek S, Weeks DE, Mardon HJ, Barlow DH, Kennedy SH, OXEGENE Collaborative Group. (2001). Linkage and association studies of the relationship between endometriosis and genes encoding the detoxification enzymes GSTM1, GSTT1 and CPY1A1. *Mol Hum Reprod,* 7(11):1073-8.

Hasan, Q, Swee T. Tan, Jason Gush, et al., (2000). Steroid Therapy of a Proliferating Hemangioma: Histochemical and Molecular Changes . *Pediatrics,* 105:1,117 -120.

Horie K, Takakura K, Imai K, Liao S, Mori T. (1992). Immunohistochemical localization of androgen receptor in the human endometrium, decidua, placenta and pathological conditions of the endometrium. *Hum Reprod,* 7: 1461-1466.

Hsieh YY, Chang C, Tsai F, Lin C, Yeh L & Peng C.(2004). Androgen Receptor Trinucleotide Polymorphism in Leiomyoma. *Journal of Assisted Reproduction and Genetics* , 21, Number 12, 453-457

Hsieh YY, Chang CC, Tsai FJ, et al. (2005). Angiotensin I converting enzyme ACE 2350*G and ACE-240*T-related genotypes and alleles are associated with higher susceptibility to endometriosis. *Mol Hum Reprod,* Jan;11(1):11-4.

Hsieh. Y Y, Chang C , Tsai F , Lin C & Tsai C. (2005). Estrogen receptor α dinucleotide repeat and cytochrome P450c17α gene polymorphisms are associated with susceptibility to endometriosis . *Fertil Steril,* 83, 3 : 567-572

Hsieh YY, Chang CC, Tsai FJ, et al. (2005). Polymorphism for transforming growth factor beta 1-509 (TGF-B1-509): association with endometriosis: *Biochem Genet,* 43 (5-6): 203-10.1 Hu W, Tay S & Zhao Y.(2006). Endometriosis-Specific Genes Identified by Real-Time Reverse Transcription-Polymerase Chain Reaction Expression Profiling of Endometriosis *Versus* Autologous Uterine Endometrium . *The Journal of Clinical Endocrinology & Metabolism* 91 , 1, 228-238

Hur SE, Lee JY, Moon HS, Chung HW. (2005). Polymorphisms of the genes encoding the GSTM1, GSTT1 and GSTP1 in Korean women: no association with endometriosis. *Mol Hum Reprod,* 11(1):15-9.

Jiang X, Morland SJ, Hitchcock A, et al. , (1998). Allelotyping of Endometriosis with Adjacent Ovarian Carcinoma Reveals Evidence of a Common Lineage , *Cancer research, 1998; 58;* 1707

Kawahara R, Matsuda M & Mori T. (2003). Increase in the number of integrinβ1-immunoreactive monocyte-lineage cells in experimentally-induced adenomyosis in mice . *Life Sciences,* 73, 7, 907-916

Kennedy SH.(1997). Is there a genetic basis to endometriosis? *Semin. Reprod. Endocrinol,* 15, 309-317.

Kennedy S. (1999). The genetics of endometriosis: *Eur J Obstet Gynecol.Reprod Biol,* 82, 129–133

Kennedy S, Bennett S & Weeks D E. (2001). Affected sib-pair analysis in endometriosis. *Hum. Reprod. Update* 7 (4): 411-418.

Kennedy, S. and Moore, J. (2003) Chronic pelvic pain. In: Waller, D. and McPherson, A. (Eds.) *Women's Health.* 5th edn. Oxford: Oxford University Press. 399-420.

Kennedy, S., Bergqvist, A., Chapron, C. et al. (2005) ESHRE guideline for the diagnosis and treatment of endometriosis. *Human Reproduction,* 20(10), 2698-2704

Keusch GT & Thea DM. (1993). Invasive and tissue damaging enteric bacterial pathogens: bloody diarrhea and dysentery. *Mechanisms of Microbial Disease.* 2nd ed. 267-272.

Kim JG, Kim H, Ku SY, et.al., (2004). Association between human alpha 2-Heremans Schmidt glycoprotein (AHSG) polymorphism and endometriosis in Korean women. *Fertil Steril,* 82(6):1,497-500.

Kim YT & Zhao M. (2005). Aberrant cell cycle regulation in cervical carcinoma. *Yonsei Med J,*31; 46(5): 597-613.

Kitawaki J , Obayashi H, Ishihara H, et al., (2001). Oestrogen receptor-alpha gene polymorphism is associated with endometriosis, adenomyosis and leiomyomata. *Hum. Reprod.* 16 (1): 51-55.

Kodati V, Govindan S, Movva S, Ponnala S and Hasan Q. (2007). Role of Shigella infection in endometriosis: A novel hypothesis. *Medical Hypotheses, 6-12*

Kodati V, P Shetty, K Vottam, S Govindan, S N Ahmad and Q Hasan. (2009). Tumor necrosis factor alpha -C850T polymorphism is significantly associated with endometriosis in Asian Indian women. *Fertil Steril, 2009; 2 april*

Lattuada D, Vigano P, Somigliana E, et al., (2004). Analysis of the codon 72 polymorphism of the TP53 gene in patients with endometriosis: *Mol Hum Reprod,* 10(9):651-4.

Lattuada D, Vigano P, Somigliani E, Odirizzi MP, Vignali M, Di Blasio AM. (2004). Androgen receptor gene cytosine, adenine, and guanine trinucleotide repeats in patients with endometriosis. *J Soc Gynecol Investig,* 11(4):237-40.

Lattuada D, Somigliani E, Vigano P, et al., (2004). Genetics of endometriosis: a role for the progesterone receptor gene polymorphism PROGINS? *Clinical Endocrinology,* 61(2):190-4.

Luokola A, Eklin K, Laiho P et al.(2001). Microsatellite marker analysis in screening for hereditary non-polyposis colorectal cancer (HNPCC). *Cancer Res.* 61: 4545-4549.

Madhavi L, Vaidya S, Movva S, Kodati VL et al. (2011). Molecular pathogenesis of endometriosis; Toll-Like Receptor - 4 A896G (D299G) polymorphism: A novel explanation. *Genetic Testing & Molecular Biomarkers* 15 (3):181-184

Markowitz S, Wang J, Myeroff L, et al., (1995). Inactivation of the type II TGF-beta receptor in colon cancer cells with microsatellite instability. *Science;* 268(5215):1336-8.

Matsuzaki S., Canis M, Vaurs-Barrière C , et al., (2004). DNA microarray analysis of gene expression profiles in deep endometriosis using laser capture microdissection. *Mol. Hum. Reprod.* 10 (10): 719-728.

Meyer, R. (1919) Ueber den stand der Frage der Adenomyositis und Adenomyome in algemeinen und insbesondere iiber Adenomyositis serosoepithelialis und Adenomyometritis sarcomatosa. *Zentralbl. Gyndkol,* 43, 745-750.

Meyer, R. (1923) Zur Frage der Urnieren-genese von Adenomyomen. *Zentral Bl. Gyndkol,* 15, 577-587.

Morizane M, Yoshida S, Nakago S, et al., (2004). No association of endometriosis with glutathione S-transferase M1 and T1 null mutations in a Japanese population. *J Soc Gynecol Investig,* 11(2):118-21.

Nakayama K, Toki T, Nikaido T, Zhai YL, Konishi I. (2001). Genetic alterations in microsatellite marker sites among tumor suppressor genes in endometriosis. *Gynecol. Obstet. Invest,* 51(4): 240-2.

Parsonnet J. (2005). Clinician-Discoverers — Marshall, Warren, and *H. pylori. N Engl J Med,* 353:2421-2423

Prowse AH, Fakis G, Manek S, et al. (2005). Allelic loss studies do not provide evidence for the "endometriosis as tumor" theory. *Fertil Steril,* 83 Suppl 1: 1134-43.

Rowe SM, Coughlan SJ, McKenna NJ, et al. (1995). Ovarian carcinoma-associated Taq1 restriction fragment length polymorphism in Intron G of the progesterone receptor gene is due to an Alu sequence insertion. *Cancer Res,* 55: 2743-5.

Roy-Engel A M,. Carroll M L, Vogel E,. et al., (2001). Alu Insertion Polymorphisms for the Study of Human Genomic Diversity. *Genetics,* 159, 279-290

Sáinz de la Cuesta R, , Izquierdo M, Cañamero M, Granizo J & Manzarbeitia F. (2004). Increased prevalence of p53 overexpression from typical endometriosis to atypical endometriosis and ovarian cancer associated with endometriosis . *Eur J Obstet & Gynecol & Reprod Biol,* 113, 1, 15, 87-93

Salyers AA & Whitt DD. (1994). Dysentery caused by Shigella species. Bacterial Pathogenesis: A Molecular Approach. *ASM Press, Washington, D.C;* Chapter. 43. 14: 169-181.

Shaik N A, Govindan S, Kodati V, Rao K P and Hasan Q. (2009). Polymorphic (CAG)n repeats in the androgen receptor gene: a risk marker for endometriosis and uterine leiomyomas. *Hematol Oncol Stem Cel Ther, 2(1): 289-293*

Sinaii N, Cleary SD, Ballweg ML, et al., (2002). High rates of autoimmune and endocrine disorders, fibromyalgia chronic fatigue syndrome and atopic diseases and among women with endometriosis: a survey analysis. *Hum Reprod,* 17: 2715-24.

Smith SK. et al. (2003). Determination of the transcript profile of human endometrium. *Mol Hum Reprod,* 9,19–33

Stefansson H, Einarsdottit A, Geirsson RT ,et al. ,(2001). Endometriosis is not associated with or linked to the GALT gene. Fertil Steril, 76 (5): 1019-22.

Strachan T & Read AP. (2004). Text book of *Human Molecular Genetics,* 3rd edition, Published by Garland Science ISBN-0-8153-4184-9, NY-USA.

Strange RC & Fryer AA. (1999). The glutathione S-transferases: influence of polymorphism on cancersusceptibility. *IARC Sci Publ,* (148):231-49.

Thomas EJ & Prentice A. (1992). The etiology and pathogenesis of endometriosis. *Reproductive Medicine review.;* 1: 21-36.

Treloar SA, Bahlo M, Ewen K, et al., (2000). Suggestive linkage for endometriosis found in genome-wide scan. *Am. J. Hum. Genet,* 67 (4S): 1764 (Abstr.)

Treloar SA, Wicks J, Nyholt DR, et al., (2005). Genomewide linkage study in 1,176 affected sister pair families identifies a significant susceptibility locus for endometriosis on chromosome 10q26. *Am J Hum Genet,* 77(3):365-76.

Tsuchiya M, Nakao H, Katoh T, et al., (2005). Association between endometriosis and genetic polymorphisms of the estradiol-synthesizing enzyme genes HSD17B1 and CYP19: *Hum Reprod,* 20(4):974-8.

Van Gorp T, Amant F , Neven P, Vergote I & Moerman P. (2004). Endometriosis and the development of malignant tumours of the pelvis. A review of literature. *Best Practice & Research Clinical Obstetrics & Gynaecology,* 18, 2, 349-371

Vierikko P, Kauppila A, Ronnemberg L & Vihko R. (1985). Steroidal regulation of endometrial tissue: lack of induction of 17β hydroxyl-steroid dehydrogenase activity by progesterone, medroxy progesterone acetate or danazol. *Fertil Steril,* 43: 218-26

Viganó P, Somigliana E, Chiodo I, Abbiati A, et al. (2006). Molecular mechanisms and biological plausibility underlying the malignant transformation of endometriosis: a critical analysis. *Hum. Reprod. Update,* 12 (1): 77-89.

Wang-Gohrke S, Chang-Claude J, Becher H, et al., (2000). Progesterone receptor gene polymorphism is associated with decreased risk for breast cancer by age 50. *Cancer Res,* 60 : 2348-50.

Wang Z , Yoshida S , Negoro K , et al., (2004). Polymorphisms in the estrogen receptor β gene but not estrogen receptor α gene affect the risk of developing endometriosis in a Japanese population. *Fertil Steril,* 81, 6, 1650-1656

Watanabe T, Imoto I, Kosugi, Y. et al., (2001). Human arylhydrocarbon receptor repressor gene (AHRR): genomic structure and analysis of polymorphism in endometriosis. *Journal of Human Genetics,* 46, 6, 342-346

Wieser F, Schneeberger C, Tong D, et al., (2002). PROGINS receptor gene polymorphism is associated with endometriosis. *Fertil Steril.* 77(2):309-12.

Jiang,X. Hitchcock,A. Bryan EJ, et al., (1996). Microsatellite Analysis of Endometriosis Reveals Loss of Heterozygosity at Candidate Ovarian Tumor Suppressor Gene Loci. *Cancer Res, 56;* 3534

Yan H, Yuan W,. Velculescu V E, Vogelstein B & . Kinzler K W,* (2002). Allelic Variation in Human Gene Expression. *Science,* 16,: 297, 5584, p. 1143

Zondervan, K T; Cardon, L R; Kennedy, S H. (2001). The genetic basis of endometriosis. *Current Opinion in Obstetrics & Gynecology,* 13 : 3, 309-314

Zondervan KT, Weeks DE, Colman R. (2004). Familial aggregation of endometriosis in a large pedigree of rhesus macaques. *Hum. Reprod,* 19: 448-55.

9

Progesterone Resistance and Targeting the Progesterone Receptors: A Therapeutic Approach to Endometriosis

Nick Pullen
Pfizer Global Research & Development, UK

1. Introduction

Endometriosis is characterised by the benign growth of endometrial glands and stroma on the surface of peritoneal tissues and other organs. It is generally regarded as an aberrant estrogen-dependent growth condition, which presents with symptoms of chronic pelvic pain, bleeding and infertility. Steroidal progestogens are already widely used in the treatment of the condition, dienogest (Visanne) the most recent of which has gained EU approval for clinical use (McCormack, 2010). Progestogens appear to work by both directly inhibiting the functional effects of estrogen on endometrial cell proliferation, and also suppressing ovarian function, to induce anovulatory amenorrhoea. The efficacy of this class of agents in patients with endometriosis, however, is relatively modest and the tolerability (breakthrough bleeding and bloating) as well as concerns on the long term safety (risk of breast cancer and thromboembolism, effect on bone mineral density) has also limited their broader utility. Progesterone receptor antagonists (PRAs) have emerged in recent years as an alternative approach to treating the disease. This class of agents has contrasting effects on reproductive function compared with progestogens. This review will focus on what we know about the PRA mechanism of action from pre-clinical in vitro and in vivo evidence and how clinical data have shaped confidence in this class of agents as a new approach to treating endometriosis symptoms and disease progression[1].

2. Progesterone receptor structure & function

The steroid hormone, progesterone, is a key modulator of normal reproductive function, including ovulation, uterine and mammary gland development and the neurobehavioral expression associated with sexual responsiveness (Clarke & Sutherland, 1990; Lydon et al., 1995). Progesterone is absolutely essential for the maintenance of pregnancy, maintaining uterine quiescence by suppressing expression of genes that mediate increased myometrial

---

[1] Zhu Y, Bond J & Thomas P (2003) Identification, classification, and partial characterization of genes in humans and other vertebrates homologous to a fish membrane progestin receptor. *Proc. Natl Acad. Sci.* USA 100(5):2237-2242.

contractility, such as the oxytocin receptor. The physiological effects of progesterone (P_4) are principally mediated by interaction with two specific intracellular receptors termed PR-A and PR-B. PR-A and PR-B are members of the nuclear receptor superfamily of transcription factors (Mangelsdorf et al., 1995; McKenna et al., 2009; O'Malley & Conneely, 1992; Tsai & O'Malley, 1994). Nuclear hormone receptors regulate gene transcription by discriminative binding to specific DNA sequences, so-called progesterone response elements (PREs) Specific interactions with co-activator and/or co-repressor proteins, induced by ligand binding, trigger interactions with the RNA polymerase complex (McKenna & O'Malley, 2001). PR-A and PR-B are expressed from a single gene as a result of transcription from two alternative promoters and translation initiation at two alternative initiation codons (Kraus et al., 1993). The human PR-A and PR-B are identical except for an additional N-terminal 164 amino acid sequence present in PR-B. Both isoforms have two activation function domains, AF-1 proximal to the DNA-binding domain, and a ligand-dependent AF-2 domain in the C terminus (Tetel et al., 1999). By virtue of the longer N-terminus, PR-B also has a unique AF-3 domain that may contribute to its differential trans-activation properties compared with PR-A (Tung et al., 2006).

Ligand binding (progesterone as well as other synthetic PR ligands such as progestogens (e.g. dienogest, tanaproget, medroxyprogesterone acetate), the progesterone receptor antagonists (PRAs, such as RU-486) and modulators (e.g. J-867)) triggers a conformational change that causes the dissociation of bound heat shock proteins, receptor phosphorylation, receptor dimerisation, nuclear translocation and DNA binding. Binding occurs at specific PRE sequences in promoters of progesterone response genes, and alters transcriptional activity, negatively or positively, depending on PRE sequence, the conformation of the ligand-bound complex and cell-specific context. In the presence of steroidal PRAs, such as RU-486, the complex becomes transcriptionally inactive due to recruitment of co-repressors such as NCoR1 (Wagner et al., 1998), whereas selective PR modulators, such as J-867, elicit a mixed agonist/antagonist response (Elger et al., 2000; Madauss et al., 2007).

Studies in mice with selective ablation of PR isoforms have revealed that PR-A is necessary for ovulation and modulates the anti-proliferative effects of progesterone in the uterus. In contrast PR-B knockout mice are fertile and sustain a normal pregnancy, but PR-B appears to be required for normal mammary gland development and function (Mulac-Jericevic & Conneely, 2005). In an attempt to understand the function of PR-B in the endometrium, one group has used PRAs and siRNA to knockdown gene expression in an immortalised human endometrial stromal cell line (Wu & Guo, 2006; Wu et al., 2008). Ablation of PR-B promoted cellular proliferation, by approximately 20% compared with control, supporting the notion that PR-B acts as a break on progesterone function. It is noteworthy that breast and endometrial malignancy is often accompanied by disruption of PR-A and PR-B expression or altered functional PR responses (Arnett-Mansfield et al., 2004; De Vivo et al., 2002; Kobayashi et al., 2010; McGowan et al., 2004), an observation which has triggered interest in the potential utility of PRAs for oncology (Fuhrmann et al., 2000; Poole et al., 2006; Tieszen et al., 2011; Wiehle et al., 2011). Recent evidence has also confirmed the existence of a functional third isoform, PR-C which lacks AF-2 and AF-3 domains and appears to act as a sink for progesterone and have a function in regulating the onset of parturition (Condon et al., 2006).

Beyond the genomic function of progesterone mediated by PR-A and PR-B, progesterone also appears to elicit non-genomic activity. Neurosteroidal function of progesterone and progesterone metabolites, such as allopregnelone (3α-hydroxy-5α-pregnan-20-one), augment GABAergic channel burst durations by increasing the opening frequency through positive allosteric modulation in the hypothalamus (Henderson, 2007). In the female rat, direct administration of allopregnelone in specific regions in the hypothalamus rapidly facilitates lordosis, suggesting a direct non-genomic effect on reproductive function. Outside of the predicted protection from catamenial exacerbation of epileptic seizures and premenstrual dysphoric disorder by neurosteroids (Biagini et al., 2010), the non-genomic effects of progesterone in reproductive function in the female human have been less well characterised. Several other reported progesterone receptors (mPR, PGRMC1 and CatSper, for instance) have also been touted to contribute to the non-genomic effects of progesterone (Dressing et al., 2011; Gellersen et al., 2009; Lishko et al., 2011; Zhu et al., 2003). Based on expression data and some functional characterisation both mPR and PGRMC1 may have a role in reproductive function and are speculated to regulate implantation and myometrial contractility. Whilst there are no evidence reported suggesting a contributing role for mPR or PGRMC1 in endometriosis, this is not the case for PR.

3. Evidence of progesterone resistance in women with endometriosis

The uterus is composed of heterogeneous cell types which undergo synchronous waves of proliferation and differentiation in response to cyclical changes in estrogen (E_2) and progesterone levels. The spatiotemporal expression of PRs in epithelial, stromal and myometrial cellular compartments are under the control of estrogen, the primary endometrial mitogen. Progesterone appears to exert proliferative function or induce differentiation depending on the cell type; on epithelia, progesterone, acting via stromal PRs, inhibits estrogen-driven cell proliferation and on stroma progesterone appears to orchestrate a more complex pattern of proliferation and differentiation.

While the actions of progesterone are critical to the establishment and maintenance of pregnancy, approximately one third of women with endometriosis also present with infertility. For some women, the loss of tubal patency, the modification of the pelvis and the inflammation associated with condition appear to be causally related to the presentation of infertility. However, the characterization of the eutopic endometrium from women with endometriosis has also revealed many defects, including altered patterns of angiogenesis, dyssynchrony with the window of implantation as well as ultra structural abnormalities which may contribute to the infertility. Supporting this, isolated endometrial stromal fibroblasts from women with endometriosis do not appear to undergo a normal decidualisation response (Aghajanova et al., 2010), suggesting an impairment of the progesterone-mediated differentiation programme. Specific alterations in the expression molecular markers of endometrial receptivity have also been widely documented, especially the integrin $\alpha_v\beta_3$, certain steroid hormone receptors and HOXA10 gene expression, the latter of which has been identified from a genome wide association study of moderate to severe endometriosis as a potential candidate disease locus with proximity to the 7p15.2 SNP association (Painter et al., 2011).

Early studies also pointed to alteration in the normal pathways of estrogen metabolism in ectopic endometrial tissue; specifically expression of 17βHSD-2, the enzyme responsible for the conversion of estradiol to estrone appears to be reduced compared with the eutopic compartment (Bulun et al., 2010; Zeitoun et al., 1998). As 17βHSD-2 is a progesterone response gene, one group has published evidence to suggest that this may be due to apparent reduction in PR levels and especially in PR-B in ectopic tissue (Attia et al., 2000; Wu et al., 2006). However, this signpost to progesterone resistance has had relatively little formal observational replication; indeed others have not been able to find evidence of alteration in the PR-A/PR-B ratio (Bergqvist & Ferno, 1993; Igarashi et al., 2005). Furthermore, decrease in PR-A mRNA and an increase in the PR-B to PR-A ratio and total PR protein levels have been detected in eutopic samples obtained from a murine endometriosis model (Lee et al., 2009). PR expression has also been found to be similarly unaltered in the eutopic endometrium of baboons with experimentally induced endometriosis compared with baseline (Fazleabas et al., 2003).

Microarray studies performed on isolated cells, eutopic/ectopic tissue biopsies and cells excised by laser capture microdissection from patients have been revealed several pathways of altered gene expression. For instance Kao et al (2002; 2003) collected biopsies from eutopic endometrium from normal women and women with endometriosis at days 8-10 after the mid-cycle LH surge and performed a microarray analysis to identify differentially expressed genes. Whilst a formal analysis of progesterone-response genes, whose expression was either elevated or suppressed in diseased versus normal tissue, was not undertaken, the expression of several progesterone response genes, including Dickkopf-1 and glycodelin, was suppressed in diseased tissues samples. The suppression of the Dickkopf-1 response has been supported by more recent studies of progesterone response in isolated human endometrial stromal fibroblasts from normal women and women with endometriosis (Aghajanova et al., 2011). In studies comparing ectopic and eutopic gene expression obtained from women with endometriosis one of the key observational fingerprints was an impairment in the normal progesterone response, especially the expression of PR, IHH, FOXO1A and Cyp26A1 amongst others (Burney et al., 2007). Relatively few genes have been qualified as progesterone responsive by testing with a PRA and this has limited larger data assignments in published microarray data. Even when microarray analysis was performed on RNA extracted from human endometrial explants cultured in the presence of E_2/P_4 and treated with RU-486, only a small population of gene expression were differentially regulated (Catalano et al., 2003). Of these, JAK1 and JNK1 appeared to be down regulated in the presence of RU-486. These observations are intriguing as JNK activity is unregulated in women with endometriosis (Uz et al., 2011) and in a *Scid* mouse experimental model of endometriosis, JNK inhibitor treatment reduces disease burden (Altan et al., 2008).

Taken together, while the data support the notion that there is an abnormal progesterone response in eutopic and ectopic endometrial compartments in women with endometriosis, it is not clear whether this is a direct effect, causally associated with infertility, or could be used for diagnostic purposes. One of the key gaps is that many of these genes have not been formally tested to be directly PR mediated, and therefore lack the qualification of alteration.

Another, somewhat controversial, observation linked with the molecular basis of progesterone resistance has been revealed from studying functional polymorphisms in the promotor region of PR. A putative functional polymorphism in the PR promoter (+331C/T; rs10895068), creates an additional TATA box that provides a unique transcriptional start site and favours increased production of PR-B relative to PR-A (De Vivo et al., 2002). Berchuck et al. (2004) first suggested a reduced risk of endometriosis associated with the T allele of the +331 variant and because of increased production of PR-B, this variant was suggested to reduce the risk of endometriosis. However the original findings suggesting that PR-B is not expressed in ectopic lesions have not had broad replication and Treloar et al. (2005) found no association with endometriosis and this variant either in a large study which included more than 900 families. Another putative functional variant in the *PGR* gene is termed the PROGINS allele. Cells prepared from the eutopic endometria of women carrying the PROGINS allele appear to respond with greater proliferative capacity to estradiol and progesterone, supporting the contention that the PROGINS polymorphism enhances the endometriosis phenotype (D'Amora et al., 2009). However while several studies have suggested that the variant increases susceptibility to endometriosis (De Carvalho et al., 2007; Lattuada et al., 2004; Wieser et al., 2002), others have not found an association (Govindan et al., 2007; Treloar et al., 2005; van Kaam et al., 2007). Therefore taken together, there is only modest supporting evidence of altered progesterone receptor expression, and progesterone resistance in contributing to endometriosis susceptibility and disease symptoms. Notwithstanding this, the current clinical utility of progesterone receptor agonists and anticipated benefit of PRAs, outweighs the confidence in PR as a therapeutic target attained from a molecular understanding of the protein and condition.

4. Discovery of small molecule modulators of PR function

The identification of drug-like, potent and selective PR antagonists has been challenging. As well as being highly lipophilic, the ligand binding sites between homologous NHRs are highly conserved and PR has the highest sequence homology with GR, AR, MR and ER (Figure 1). Early classes of anti-progestagens were poorly selective, yet some, such as gestrinone, still found clinical utility in the treatment of endometriosis (Cornillie et al., 1986; Coutinho, 1982). Furthermore, the ligand binding domains of PR-A and PR-B are identical and yet several in vitro and in vivo lines of evidence suggest that the effects of progesterone on transcriptional activation and repression by PR-A and PR-B are different (Conneely et al., 2001; Tung et al., 2006). To date, however, there are no agonist or antagonist agents that have been characterised with selectivity for PR-A over PR-B or vice versa.

The development of selective and safe steroidal PRAs has been challenging, both due to reported hepatoxicity as well as potential dose-limiting anti-glucocorticoid effects, due to lack of selectivity (Robertson et al., 1999). More recently, an additional concern has emerged following histological evaluations of subjects dosed for more than 3 months on steroidal PRAs. The endometrium of these individuals undergoes a characteristic cystic histological change which may be difficult to distinguish from endometrial hyperplasia without specialist evaluation (Ioffe et al., 2009; Mutter et al., 2008; Williams et al., 2007).

Mifepristone/RU-486, the founding member of the steroidal class of PRAs, was originally produced by Roussel-Uclaf and licensed for use for medical abortion and as an emergency contraceptive. The in vivo pharmacokinetic/pharmacodynamic profile of RU-486 is challenging to model as RU-486 generates a large number of pharmacologically active metabolites (Heikinheimo et al., 1987). Since its identification, >100 related analogues, principally by modifying the C-11 and/or C-17 positions of the steroid ring, have been synthesized and have shown all degrees of anti-progestagenic activity. The pharmacological profile of these examples range from pure antagonists, such as RU-486 to those with mixed antagonist/agonist activity, such as J-867 (Table 1).

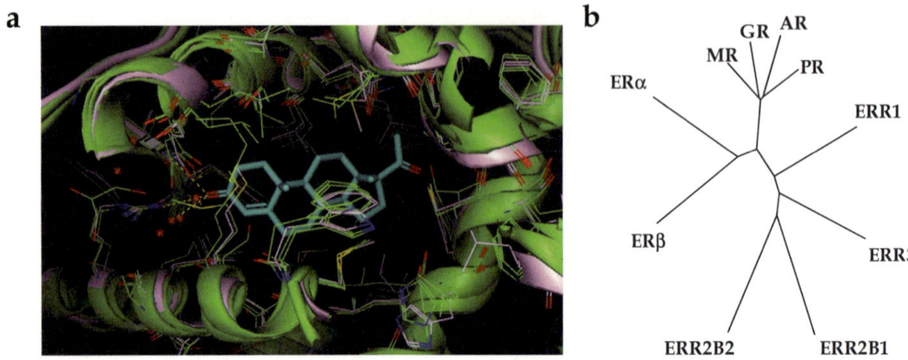

Fig. 1. (a) X-ray structure of progesterone (cyan) bound to the PR ligand binding pocket (pink) (Williams & Sigler, 1998) and overlaid with the x-ray co-ordinates of GR, MR and AR (in green) to illustrate the high degree of structural similarity between homologous NHRs (b) Phylogentic tree illustrating the sequence similarity of homologous NHRs with PR.

More recently, several alternative non-steroidal chemical PRA scaffolds have been published. These might have advantages over the steroidal templates due to simpler synthetic route, and potential for greater selectivity and metabolic stability compared with steroidal templates (Dack et al., 2010; Fensome et al., 2008; Terefenko et al., 2005; Zhang et al., 2002),. With a few exceptions, these classes of agents tend to mimic the steroid A ring ketone with a cyanoaryl group isostere, as is also seen with tanaproget, the non-steroidal progestogen (Fensome et al., 2005).

Steroidal PRAs have been characterised as facilitating PR dimerisation and nuclear translocation, but induce a conformation of the DNA-bound complex which recruits co-repressors to directly shutdown transcriptional PRE activity and other transcriptional promoters by trans-repression. The pharmacological profile of the non-steroidal compounds appears to be subtly different from steroidal examples (Howe et al., 2011; Zhang et al., 2007). In vitro pharmacological profiling of PRA-910 and PF-02413873 has indicated that at low concentrations the compounds inhibit the expression of progesterone-reporter genes, but at high concentrations, they induce agonism. For PF-02413873, the inhibition of progesterone-reporter gene expression appears to be due to blocking PR nuclear translocation and then at high concentrations PF-02413873 facilitates it, recruits co-activators and induces gene transcription.

Compound	Structure	Pharmacology data	In vivo observations	Reference
Non-steroidal PRAs				
PF-02367982	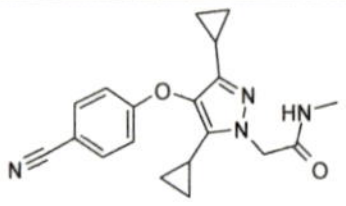	PR binding K_i=76 nM; functional IC_{50}=40.3 nM >3000x functional selectivity over GR, AR, MR	Dose dependent inhibition of arborisation of the immature rabbit and luteal phase endometrium of the intact macaque	(de Giorgio-Miller et al., 2008)

Table 1. Pharmacological properties of key non-steroidal and steroidal PRAs [1] In these assays, the activity of RU-486 was PR binding IC_{50}=9 nM; T47D IC_{50}=7.6 nM; GR binding IC_{50}=10 nM; IC_{50}=5.9 nM; AR binding IC_{50}=45 nM; [2] In these assays, the activity of RU-486 was PR binding IC_{50}=0.028 nM; GR binding IC_{50}=2.2 nM; AR binding IC_{50}=10 nM

PF-02413873	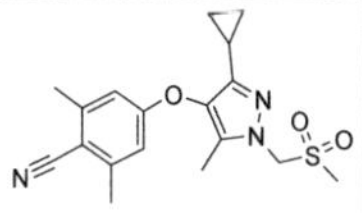	PR binding K_i=2.6 nM; functional K_i=9.7 nM; pK_B= 8.0 [Agonist format: ~25% activation at 10 µM] AR binding IC_{50}=2100 nM; functional K_i=1130 nM MR functional K_i=307 nM GR binding K_i=410 nM; functional K_i=2710 nM	Dose dependent inhibition in functionalis thickness & BrdU incorporation of follicular phase macaque endometrium; maximum effects at 10 mg/kg (p.o, *b.i.d*)	(Howe et al., 2011)
PRA-910	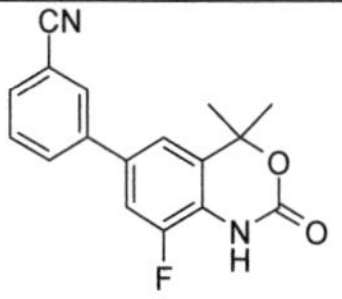	PR binding Kd=4.4 nM; functional 14 nM [Agonist format: ~60-70% activation at 0.1 µM AR binding IC_{50}=1292 nM GR binding IC_{50}=1756 nM MR binding IC_{50}=2369 nM ER binding IC_{50} >10000 nM	Dose dependent inhibition of the P_4-induced rat decidual response (mean ED_{50} =0.3 mg/kg) with no evidence of agonism at 10 mg/kg. 5 mg/kg reduced BrdU incorporation in the E_2/OVX macaque, but no effect on endometrial thickness c.f. control	(Zhang et al., 2002; 2007)
WAY-255348	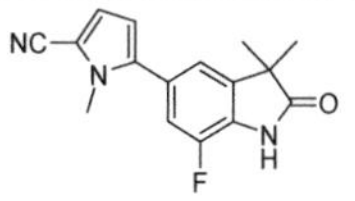	PR binding IC_{50}=5 nM; functional IC_{50}=5 nM AR functional IC_{50}=196 nM MR functional IC_{50}=3700 nM >No significant activity at GR, ER	Inhibition of P_4-induced rat decidual response (ED_{50} = 0.3 mg/kg). Dose dependent inhibition of ovulation in the macaque. All the animals treated at 10 mg/kg had thin-atrophied endometria	(Fensome et al., 2008)
Steroidal PRAs				
RU-486 / mifepristone	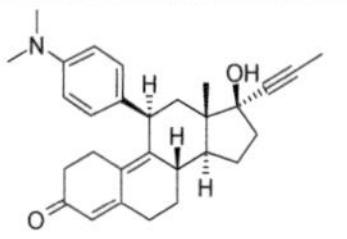	PR binding K_i=0.5 nM; T47D IC_{50}=0.2 nM AR functional C_{50}=20 nM GR binding K_i=1.4 nM; Functional IC_{50}=3 nM MR functional IC_{50}=3 nM	Dose dependent induction of menses in intact and E_2/P_4 artificially cycled macaque. Inhibition of ovulation and endometrial proliferation. ~75% reduction in peritoneal disease volume in a surgical model of endometriosis in the macaque	(de Giorgio-Miller et al., 2008; Grow et al., 1996; Slayden & Brenner, 1994; Slayden et al., 2001; Wolf et al., 1989)

Table 1. (continuation) Pharmacological properties of key non-steroidal and steroidal PRAs[1] In these assays, the activity of RU-486 was PR binding IC_{50}=9 nM; T47D IC_{50}=7.6 nM; GR binding IC_{50}=10 nM; IC_{50}=5.9 nM; AR binding IC_{50}=45 nM; [2] In these assays, the activity of RU-486 was PR binding IC_{50}=0.028 nM; GR binding IC_{50}=2.2 nM; AR binding IC_{50}=10 nM

CDB-4124 / proellex	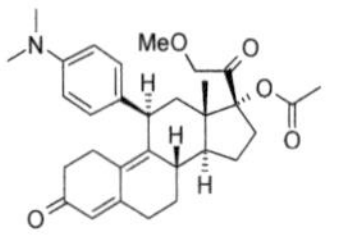	PR binding IC_{50}=19 nM; T47D functional IC_{50}=11 nM[1] GR binding IC_{50}=17 nM IC_{50}=130 nM AR binding IC_{50}=288 nM	Dose dependent suppressed cell proliferation and tumour latency in a N-methyl-N-nitrosourea-induced mammary carcinogenesis rat model	(Attardi et al., 2002; Brenner et al., 2010; Wiehle et al., 2011)
CDB-2914 / ulipristal	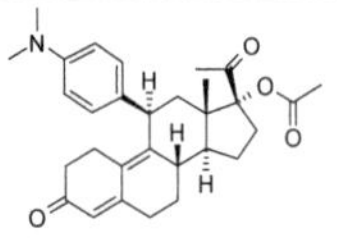	PR binding IC_{50}=7 nM; T47D functional IC_{50}=7 nM GR binding IC_{50}=18 nM; functional IC_{50}=73.8 nM AR binding IC_{50} = 65 nM[1]	Intrauterine delivery of CDB-2914 suppressed endometrial growth and menstruation in artificially cycled Rhesus macaques	(Attardi et al., 2002; Brenner et al., 2010; Gainer & Ulmann, 2003)
ZK-230211 / linaprostone	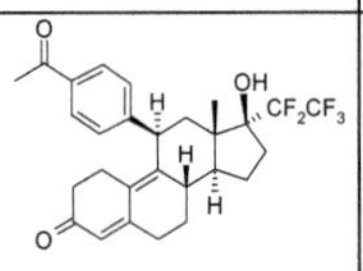	PR binding IC_{50} = 0.0036 nM GR binding IC_{50} = 16 nM AR binding IC_{50} = 54 nM[2]	Dose dependent interruption of pregnancy in the rat and reduction in tumour mass in a DMBA-induced rat mammary tumour model. Dose dependent inhibition of endometrial growth in the macaque	(Afhüppe et al., 2010; Fuhrmann et al., 2000; Slayden et al., 2001)
J-867 / asoprisnil	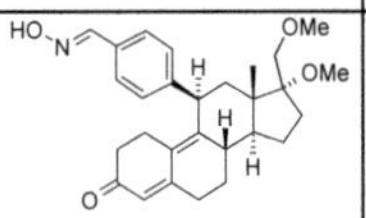	PR functional IC_{50}=0.2 nM AR functional IC_{50}=6.1 nM GR functional IC_{50}=85 nM MR functional IC_{50}=1.6 μM ER functional IC_{50}= 1.9 μM	Partial agonist properties in McPhail's assay. Marginal labour-inducing activity during mid-pregnancy and ineffective in inducing preterm parturition in the guinea pig. Abolition of menstrual cyclicity and induction of endometrial atrophy in the macaque	(DeManno et al., 2003; Elger et al., 2000; Fensome et al., 2008)
ORG-31710	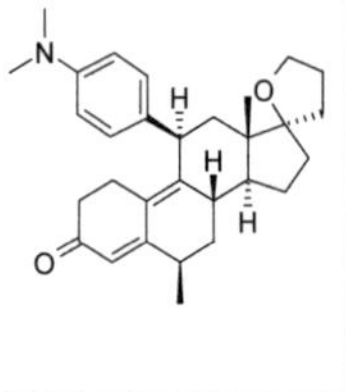	PR relative binding affinity equivalent to RU-486. 30 fold lower GR relative binding affinity c.f. RU-486	ORG-31710 administered with desogestrel reduced the incidence of unscheduled vaginal bleeding c.f. desogestrel alone in the macaque	(Kloosterboer et al., 1994; 2000; Verbost et al., 2005)

Table 1. (continuation) Pharmacological properties of key non-steroidal and steroidal PRAs [1] In these assays, the activity of RU-486 was PR binding IC_{50}=9 nM; T47D IC_{50}=7.6 nM; GR binding IC_{50}=10 nM; IC_{50}=5.9 nM; AR binding IC_{50}=45 nM; [2] In these assays, the activity of RU-486 was PR binding IC_{50}=0.028 nM; GR binding IC_{50}=2.2 nM; AR binding IC_{50}=10 nM

ZK-98299 / Onapristone	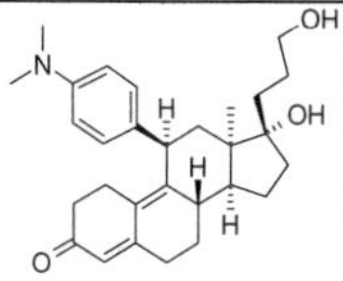	PR relative binding affinity equivalent to RU-486	Inhibition of arborisation of the immature rabbit. Reduction in cell proliferation of cells in ectopic lesion in a rat endometriosis model. Inhibition of ovulation and endometrial growth in monkeys	(Elger et al., 2000; Gopalkrishnan et al., 2003; Ishwad et al., 1993; Stoeckemann et al., 1995)
ZK-137316		PR relative binding affinity equivalent to RU-486	Inhibition of arborisation of the immature rabbit. Reduction in cell proliferation of cells in ectopic lesion in a rat endometriosis model. Inhibition of ovulation and endometrial growth in macaques.	(Borman et al., 2003; Slayden et al., 1998; 2001; Slayden & Brenner, 2003; Stoeckemann et al., 1995; Zelinski-Wooten et al., 1998)

Table 1. (continuation) Pharmacological properties of key non-steroidal and steroidal PRAs [1] In these assays, the activity of RU-486 was PR binding IC_{50}=9 nM; T47D IC_{50}=7.6 nM; GR binding IC_{50}=10 nM; IC_{50}=5.9 nM; AR binding IC_{50}=45 nM; [2] In these assays, the activity of RU-486 was PR binding IC_{50}=0.028 nM; GR binding IC_{50}=2.2 nM; AR binding IC_{50}=10 nM

5. Pre-clinical effects of PR antagonists in pre-clinical models

The study of the effects of PRAs in pre-clinical models has shed light on the site of and mechanism of action of PRAs in normal reproductive physiology and disease. The classical models for quantifying PRA activity are the modified assay in juvenile rabbits according to McPhail (McPhail, 1933), the induction of luteolysis in the guinea pig (Elger et al., 2000) and the inhibition of decidualisation in the rat. For the purposes of this review, I have focussed on the pre-clinical models which have been used to support a role for PR in the pathogenesis and treatment of endometriosis, principally focussing on studies in the rodent and macaque. Many data have been acceded from studies in the normal animal, but several experimental models of endometriosis have been also developed in normal as well as immune compromised rodents and non-human primates (D'Hooghe et al., 2009; Grummer, 2006; Laschke & Menger, 2007). In these models, cystic ectopic endometrial lesions develop following the transplantation of syngeneic or human uterine endometrial tissue under the control of ovarian estradiol. Measuring temporal changes in the size of these lesions and their proliferative capacity as well other aspects of the disease presentation is a powerful pre-clinical yardstick for testing the efficacy of experimental drugs.

5.1 Rodent

Mouse knockout studies have elegantly described differences in the function of PR-A and PR-B. Both PR null mutation (PRKO) and selective disruption of the PR-A isoform (PRAKO)

in the mouse leads to a failure of ovulation due to disabled follicular rupture in response to gonadotrophin stimulation (Lydon et al., 1995; Mulac-Jericevic & Conneely, 2005). The histological characterisation of uteri from PRKO mice confirmed extensive epithelial hyperplasia (Lydon et al., 1995). In contrast, the stromal compartment was distinctly oedematous and infiltrated with neutrophils and macrophages. While these data strongly support the notion of PR in suppressing ER function in the uterus, the cystic dilation, epithelial hyperplasia and associated inflammation are also histological hallmarks of endometriosis, especially those characterised in rodent disease models (Bruner et al., 1997; Grummer, 2006; Hull et al., 2003; Vernon & Wilson, 1985). The endometrial epithelial hyperplasia observed in the uteri of PRAKO mice was similar to that observed for PRKO mice suggesting that PR-B is unable to compensate for the loss of PR-A (Mulac-Jericevic et al., 2000). In contrast, ovarian and uterine response to E_2/P_4 appear to be normal in PR-B knockout mice, whereas mammary lobuloalveolar development was markedly reduced due to decreased ductal and alveolar epithelial cell proliferation (Mulac-Jericevic et al., 2003). Taken together these findings demonstrate the extremely important role PR plays in regulating ovarian function and spatiotemporal cell growth in different tissue compartments in response to E_2/P_4 in the mouse.

PRKO mice have been used to explore the role of PR in the development and growth of ectopic lesions in a syngenic mouse model of endometriosis (Fang et al., 2004). In this study, the volumes of PRKO lesions collected from animals treated with E_2 were approximately 20% larger than those from corresponding wild-type animals. Additionally, the effects of P_4 on PRKO lesions were ablated compared with those from wild-type animals, underscoring the important role that PR plays in regulating E_2-dependent cell proliferation in the rodent.

Whilst the evaluation of gene ablation on eutopic and ectopic endometrial cell growth has been revealing, the studies of pharmacological modulation contrast these observations to a certain extent as both progestogens and PRAs reduce ectopic endometrial cell proliferation and disease burden in pre-clinical rodent models of endometriosis (Bruner-Tran et al., 2006; Chwalisz et al., 1998; Katayama et al., 2010; Katsuki et al., 1998; Stoeckemann et al., 1995). An explanation of this phenomenon compared with the phenotype of PRKO animals has been revealed by studies with PRAs in the non-human primate.

5.2 Macaque

Given the evolutionary and physiological proximity of the macaque menstrual cycle with the human, many groups have evaluated the role of PR and the effects of PRAs on the macaque endometrium. Most data revealing the effect of PRAs on the endometrium have come from studies evaluating the effects of steroidal PRAs. When administered acutely after the mid-cycle LH surge, or during the progesterone phase in artificially cycled animals, PRAs impair the effects of progesterone on endometrial arborisation and induce an early menstruation. In the intact macaque, animals undergo an anovulatory amenorrhoea under the influence of continuous steroidal PRA exposure (Brenner et al., 2010; Slayden et al., 2001). In these animals, the endometrium is characterised by decreased wet weight, thickness and mitotic activity. The endometrium undergoes a characteristic atrophy and compaction of the stroma, glandular apoptosis as well as degeneration of the endometrial spiral arterioles. These effects are characteristically anti-estrogenic in nature, and yet the effects occur in the presence of mid-follicular levels of E_2, levels that should be sufficient to facilitate endometrial growth. Studies in ovariectomised (OVX) and E_2-supplemented macaques, have been perhaps even more revealing with respect to the mechanism driving this effect, especially the direct as well as indirect effects of PRAs on the hypothalamic-pituitary-gonadal axis and endometrium. Firstly, RU-486 has been shown to suppress the estrogen-induced LH surge in the OVX macaque (Wolf et al., 1989), underwriting a role for PR in regulating the hypothalamic-pituitary axis in higher species as suggested by early studies in knockout mice (Conneely et al., 2001). Furthermore, as RU-486 does not appear to blunt GnRH-induced LH secretion in the macaque (Heikinheimo et al., 1995), this has suggested that PRAs directly block ovarian folliculogenesis. In intact macaques with PRA doses that are too low to block ovulation or in the OVX/E_2 macaque, steroidal PRAs that include can also directly suppress the effects of estrogen on the endometrium by inhibiting cell proliferation and thickness suggesting that PR regulates reproductive function at multiple points (Brenner et al., 2010; DeManno et al., 2003; Hodgen et al., 1994; Ishwad et al., 1993; Slayden et al., 1998; 2001; 2006; Wolf et al., 1989; Zelinski-Wooten et al., 1998).

While many studies have been commonly undertaken by oral or systemic administration of PRAs, principally RU-486, some studies have also been undertaken by local, intrauterine administration, such as those with CDB-2914 and ZK-230211(Brenner et al., 2010; Nayak et al., 2007). In each case, the intrauterine administration resulted in the characteristic inhibition of normal menstrual bleeding, atrophy of endometrial spiral arterioles and functionalis thickness, consistent with observations from systemic administration (Figure 2). Unfortunately neither of these studies were supported with a confirmation of drug exposure, comparing the local versus systemic exposure to demonstrate that the effects were mediated by a local site of action and not an indirect effect. Nonetheless the data support others which suggest that PRAs can work locally to block estrogen effects on endometrial growth in the macaque.

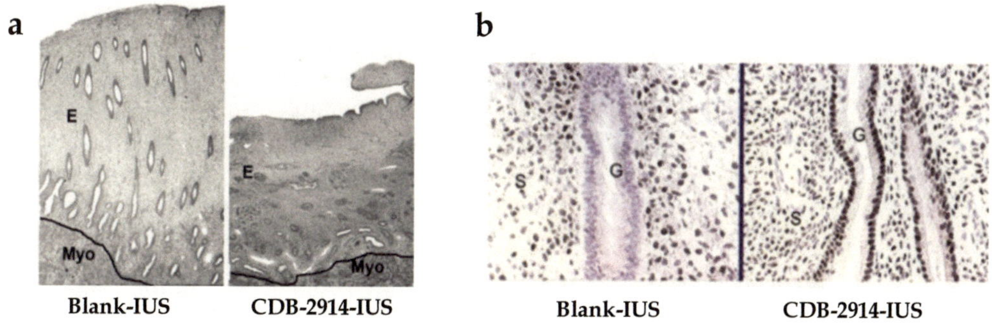

Fig. 2. (a) Induction of endometrial atrophy by CDB-2914-intrauterine system (IUS) versus blank-IUS (taken from (Brenner et al., 2010) with permission); E, endometrium; Myo, myometrium (original magnification ×25). (b) AR staining on endometrial tissue samples taken from macaques treated with CDB-2914-IUS or blank-IUS (original magnification ×340).

The mechanism of attenuation of estradiol effects on the endometrium is not well understood, and although steroidal PRAs appear to block cell proliferation in various *in vitro* cell-based systems, the concentrations needed for this effect are considerably greater than those which elicit the effect *in vivo* (Freeburg et al., 2009a; Goyeneche et al., 2007; Murphy et al., 2000; Ohara et al., 2007; Wu & Guo, 2006). One clue to a potential mechanism has emerged from observations of elevated endometrial androgen receptor (AR) expression (Narvekar et al., 2004; Slayden & Brenner, 2003) following PRA administration and the known effects of AR modulators (e.g. danazol) on endometrium (Rose et al., 1988).

These observations have been functionally evaluated further (Slayden & Brenner, 2003) in which OVX/E_2 macaques were continuously treated with ZK-137316 or together with the AR antagonist, flutamide, for 28 days. Flutamide reversed the inhibitory effects of ZK-137316 on the E_2/OVX endometrium, restoring levels of endometrial proliferation and thickness to control levels (Table 2).

	E_2 alone	E_2/ZK-137316 (0.1 mg/kg i.m.)	E_2/ZK-137316 (0.1 mg/kg i.m.) + Flutamide (2 mg/kg s.c.)
Weight (mg)	360 ± 32	64 ± 10^b	265 ± 92
Thickness (mm)	3.3 ± 0.4	1.1 ± 0.3^b	2.2 ± 0.6
Stromal compaction^c	45.5 ± 3.4	142.3 ± 63.7^b	54.0 ± 4.6
Mitotic index^d	6.3 ± 0.6	0.3 ±0.3^b	5.2 ± 3.8

Table 2. Morphometric assessment of androgen receptor blockade of ZK-137316 effects on OVX/E_2 macaques^a (Adapted from (Slayden & Brenner, 2003)) ^{a}All values represent mean ± SE; ^{b}*p*<0.05 compared with values in the same row; ^{c}stromal cells/10,000 μm^2; ^{d}mitotic cells/1000 epithelial cells

That flutamide did not appear to inhibit the PR activity of ZK-137316 (i.e. ZK-137316-induced menstruation in E_2/P_4 artificially cycled animals in the presence of flutamide), suggested that the endometrial anti-proliferative effects of steroidal PRAs like ZK-137316 are mediated by a mechanism involving AR. However, despite this extremely important observation, the seminal Slayden publication has not been followed up further. For instance, it is not clear what ligand is driving the AR effect, as testosterone levels do not appear to be altered in ZK-137316 treated animals, or how the signal is transduced through AR; if it is genomic or non-genomic. If AR is inducing a genomic effect, what are the transcripts that are altered and confer the inhibitory effect on PRA? Other important and, as yet, unaddressed questions also include whether these effects are only manifested only by the steroidal class of PRAs, but the observation that RU-486 can elevate endometrial AR expression in women goes some way to understanding the translational significance of the macaque findings (Narvekar et al., 2004).

Non-steroidal classes of PRAs have also been studied in a similar way in the macaque. Of the novel class of cyanophenoxypyrazoles, PF-02367982 dose-dependently inhibited the progesterone-mediated aborisation of the endometrium and delayed menses induction when dosed for 20 days from the start of the menstrual cycle. PF-02367982 also increased AR protein expression in a similar manner to that observed by RU-486 and the non-steroidal PRA, WAY-255348 (de Giorgio-Miller et al., 2008; Fensome et al., 2008). These data are consistent with other non-steroidal PRAs that have been assessed, such as WAY-255348 (Fensome et al., 2008). More recently, PF-02413873 a more potent PRA than PF-02367982 (Table 1) has been shown to reduce endometrial cell proliferation and thickness in intact macaques dosed for 10 days from the start of menstruation (Howe et al., 2011). In this study, however, AR expression was not appreciably altered with PF-02413873 treatment compared with RU-486. While this may be, in part, due to the timepoint for the comparison and assessment, PF-02413873 also appears to have a different pharmacological profile from RU-486 and other steroidal PRAs.

While these interesting observations are important in the context of normal endometrial physiology, few studies have been undertaken in macaques with endometriosis to build translational understanding to disease. Menstruating primates, such as the baboon and the macaque, develop spontaneous endometriosis and ectopic lesions that are histologically identical to the human disease (D'Hooghe et al., 2009). For many researchers, the proximity of this model to the human condition has made this the model of choice for the assessment of interventional agents the endometriosis. Spontaneous disease is acquired with a similar time course as experienced by the human female, developing slowly over a period of years and is not easily diagnosed without laparoscopy. Consequently, researchers have used intraperitoneal inoculation of autologous menstrual or endometrial tissue to develop an experimental model of endometriosis that is similar to that observed in women.

The only study evaluating the effect of a steroidal PRA, RU-486, in a non-human primate model of endometriosis was reported by Grow *et al* (1996). This study was undertaken in a surgical induction model of endometriosis and disease allowed to develop prior to dosing. A baseline measure of burden (peritoneal lesion area) was undertaken and then macaques were treated with either RU-486, leuprolide or vehicle for one year. Both RU-486 and leuprolide induced an anovulatory amenorrhoea and reduced peritoneal disease levels to a similar levels, $\geq$75%, compared with the vehicle control group. The authors additionally evaluated the effect of RU-486 and leuprolide on bone mineral density as revealed by dual x-ray absorptiometry. Consistent with the post-menopausal levels of E_2 achieved, leuprolide induced a 0.035 g/cm^2 reduction in bone mass compared with +0.1 g/cm^2 for vehicle control and +0.25 g/cm^2 for the RU-486 treated animals. These data support earlier observations that steroidal PRAs are able to suppress endometrial cell growth whilst maintaining bone-sparing mid-follicular levels of E_2 (Heikinheimo et al., 1995).

6. Clinical evaluation in healthy women and women with endometriosis

RU-486 was originally developed for emergency contraception, however early observations with lower doses than those used clinically, indicated that when given acutely during the luteal phase, RU-486 would facilitate the onset of menstruation by the upregulation of endometrial prostaglandins and given chronically, RU-486 would delay menses (Hapangama et al., 2002; Shoupe et al., 1987). The effects of RU-486 on the ovarian cycle and endometrium appear to be dose dependent, that is low doses interfere with estrogen function and disrupt endometrial growth (Croxatto et al., 1993; Narvekar et al., 2004), but higher doses additionally suppress follicular development by impairing gonadotrophin secretion (Gemzell-Danielsson et al., 1996; Liu et al., 1987; Spitz et al., 1993; 1994). These observations strike a resounding chord with those data acceded in the macaque described earlier. The potential value of PRAs as alternative contraceptives to current combined or progestin-only pills have been long recognised and evaluated in a number of different dosing and delivery strategies (Baird et al., 2003; Brown et al., 2002; Chabbert-Buffet et al., 2007; Heikinheimo et al., 2007; Lakha et al., 2007; Nayak et al., 2007). Whilst no pregnancies were reported after 200 months in women who received 2-5 mg RU-486 daily (Brown et al., 2002), lower doses appeared to be less effective (Croxatto et al., 1998). Similar observations on the suppression of ovulation and the normal menstrual cycle have also been made with other PR-As such as a onapristone, J-876 as well as CDB-2914 (Chabbert-Buffet et al., 2007; Chwalisz et al., 2005a; Katkam et al., 1995; Stratton et al., 2000). The utility of PRAs as a new class of oral contraceptives has still not been fully exploited and this feature alone is anticipated to have potential benefit in endometriosis patients by reducing cyclical menstrual pain.

Intrauterine delivery (IUD) of progestogens (levonorgestrel/Mirena) is an effective way of administering durable contraceptive exposures of drug and to bypass systemic side effects. IUD studies with PRAs in the macaque have also been followed up with a single human study. The study compared levonorgestrel with an IUD releasing ZK-230211. The dose of ZK-230211 was selected based on an equivalent IUD dose of ZK-230211 that suppressed ovulation and menstruation in the macaque (Heikinheimo et al., 2007). In contrast to the data acceded in the macaque, however, the ZK-230211 IUD did not appreciably alter bleeding patterns suggesting that either the local drug exposure was insufficient or that there are translational differences between the macaque and human.

Increasingly, however, the endometrial effects of PRAs have been subject to concern due observed histological changes in the endometrium with chronic exposure. In the past, endometrial hyperplasia has been reported as a safety concern with chronic use of RU-486 (Newfield et al., 2001). Recent, detailed histological analyses of endometrial biopsies from patients exposed to steroidal PRA for more than 3 months have indicated that these agents produce a slightly thickened endometrium with cystically dilated endometrial glands (Ioffe et al., 2009; Mutter et al., 2008; Williams et al., 2007). The appearance of glandular epithelium appears to change with dose and exposure duration, from inactive/non-mitotic to non-physiologic combinations of features usually seen separately in normal proliferative and secretory endometrium. These alterations do not appear to be limited to the glands only, as thick-walled vessels most commonly seen in endometrial polyps, become more widely distributed throughout the endometrium. Whether these effects on the endometrium are mediated by the unopposed effects of persistent follicular phase levels of estradiol, the pharmacological class or some non-specific effect of PRAs on the endometrium is not clear, but this appears to be a common feature of all steroidal PRAs assessed so far. Individuals on prolonged exposure to asoprisnil/J-867 were at a higher risk of developing endometrial changes sufficient to raise concern with regulatory authorities indicates that more research is needed to understand the phenomenon of PRA associated endometrial changes and whether this might be in part mitigated by an alternative dosing regimen from continuous dosing (Baird et al., 2003).

The first evidence that PRAs such as RU-486 would have a potential benefit in women with endometriosis was published by Kettel and co-workers (1991; 1994; 1996; 1998). The incentive for these early investigational studies was the clinical observation that RU-486 could block follicular maturation and ovulation when given early in the menstrual cycle, disrupt endometrial integrity when administered in the luteal phase and induce an anovulatory amenorrhoea when administered continuously. However, even earlier studies than those conducted with RU-486, indicated the potential utility of treating women with endometriosis with an anti-progestin (Coutinho, 1982). In this small open-label study, 20 patients with endometriosis were subjected to 6 months of continuous treatment with gestrinone (5 mg/twice weekly), a reportedly mixed antagonist with anti-progestogenic activity. All subjects became amenorrhoeic and had reportedly dramatic improvements in dyspareunia symptoms and fertility outcomes. Whilst no visualisation of the change in the disease burden was made in this study, this assessment was followed up by others (Cornillie et al., 1986) and incorporated as part of the validation work performed by Kettel and co-workers with RU-486. In these studies, doses of RU-486 were carefully selected to avoid the known anti-glucocorticoid effects. Treatment of women with endometriosis with a daily dose of 5-100 mg for 3-6 months resulted in durable inhibition of the normal menstrual cycle (although not optimal for the 5 mg dose) and a suppression in ovarian hormone levels consistent with a block on folliculogenesis. Endometriosis-associated pain scores and American Fertility Scores determined by laparoscopic examination also decreased from baseline (Kettel et al., 1994; 1996; 1998; Murphy et al., 1995). These preliminary studies were not able to rule out the possibility that the visible changes in disease burden were secondary to the absence of ovarian hormone cyclicity; indeed this is still not known. From a safety perspective, there was no suppression of cortisol levels, indicative of anti-glucocorticoid effects. Serum estradiol concentrations were also maintained at a mid-follicular level which preserved femur and lumbar spinal bone mineral density (Kettel et al., 1996). These bone safety data are consistent with those reported in the cynomolgus macaque and contrast clinical observations of GnRH receptor agonists (Grow et al., 1996).

Asoprisnil has also been compared with placebo for treatment of pain in laparoscopically diagnosed endometriosis in a randomized, controlled trial. Whilst the results of this study were reported as an abstract only, a significant decrease in daily pain scores with all doses of asoprisnil (5, 10 or 25 mg) compared with placebo was noted (Chwalisz et al., 2005b). Intriguing as these data are, there has been a compelling lack of replication studies from double blinded, randomised and controlled trials in women with endometriosis, using empirical and objective outcome measures approved by regulatory bodies. This lack of evidence may be in part due to the level of investment needed for such an old drug as RU-486, or concerns over the safety of continuously administered RU-486 or PRAs like it. CDB-4124 is currently in development for the treatment of endometriosis and uterine fibroids and data are anticipated on its clinical efficacy/safety profile.

In contrast to the relatively large wealth or reported data with steroidal PRAs, there is only a single study evaluating the effects of a non-steroidal PRA, PF-02413873, in healthy female subjects (Howe et al., 2011). When orally dosed to healthy female volunteers, daily from the first day of the menstrual cycle, PF-02413873 blocked the mid-cycle LH surge and endometrial growth (Figure 3).

Whilst PF-02413873 development for endometriosis was curtailed due to a high incidence of idiosyncratic maculopapular rash, PF-02413873 proves the principle that a non-steroidal PRA can similarly block the effects of follicular hormones on endometrial growth as steroidal PRAs. Further data are needed to determine whether the histological changes encountered by the class of steroidal PRAs endometrial are similarly manifested by the non-steroidal PRA class.

Given the anti-proliferative effects observed in vitro and in vivo for PRAs (Freeburg et al., 2009b; Goyeneche et al., 2007; Ohara et al., 2007; Poole et al., 2006; Tieszen et al., 2011), the broader utility of this class in treating other benign and malignant growth conditions has not gone unnoticed (Chwalisz et al., 2007; Robertson et al., 1999; Rocereto et al., 2000; Wilkens et al., 2008). In the closely related condition of uterine fibroids, small studies have demonstrated a reduction in myoma volume and uterine bleeding with asoprisnil and RU-486 (Chabbert-Buffet et al., 2005; DeManno et al., 2003; Fiscella et al., 2006). Larger studies have been completed for asoprisnil. In one randomized, controlled trial, 129 women with at least 1 fibroid greater than 3 cm in diameter or a uterine volume twice the normal (>200 cm^3) were treated for up to 3 months with asoprisnil (5, 10, or 25 mg) or placebo (Chwalisz et al., 2007). Significant reduction in uterine fibroid volume was noted by week 4 and persisted through the end of the study in a dose-dependent fashion.

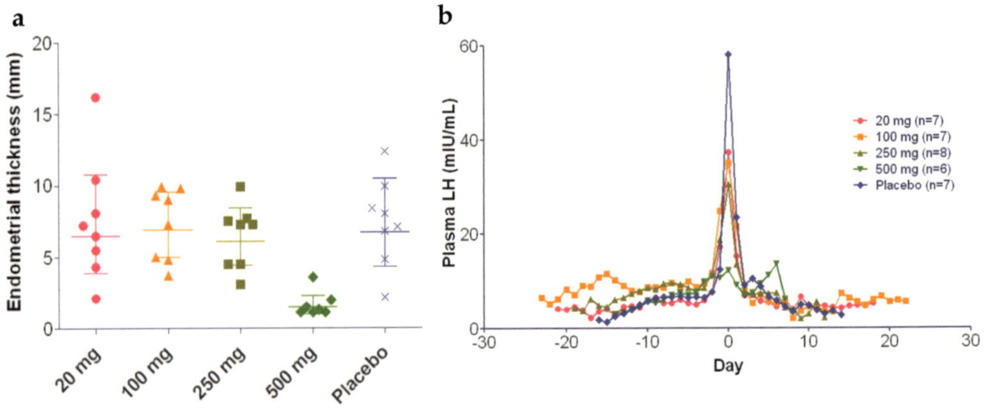

Fig. 3. Effect of escalating multiple dose of PF-02413873 on endometrial thickness (mm) (a) and the mid cycle LH surge (mIU/mL) (b) in healthy women compared with placebo (Howe et al., 2011)

7. Conclusion

There are compelling pre-clinical and clinical evidence to suggest that as well as directly antagonising the effect of progesterone, PRAs also functionally antagonise the effects of estrogen on the endometrium. This coupled with the suppression of ovarian folliculogenesis induces anovulatory amenorrhoea. Evaluation of the PR axis in animal models of endometriosis has suggested that PRAs can suppress the growth of ectopic endometriotic lesions. The mechanism driving this effect is still not clear, but it sufficient to maintain ovarian activity and estradiol levels adequately to protect bone as well as other potential post-menopausal symptoms more commonly encountered with ovarian suppression. In women with endometriosis, the data available from small clinical evaluations, strongly suggest that PRA treatment reduces disease symptoms, whilst maintaining normal levels of bone mineral density. Further clinical evaluation in larger randomised, placebo controlled and blinded studies are warranted, both to underscore the clinical benefit as well as understand the safety of the mechanism compared with existing standard of care therapy (endometrial, cardiovascular and bone safety, in particular). The medicinal chemistry challenge in designing potent, selective and safe PRAs is not inconsiderable, especially given the large number of examples whose clinical development have been curtailed (e.g. onapristone, PF-02413873, asoprisnil). However, the clinical evidence observed so far provides strong confidence that the class could have utility as a chronic treatment for endometriosis as well as a range of other gynaecological indications and malignant conditions.

8. References

Afhüppe W, Beekman JM, Otto C, Korr D, Hoffmann J, Fuhrmann U & Möller C (2010) In vitro characterization of ZK 230211--A type III progesterone receptor antagonist with enhanced antiproliferative properties. *J Steroid Biochem Mol Biol* 119(1-2):45-55.

Aghajanova L, Horcajadas JA, Weeks JL, Esteban FJ, Nezhat CN, Conti M & Giudice LC (2010) The protein kinase A pathway-regulated transcriptome of endometrial stromal fibroblasts reveals compromised differentiation and persistent proliferative potential in endometriosis. *Endocrinology* 151(3):1341-1355.

Aghajanova L, Tatsumi K, Horcajadas JA, Zamah AM, Esteban FJ, Herndon CN, Conti M & Giudice LC (2011) Unique transcriptome, pathways, and networks in the human endometrial fibroblast response to progesterone in endometriosis. *Biol Reprod* 84(4):801-815.

Altan M, Bruner-Tran KL, Osteen K & Palmer S (2008) JNK Inhibitor AS-01 Causes Regression of Endometriosis and Suppression of Inflammatory Cytokines and Tissue Remodeling Enzymes. *Biol Reprod* 78(169):486.

Arnett-Mansfield RL, DeFazio A, Mote PA & Clarke CL (2004) Subnuclear distribution of progesterone receptors A and B in normal and malignant endometrium. *J Clin Endocrinol Metab* 89(3):1429-1442.

Attardi BJ, Burgenson J, Hild SA, Reel JR & Blye RP (2002) CDB-4124 and its putative monodemethylated metabolite, CDB-4453, are potent antiprogestins with reduced antiglucocorticoid activity: in vitro comparison to mifepristone and CDB-2914. *Mol Cell Endocrinol* 188(1-2):111-123.

Attia GR, Zeitoun K, Edwards D, Johns A, Carr BR & Bulun SE (2000) Progesterone receptor isoform A but not B is expressed in endometriosis. *J Clin Endocrinol Metab* 85(8):2897-2902.

Baird DT, Brown A, Cheng L, Critchley HO, Lin S, Narvekar N & Williams AR (2003) Mifepristone: a novel estrogen-free daily contraceptive pill. *Steroids* 68(10-13):1099-1105.

Berchuck A, Schildkraut JM, Wenham RM, Calingaert B, Ali S, Henriott A, Halabi S, Rodriguez GC, Gertig D, Purdie DM, Kelemen L, Spurdle AB, Marks J & Chenevix-Trench G (2004) Progesterone receptor promoter +331A polymorphism is associated with a reduced risk of endometrioid and clear cell ovarian cancers. *Cancer Epidemiol Biomarkers Prev* 13(12):2141-2147.

Bergqvist A & Ferno M (1993) Estrogen and progesterone receptors in endometriotic tissue and endometrium: comparison according to localization and recurrence. *Fertil Steril* 60(1):63-68.

Biagini G, Panuccio G & Avoli M (2010) Neurosteroids and epilepsy. *Curr Opin Neurol* 23(2):170-176.

Borman SM, Chwalisz K, Stouffer RL & Zelinski-Wooten MB (2003) Chronic low-dose antiprogestin impairs preimplantation embryogenesis, but not oocyte nuclear maturation or fertilization in rhesus monkeys. *Steroids* 68(10-13):1041-1051.

Brenner RM, Slayden OD, Nath A, Tsong YY & Sitruk-Ware R (2010) Intrauterine administration of CDB-2914 (Ulipristal) suppresses the endometrium of rhesus macaques. *Contraception* 81(4):336-342.

Brown A, Cheng L, Lin S & Baird DT (2002) Daily low-dose mifepristone has contraceptive potential by suppressing ovulation and menstruation: a double-blind randomized control trial of 2 and 5 mg per day for 120 days. *J Clin Endocrinol Metab* 87(1):63-70.

Bruner-Tran KL, Zhang Z, Eisenberg E, Winneker RC & Osteen KG (2006) Down-regulation of endometrial matrix metalloproteinase-3 and -7 expression in vitro and therapeutic regression of experimental endometriosis in vivo by a novel nonsteroidal progesterone receptor agonist, tanaproget. *J Clin Endocrinol Metab* 91(4):1554-1560.

Bruner KL, Matrisian LM, Rodgers WH, Gorstein F & Osteen KG (1997) Suppression of matrix metalloproteinases inhibits establishment of ectopic lesions by human endometrium in nude mice. *J Clin Invest* 99(12):2851-2857.

Bulun SE, Cheng YH, Pavone ME, Yin P, Imir G, Utsunomiya H, Thung S, Xue Q, Marsh EE, Tokunaga H, Ishikawa H, Kurita T & Su EJ (2010) 17Beta-hydroxysteroid dehydrogenase-2 deficiency and progesterone resistance in endometriosis. *Semin Reprod Med* 28(1):44-50.

Burney RO, Talbi S, Hamilton AE, Vo KC, Nyegaard M, Nezhat CR, Lessey BA & Giudice LC (2007) Gene expression analysis of endometrium reveals progesterone resistance and candidate susceptibility genes in women with endometriosis. *Endocrinology* 148(8):3814-3826.

Catalano RD, Yanaihara A, Evans AL, Rocha D, Prentice A, Saidi S, Print CG, Charnock-Jones DS, Sharkey AM & Smith SK (2003) The effect of RU486 on the gene expression profile in an endometrial explant model. *Mol Hum Reprod* 9(8):465-473.

Chabbert-Buffet N, Meduri G, Bouchard P & Spitz IM (2005) Selective progesterone receptor modulators and progesterone antagonists: mechanisms of action and clinical applications. *Hum Reprod Update* 11(3):293-307.

Chabbert-Buffet N, Pintiaux-Kairis A & Bouchard P (2007) Effects of the progesterone receptor modulator VA2914 in a continuous low dose on the hypothalamic-pituitary-ovarian axis and endometrium in normal women: a prospective, randomized, placebo-controlled trial. *J Clin Endocrinol Metab* 92(9):3582-3589.

Chwalisz K, Stockemann K, Fritzemeier KH & Fuhrmann U (1998) Modulation of oestrogenic effects by progesterone antagonists in the rat uterus. *Hum Reprod Update* 4(5):570-583.

Chwalisz K, Elger W, Stickler T, Mattia-Goldberg C & Larsen L (2005a) The effects of 1-month administration of asoprisnil (J867), a selective progesterone receptor modulator, in healthy premenopausal women. *Hum Reprod* 20(4):1090-1099.

Chwalisz K, Perez MC, Demanno D, Winkel C, Schubert G & Elger W (2005b) Selective progesterone receptor modulator development and use in the treatment of leiomyomata and endometriosis. *Endocr Rev* 26(3):423-438.

Chwalisz K, Larsen L, Mattia-Goldberg C, Edmonds A, Elger W & Winkel CA (2007) A randomized, controlled trial of asoprisnil, a novel selective progesterone receptor modulator, in women with uterine leiomyomata. *Fertil Steril* 87(6):1399-1412.

Clarke CL & Sutherland RL (1990) Progestin regulation of cellular proliferation. *Endocrine Rev* 11(2):266-300.

Condon JC, Hardy DB, Kovaric K & Mendelson CR (2006) Up-Regulation of the Progesterone Receptor (PR)-C Isoform in Laboring Myometrium by Activation of Nuclear Factor-κB May Contribute to the Onset of Labor through Inhibition of PR Function. *Molecular Endocrinology* 20(4):764-775.

Conneely OM, Mulac-Jericevic B, Lydon JP & De Mayo FJ (2001) Reproductive functions of the progesterone receptor isoforms: lessons from knock-out mice. *Mol Cell Endocrinol* 179(1-2):97-103.

Cornillie FJ, Brosens IA, Vasquez G & Riphagen I (1986) Histologic and ultrastructural changes in human endometriotic implants treated with the antiprogesterone steroid ethylnorgestrienone (gestrinone) during 2 months. *Int J Gynecol Pathol* 5(2):95-109.

Coutinho EM (1982) Treatment of endometriosis with gestrinone (R-2323), a synthetic antiestrogen, antiprogesterone. *Am J Obstet Gynecol* 144(8):895-898.

Croxatto HB, Salvatierra AM, Croxatto HD & Fuentealba B (1993) Effects of continuous treatment with low dose mifepristone throughout one menstrual cycle. *Hum Reprod* 8(2):201-207.

Croxatto HB, Salvatierra AM, Fuentealba B & Massai R (1998) Contraceptive potential of a mifepristone-nomegestrol acetate sequential regimen in women. *Hum Reprod* 13(12):3297-3302.

D'Amora P, Maciel TT, Tambellini R, Mori MA, Pesquero JB, Sato H, Girao MJ, Guerreiro da Silva ID & Schor E (2009) Disrupted cell cycle control in cultured endometrial cells from patients with endometriosis harboring the progesterone receptor polymorphism PROGINS. *Am J Pathol* 175(1):215-224.

D'Hooghe TM, Kyama CM, Chai D, Fassbender A, Vodolazkaia A, Bokor A & Mwenda JM (2009) Nonhuman primate models for translational research in endometriosis. *Reprod Sci* 16(2):152-161.

Dack KN, Skerratt S, Johnson PS, Bradley PA & Marsh IR (2010) Optimisation of a pyrazole series of progesterone antagonists; Part 1. *Bioorg Med Chem Lett* 20(11):3384-3386.

De Carvalho CV, Nogueira-De-Souza NC, Costa AM, Baracat EC, Girao MJ, D'Amora P, Schor E & da Silva ID (2007) Genetic polymorphisms of cytochrome P450cl7alpha (CYP17) and progesterone receptor genes (PROGINS) in the assessment of endometriosis risk. *Gynecol Endocrinol* 23(1):29-33.

de Giorgio-Miller A, Bungay P, Tutt M, Owen J, Goodwin D & Pullen N (2008) The translational pharmacology of a novel, potent, and selective nonsteroidal progesterone receptor antagonist, 2-[4-(4-cyano-phenoxy)-3,5-dicyclopropyl-1H-pyrazol-1-yl]-N-methylacetamide (PF-02367982). *J Pharmacol Exp Ther* 327(1):78-87.

De Vivo I, Huggins GS, Hankinson SE, Lescault PJ, Boezen M, Colditz GA & Hunter DJ (2002) A functional polymorphism in the promoter of the progesterone receptor gene associated with endometrial cancer risk. *Proc Natl Acad Sci U S A* 99(19):12263-12268.

DeManno D, Elger W, Garg R, Lee R, Schneider B, Hess-Stumpp H, Schubert G & Chwalisz K (2003) Asoprisnil (J867): a selective progesterone receptor modulator for gynecological therapy. *Steroids* 68(10-13):1019-1032.

Dressing GE, Goldberg JE, Charles NJ, Schwertfeger KL & Lange CA (2011) Membrane progesterone receptor expression in mammalian tissues: A review of regulation and physiological implications. *Steroids* 76(1-2):11-17.

Elger W, Bartley J, Schneider B, Kaufmann G, Schubert G & Chwalisz K (2000) Endocrine pharmacological characterization of progesterone antagonists and progesterone receptor modulators with respect to PR-agonistic and antagonistic activity. *Steroids* 65(10-11):713-723.

Fang Z, Yang S, Lydon JP, DeMayo F, Tamura M, Gurates B & Bulun SE (2004) Intact progesterone receptors are essential to counteract the proliferative effect of estradiol in a genetically engineered mouse model of endometriosis. *Fertil Steril* 82(3):673-678.

Fazleabas AT, Brudney A, Chai D, Langoi D & Bulun SE (2003) Steroid receptor and aromatase expression in baboon endometriotic lesions. *Fertil Steril* 80 (Suppl 2):820-827.

Fensome A, Bender R, Chopra R, Cohen J, Collins MA, Hudak V, Malakian K, Lockhead S, Olland A, Svenson K, Terefenko EA, Unwalla RJ, Wilhelm JM, Wolfrom S, Zhu Y, Zhang Z, Zhang P, Winneker RC & Wrobel J (2005) Synthesis and structure-activity relationship of novel 6-aryl-1,4-dihydrobenzo[d][1,3]oxazine-2-thiones as progesterone receptor modulators leading to the potent and selective nonsteroidal progesterone receptor agonist tanaproget. *J Med Chem* 48(16):5092-5095.

Fensome A, Adams WR, Adams AL, Berrodin TJ, Cohen J, Huselton C, Illenberger A, Kern JC, Hudak VA, Marella MA, Melenski EG, McComas CC, Mugford CA, Slayden OD, Yudt M, Zhang Z, Zhang P, Zhu Y, Winneker RC & Wrobel JE (2008) Design, synthesis, and SAR of new pyrrole-oxindole progesterone receptor modulators leading to 5-(7-fluoro-3,3-dimethyl-2-oxo-2,3-dihydro-1H-indol-5-yl)-1-methyl-1H-pyrrole-2-c arbonitrile (WAY-255348). *J Med Chem* 51(6):1861-1873.

Fiscella K, Eisinger SH, Meldrum S, Feng C, Fisher SG & Guzick DS (2006) Effect of mifepristone for symptomatic leiomyomata on quality of life and uterine size: a randomized controlled trial. *Obstet Gynecol* 108(6):1381-1387.

Freeburg EM, Goyeneche AA, Seidel EE & Telleria CM (2009a) Resistance to cisplatin does not affect sensitivity of human ovarian cancer cell lines to mifepristone cytotoxicity. *Cancer Cell Int* 9:4.

Freeburg EM, Goyeneche AA & Telleria CM (2009b) Mifepristone abrogates repopulation of ovarian cancer cells in between courses of cisplatin treatment. *Int J Oncol* 34(3):743-755.

Fuhrmann U, Hess-Stumpp H, Cleve A, Neef G, Schwede W, Hoffmann J, Fritzemeier KH & Chwalisz K (2000) Synthesis and biological activity of a novel, highly potent progesterone receptor antagonist. *J Med Chem* 43(26):5010-5016.

Gainer EE & Ulmann A (2003) Pharmacologic properties of CDB(VA)-2914. *Steroids* 68(10-13):1005-1011.

Gellersen B, Fernandes MS & Brosens JJ (2009) Non-genomic progesterone actions in female reproduction. *Hum Reprod Update* 15(1):119-138.

Gemzell-Danielsson K, Westlund P, Johannisson E, Swahn ML, Bygdeman M & Seppala M (1996) Effect of low weekly doses of mifepristone on ovarian function and endometrial development. *Hum Reprod* 11(2):256-264.

Gopalkrishnan K, Katkam RR, Sachdeva G, Kholkute SD, Padwal V & Puri CP (2003) Effects of an Antiprogestin Onapristone on the Endometrium of Bonnet Monkeys: Morphometric and Ultrastructural Studies. *Biol Reprod* 68(6):1959-1967.

Govindan S, Ahmad SN, Vedicherla B, Kodati V, Jahan P, Rao KP, Ahuja YR & Hasan Q (2007) Association of progesterone receptor gene polymorphism (PROGINS) with endometriosis, uterine fibroids and breast cancer. *Cancer Biomark* 3(2):73-78.

Goyeneche AA, Caron RW & Telleria CM (2007) Mifepristone inhibits ovarian cancer cell growth in vitro and in vivo. *Clin Cancer Res* 13(11):3370-3379.

Grow DR, Williams RF, Hsiu JG & Hodgen GD (1996) Antiprogestin and/or gonadotropin-releasing hormone agonist for endometriosis treatment and bone maintenance: a 1-year primate study. *J Clin Endocrinol Metab* 81(5):1933-1939.

Grummer R (2006) Animal models in endometriosis research. *Hum Reprod Update* 12(5):641-649.

Hapangama DK, Critchley HO, Henderson TA & Baird DT (2002) Mifepristone-induced vaginal bleeding is associated with increased immunostaining for cyclooxygenase-2 and decrease in prostaglandin dehydrogenase in luteal phase endometrium. *J Clin Endocrinol Metab* 87(11):5229-5234.

Heikinheimo O, Kontula K, Croxatto H, Spitz I, Luukkainen T & Lahteenmaki P (1987) Plasma concentrations and receptor binding of RU 486 and its metabolites in humans. *J Steroid Biochem* 26(2):279-284.

Heikinheimo O, Gordon K, Lahteenmaki P, Williams RF & Hodgen GD (1995) Antiovulatory actions of RU 486: the pituitary is not the primary site of action in vivo. *J Clin Endocrinol Metab* 80(6):1859-1868.

Heikinheimo O, Vani S, Carpén O, Tapper A, Härkki P, Rutanen E-M & Critchley H (2007) Intrauterine release of progesterone antagonist ZK230211 is feasible and results in novel endometrial effects: a pilot study. *Hum Reprod* 22(9):2515-2522.

Henderson LP (2007) Steroid modulation of GABAA receptor-mediated transmission in the hypothalamus: Effects on reproductive function. *Neuropharmacology* 52(7):1439-1453.

Hodgen GD, van Uem JF, Chillik CF, Danforth DR, Wolf JP, Neulen J, Williams RF & Chwalisz K (1994) Non-competitive anti-oestrogenic activity of progesterone antagonists in primate models. *Hum Reprod* (Suppl 1):77-81.

Howe DC, Mount NM, Bess K, Brown AN, Bungay P, Gilbson KR, Hawcock T, Richard J, Jones G, Walley R, McLeod A, Apfeldorfer CS, Ramsey S, Tweedy S & Pullen N (2011) The translational efficacy of a non-steroidal progesterone receptor antagonist, 4-[3-cyclopropyl-1-(mesylmethyl)-5-methyl-1H-pyrazol-4-yl]oxy,-2,6-dimethylbenzonitrile (PF-02413873), on endometrial growth in macaque and human. *J Pharmacol Exp Ther* 339(2):642-653

Hull ML, Charnock-Jones DS, Chan CL, Bruner-Tran KL, Osteen KG, Tom BD, Fan TP & Smith SK (2003) Antiangiogenic agents are effective inhibitors of endometriosis. *J Clin Endocrinol Metab* 88(6):2889-2899.

Igarashi TM, Bruner-Tran KL, Yeaman GR, Lessey BA, Edwards DP, Eisenberg E & Osteen KG (2005) Reduced expression of progesterone receptor-B in the endometrium of women with endometriosis and in cocultures of endometrial cells exposed to 2,3,7,8-tetrachlorodibenzo-p-dioxin. *Fertil Steril* 84(1):67-74.

Ioffe OB, Zaino RJ & Mutter GL (2009) Endometrial changes from short-term therapy with CDB-4124, a selective progesterone receptor modulator. *Mod Pathol* 22(3):450-459.

Ishwad PC, Katkam RR, Hinduja IN, Chwalisz K, Elger W & Puri CP (1993) Treatment with a progesterone antagonist ZK 98.299 delays endometrial development without blocking ovulation in bonnet monkeys. *Contraception* 48(1):57-70.

Kao LC, Tulac S, Lobo S, Imani B, Yang JP, Germeyer A, Osteen K, Taylor RN, Lessey BA & Giudice LC (2002) Global gene profiling in human endometrium during the window of implantation. *Endocrinology* 143(6):2119-2138.

Kao LC, Germeyer A, Tulac S, Lobo S, Yang JP, Taylor RN, Osteen K, Lessey BA & Giudice LC (2003) Expression profiling of endometrium from women with endometriosis reveals candidate genes for disease-based implantation failure and infertility. *Endocrinology* 144(7):2870-2881.

Katayama H, Katayama T, Uematsu K, Hiratsuka M, Kiyomura M, Shimizu Y, Sugita A & Ito M (2010) Effect of dienogest administration on angiogenesis and hemodynamics in a rat endometrial autograft model. *Hum Reprod* 25(11):2851-2858.

Katkam RR, Gopalkrishnan K, Chwalisz K, Schillinger E & Puri CP (1995) Onapristone (ZK 98.299): a potential antiprogestin for endometrial contraception. *Am J Obstet Gynecol* 173(3 Pt 1):779-787.

Katsuki Y, Takano Y, Futamura Y, Shibutani Y, Aoki D, Udagawa Y & Nozawa S (1998) Effects of dienogest, a synthetic steroid, on experimental endometriosis in rats. *Eur J Endocrinol* 138(2):216-226.

Kettel LM, Murphy AA, Mortola JF, Liu JH, Ulmann A & Yen SS (1991) Endocrine responses to long-term administration of the antiprogesterone RU486 in patients with pelvic endometriosis. *Fertil Steril* 56(3):402-407.

Kettel LM, Murphy AA, Morales AJ & Yen SS (1994) Clinical efficacy of the antiprogesterone RU486 in the treatment of endometriosis and uterine fibroids. *Hum Reprod* (Suppl 1):116-120.

Kettel LM, Murphy AA, Morales AJ, Ulmann A, Baulieu EE & Yen SS (1996) Treatment of endometriosis with the antiprogesterone mifepristone (RU486). *Fertil Steril* 65(1):23-28.

Kettel LM, Murphy AA, Morales AJ & Yen SS (1998) Preliminary report on the treatment of endometriosis with low-dose mifepristone (RU 486). *Am J Obstet Gynecol* 178(6):1151-1156.

Kloosterboer HJ, Deckers GH & Schoonen WG (1994) Pharmacology of two new very selective antiprogestagens: Org 31710 and Org 31806. *Hum Reprod* 9 (Suppl 1):47-52.

Kloosterboer HJ, Deckers GH, Schoonen WGEJ, Hanssen RGJM, Rose UM, Verbost PM, Hsiu JG, Williams RF & Hodgen GD (2000) Preclinical experience with two selective progesterone receptor modulators on breast and endometrium. *Steroids* 65(10-11):733-740.

Kobayashi S, Stice JP, Kazmin D, Wittmann BM, Kimbrel EA, Edwards DP, Chang CY & McDonnell DP (2010) Mechanisms of progesterone receptor inhibition of inflammatory responses in cellular models of breast cancer. *Mol Endocrinol* 24(12):2292-2302.

Kraus WL, Montano MM & Katzenellenbogen BS (1993) Cloning of the rat progesterone receptor gene 5'-region and identification of two functionally distinct promoters. *Mol Endocrinol* 7(12):1603-1616.

Lakha F, Ho PC, Van der Spuy ZM, Dada K, Elton R, Glasier AF, Critchley HO, Williams AR & Baird DT (2007) A novel estrogen-free oral contraceptive pill for women: multicentre, double-blind, randomized controlled trial of mifepristone and progestogen-only pill (levonorgestrel). *Hum Reprod* 22(9):2428-2436.

Laschke MW & Menger MD (2007) In vitro and in vivo approaches to study angiogenesis in the pathophysiology and therapy of endometriosis. *Hum Reprod Update* 13(4):331-342.

Lattuada D, Somigliana E, Vigano P, Candiani M, Pardi G & Di Blasio AM (2004) Genetics of endometriosis: a role for the progesterone receptor gene polymorphism PROGINS? *Clin Endocrinol (Oxf)* 61(2):190-194.

Lee B, Du H & Taylor HS (2009) Experimental murine endometriosis induces DNA methylation and altered gene expression in eutopic endometrium. *Biol Reprod* 80(1):79-85.

Lishko PV, Botchkina IL & Kirichok Y (2011) Progesterone activates the principal Ca2+ channel of human sperm. *Nature* 471(7338):387-391.

Liu JH, Garzo G, Morris S, Stuenkel C, Ulmann A & Yen SS (1987) Disruption of follicular maturation and delay of ovulation after administration of the antiprogesterone RU486. *J Clin Endocrinol Metab* 65(6):1135-1140.

Lydon JP, DeMayo FJ, Funk CR, Mani SK, Hughes AR, Montgomery CAJ, Shyamala G, Conneely OM & O'Malley BW (1995) Mice lacking progesterone receptors exhibit pleiotropic reproductive abnormalities. *Genes & Dev* 9(18):2266-2278.

Madauss KP, Grygielko ET, Deng SJ, Sulpizio AC, Stanley TB, Wu C, Short SA, Thompson SK, Stewart EL, Laping NJ, Williams SP & Bray JD (2007) A structural and in vitro characterization of asoprisnil: a selective progesterone receptor modulator. *Mol Endocrinol* 21(5):1066-1081.

Mangelsdorf DJ, Thummel C, Beato M, Herrlich G, Schutz G, Umesono K, Blumberg B, Kastner P, Mark M, Chambon P & Evans RM (1995) The nuclear receptor superfamily: the second decade. *Cell* 83(6): 835-839.

McCormack PL (2010) Dienogest: a review of its use in the treatment of endometriosis. *Drugs* 70(16):2073-2088.

McGowan EM, Saad S, Bendall LJ, Bradstock KF & Clarke CL (2004) Effect of progesterone receptor a predominance on breast cancer cell migration into bone marrow fibroblasts. *Breast Cancer Res Treat* 83(3):211-220.

McKenna NJ & O'Malley BW (2001) Nuclear Receptors, Coregulators, Ligands, and Selective Receptor Modulators. *Ann N Y Acad Sci* 949(1):3-5.

McKenna NJ, Cooney AJ, DeMayo FJ, Downes M, Glass CK, Lanz RB, Lazar MA, Mangelsdorf DJ, Moore DD, Qin J, Steffen DL, Tsai M-J, Tsai SY, Yu R, Margolis RN, Evans RM & O'Malley BW (2009) Minireview: Evolution of NURSA, the Nuclear Receptor Signaling Atlas. *Mol Endocrinol* 23(6):740-746.

McPhail MK (1933) Capacity of the uterus of the rabbit to respond to prolonged luteal activity. *J Physiol* 79(1):118-120.

Mulac-Jericevic B, Mullinax RA, DeMayo FJ, Lydon JP & Conneely OM (2000) Subgroup of Reproductive Functions of Progesterone Mediated by Progesterone Receptor-B Isoform. *Science* 289(5485):1751-1754.

Mulac-Jericevic B, Lydon JP, DeMayo FJ & Conneely OM (2003) Defective mammary gland morphogenesis in mice lacking the progesterone receptor B isoform. *Proc Natl Acad Sci U S A* 100(17):9744-9749.

Mulac-Jericevic B & Conneely OM (2005) Reproductive tissue-selective actions of progesterone receptors. *Ernst Schering Res Found Workshop* 52:19-37.

Murphy AA, Kettel LM, Morales AJ, Roberts V, Parmley T & Yen SS (1995) Endometrial effects of long-term low-dose administration of RU486. *Fertil Steril* 63(4):761-766.

Murphy AA, Zhou MH, Malkapuram S, Santanam N, Parthasarathy S & Sidell N (2000) RU486-induced growth inhibition of human endometrial cells. *Fertil Steril* 74(5):1014-1019.

Mutter GL, Bergeron C, Deligdisch L, Ferenczy A, Glant M, Merino M, Williams AR & Blithe DL (2008) The spectrum of endometrial pathology induced by progesterone receptor modulators. *Mod Pathol* 21(5):591-598.

Narvekar N, Cameron S, Critchley HO, Lin S, Cheng L & Baird DT (2004) Low-dose mifepristone inhibits endometrial proliferation and up-regulates androgen receptor. *J Clin Endocrinol Metab* 89(5):2491-2497.

Nayak NR, Slayden OD, Mah K, Chwalisz K & Brenner RM (2007) Antiprogestin-releasing intrauterine devices: a novel approach to endometrial contraception. *Contraception* 75(6, Supplement 1):S104-S111.

Newfield RS, Spitz IM, Isacson C & New MI (2001) Long-term mifepristone (RU486) therapy resulting in massive benign endometrial hyperplasia. *Clin Endocrinol (Oxf)* 54(3):399-404.

O'Malley BW & Conneely OM (1992) Orphan receptors: in search of a unifying hypothesis for activation. *Mol Endocrinol* 6(12):1359-1361.

Ohara N, Morikawa A, Chen W, Wang J, DeManno DA, Chwalisz K & Maruo T (2007) Comparative effects of SPRM asoprisnil (J867) on proliferation, apoptosis, and the expression of growth factors in cultured uterine leiomyoma cells and normal myometrial cells. *Reprod Sci* 14(8 Suppl):20-27.

Painter JN, Anderson CA, Nyholt DR, Macgregor S, Lin J, Lee SH, Lambert A, Zhao ZZ, Roseman F, Guo Q, Gordon SD, Wallace L, Henders AK, Visscher PM, Kraft P, Martin NG, Morris AP, Treloar SA, Kennedy SH, Missmer SA, Montgomery GW & Zondervan KT (2011) Genome-wide association study identifies a locus at 7p15.2 associated with endometriosis. *Nat Genet* 43(1):51-54.

Poole AJ, Li Y, Kim Y, Lin SC, Lee WH & Lee EY (2006) Prevention of Brca1-mediated mammary tumorigenesis in mice by a progesterone antagonist. *Science* 314(5804):1467-1470.

Robertson JF, Willsher PC, Winterbottom L, Blamey RW & Thorpe S (1999) Onapristone, a progesterone receptor antagonist, as first-line therapy in primary breast cancer. *Eur J Cancer* 35(2):214-218.

Rocereto TF, Saul HM, Aikins JA, Jr. & Paulson J (2000) Phase II study of mifepristone (RU486) in refractory ovarian cancer. *Gynecol Oncol* 77(3):429-432.

Rose GL, Dowsett M, Mudge JE, White JO & Jeffcoate SL (1988) The inhibitory effects of danazol, danazol metabolites, gestrinone, and testosterone on the growth of human endometrial cells in vitro. *Fertil Steril* 49(2):224-228.

Shoupe D, Mishell DR, Jr., Page MA, Madkour H, Spitz IM & Lobo RA (1987) Effects of the antiprogesterone RU 486 in normal women. II. Administration in the late follicular phase. *Am J Obstet Gynecol* 157(6):1421-1426.

Slayden OD & Brenner RM (1994) RU 486 action after estrogen priming in the endometrium and oviducts of rhesus monkeys (Macaca mulatta). *J Clin Endocrinol Metab* 78(2):440-448.

Slayden OD, Zelinski-Wooten MB, Chwalisz K, Stouffer RL & Brenner RM (1998) Chronic treatment of cycling rhesus monkeys with low doses of the antiprogestin ZK 137 316: morphometric assessment of the uterus and oviduct. *Hum Reprod* 13(2):269-277.

Slayden OD, Chwalisz K & Brenner RM (2001) Reversible suppression of menstruation with progesterone antagonists in rhesus macaques. *Human Reprod* 16(8):1562-1574.

Slayden OD & Brenner RM (2003) Flutamide counteracts the antiproliferative effects of antiprogestins in the primate endometrium. *J Clin Endocrinol Metab* 88(2):946-949.

Slayden OD, Zelinski MB, Chwalisz K, Hess-Stumpp H & Brenner RM (2006) Chronic progesterone antagonist-estradiol therapy suppresses breakthrough bleeding and endometrial proliferation in a menopausal macaque model. *Hum Reprod* 21(12):3081-3090.

Spitz IM, Croxatto HB, Salvatierra AM & Heikinheimo O (1993) Response to intermittent RU486 in women. *Fertil Steril* 59(5):971-975.

Spitz IM, Croxatto HB, Lahteenmaki P, Heikinheimo O & Bardin CW (1994) Effect of mifepristone on inhibition of ovulation and induction of luteolysis. *Hum Reprod* 9 (Suppl 1):69-76.

Stoeckemann K, Hegele-Hartung C & Chwalisz K (1995) Effects of the progesterone antagonists onapristone (ZK 98 299) and ZK 136 799 on surgically induced endometriosis in intact rats. *Hum Reprod* 10(12):3264-3271.

Stratton P, Hartog B, Hajizadeh N, Piquion J, Sutherland D, Merino M, Lee YJ & Nieman LK (2000) A single mid-follicular dose of CDB-2914, a new antiprogestin, inhibits folliculogenesis and endometrial differentiation in normally cycling women. *Hum Reprod* 15(5):1092-1099.

Terefenko EA, Kern J, Fensome A, Wrobel J, Zhu Y, Cohen J, Winneker R, Zhang Z & Zhang P (2005) SAR studies of 6-aryl-1,3-dihydrobenzimidazol-2-ones as progesterone receptor antagonists. *Bioorg Med Chem Lett* 15(15):3600-3603.

Tetel MJ, Giangrande PH, Leonhardt SA, McDonnell DP & Edwards DP (1999) Hormone-Dependent Interaction between the Amino- and Carboxyl-Terminal Domains of Progesterone Receptor in Vitro and in Vivo. *Mol Endocrinol* 13(6):910-924.

Tieszen CR, Goyeneche AA, Brandhagen BN, Ortbahn CT & Telleria CM (2011) Antiprogestin mifepristone inhibits the growth of cancer cells of reproductive and non-reproductive origin regardless of progesterone receptor expression. *BMC Cancer* 11:207.

Treloar SA, Zhao ZZ, Armitage T, Duffy DL, Wicks J, O'Connor DT, Martin NG & Montgomery GW (2005) Association between polymorphisms in the progesterone receptor gene and endometriosis. *Mol Hum Reprod* 11(9):641-647.

Tsai M-J & O'Malley BW (1994) *Mechanism of steroid hormone regulation of gene transcription (molecular biology intelligence unit).* R.G. Landes Co., Austin, TX.

Tung L, Abdel-Hafiz H, Shen T, Harvell DME, Nitao LK, Richer JK, Sartorius CA, Takimoto GS & Horwitz KB (2006) Progesterone Receptors (PR)-B and -A Regulate Transcription by Different Mechanisms: AF-3 Exerts Regulatory Control over Coactivator Binding to PR-B. *Mol Endocrinol* 20(11):2656-2670.

Uz Y, Murk W, Bozkurt I, Kizilay G, Arici A & Kayisli U (2011) Increased c-Jun N-terminal kinase activation in human endometriotic endothelial cell. *Histochem & Cell Biol* 135 (1):83-91.

van Kaam KJ, Romano A, Schouten JP, Dunselman GA & Groothuis PG (2007) Progesterone receptor polymorphism +331G/A is associated with a decreased risk of deep infiltrating endometriosis. *Hum Reprod* 22(1):129-135.

Verbost PM, Hanssen RG, Korver GH & Mulders TM (2005) ORG 33628 and ORG 31710 to control vaginal bleeding in progestin-only contraceptive regimens. *Semin Reprod Med* 23(1):101-111.

Vernon MW & Wilson EA (1985) Studies on the surgical induction of endometriosis in the rat. *Fertil Steril* 44(5):684-694.

Wagner BL, Norris JD, Knotts TA, Weigel NL & McDonnell DP (1998) The nuclear corepressors NCoR and SMRT are key regulators of both ligand- and 8-bromo-cyclic AMP-dependent transcriptional activity of the human progesterone receptor. *Mol Cell Biol* 18(3):1369-1378.

Wiehle R, Lantvit D, Yamada T & Christov K (2011) CDB-4124, a progesterone receptor modulator, inhibits mammary carcinogenesis by suppressing cell proliferation and inducing apoptosis. *Cancer Prev Res (Phila)* 4(3):414-424.

Wieser F, Schneeberger C, Tong D, Tempfer C, Huber JC & Wenzl R (2002) PROGINS receptor gene polymorphism is associated with endometriosis. *Fertil Steril* 77(2):309-312.

Wilkens J, Chwalisz K, Han C, Walker J, Cameron IT, Ingamells S, Lawrence AC, Lumsden MA, Hapangama D, Williams AR & Critchley HO (2008) Effects of the selective progesterone receptor modulator asoprisnil on uterine artery blood flow, ovarian activity, and clinical symptoms in patients with uterine leiomyomata scheduled for hysterectomy. *J Clin Endocrinol Metab* 93(12):4664-4671.

Williams AR, Critchley HO, Osei J, Ingamells S, Cameron IT, Han C & Chwalisz K (2007) The effects of the selective progesterone receptor modulator asoprisnil on the morphology of uterine tissues after 3 months treatment in patients with symptomatic uterine leiomyomata. *Hum Reprod* 22(6):1696-1704.

Williams SP & Sigler PB (1998) Atomic structure of progesterone complexed with its receptor. *Nature* 393(6683):392-396.

Wolf JP, Hsiu JG, Anderson TL, Ulmann A, Baulieu EE & Hodgen GD (1989) Noncompetitive antiestrogenic effect of RU 486 in blocking the estrogen-stimulated luteinizing hormone surge and the proliferative action of estradiol on endometrium in castrate monkeys. *Fertil Steril* 52(6):1055-1060.

Wu Y & Guo SW (2006) Inhibition of proliferation of endometrial stromal cells by trichostatin A, RU486, CDB-2914, N-acetylcysteine, and ICI 182780. *Gynecol Obstet Invest* 62(4):193-205.

Wu Y, Strawn E, Basir Z, Halverson G & Guo SW (2006) Promoter hypermethylation of progesterone receptor isoform B (PR-B) in endometriosis. *Epigenetics* 1(2):106-111.

Wu Y, Shi X & Guo SW (2008) The knockdown of progesterone receptor isoform B (PR-B) promotes proliferation in immortalized endometrial stromal cells. *Fertil Steril* 90(4):1320-1323.

Zeitoun K, Takayama K, Sasano H, Suzuki T, Moghrabi N, Andersson S, Johns A, Meng L, Putman M, Carr B & Bulun SE (1998) Deficient 17beta-hydroxysteroid dehydrogenase type 2 expression in endometriosis: failure to metabolize 17beta-estradiol. *J Clin Endocrinol Metab* 83(12):4474-4480.

Zelinski-Wooten MB, Chwalisz K, Iliff SA, Niemeyer CL, Eaton GG, Loriaux DL, Slayden OD, Brenner RM & Stouffer RL (1998) A chronic, low-dose regimen of the antiprogestin ZK 137 316 prevents pregnancy in rhesus monkeys. *Hum Reprod* 13(8):2132-2138.

Zhang P, Terefenko EA, Fensome A, Wrobel J, Winneker R, Lundeen S, Marschke KB & Zhang Z (2002) 6-Aryl-1,4-dihydro-benzo[d][1,3]oxazin- 2-ones: a novel class of potent, selective, and orally active nonsteroidal progesterone receptor antagonists. *J Med Chem* 45(20):4379-4382.

Zhang Z, Lundeen SG, Slayden O, Zhu Y, Cohen J, Berrodin TJ, Bretz J, Chippari S, Wrobel J, Zhang P, Fensome A, Winneker RC & Yudt MR (2007) In vitro and in vivo characterization of a novel nonsteroidal, species-specific progesterone receptor modulator, PRA-910. *Ernst Schering Found Symp Proc* 1:171-197.

Zhu Y, Bond J & Thomas P (2003) Identification, classification, and partial characterization of genes in humans and other vertebrates homologous to a fish membrane progestin receptor. *Proc Natl Acad Sci U S A* 100(5):2237-2242.

10

Endometriosis and Angiogenic Factors

P. G. Artini, M. Ruggiero, F. Papini, G. Simi, V. Cela and A. R. Genazzani
Department of Gynecology and Obstetrics University of Pisa, Pisa, Italy

1. Introduction

Little is known about the pathogenesis of endometriosis. The prevailing hypothesis is that following retrograde menstruation, uterine endometrial tissue attaches, invades the peritoneal surface, and becomes vascularized.

The development of new blood vessels represents a crucial step during the establishment of endometriosis because endometriotic implants require neovascularization to guarantee oxygen and essential nutrient supply (Groothuis et al., 2005; McLaren, 2000). The interaction between the ectopic endometrium and the peritoneal tissue is a prerequisite for the induction of angiogenesis and the maintenance of endometriosis

At least, three processes appear to be critical to the establishment of endometriosis, according to the implantation theory: invasiveness, tissue remodeling and interactions between the ectopic endometrium and the surrounding peritoneal tissues (Giudice et al., 2008).

The establishment of endometriotic lesions needs a cascade of neoangiogenic factor, like the vasculatr endothelial factor, cytokines and metalloproteinases: this complex interrelation between factors permit sprouting of capillaries from pre-existing vessels and the subsequent supply for the development of ectopic implants (Hyder and Stancel, 1999).

2. Vascular endothelial growth factors family

2.1 Vascular Endothelial Growth Factor(VEGF)

2.1.1 VEGF family and its receptors

Vascular endothelial growth factors are important signaling proteins involved in both vasculogenesis (the *de novo* formation of the embryonic circulatory system) and angiogenesis (the growth of blood vessels from pre-existing vasculature). VEGF family comprises seven members: VEGF-A, VEGF-B, VEGF-C, VEGF-D, VEGF-E, VEGF-F, and PlGF. All members have a common VEGF homology domain. This core region is composed of a cystine knot motif, with eight invariant cysteine residues involved in inter- and intramolecular disulfide bonds at one end of a conserved central four-stranded-sheet within each monomer, which dimerize in an antiparallel, side-by-side orientation (Neufeld G, wt al 1999).

The human *VEGF* gene (*VEGFA*, OMIM 192240) is located on chromosome 6p12 (Zhao Z, et al 2008).

Vascular endothelial growth factor (VEGF) is one of the most potent and specific angiogenic factors. When VEGF binds to its targeted receptor, the VEGF receptor activation leads to a rapid increase in intracellular Ca2+ and inositol triphosphate concentrations in endothelial cells. The basic physiological function of VEGF is to induce angiogenesis, which allows the endometrium to repair itself following menstruation. It also modulates the characteristics of the newly formed vessels by controlling the microvascular permeability and permitting the formation of a fibrin matrix for endothelial cell migration and proliferation. This modulation may be responsible for local endometrial edema, which helps prepare the endometrium for embryo implantation. In endometriosis patients, VEGF is localized in the epithelium of endometriotic implants, particularly in hemorrhagic red implants. Moreover, the concentration of VEGF is increased in the PF of endometriosis patients. The exact cellular sources of VEGF in PF have not yet been precisely defined. Although evidence suggests that endometriotic lesions themselves produce this factor, activated peritoneal macrophages also can synthesize and secrete VEGF.

In women, physiological neoangiogensis is presented during the female reproductive cycle. VEGF-A is important in luteal angiogenesis. VEGF-A mRNA or protein is detectable in the granulosa cells of primordial and primary follicles, as they progressively become localized to the granulosa surrounding the oocyte and theca cells of the preovulatory follicle. After ovulation, VEGF-A mRNA and protein expression are observed in granulosa-derived luteal cells. VEGF-A expression in the corpus luteum appears highest early in the luteal phase and declines after the mid-luteal phase, with little or no expression in the late corpus luteum (Fraser HM, et al 2000). Gonadotrophic hormones, particularly luteinizing hormone (LH), appear to be major regulators of angiogenesis in the ovary (Hyder SM. Et al, 1999). The LH-stimulated luteinization of granulosa cells at the time of ovulation is associated with enhanced VEGF-A expression.

When VEGF is overexpressed, it can contribute to disease. Three VEGF tyrosine kinase receptors have been identified: The fms-like tyrosine kinase Flt-1 (VEGFR-1/Flt-1), the kinase domain region, also referred to as fetal liver kinase (VEGFR-2/KDR/Flk-1), and Flt-4 (VEGFR-3). Each receptor has seven immunoglobulinlike domains in the extracellular domain, a single transmembrane region, and a consensus tyrosine kinase sequence interrupted by a kinase insert domain (Ortega N et al, 1999). Binding its receptors R1, VEGF regulates development of tubular capillaries; binding R2 receptor, it promotes mesodermic cells differentiation into endothelial cells. In vivo and in vitro experiments indicate that steroid hormones, hypoxia and nitric oxide are potent inducers of vascular endothelial growth factor gene expression by enhancing hypoxia inducible factor 1-α activity and by the activation of the AKT/protein kinase B pathway (Kimura H, et al 2006).

2.1.2 VEGF role in endometriosis

Although the aetiology of endometriosis is unknown, it is generally accepted that the condition is a result of the implantation of exfoliated endometrium, deposited in the peritoneal cavity following retrograde menstruation (Sampson J 1927). When the exfoliated endometrium enters the peritoneal cavity and becomes attached to the mesothelial layer through attachment proteins like the cadherins, a process of angiogenesis is essential for further implantation and the development of peritoneal endometriosis (Nisolle M et al 1993). Angiogenesis is a fundamental process by which new blood vessels are formed and is considered as a major process in the pathogenesis of endometriosis. It is dependent on soluble factors released from cells. Many factors are involved in this complex mechanism, including FGF-a, FGF- b, PD-ECGF and VEGF, stimulate vascular endothelial cell growth *in vitro* and angiogenesis *in vivo* (Gordon J. Et al, 1995).

The development and maintenance of endometriosis is dependent on the recruitment of blood vessels to the endometriotic lesions from pre-existing ones to guarantee oxygen and essential nutrient supply. It has been shown that those endometriotic lesions recruit blood vessels by inducing angiogenesis. In a rat model, analyses of the assessed microvessel density demonstrated that angiogenesis is higher in ectopic endometriotic lesions compared with the eutopic endometrium (Machado DE et al, 2010).

Promoting angiogenesis, VEGF is involved in the etiology but also in the maintenance of peritoneal endometriosis. The endometrial tissue that has been migrated into the peritoneal space develops different angiogenic properties and invasive patterns, which could have a role in the implantation in the peritoneum of the pelvic cavity. It is likely that the action of VEGF in the implant of endometrial ectopic cells is to promote the differentiation of mesodermic cells into endothelial cells and to regulate the tubular capillary formation (Di Carlo C. Et al 2009).

VEGF-A is localized predominantly in the glandular epithelium of endometriosis lesions. Peritoneal fluid concentrations of VEGF have been demonstrated to be significantly higher in women with endometriosis than in the control patient and a positive correlation between the severity of endometriosis and the concentrations of VEGF in peritoneal fluid has been observed. Peritoneal fluid itself induced higher expression of the protein participating in the establishment and persistence of peritoneal endometriosis (Fasciani G. Et al, 2000).

In patients with endometriosis, high concentrations of VEGF in cystic and peritoneal fluids may be ascribed to a state of inflammation, where macrophages, which are the main source of this growth factor, play a central role.

It has been shown that cytokines released from immune cells play an important role in the pathogenesis of endometriosis, and many of these cytokines possess angiogenic activity. Pelvic implants and peritoneal fluid macrophages are the most likely source of VEGF-A in peritoneal fluid. McLaren (McLaren J, et al 2006) showed that peritoneal fluid macrophages express receptors for steroid hormones and secrete VEGF-A in response to ovarian steroids. The VEGF receptors VEGFR-1 and VEGFR-2 were also detected, suggesting an autocrine regulation. Peritoneal macrophages and activated lymphocytes seem to play an integral role in the secretion of proinflammatory/proangiogenic cytokines resulting in upregulation of VEGF from infiltrating neutrophils and macrophages (Machado DE et al, 2010).

Ovarian endometriotic cysts also over express VEGF in their cystic fluid with respect to follicular and serous cysts and to a similar degree as ovarian cystadenocarcinoma and a negative or positive correlation of VEGF expression has been reported with cyst diameter.

In ovary the process of angiogenesis is characterized by the existence of complex interrelations between the cell components of the ovarian cyst: diffuse VEGF expression in epithelial cells was associated with larger cysts; high VEGF expression in capsular fibroblast was associated with bilateral cysts; and expression of VEGF was found to be related in epithelial cells, capsular fibroblast and vessels, suggesting that neoangiogenesis might especially affect the outer cell cyst wall, thus contributing to cyst growth.(Goteri G. et al,

2004). The inner layers of cysts are characterized by high microvessel density but low expression of VEGF, whereas in the outer fibrosclerotic capsule, the vessels were less abundant, but Had a higher expression of VEGF and survive, thus activated to proliferate and protected from programmed cells death. Angiogenesis mediated by VEGF in the outer capsule contributed to the cyst growth and to the fibrosing process of adhesion (Goteri G. et al 2010). Antiangiogenetic drugs could act on the capsular vasculature and block the growth of ovarian cyst. The high VEGF levels could provoke an increase in the subperitoneal vascular network and facilitate implantation and viability of endometrial cells in the retroperitoneal space. Concerning sVEGFR-1, the highest levels of this protein were found in peritoneal fluids and cystic fluids of endometriosis patients with respect to both benign and malignant serous cysts. The soluble form of VEGFR-1, as already stated, should function as a modulator of VEGF's angiogenic activity. For this reason, it seems that sVEGFR-1 is secreted in proportionate amounts as VEGF itself. In benign cyst and peritoneal fluids, VEGF and sVEGFR-1 concentrations are proportionately low, while in endometriosis cyst and peritoneal fluids, VEGF and its soluble receptor are both expressed in much higher concentrations. Endothelial sVEGFR-1 is also known to be up-regulated by its ligand, VEGF-A, and the high levels of VEGF-A found in endometriomata compared with cystadenomas are likely to further contribute to up-regulation of sVEGFR-1. On the other hand, in patients affected by cystadenocarcinomas, there was discordance between the levels of VEGF and the levels of sVEGFR-1 in both cyst and peritoneal fluids. In fact, in malignant processes there seems to be an imbalance between pro-angiogenetic factors, represented by VEGF, and anti-angiogenetic factors, represented by sVEGFR-1, leading to a disordered and exaggerated formation of blood vessels (Artini PG et al, 2008).

The microenvironment of endometriosis is a locale of important secretion of angiogenic factors that play a key role in the establishment and maintenance of endometriotic lesions, and suggest that the balance of these local pro-antiangiogenic factors and cytokines may determine whether endometriotic lesions develop and grow.

2.1.3 Genetic polymorphisms of VEGF genes

An important aspect of the correlation between endometriosis and VEGF, also for possible future therapeutic application is that the polymorphisms in vascular endothelial growth factor gene are associated with the risk of familial endometriosis. The human *VEGF* gene (*VEGFA*, OMIM 192240) is located on chromosome 6p12 (Zhao Z, et al 2008). *VEGF* messenger ribonucleic acid and protein were significantly higher in women with endometriosis, which supported a key role for *VEGF* in the pathological angiogenesis in endometriosis (Gilabert-Estelles J, 2007). In particular several transcription factor-binding sites are found in the VEGF 5′ -untranslated region and variation within the region increases the transcriptional activity. A single family in two generations with four members who have histologically proven endometriosis showed that the circulating levels of *VEGF* were higher than the healthy control group, indicating a role for *VEGF* in disease susceptibility (Simpson JL et al 2003). In Chinese patients, the T allele of the *VEGF* gene −60 T/C (rs833061) polymorphism was associated with a higher risk of endometriosis. Study of the *VEGF* +405 G/C (rs2010963) polymorphism in a Korean population showed that the SNP was associated with the risk of advanced stage endometriosis. The analysis of both SNPs in an Indian population identified a haplotype associated with endometriosis In addition, the analysis of *VEGF* −460 T/C (rs833061), +405 G/C (rs2010963) and +936 C/T (rs3025039) polymorphisms in 147 endometriosis cases and 181 controls found a positive association between stages III–IV disease and the *VEGF* +936 T allele in a Japanese population. (Zhao Z, et al 2008). The first reported study in a Caucasian population of +405 G/C (rs2010963) in 203 Italian women affected with endometriosis and 140 controls reported a weak association of the C allele with endometriosis (Gentilini D et al, 2008).

2.1.4 Therapeutical approach

Therapy of endometriosis consists of surgical removal of implants or medical treatment such as analogues of Gonadotrophin releasing hormone or oral contraceptive or progestins. This therapeutic approach has been shown to be of limited benefit so new approaches need to be developed. Considering the importance of angiogenesis in developing and maintaining disease, and the role of vascular endothelial growth factor, anti-angiogenetic drugs could be very important.

Romidepsin, the Histone deacetylase (HDC) inhibitor, modulates the expression of a variety of genes by alteriting gormatin structure. It has been recently shown to inhibit proliferation and activate apoptosis in human epithelial endometriotic cells. In particle Imesch demonstrated that his epigenetically acting drug inhibits VEGF transcription at low nanomolar concentration with high efficency. It works at the transcriptional level down regulated VEGF expression. Romidepsin reduced the level of HIF-α protein, indicating that VEGF mRNA expression may be related to the reduction of HIF-α protein levels. The issue of whether VEGF transcription is the primary target of romidepsin or if it acts preventing deacytalation of HIF-α, must still be solved. However Romidepsin, acting at a transcriptional level, could be more effective than other angiogenetic drugs, which inhibit the VEGF active form in targeting angiogenesis, and it can be considered a novel therapeutic candidate to counter endometriosis (Imesch P et al, 2011).

Gonadotrophin- releasing hormone agonist (GnHRa I) have been applied with success, in the treatment of endometriosis combined with the laparoscopic surgery. It leads to a reduction of ovarian hormone levels, to atrophy of endometriotic implants and it has anti-proliferation and apoptotic effects. It reduce VEGF expression and it has been seen that after GnRHa treatment the concentration in peritoneal fluid of VEGF are significantly lower New molecule GnRHa II has been studied. Fengying et al demonstarted that this molecule can dose-dependently reduce VEGF protein secreted by ectopic and eutopic endometrial stromal cells cultured in vitro, and the inhibition effect is stronger than that of GnRHa I. GnRH II may reduce the secretion also of immune factors such as interleukin-8 and cyclooxigenase 2 relating to the incidence of endometriosis, suggesting for a anti-proliferation and anti-inflammatory effect on endometrial cells (Fengying, H et al 2010).

Yilmaz showed (Yilmaz B et al, 2010.) the effect of metformin of endometriosis implants for his antioxidant characteristics and the beneficial effects on VEGF, and matrix metalloproteinases. In particular it reduces endometriotic implants in rats reducing VEGF levels.

Molecular therapies have been proposed as a treatment alternative for recurrent endometriosis. The use of concitionally replicative adenovirus (CRADs) has been explored for the therapy of disease. In particular Adenovirus constructed with the VEGF promoter controlling the expression of a marker gene have been evaluated in vitro culture of endometriotic cells. AdVEGFE1 replicates in a short-term culture of purified ectopic endometriosis cells. The virus induces apoptosis in endometriotic cells in vitro (Rein DT. Et al, 2010). Ad VEGFE1 allowed specific replication and efficient killing of endometriotic cells.

Another approach, which has been recently been published (Essam –Eldin R et al, 2008) is the transfection of endometriotic cells by dominant negative estrogen receptor gene via Ad vector. Dominant negative mutants of the estrogen receptor are altered estrogen receptors forms that are unable to activate transcription of estrogen-responsive genes when estradiol binds them, resulting in decreased cell proliferation and increased apoptosis.

2.2 Endocrine Gland derived Vascular Endothelial Growth Factor (EG-VEGF)

Human endocrine gland derived vascular endothelial growth factor is a secreted angiogenetic mitogen growth factor expressed in the steroidogenic glands, ovary, testis, adrenal and placenta. It induces proliferation, migration and fenestration (formation of membrane discontinue) in capillary endothelial cells derived from endocrine glands. Human EG-VEGF is a 9.6 kDa protein consisting of 86 amino acid residues. Endocrine gland-derived VEGF (EG_VEGF) belongs to the prokineticin family. It is also known as prokineticn 1 (PK1). Although EG- VEGF is structurally distinct from VEGF, they induce similar angiogenic response in the ovary. The EG- VEGF acts through G-protein couplesd receptors, pkr1.

EG-VEGF was found to be expressed in non-endocrine tissues including endometrium: in human, it is highly expressed during the secretory phase of the menstrual cycle, when angiogenesis occurs. Lee et al evaluated the expression of EG-VEGF and its receptors in eutopic and ectopic endometrial tissues. A significant increase in molecule expression was found in the stromal cells of ectopic endometrium. It is possible that the stromal cells may synthesize EG-VEGF or that it is synthesize in the epithelial cells but is accumulated in the extracellular matrix of stroma. The endocrine gland-vascular endothelial growth factor, through its heparin- binding domain can, as VEGF, accumulated in the extracellular matrix (Lee K et al, 2010).

3. Cytokynes (IL-1, IL-6, IL-8, TNF- a)

Cytokines are small cell-signaling protein molecules that are secreted by several cells types and are a category of signaling molecules used extensively in intercellular communication. Cytokines can be classified as proteins, peptides, or glycoproteins; the term "cytokine" encompasses a large and diverse family of regulators produced throughout the body by cells of diverse embryological origin (Gilman et al., 2001). Virtually all nucleated cells, but especially endo/epithelial cells and resident macrophages (many near the interface with the external environment) are potent producers of IL-1, IL-6, and TNF-α (Boyle, 2005) .Studies have reported elevated levels of several cytokines in the peritoneal fluid of women with endometriosis, thus implicating these proteins in the development and progression of endometriosis and endometriosis-associated infertility (Koninckx et al.,1998); (Harada et al.,2001); (Bedaiwy et al., 2003); (Kalu et al., 2007). Peritoneal fluid is derived from plasma transudate and ovarian exudates and in a small part from secretions of the mesothelial surface and tubal luminal fluid. Some studies suggest that the peritoneal fluid of women with endometriosis contains an increased number of activated macrophages and other immune cells that secrete various local products, such as growth factors and cytokines, which exert a paracrine action on endometriotic cells. (Harada et al., 2001)

3.1 Cytokines and pathogenesis of endometriosis

Studies have shown the role of some cytokines in the implantation of ectopic endometrial tissue, and its progression and infiltration. In the implantation and growth of ectopic tissue, a primary role was attributed to several cytokines contained in the peritoneal fluid including interleukin IL-1,IL-6, IL-8, IL-12 and tumor necrosis factor-a (TNF-a) (Arici et al.,1996); (Iwabe et al., 1998); (Ho et al.,1997) Normally, peritoneal fluid contains leukocytes in concentrations of 0.5 to 2.0 3 106/mL, of which approximately 85% are macrophages (Syrop et al., 1987). Halme et al., (Halme et al.,1984) postulated that peritoneal macrophage activation may be a central contributor to the pathogenesis of endometriosis and activated macrophages in the peritoneal cavity of women with endometriosis (Vinatier et al., 1996) are potent producers of cytokines (Halme, 1989) ;(Fakih et al., 1987); (Rana et al., 1996). Thus, peritoneal fluid contains a rich cocktail of cytokines. Cytokines play a major role in the initiation, propagation, and regulation of immune and inflammatory responses. Immune cell activation results in a burst and cascade of inflammatory cytokines. These cytokines have pleiotropic and redundant activities that culminate in recruitment of numerous cell types to the site of inflammation (Harada et al, 2001). More, cytokines may regulate the actions of leukocytes in the peritoneal fluid or may act directly on ectopic endometrium, where they may play various roles in the pathogenesis and pathophysiology of endometriosis. Increased levels of cytokines in the peritoneal fluid of women with endometriosis may reflect increased synthesis of cytokines by peritoneal macrophages, lymphocytes, ectopic endometrial implants, or mesothelial cells of the peritoneum, all of which can produce cytokines (Tabibzadeh et al., 1989) ; (Betjes et al., 1993). The main source of cytokines is thought to be the macrophages, which originate in bone marrow, circulate as monocytes, and migrate to various body cavities. It seems that the cytokines playing the most important role in the endometriosis are : IL-1, IL-6, IL-8,IL-12, TNF- α.

- **Interleukin-1 (IL1)** is one of the major proinflammatory cytokine found in the peritoneal fluid of women with endometriosis (Mori et al., 1991); (Taketani et al., 1992); (Fakih et al., 1987). This multifunctional cytokine was shown to stimulate the production of angiogenic factors by ectopic endometrial cells and therefore play a role in ectopic endometrial cell growth (Lebovic et al., 2000). Other studies pointed to a possible role for IL1 in endometriosis-associated infertility (Fakih et al.,1987); (Sueldo et al.,1990). Both ectopic and eutopic endometrial cells of women with endometriosis display an increased sensitivity to IL1, which results in an enhanced production of angiogenic, growth, and proinflammatory factors (Lebovic et al., 2000); (Akoum et al., 1995); (Akoum et al.,2002).Some previous studies showed that the increased endometrial and endometriotic cell responsiveness to IL1 may in part be due to a deficiency in the expression of interleukin-1 receptor type II (IL1R2) revealed in eutopic and ectopic endometrial tissues (Akoum et al., 2001);(Kharfi et al.,2002). The soluble IL1R2 levels were found to be reduced in the peripheral blood of women with endometriosis, which may account for the activation of peripheral blood monocytes in them (Kharfi et al., 2002). More, the IL1R2 has no signaling properties in contrast to the functional signaling IL1R1, which mediates cell activation by IL1 (Bossu et al., 1995); (Dinarello 2004); (Colotta et al.,1993). However, the membrane form of this receptor and the soluble form, which is shed by proteolysis from the cell surface (Cui et al.,2003); (Orlando et al.,1997), bind to IL1 and with higher affinity to IL1b, which is the circulating and the preferential ligand for IL1R2, in particular for its soluble form (Bossu et al., 1995). This inhibits the interaction of

IL1 with its functional receptor type I and, consequently, IL1-mediated cell activation (Bossu et al., 1995); (Colotta et al.,1993); (Subramaniam et al., 2004);(Symons et al, 1995). Akoum et al. (Akoum et al., 2008) showed an imbalance in IL1/soluble IL1R2 levels in women with endometriosis suffering from infertility and pelvic pain and a relationship with endometriosis initial stages and infertility. This is in keeping with other findings showing a reduced expression of IL1R2 in the eutopic endometrial tissue of women with endometriosis, particularly in those who were infertile, and provide evidence for a deficiency in the regulation of IL1 actions at the local peritoneal level in initial endometriosis stages, which may result in increased cell reactivity and contribute to endometriosis development and the manifestation of its clinical symptoms.

- **Interleukin-6 (IL-6)** is a pleiotropic cytokine that is produced by a variety of cell types, including monocytes, lymphocytes, fibroblasts, endothelial cells, and mesangial cells. It is said to mediate numerous physiological and pathogenic processes and acts on a wide variety of cells. IL-6 may also have important functions in reproductive physiology, including the regulation of ovarian steroid production, folliculogenesis and early events related to implantation. (Jacobs et al.,1992); (Akoum et al., 1996). Both eutopic and ectopic endometrium are known to produce IL-6 (Harada et al., 1997). Infact IL-6 belongs to the group of cytokines produced in increased amount by endometriotic cells both in basal and cytokine-stimulated conditions (Akoum et al., 1996), (Tsudo et al., 2000). IL-6 in turn is able to increase the secretion of several other cytokines and promotes the activation of immune cells (Iwabe et al., 2002).Examining eutopic endometrium from patients with endometriosis , it was found an increased basal- and IL-1b stimulated production of IL-6 compared with patients without endometriosis. This suggests that the endometrial cells of women who develop endometriosis may function differently from those in women who do not develop this condition. Endometrial stromal cells were considered the critical cells in endometrial attachment to the mesothelial surface of the peritoneum and that endometrial epithelial cells fail to attach to the mesothelium (Scott et al., 1953). It has also been suggested that cellular adhesion itself stimulates chemokine expression (Smith et al.,1997). More interestingly IL-6 family cytokines, such as IL-6, IL-11, leukemia inhibitory factor, and oncostatin M, were shown to be potent stimulators of aromatase expression in adipose stromal cells in culture (Zhao et al.,1995). Yoshioka et al. (Yoshioka et al.,1999) reported that IL-6 inhibits proliferation of endometrial stromal cells derived from the secretory phase but not from the proliferative phase. In contrast, negative regulation by IL-6 was not observed in the stromal cells of endometriotic tissues, suggesting that the biological characteristics of endometriotic cells differ from those of eutopic endometrial cells. Bedaiwy et al. (Bedaiwy et al., 2002) reported that serum IL-6 and peritoneal fluid TNF- α, could be used to discriminate between patients with and without endometriosis with a high degree of sensitivity and specificity. On the other hand, other authors, such as Kalu (Kalu et al, 2007) have failed to confirm this. They did not find any significant differences in the concentration of IL-6 in the sera of women in the two groups and more, they try to explain this result, considering that the measurement of cytokine concentrations is complicated by the fact that they have very short half-lives and are never produced in isolation, but as a mixture which may have similar or opposing effects. So, it is possible that the circulating IL-6, IL-1 b, and TNF- α found by some investigators may be non-functional or antagonized by anti-inflammatory cytokines or cytokine inhibitors. While this may also be true of peritoneal fluid cytokines, the presence of activated macrophages does suggest that at least some of the cytokines are functionally active.

- **Interleukin-8 (IL-8)** is a potent angiogenic cytokine produced by mesothelial cells, macrophages, and endometrial and other cells. Its concentration in the peritoneal fluid of patients with red endometriosis is found to increase as the size and number of active lesions increase (Iwabe et al.,1998). It stimulates adhesion of endometrial stromal cells to extracellular matrix proteins, matrix metalloproteinase activity and endometrial stromal cell proliferation in a dose-dependent manner, all of which can help to promote the implantation and growth of ectopic endometrium (Garcia-Velasco et al.,1999); (Ryan et al.,1995); (American Society for Reproductive Medicine, 1997); (Harada et al.,1997); (Punnonen et al.,1996); (Jolicoeur et al., 1998); (Akoum et al.,2000); (Pizzo et al., 2002) ; (Arci et al., 1998).

- Arici et al. reported that IL-8 is produced in the human endometrium in vivo, mainly in glandular cells (Arici A, et al.,.) and that this interleukin induces proliferation of endometrial stromal cell as a potential autocrine growth factor (Arici et al., 1998). Iwabe et al. (Iwabe et al.,1998) also found that peritoneal fluid levels of IL-8 significantly enhanced proliferation of stromal cells derived from ovarian endometriomas. Expression of IL-8 receptor type A messenger RNA was detected in endometriotic stromal cells These results suggest that IL-8 may promote the progression of endometriosis.

- **Tumor necrosis factor** α (**TNF-** α is a cytokine involved in systemic inflammation and is a member of a group of cytokines that stimulate the acute phase reaction. The primary role of TNF is in the regulation of immune cells. TNF is able to induce apoptotic cell death, to induce inflammation and to inhibit tumorigenesis and viral replication. It is considered the most representative cytokine involved in the pathogenesis of endometriosis: a clear positive association between the content of TNF- α in peritoneal fluid and the severity of endometriosis has been demonstrated (Overton et al.,1996). Numerous studies indicate that both activated macrophages and the ectopic endometrium itself are responsible for the abnormal production of TNF- α in the peritoneal fluid and that this cytokine is involved in the proliferation of endometriotic stromal cells (Iwabe et al., 2000). It acts through both direct and indirect mechanisms, and by mediating the proliferative effect of IL-8 (Sakamoto Y et al., 2003). Moreover, gene and protein expression of IL-8 in the stromal cells of endometriotic tissues are up-regulated by TNF- α (Iwabe et al., 2000), and TNF- α stimulates the proliferation of the endometriotic stromal cells. This stimulatory effect of TNF- α was abolished by adding anti-TNF- α antibody or anti-IL-8 antibody. Therefore, TNF- α may act on stromal cells by mediating the proliferative effects of IL-8. Expression of type I and type II receptors for TNF- α was observed in endometriotic stromal cells. This evidence suggests that TNF- α action mediated by IL-8 may not only be an initiating factor that facilitates adhesion of endometrial cells to the peritoneum but may also contribute to development and progression of endometriosis. Thus, the differential response of endometrial cells to TNF- α in women with and without endometriosis may reflect differential regulation of TNF-receptor expression or signaling by this cytokine. Braun et al. (Braun et al., 2002) published data suggesting that in women without endometriosis, endometrial cells do not implant in ectopic locations because normal apoptotic mechanisms are activated by TNF- α through the TNFR1 receptor and because the proliferation enhancing effects of TNF- α are inhibited by down-regulation of the TNFR2 receptor. Disruption or dysregulation of the normal, cyclical expression of these two TNF- α receptors on endometrium from women with endometriosis could create cells that can grow in the presence of high concentrations of TNF- α a possibility for which evidence is avalaible (Ding et al.,2000). Harada et al. (Harada et al., 1997) and Iwabe et al. (Iwabe et al.,1998) found that the extent of superficial red endometriotic lesions was related to increased levels of IL-6, IL-8, and TNF- α in the peritoneal fluid. Red lesions, such as red flame-like lesions, gland-like lesions, and red vesicles, were classified as active lesions of endometriosis because angiogenesis is more pronounced in red lesions than in black or white lesions (Wiegerick et al.,1993) and because early red lesions invade extracellular matrix (Spuijbroek et al.,1992). Braun et al. (Braun et al., 2002) also suggested that ectopic growth of endometrial cells and the physiological consequences of that growth in women with endometriosis may be retarded by agents that block the effects of TNF- α. Presumably, this could be achieved by blocking TNF- α production (e.g., administration of pentoxifylline or ciprofloxacin) or by blocking the effects of TNF- α on target tissues (e.g., administration of etanercept). The attenuation of the proliferation-enhancing activity in peritoneal fluid from women with endometriosis by etanercept that the athors observed, and results in an animal model of endometriosis using a recombinant human TNF-binding protein (D'Antonio et al., 2000;), support this idea. Blocking the effects of TNF- α on target tissues might be especially appropriate in patients with extensive or intractable disease and might be useful in the postsurgical adjuvant setting to reduce the likelihood of recurrence. Given the potential of TNF- α to play a prominent role in both the etiology and the pathogenicity of endometriosis, studies of such treatment are warranted

- **Interleukin-12 (IL-12)** is naturally produced by dendritic cells (Kaliński Pet al., 1997), macrophages and human B-lymphoblastoid cells in response to antigenic stimulation. It is known as a T cell-stimulating factor, which can stimulate the growth and function of T cells. It stimulates the production of interferon-gamma (IFN-γ) and tumor necrosis factor-alpha (TNF-α) from T and natural killer (NK) cells, and reduces IL-4 mediated suppression of IFN-γ. It acts on T and NK cells, inducing cytokine production, enhancing NK cell cytotoxic activity, and finally favoring generation of Th1 cell response, (Kobayashi et al., 1989) ;(Wysocka et al., 1995) so it seems to play an important role, in the controll of the endometriosis. Harada et al., (Harada et al.,2001)demonstrated that the concentrations of IL-12 in the peritoneal fluid are low, but detectable, regardless of the presence or absence of endometriosis (Zeyneloglu et al., 1998). Administration of IL-12 significantly prevented ectopic endometrial implantation in a murine model of endometriosis (Somigliana et al.,1999). A direct growth inhibitory effect on endometrial cells seems unlikely because endometrial cells do not express receptors for IL-12. A potential explanation for these results is that IL-12 enhances the growth and augments the cytolytic activity of both NK and T cells. These data support the idea that manipulation of cytokine activity in the peritoneal fluid is a novel management approach to controlling the establishment of endometriosis.

3.2 Cytokines and endometriosis related to infertility

Muscato et al. (Muscato et al., 1982) demonstrated that peritoneal macrophages phagocytized sperm in vitro and that macrophages from women with endometriosis were more active than those from women without the disease. Peritoneal fluid diffusing into the tubal and endometrial environment may affect sperm and their interaction with the oocyte. Studies showed that the peritoneal fluid of patients with endometriosis has detrimental effects on sperm function. Sperm motility (Curtis et al., 1993) ;(Drudy et al., 1994), acrosome reaction (Arumugam et al.,1994), gamete interaction (Coddington et al, 1992.), and ovum capture by tubal fimbriae (Suginami et al., 1988) have been studied. Aeby et al. (Aeby et al.,1996), using a penetration assay, showed that peritoneal fluid from patients with endometriosis impaired gamete interaction. In their study, the mean number of eggs penetrated by sperm mixed with peritoneal fluid from patients with endometriosis was significantly less than that observed in controls. These data suggest that substances in the peritoneal fluid of patients with endometriosis contribute to infertility by impairing sperm function. Peritoneal fluid from patients with endometriosis has frequently been shown to be toxic to the preimplantation embryo. A study demonstrated that medical treatment of endometriosis eliminated the embryotoxicity of the peritoneal fluid (Keenan et al.,1995). In this study, the levels of IL-1 and TNF- α were markedly reduced in the peritoneal fluid of women who had undergone medical treatment (danazol or intranasal buserelin for 4 to 6 months) of endometriosis. This finding supports the hypothesis that increased levels of cytokines in peritoneal fluid may be involved in the pathogenesis of endometriosis-associated infertility. One study demonstrated that the addition of human recombinant IL-6 to culture medium suppressed the rate of blastocyst formation of mouse embryos (Harada et al., 1997), suggesting that increased IL-6 in the peritoneal fluid of endometriosis patients may contribute to infertility by adversely affecting embryonic development. Moreover, other authors (Minici et al., 2008) showed that in endometriosis, the milieu surrounding the uterine cavity may be involved in impaired eutopic endometrial stromal cell decidualization, partially due to increased peritoneal levels of TNF- α. So they concluded that in endometriosis either intrinsic defects of endometrial stromal cell differentiation or the biochemical environment of the uterine cavity could concur to compromise the normal decidualization required for optimal implantation.

In conclusion, cytokines, which are produced by many cell types in peritoneal fluid, play a diverse role in constructing the peritoneal environment that induces the development and progression of endometriosis and endometriosis-associated infertility.

Intense basic research into the specific role of these cells and soluble factors may improve our understanding of endometriosis and result in novel therapies for endometriosis.

4. Transforming growth factor beta (TGF-ß)

Transforming growth factor beta (TGF-β) is a protein that controls proliferation, cellular differentiation and other functions in most cells. TGF-β is a secreted protein that exists in at least five isoforms called TGF- ß 1, TGF- ß 2 and TGF- ß 3. It was also the original name for TGF- ß 1, which was the founding member of this family. TGF-beta acts as an antiproliferative factor in normal epithelial cells and at early stages of oncogenesis. Some cells that secrete TGF- ß also have receptors for TGF- ß. This is known as autocrine signalling. Cancerous cells increase their production of TGF-β, which also acts on surrounding cells.Oosterlynck et al. (Oosterlynck et al.,1994) found increased TGF-b activity in the peritoneal fluid of women with endometriosis. Transforming growth factor-b may be a cytokine that inhibits NK activity in the peritoneal fluid of women with endometriosis (Oosterlynck et al.,1994). It may play a major role in the biological processes leading to establishment and maintenance of endometriosis., in fact TGF- ß is implicated in the gene expression, cell motility, proliferation, apoptosis, differentiation, immune responses and tumorigenesis (Derynck et al., 2001). TGF-b is abundantly and differentially expressed in the endometrium and is secreted by endometrial cells and macrophages into the uterine fluid where interaction with the preimplantation embryo is suspected (Jones et al., 2006).

Secretion of TGF-b into peritoneal fluid of women suffering from endometriosis suggests that they may be crucial in establishment and/or maintenance of endometriosis. Omwandho et al., showed that all TGF- ß and their high-affinity receptors were stage-specifically expressed in the human endometrium with highest levels around menstruation . Many researchers have reported staining of TGF-b1 and 3 in stromal and glandular cells (Chegini et al., 1994); (Gold et al., 1994) ; (Johnson et al., 2005) ; (Komiyama et al., 2007); (Gaide Chevronnay et al., 2008) and for TGF-b1 also in nerve fibres (Tamburro et al., 2003) and inflammatory cells specially in macrophages (Chegini et al., 1994); (Tamura et al., 1999); (Komiyama et al., 2007). TGF- ß 2 is more strongly expressed in stromal compared with glandular cells (Gold et al., 1994); (Bruner et al., 1995); (Gaide Chevronnay et al., 2008), although opposite staining intensity has been reported (Chegini et al., 1994). Localization of TbRII and RI was observed in both cellular compartments of the endometrium (Chegini et al., 1994; (Gaide Chevronnay et al., 2008) with stronger expression of TbRII than TbRI (Gaide Chevronnay et al., 2008) suggesting that TbRI might be a limiting factor for signal transduction in the endometrium or during endometriosis. TGF-b1 was found in the stromal cells (Johnson et al., 2005) and expression increased in the epithelial cells of endometriotic cysts (Tamura et al., 1999) and endometriotic nerve fibers (Tamburro et al., 2003). The TGF-b signal transducers Smad3, pSmad3, Smad4 (SMADs are intracellular proteins that transduce extracellular signals from TGF beta ligands to the nucleus where they activate downstream TGF- ß gene transcription) and the inhibitory Smad7 proteins were also observed in the endometrial stromal and epithelial cells (Luo et al., 2003). These observation suggest a role of the TGF- ß s in the normal function of the human endometrium. In fact is well known that TGF- ß sprevent the breakdown of the endometrial tissue (Tabibzadeh, 2002). This assumption is based on the observation that Lefty-2/EBAF (endometrial bleeding associated factor), a member of the TGF-b family, is dramatically up-regulated during endometriosis (Kothapalli et al., 1997) and antagonized TGF- ß signaling by inhibiting phosphorylation of Smad2 downstream of the TbRI (Ulloa et al., 2001). That Lefty-2 was noticeably more abundant in patients with endometriosis who did not conceive compared with those who became pregnant, suggested a role in implantation (Tabibzadeh et al., 2000). More, it has been shown that TGF- ß 1also induces contractions of decidual stromal cells (Kimatrai et al., 2003) and inhibits motility of stromal endometrial cells (Nasu et al., 2005).It is important to show how TGF- ß 1stimulated DNA synthesis in epithelial cells at low concentrations, but inhibited DNA synthesis at higher concentrations in women with and without endometriosis (Meresman et al., 2003). Additional evidence showed that TGF- ß 1induces expression of FasL mRNA and protein in endometrial stromal cells (Garci-Velasco et al., 1999), possibly preventing apoptosis during transit to the peritoneal cavity. Another very important analysis showed that TGF- ß 1represses the immune system (Shull et al., 1992) and the escape from immune surveillance is also important for adhesion of endometriotic cells in the peritoneum. Finally TGF- ßs participate in the initiation of menstruation via vasoconstriction, in menstrual tissue repair and in endometriosis. In a classic experiment, Luo et al. (2003b) demonstrated that the pretreatment with a GnRH antaonist resulted in further suppression of Smad3 in endometrial stromal cells but co-treatment with GnRH and TGF- ß 1or pretreatment with TbRII antisense partially inhibited TGF- ß 1-activated Smad3. Taken collectively, these observations suggest that GnRH may prevent endometriosis by altering expression and activation of Smads and interrupting TGF- ß receptor signaling.

5. Plasminogen activator (uPA) and matrix metalloproteinase systems (MMS)

5.1 Plasminogen activator system (PA)

The PA system includes a wide cluster of proteolytic enzymes for plasmin generation. Plasminogen is activated to plasmin by two types of activators, urokinase-type PA (uPA) and tissue- type PA (tPA). Whereas tPA is involved in the role in the control of intravascular fibrin degradation, uPA is mainly implicated in cellular proteolysis and migration. The activity of the PAs is regulated by specific PA inhibitors (PAIs). (Kruithof et al., 1995; Grancha et al., 1996; Heeb et al., 1987).

The PA system and its specific plasminogen activator inhibitors (PAIs) exert physiological and pathophysiological functions such as fibrinolysis, tissue remodelling and tumor invasion, signal transduction, cell adherence and cell migration (Harbeck et al., 2001).

Fernández-Shaw et al., firstly reported high levels of urokinase and plasminogen in ectopic endometrium as a more invasive nature of the endometriotic implants in the peritoneal cavità (Fernández-Shawet al., 1995); afterwards, Sillem confirmed an altered activation of plasminogen in endometrium from women with endometriosis that could lead to a higher proteolytic potential of retrogradely menstruated endometrial fragments with consecutive development of endometriotic foci (Sillem et al., 1997).

In situ hybridization studies performed by Bruse et al. showed that uPA mRNA seems to be up-regulated in both endometriotic glands and endometrial stroma from women with endometriosis (Bruse et al., 2005).

Moreover, Lembessis and coworkers reported an increase in uPA mRNA expression in endometriotic lesions compared to eutopic endometrium (Lembessis et al. (2003).

Despite contrasting data in vitro culture model (Guan et al., 2002) ; recently, Cosin reported an increase in uPA antigenic levels in endometrium from women with endometriosis (Cosin et al., 2010)

In relation to PA levels in eutopic endometrium from women with endometriosis, it has been suggested that a higher concentration of uPA in the endometrium might result in endometrial fragments with a higher potential to degrade the extracellular matrix after the implantation at ectopic sites (Spuijbroek et al., 1992; Bruse et al., 1998, 2004; Kobayashi, 2000).

5.2 Matrix metalloproteinase systems (MMPs)

Matrix metalloproteinases (MMPs) are a class of zinc-dependent endopeptidases involved in extracellular matrix remodelling (Matrisian, 1992).

Members of this family share high level of structural analogy and are secreted by several cell types as zymogens. In relation to substrate preference and protein-domain considerations, MMP family members have been categorized into subgroups that include gelatinases, stromelysins, collagenases, membrane-type (MT)-MMPs and 'other MMPs'.

The activity of metalloproteinases is tightly regulated,as these molecules are potent proteolytic enzymes, at differente steps: transcriptional level (by cytokines, chemicals, and growth factors), post-translation modification and by a family of inhibitors: the tissue inhibitors of metalloproteinases or TIMPs (Matrisian, 1990).

Elevated cytokines may play a role in the establishment of ectopic endometrium in the peritoneal cavity by stimulating MMPs to remodel the mesothelial lining of the peritoneum thus allowing for tissue invasion.

MMPs are stimulated by cytokines and also by the protein Extracellular Matrix Metalloproteinase Inducer (EMMPRIN). Braundmeier et al., showed that IL-1beta stimulated MMP-1 protein secretion and mRNA levels in a time dependent manner ($P < 0.05$), MMP-2 mRNA in a time dependent manner and MMP-3 in a time and dose dependent manner. TNF-alpha stimulated MMP-1 and -3 protein secretion in a time dependent manner and stimulated MMP-1, -2 and -3 mRNA levels in a time dependent manner). Neither IL-1beta nor TNF-alpha treatment affected MMP-2 protein secretion. TGF-beta-1 inhibited MMP-1 and MMP-2 mRNAs at the highest treatment dose after 24 hr but there was no effect on protein secretion. TGF-beta-1 exerted no effect on MMP-3 mRNA or protein secretion (Braundmeier et al., 2010).

MMPs have been implicated in the endometrial remodelling during the menstrual cycle with higher levels during menstrual and proliferative phases and decreased levels during the secretory phase (Salamonsen and Woolley, 1996);

Montly, in the absence of pregnancy, degradation of the ECM is a critical step in the initiation of tissue breakdown that leads to menstruation (Marbaix *et al.*, 1996; Salamonsen and Woolley, 1996).

During the proliferative phase of the natural cycle, MMP-1, MMP-3 and MMP-9 are downregulated in the stroma (Hulboy *et al.*, 1997), presumably to allow endometrial stable growth. The expression of MMPs then decline in the early secretory phase and then increase during the late secretory phase in anticipation of the next proliferative phase. These modification are related to serum progesterone levels, which has led to the suggestion that endometrial expression of MMPs is under gonadal steroid hormone control. Critically, MMP-9 expression is highest in the menstrual phase endometrium when tissue breakdown occurs.

Moreover, several repots suggest that these proteases are also involved in the ectopic invasion of endometriotic cells associated with endometriosis (Cox et al., 2001).

Deregulation of peritoneal fluid cytokines levels of women with endometriosis show indicate that an altered immune system may play an important role in the pathogenesis of endometriosis. The invasion of ectopic endometrium into peritoneal mesothelium, in association of different angiogenic factors, requires matrix metalloproteinases (MMPs) for tissue remodeling. Several MMPs are differentially expressed in human uterine endometrium with menstrual endometrium showing the highest level of expression. (Braundmeier et al., 2010)

MMP systems closely interact with PA system, because plasmin is an active enzyme, which degrades a variety of extracellular matrix proteins and activates MMPs and growth factors (Murphy et al., 2000).

The catalytic domains of all MMPs share high amino acid similarity and their active sites are extensively conserved (Lauer-Fields et al., 2009). As a consequence, differenciate between different MMPs activities is extraordinarily difficult. However, some members of these proteases showed a role in the pathogenesis of endometriosis.

Matrix metalloproteinase 7 (MMP7): MMP7 is secreted mostly from the endometrial epithelium cells during the receptive phase localized to endometrial glandular and luminal epithelium (Yanaihara et al., 2004; Zhang et al., 2005)

Moreover, MMP-7 has been shown to be the dominant metalloproteinase during the initial development of endometriosis in a baboon model (Fazleabas et al., 2002). In addition, a recent study clearly demonstrated that MMP-7 mRNA was identified in host peritoneal tissues during the development of endometriosis in a nude mouse model (Hull et al., 2008)

MMP-7 protein expression in epithelial cells was significantly higher in red peritoneal lesions compared with that of deep infiltrating endometriosis, ovarian endometriosis and black peritoneal lesions, in all phases of the menstrual cycle. MMP-7 protein expression may be down-regulated during the evolution of peritoneal endometriotic implants, as active red lesions transition into inactive black lesions (Matsuzaki et al., 2010).

Matrix metalloproteinase 5 (MMP5): The strongest MMP5 staining was seen in luminal epithelial cells, whereas endometrial glands frequently showed partial expression.

Both the gene chip expression analyses as well as PCR indicated strongly elevated transcript levels in most peritoneal endometriosis lesions. Moreover enhanced MT5-MMP expression has been detected in the eutopic endometrium from patients suffering from endometriosis. (Gaetje et al., 2007)

Matrix metalloproteinase 3 (MMP3): IMMP-3 is hormonally regulated during the menstrual cycle, with the highest levels of expression occurring during menses local regulation that is absent in the in vitro cultures. (Hulboy et al., 1997;.)

MMP-3 has not been well studied in endometriosis, however, studies suggest that retrogradely shed menstrual fragments, the putative precursors of endometriotic lesions, express high levels of MMP- 3 (Koks et al., 2000).

Cox et al, demonstrated in a rat model that elevated MMP-3 expression by endometrial tissue leads to the establishment and progression of ectopic endometrial tissue growth. (KE. Cox, et al., 2001).

Significant expression differences were obtained for MMP3 in the ovarian endometriomas. The deregulation of the different genes, included MMP3 genes, may be responsible for the loss of cellular homeostasis in endometriotic lesions (Meola et al., 2010)

Matrix metalloproteinase 2 (MMP): Overexpression of stromal MMP-2 may play a role in the development of adenomyosis (Tokyol et al., 2009)

Matrix metalloproteinase 9 (MMP9): Eutopic endometrium of women with endometriosis compared with normal women showed an increased release of MMP-9, and a decreased release of its natural inhibitor, TIMP-1, at both the protein and the mRNA levels (Chen *et al.* 2004; Collette et al., 2004; Collette et al., 2006).

5.2.1 Genetic polymorphism of MMPs family

Genetic polymorphisms located in the promoter region of the MMP genes could lead to increased gene expression and could be associated with predisposition to endometriosis (Ye, 2006). Nevertheless, the genetic susceptibility of endometriosis in relation to MMPs polymorphism is very complex, because for several polymorphisms, allele frequencies were found to be significantly different according to ethnic origin (MMP2.1, MMP2.2, MMP3 and MMP12).

Borghese et al., investigated the role of MMP1, MMP2, MMP3, MMP7, MMP12 and MMP13 polymorphisms as endometriosis risk factors in a case – control study of patients affected by superficial, deep infiltrating or endometrioma in the Caucasian population. The study found a potential role for MMP12 -82 A/G and MMP13 -77 A/G combined polymorphisms, which modulate transcriptional activity, in superficial endometriosis. As no association was found with deep infiltrating endometriosis, this combination of polymorphisms might protect from a more in-depth penetration of tissues (Borghese et al., 2008). On the other hand, they did not find any correlation between endometriosis and MMP1, MMP2, MMP3, MMP7 polymorphism (Borghese et al., 2008). Data regarding the lack of association between MMP-1 e MMP-3 polymorphism and endometriosis susceptibility were confirmed in another study concerning the Italian population (Ferrari et al., 2006).

A case-control study in women of caucasian origin, evaluated the potential associations of MMP-2 and MMP-9 gene promoter region polymorphisms as well as MMP-2 promoter haplotypes with susceptibility to endometriosis. The results demonstrated that polymorphisms in MMP-2 (-735 C/T) and MMP-9 (-1562 C/T) were associated with elevated risk of endometriosis and that certain MMP-2 promoter haplotypes were more common in control group (Saare et al., 2010).

A genetic study regarding North Chinese women on three polymorphisms in the MMP-2 (MMP-2; -1306C-->T and -735C-->T) and TIMP-2 (TIMP-2; -418G-->C) genes found that the TIMP-2 -418C/C homozygote may be a protective factor against the development of endometriosis (Kang et al., 2008). A analogous study in the same population showed that MMP-7-181A/G polymorphism has a potential to be a susceptibility factor for endometriosis and adenomyosis while MMP-9-1562C/T polymorphism may not provide a useful marker to predict susceptibility to endometriosis and adenomyosis (Shan et al., 2006). On the other hand, an increase in the distribution of the MMP-9R279Q/P574R (2678G>A/4859C>G) and -1562C>T/R668Q (-1562C>T/5546G>A) haplotypes was significantly associated with endometriosis (Han et al., 2009).

5.2.2 Relevance of MMPs serum/urinary levels as diagnostic markers

The balance between MMPs and their inhibitors is preserved in the serum of women with endometriosis; however MMP-3 mRNA seems to be a promising peripheral blood marker that discriminates between patients with endometriosis and healthy subjects. Circulating mRNA for MMP-3 is significantly higher in patients with endometriosis than in control patients, regardless of the degree of severity. (De Sanctis et al., 2010).

Conversely, the clinical relevance of MMP-2 and MMP-9 as markers of endometriosis is controversial; some data report that serum concentrations of MMP-2, MMP-9, TIMP-1 and TIMP-2 cannot be considered to represent a valid measure of the severity of endometriosis

(Salata et al., 2008; De Sanctis et al., 2010). On the other hand a prospective, blinded, longitudinal study show that MMP-2, MMP-9, and MMP-9/neutrophil gelatinase-associated lipocalin were significantly more likely to be detected in the urine of patients with endometriosis than in controls (Beker et al. 2010).

Bruner-Tran et al. described progesterone treatment inhibits expression of MMP-3 and -7 in human endometrium and prevents the establishment of ectopic lesions in a nude mouse model (Bruner-Tran et al., 2002).

A study concerning human endometrium intraperitoneally transplanted into nude mice, demonstrated a significant suppression of MMP-2 transcription by all progestins tested, and a significant down-regulation of MMP-3 by dydrogesterone (Mönckedieck et al., 2009).

In conclusion, angiogenesis is proposed as an important mechanism for the pathogenesis of endometriosis. Different evidences support the hypothesis that the endometrium of women with endometriosis has an increased capacity to proliferate, implant and grow in the peritoneal cavity. Further studies are needed to better understand critical steps of the pathogenesis of endometriosis; nevertheless excessive endometrial angiogenesis suggests novel new medical treatments.

6. References

Aeby TC, Huang T, Nakayama RT. The effect of peritoneal fluid from patients with endometriosis on human sperm function in vitro. Am J Obstet Gynecol 1996;174:1779–85

Akoum A, Jolicoeur C, Boucher A. Estradiol amplifies interleukin-1 induced monocyte chemotactic protein-1 by ectopic endometrial cells of womenwith endometriosis. J Clin Endocrinol Metab 2000; 85: 896–904.

Akoum A, Jolicoeur C, Kharfi A, Aube M. Decreased expression of the decoy interleukin-1 receptor type II in human endometriosis. Am J Pathol 2001;158:481–9.

Akoum A, Lemay A, Brunet C, Hebert J. Cytokine-induced secretion of monocyte chemotactic protein-1 by human endometriotic cells in culture. The Groupe d'Investigation en Gynecologie. Am J Obstet Gynecol 1995;172:594–600.

Akoum A, Lemay A, Maheux R. Estradiol and interleukin-1beta exert a synergistic stimulatory effect on the expression of the chemokine regulated upon activation, normal T cell expressed, and secreted in endometriotic cells. J Clin Endocrinol Metab 2002;87:5785–92.

Akoum A, Lemay A, Paradis L, Rheault N, Maheux R. Secretion of interleukine-6 by human endometriotic cells and regulation by proinflammatory cytokines and sex steroids. Hum Reprod 1996; 11: 2269–2275.

Akoum A, Mahera Al-Akoum, Andre Lemay, Rodolphe Maheux,Mathieu Leboeuf. Imbalance in the peritoneal levels of interleukin 1 and its decoy inhibitory receptor type II in endometriosis nwomen with infertility and pelvic pain. Fertility and Sterility 2008; 89, 6.

American Society for Reproductive Medicine. Revised American Society for Reproductive Medicine classification of endometriosis. Fertil Steril 1997; 67: 817–821.

Arci A, Seli E, Zeyneloglu HB, Senturk LM, Oral E, Olive DL. Interleukin-8 induces proliferation of endometrial stromal cells: a potential autocrine growth factor. J Clin Endocrinol Metab 1998; 83: 1201–1205.

Arici A, Tazuke SI, Attar E, Kliman HJ, Olive DL. Interleukin-8 concentration in peritoneal fluid of patients with endometriosis and modulation of interleukin-8 expression in human mesothelial cells. Mol Hum Reprod 1996;2:40–45. 28.

Arumugam K. Endometriosis and infertility: raised iron concentration in the peritoneal fluid and its effect on the acrosome reaction. Hum Reprod 1994;9:1153–7.

Becker CM, Louis G, Exarhopoulos A, Mechsner S, Ebert AD, Zurakowski D, Moses MA. Matrix metalloproteinases are elevated in the urine of patients with endometriosis. Fertil Steril. 2010 Nov;94(6):2343-6. Epub 2010 Apr 7.

Bedaiwy MA, Falcone T, Sharma RK et al. Prediction of endometriosis with serum and peritoneal markers: a prospective controlled trial. Hum Reprod 2002; 17: 426– 431

Betjes MGH, Tuk CW, Struik DG, Kredict RT, Arisz L, Hart M, et al. Interleukin-8 production by human peritoneal mesothelial cells in response to tumor necrosis factor-a, interleukin-1, and medium conditioned by macrophages co-cultured with Staphylococcus epidermidis. J Infect Dis 1993;168:1202–10.

Borghese B, Chiche JD, Vernerey D, Chenot C, Mir O, Bijaoui G, Bonaiti-Pellié C, Chapron C. Genetic polymorphisms of matrix metalloproteinase 12 and 13 genes are implicated in endometriosis progression. Hum Reprod. 2008 May;23(5):1207-13. Epub 2008 Feb 28.

Bossu P, Visconti U, Ruggiero P, Macchia G, Muda M, Bertini R, et al. Transfected type II interleukin- 1 receptor impairs responsiveness of human keratinocytes to interleukin- 1. Am J Pathol 1995;147:1852–61.

Boyle, J. J. . Macrophage activation in atherosclerosis: pathogenesis and pharmacology of plaque rupture. Curr Vasc Pharmacol, 3(1), 63-68. (2005)

Braun D.P., Jianchi Ding, W. Paul Dmowski. Peritoneal fluid–mediated enhancement of eutopic and ectopic endometrial cell proliferation is dependent on tumor necrosis factor-□ in women with endometriosis . Fertil Steril, 78,4,OCTOBER 2002

Braundmeier AG, Fazleabas AT, Nowak RA. Extracellular matrix metalloproteinase inducer expression in the baboon endometrium: menstrual cycle and endometriosis. Reproduction 2010 Dec;140(6):911-20. Epub 2010 Sep 14.

Bruner KL, Rodgers WH, Gold LI, Korc M, Hargrove JT, Matrisian LM, Osteen KG. Transforming growth factor-b mediates the progesterone suppression of an epithelial metalloproteinase by adjacent stroma in the human endometrium. Proc Natl Acad Sci USA 1995;92:7362–7366

Bruner-Tran KL, Eisenberg E, Yeaman GR, Anderson TA, McBean J, Osteen KG Steroid and cytokine regulation of matrix metalloproteinase expression in endometriosis and the establishment of experimental endometriosis in nude mice. *J Clin Endocrinol Metab* 2002;87:4782-4791.

Bruse C, Gan Y, Carlberg M, Carlström K, Bergqvist A. Basal release of urokinase plasminogen activator, plasminogen activator inhibitor-1, and soluble plasminogen activator receptor from separated and cultured endometriotic and endometrial stromal and epithelial cells. Fertil Steril. 2005 Apr;83 Suppl 1:1155-60

Chegini N, Zhao Y, Williams RS, Flanders KC. Human uterine tissue throughout the menstrual cycle expresses transforming growth factor-b1 (TGFb1), TGFb2, TGFb3, and TGFb type II receptor messenger ribonucleic acid and protein and contains [125I]TGFb1-binding sites. Endocrinology 1994;135:439–449.

Chen QH, Qu JY, Xu YY, Qiu NX, Zhuang YZ, Zhong S, Fang QQ [Expressions of matrix metalloproteinase-9 and tissue inhibitor of metalloproteinase-1 in ectopic and eutopic endometrium]. *Zhonghua Fu Chan Ke Za Zhi* 2004;39:809-812.

Collette T, Bellehumeur C, Kats R, Maheux R, Mailloux J, Villeneuve M, Akoum A. Evidence for an increased release of proteolytic activity by the eutopic endometrial tissue in women with endometriosis and for involvement of matrix metalloproteinase-9. *Hum Reprod* 2004;19:1257-1264.

Collette T, Maheux R, Mailloux J, Akoum A Increased expression of matrix metalloproteinase-9 in the eutopic endometrial tissue of women with endometriosis. *Hum Reprod.* 2006 Dec;21(12):3059-67. Epub 2006 Jul 31.

Colotta F, Re F, Muzio M, Bertini R, Polentarutti N, Sironi M, et al. Interleukin-1 type II receptor: a decoy target for IL-1 that is regulated by IL-4. Science 1993;261:472–5.

Cosín R, Gilabert-Estellés J, Ramón LA, Gómez-Lechón MJ, Gilabert J, Chirivella M, Braza-Boïls A, España F, Estellés A.Influence of peritoneal fluid on the expression of angiogenic and proteolytic factors in cultures of endometrial cells from women with endometriosis. Hum Reprod. 2010 Feb;25(2):398-405. Epub 2009 Nov 26.

Cox KE, Piva M and Sharpe-Timms KL (2001) Differential regulation of matrix metalloproteinase-3 gene expression in endometriotic lesions compared with endometrium. Biol Reprod 65,1297 - 1303.

Cui X, Rouhani FN, Hawari F, Levine SJ. Shedding of the type II IL-1 decoy receptor requires a multifunctional aminopeptidase, aminopeptidase regulator of TNF receptor type 1 shedding. J Immunol 2003;171: 6814–9.

Curtis P, Jackson AE. Adverse effects on sperm movement characteristics in women with minimal and mild endometriosis. Br J Obstet Gynecol 1993;100:165–9.

D'Antonio M, Martelli F, Peano S, Papoian R, Borrelli F. Ability of recombinant human TNF binding protein-1 (r-hTBP-1) to inhibit the development of experimentally-induced endometriosis in rats. J Reprod Immunol 2000;48:81–98.

Daniel T. Rein M.D. Torsten Schmidt M.D., et al (2010) Treatment of endometriosis with a VEGF-targeted conditionally replicative adenovirus. Fertil Steril Vol93 (8): 2687-2694

De Sanctis P, Elmakky A, Farina A, Caramelli E, Seracchioli R, Mabrouk M, Mignemi G, Venturoli S, Villa G, Guerrini M, Manuzzi L, Montanari G, Valvassori L, Zucchini C. Matrix metalloproteinase-3 mRNA: a promising peripheral blood marker for diagnosis of endometriosis. Gynecol Obstet Invest. 2011;71(2):118-23. Epub 2010 Dec 9.

Derynck R, Akhurst RJ, Balmain A. TGF-b signaling in tumor suppression and cancer progression. Nat Genet 2001;29:117–129.

Di Carlo C, Bonifacio M, Tommaselli G et al (2009). Metalloproteinases, vascular endothelial growth factor and angiopoietin 1 and 2 in eutopic and ectopic endometrium. *Fertil Steril* 91:2316-2323.

Dinarello CA. Therapeutic strategies to reduce IL-1 activity in treating local and systemic inflammation. Curr Opin Pharmacol 2004;4:378–85.

Ding J, Shen M, Gogacz M, Braun DP, Rana N, Dmowski WP. Endometrial apoptosis is inhibited in vitro by TNF-alfain women with endometriosis and is stimulated by TNF-alfa in healthy women. J Soc Gynecol Invest 2000; 47:218A.

Drudy L, Lewis SEM, Kinsella CB, Harrison RF, Thompson W. The influence of peritoneal fluid from patients with minimal stage or treated endometriosis on sperm motility parameters using computerassisted semen analysis. Hum Reprod 1994;9:2418 -23

Essam-Eldin R. Othman M.D , Salama Salama Ph.D., Nahed Ismail Ph.D., M.D. and Ayman Al-Hendy Ph.D., M.D. (2007)Toward gene therapy of endometriosis: adenovirus-mediated delivery of dominant negative estrogen receptor genes inhibits cell proliferation, reduces cytokine production, and induces apoptosis of endometriotic cells. Fertility and Sterility Volume 88, Issue 2, , Pages 462-471

Fakih H, Baggett B, Holtz G, Tsang K-Y, Lee JC, Williamson HO. Interleukin-1: possible role in the infertility associated endometriosis. Fertil Steril 1987;47:213–7.

Fasciani A., D'Ambrogio G., Monti M., Bocci G, Genazzani A.R., Artini P.G. (2000) High concentration of the vascular endothelial growth factor and interleukin-8 in ovarian endometrioma. Mol.Hum. Reprod. Vol 6., n°1:50-54

Fazleabas AT, Brudney A, Gurates B, Chai D, Bulun S. A modified baboon model for endometriosis. Ann N Y Acad Sci 2002;955:308 - 317.).

Fengying, H, Qiuhong L, Huaping w et al (2010). Effect of Gnrh II on secretion of VEGF by eutopic and ectopic endometrial stromal cells of endometriosis patients. J Cent South Univ (Med Sci) 35(5)

Fernández-Shaw S, Marshall JM, Hicks B, Barlow DH, Starkey PM. Plasminogen activators in ectopic and uterine endometrium. Fertil Steril. 1995 Jan;63(1):45-51.

Ferrari MM, Biondi ML, Rossi G, Grijuela B, Gaita S, Perugino G, Viganò P. Analysis of two polymorphisms in the promoter region of matrix metalloproteinase 1 and 3 genes in women with endometriosis. Acta Obstet Gynecol Scand. 2006;85(2):212-7.

Fraser HM and Lunn SF (2000) Angiogenesis and its control in the female reproductive system. *Br Med Bull* 56:787–797.

Gaetje R, Holtrich U, Engels K, Kourtis K, Cikrit E, Kissler S, Rody A, Karn T, Kaufmann M. Expression of membrane-type 5 matrix metalloproteinase in human endometrium and endometriosis. Gynecol Endocrinol. 2007 Oct;23(10):567-73.

Gaide Chevronnay HP, Cornet PB, Delvaux D, Lemoine P, Courtoy PJ, Henriet P, Marbaix E. Opposite regulation of transforming growth factor-b2 and -b3 expression in the human endometrium. Endocrinology 2008; 149:1015–1025

Garcia-Velasco JA, Arici A, Zreik T, Naftolin F, Mor G. Macrophagederived growth factors modulate Fas ligand expression in cultured endometrial stromal cells: a role in endometriosis. Mol Hum Reprod 1997;5:642–650.

Garcia-Velasco JA, Arici A. Interleukin-8 stimulates the adhesion of endometrial stromal cells to fibronectin. Fertil Steril 1999; 72: 336–340.

Gentilini D, Somigliana E, Vigano P, et al (2008). The vascular endothelial growth factor +405G>C polymorphism in endometriosis. *Hum Reprod.* 23:211-215.

Gilabert-Estelles J, Ramon LA, Espana F et al. (2007) Expression of angiogenic factors in endometriosis: relationship to fibrinolytic and metalloproteinase systems. *Hum Reprod*, 22:2120-2127.

Giudice LC, Kao LC. Endometriosis (review). Lancet 2004; 364:1789 - 1799.; Hull ML, Escareno CR, Godsland JM, Doig JR, Johnson CM, Phillips SC, Smith SK, Tavare S,

Print CG, Charnock-Jones DS. Endometrial-peritoneal interactions during endometriotic lesion establishment. Am J Pathol 2008;173:700 - 715).

Gilman A, Goodman LS, Hardman JG, Limbird LE Goodman & Gilman's the pharmacological basis of therapeutics. New York: McGraw-Hill. ISBN 0-07-135469-7. (2001).

Gold LI, Saxena B, Mittal KR, Marmor M, Goswami S, Nactigal L, Korc M, Demopoulos RI. Increased expression of transforming growth factorb isoforms and basic fibroblast growth factor in complex hyperplasia and adenocarcinoma of the endometrium: evidence for paracrine and autocrine action. Cancer Res 1994;54:2347–2358.

Gordon, J., Shifren, J., Foulk, R. et al. (1995) Angiogenesis in the human female reproductive tract. *Obstet. Gynecol. Surv.*, 50, 688–697.

Goteri G, Lucarini G, Filosa A et al (2004) Immunoistochimical analysis of vascular endothelial growth factor cellular expression in ovarian endometrioma. *Fertil Steril* 81: 1528-1533

Goteri G, Lucarini G, Zizzi A, et al (2010) Proangiogenetic molecole, hypoxia-inducible factor 1-α and nitric oxide synthase isoforms in ovarian endometirotic cyst. *Virchows Arch* 456: 703-710.

Grancha S, Estelles A, Gilabert J, Chirivella M, Espana F, Aznar J and Loskutoff DJ (1996) Decreased expression of PAI-2 mRNA and protein in pregnancies complicated with intrauterine fetal growth retardation. Thromb Haemostas 76,761 - 767.

Groothuis PG, Nap AW, Winterhager E, Grümmer R. Vascular development in endometriosis Angiogenesis. 2005;8(2):147-56. Epub 2005 Oct 7. Review.

Guan YM, Carlberg M, Bruse C, Carlström K, Bergqvist A. Effects of hormones on uPA, PAI-1 and suPAR from cultured endometrial and ovarian endometriotic stromal cells. Acta Obstet Gynecol Scand. 2002 May;81(5):389-97.);

Halme J, Becker S, Wing R. Accentuated cyclic activation of peritoneal macrophages in patients with endometriosis. Am J Obstet Gynecol 1984;148:85–90

Halme J. Release of tumor necrosis factor-a by human peritoneal macrophages in vivo and vitro. Am J Obstet Gynecol 1989;161:1718– 25.

Han YJ, Kim HN, Yoon JK, Yi SY, Moon HS, Ahn JJ, Kim HL, Chung HW.

Haplotype analysis of the matrix metalloproteinase-9 gene associated with advanced-stage endometriosis. Fertil Steril. 2009 Jun;91(6):2324-30. Epub 2008 Jun 12.

Harada T, Enatsu A, Yoshida S et al. Increased interleukin-6 levels in peritoneal fluid of infertile patients with active endometriosis. Am J Obstet Gynecol 1997; 176: 593-597.

Harada T, Iwabe T, Terakawa N. Role of cytokines in endometriosis. Fertil Steril 2001;76:1-10.

Harada T, Terakawa N. Cytokines in peritoneal fluid from women with active endometriosis. In: Minaguchi H, Sugimoto O (eds). Endometriosis today. New York: Parthenon, 1997:144–8.

Harada T, Yoshioka H, Yoshida S, Iwabe T, Onohara Y, Tanikawa M, et al. Increased interleukin-6 levels in peritoneal fluid of infertile patients with active endometriosis. Am J Obstet Gynecol 1997;176: 593–7.

Harbeck N, Kruger A, Sinz S, Kates RE, Thomssen C, Schmitt M and Janicke F (2001) Clinical relevance of the plasminogen activator inhibitor type 1—a multifaceted proteolytic factor. Onkologie 24,238 - 244.

Heeb MJ, Espana F, Geiger M, Collen D, Stump DC and Griffin JH (1987) Immunological identity of heparine dependent plasma and urinary protein C inhibitor and plasminogen activator inhibitor-3. J Biol Chem 262, 15813 - 15816.

Hyder SM, Stancel GM. Regulation of angiogenic growth factors in the female reproductive tract by estrogens and progestins. Mol Endocrinol. 1999 Jun;13(6):806-11. Review.

Ho HN, Wu MY, Chao KH, Chen CD, Chen SU, Yang YS. Peritoneal interleukin-10 increases with decrease in activated CD4þ T lymphocytes in women with endometriosis. Hum Reprod 1997;12:2528–2533.]

Hodgen GD. Peritoneal fluid from patients with endometriosis decreases sperm binding to the zona pellucida in the hemizona assay: a preliminary report. Fertil Steril 1992;57:783- 6.

Hulboy DL, Rudolph LA, Matrisian LM. Matrix metalloproteinases as mediators of reproductive function. Mol Hum Reprod 1997; 3:27- 45.

Hull ML, Escareno CR, Godsland JM, Doig JR, Johnson CM, Phillips SC, Smith SK, Tavare S, Print CG, Charnock-Jones DS. Endometrial-peritoneal interactions during endometriotic lesion establishment. Am J Pathol 2008;173:700 - 715.

Hyder SM, Stancel GM (1999) Regulation of angiogenic growth factors in the female r eproductive tract by estrogens and progestins. *Mol Endocrinol* 13:806–811.

Imesch P, Samartzis E, Schneider M et al (2011).Inhibition of transcription, expression, and secretion of the vascular epithelial growth factor in human epithelial endoemtriotic cells by romidepsin. Fertil Steril. 95(5):1580-1583.

Iwabe T, Harada T, Terakawa N. Role of cytokines in endometriosis-associated infertility. Gynecol Obstet Invest 2002;53(Suppl 1):19–25.

Iwabe T, Harada T, Tsudo T, Nagano Y, Tanikawa M, Terakawa N. Tumor necrosis factor-a promotes proliferation of the endometrio tic stromal cells by inducing interleukin-8 gene and protein expression. J Clin Endocrinol Metab 2000;85:824 -9

Iwabe T, Harada T, Tsudo T, Tanikawa M, Onohara Y, Terakawa N. Pathogenetic significance of increased levels of interleukin-8 in peritoneal fluid of patients with endometriosis. Fertil Steril 1998;69:924- 30.

Jacobs AL, Sehgal PB, Julian J, Carson DD. Secretion and hormonal regulation of interleukine-6 production by mouse uterine stromal and polarized epithelial cells cultured in vitro. Endocrinology 1992; 131: 1037–1045.

Johnson MC, Torres M, Alves A, Bacallao K, Fuentes A, Vega M, Boric MA. Augmented cell survival in eutopic endometrium from women with endometriosis: expression of c-myc, TGF-beta1 and bax genes. Reprod Biol Endocrinol 2005;3:45.

Jolicoeur C, Boutouil M, Drouin R, Paradis I, Lemay A, Akoum A. Increase expression of monocyte protein-1 in the endometrium of women with endometriosis. Am J Pathol 1998; 152: 125–133.

Jones RL, Stoikos C, Findlay JK, Salamonsen LA. TGF-ß superfamily expression and actions in the endometrium and placenta. Reproduction 2006;132:217–232.

Kaliński P, Hilkens CM, Snijders A, Snijdewint FG, Kapsenberg ML (1997). "IL-12-deficient dendritic cells, generated in the presence of prostaglandin E2, promote type 2 cytokine production in maturing human naive T helper cells". J. Immunol. 159 (1): 28–35.

Kalu E, Nazira Sumar, Theodoros Giannopoulos, Pinika Patel, Carolyn Croucher, Elizabeth Sherriff,Amolak Bansal. Cytokine profiles in serum and peritoneal fluid from infertile women with and without endometriosis. J. Obstet. Gynaecol. Res. Vol. 33, No. 4: 490–495, August 2007

Kang S, Zhao XW, Wang N, Chen SC, Zhou RM, Li Y. Association of polymorphisms of the MMP-2 and TIMP-2 genes with the risk of endometriosis in North Chinese women. Fertil Steril. 2008 Nov;90(5):2023-9. Epub 2008 Jan 4.

Keenan JA, Chen TT, Chadwell NL, Torry DS, Caudle MR. IL-1 beta, TNF-alpha, and IL-2 in peritoneal fluid and macrophage-conditioned media of women with endometriosis. Am J Reprod Immunol 1995;34: 381–5

Kharfi A, Akoum A. Soluble interleukin-1 receptor type II blocks monocyte chemotactic protein-1 secretion by U937 cells in response to peripheral blood serum of women with endometriosis. Fertil Steril 2002;78: 836–42.).

Kharfi A, Boucher A, Akoum A. Abnormal interleukin-1 receptor type II gene expression in the endometrium of women with endometriosis. Biol Reprod 2002;66:401–6.

Kimatrai M, Oliver C, Abadia-Molina AC, Garcia-Pacheco JM, Olivares EG. Contractile activity of human decidual stromal cells. J Clin Endocrinol Metab 2003;88:844–849

Kimura H, Weisz A, Ogura T, Hitomi H, Kuraschima Y, Hashimoto K et al. (2001) Identification of hypoxia-inducible factor-1 ancillaty sequence and its function in vascular endothelial growth factor gene induction by hypoxia and nitric oxide. *J. Biol. Chem* 276:2292-2298.

Kobayashi M, Fitz L, Ryan M, Hewick RM, Clark SC, Chan S, et al. Identification and purification of natural killer cell stimulatory factor (NKSF), a cytokine with multiple biologic effects on human lymphocytes. J Exp Med 1989;170:827- 45.

Koks CA, Groothuis PG, Slaats P, Dunselman GA, de Goeij AFPM, Evers JLH. Matrix metalloproteinases and their tissue inhibitors in antegradely shed menstruum and peritoneal fluid. Fertil Steril 2000; 73:604 -612.

Komiyama S, Aoki D, Komiyama M, Nozawa S. Local activation of TGF-beta1 at endometriosis sites. J Reprod Med 2007;52:306–312.

Koninckx et al., 1998, 1999; Harada et al., 2001; Braun et al., 2002; Bedaiwy and Falcone, 2003; Kalu et al., 2007

Kothapalli R, Buyuksal I, Wu SQ, Chegini N, Tabibzadeh S. Detection of ebaf, a novel human gene of the transforming growth factor beta superfamily association of gene expression with endometrial bleeding.J Clin Invest 1997;99:2342–2350.

Kruithof EKO, Baker MS and Bunn CL (1995) Biological and clinical aspects of plasminogen activator inhibitor type 2. Blood 86,4007 - 4024.Gynecol Reprod Biol 95,167 - 174.

Lauer-Fields, J. L., Chalmers, M. J., Busby, S. A., Minond, D., Griffin, P. R., and Fields, G. B. (2009) Identification of specific hemopexin-like domain residues that facilitate matrix metalloproteinase collagenolytic activity. J Biol Chem 284, 24017-24024

Lebovic DI, Bentzien F, Chao VA, Garrett EN, Meng YG, Taylor RN. Induction of an angiogenic phenotype in endometriotic stromal cell cultures by interleukin-1beta. Mol Hum Reprod 2000;6:269–75.

Lee K, Lee Y, Chan R, et al (2010). Up-regulation of endocrine gland-derived vascular endothelial growth factor but not vascular endothelial growth factor but not vascular endothelial growth factor in human ectopic endometriotic tissue. *Fertil Steril* 4:1053-1060.

Lembessis P, Milingos S, Michalas S, Milingos D, Creatsas G, Sourla A, Koutsilieris M.Urokinase-type plasminogen activator and insulin-like growth factor-binding protein 3 mRNA expression in endometriotic lesions and eutopic endometrium: implications for the pathophysiology of endometriosis. Ann N Y Acad Sci. 2003 Nov;997:223-8.

Luo X, Xu J, Chegini N. The expression of Smads in human endometrium and regulation and induction in endometrial epithelial and stromal cells by transforming growth factor-b. J Clin Endocrinol Metab 2003; 88:4967–4976.

Machado DE, Berardo PT, Palmero CY, Nasciutti LE (2010). Higher express of vascular endothelial growth factor (VEGF) and its receptor VEGFR-2 (Flk-1) and metalloproteinase-9 (MMP-9) in a rat model of peritoneal endometirosis is similar to cancer. *Journal of Experiment &Clinical Cancer Resarch*, 29:4

Marbaix E, Kokorine I, Donnez J, Eeckhout Y and Courtoy PJ (1996) Regulation and restricted expression of interstitial collagenase suggest a pivotal

Matrisian LM (1990) Metalloproteinases and their inhibitors in matrix remodelling. Trends Genet 12,121 - 125.

Matrisian LM (1992) The matrix-degrading metalloproteinases. BioEssays 14,455 - 463.

Matsuzaki S, Maleysson E, Darcha C. Analysis of matrix metalloproteinase-7 expression in eutopic and ectopic endometrium samples from patients with different forms of endometriosis. Hum Reprod. 2010 Mar;25(3):742-50. Epub 2009 Dec 10.

McLaren, J., Prentice, A., Charnock-Jones, D.S. et al. (1996a) Vascular endothelial growth factor is produced by peritoneal fluid macrophages in endometriosis and is regulated by ovarian steroids. *J. Clin. Invest.*, 98, 482–489.

McLaren J (2000) Vascular endothelial growth factor and endometriotic angiogenesis. Hum Reprod Update. Jan-Feb;6(1):45-55. Review.

Meola J, Rosa e Silva JC, Dentillo DB, da Silva WA Jr, Veiga-Castelli LC, Bernardes LA, Ferriani RA, de Paz CC, Giuliatti S, Martelli L. Differentially expressed genes in eutopic and ectopic endometrium of women with endometriosis. Fertil Steril. 2010 Apr;93(6):1750-73. Epub 2009 Feb 6.

Meresman GF, Bilotas M, Buquet RA, Baranao RI, Sueldo C, Tesone M. Gonadotropin-releasing hormone agonist induces apoptosis and reduces cell proliferation in eutopic endometrial cultures from women with endometriosis. Fertil Steril 2003;80(Suppl. 2):702–707.

Minici F, Tiberi F, Tropea A, Orlando M , Gangale M.F.,Romani F , Campo S , A Bompiani , A Lanzone , Apa R .Endometriosis and human infertility: a new investigation into the role of eutopic endometrium Hum Repr ;23,3;530–537, 2008

Mönckedieck V, Sannecke C, Husen B, Kumbartski M, Kimmig R, Tötsch M, Winterhager E, Grümmer R. Progestins inhibit expression of MMPs and of angiogenic factors in human ectopic endometrial lesions in a mouse model. Mol Hum Reprod. 2009 Oct;15(10):633-43. Epub 2009 Aug 11

Mori H, Sawairi M, Nakagawa M, Itoh N,Wada K, Tamaya T. Peritoneal fluid interleukin-1 beta and tumor necrosis factor in patients with benign gynecologic disease. Am J Reprod Immunol 1991;26:62–7.

Murphy G, Kna ¨ uper V, Atkinson A, Gavrilovic J and Edwards D (2000) Cellular mechanisms for focal proteolysis and the regulation of the microenvironment. Fibrinolysis Proteolysis 14,165 – 174.

Muscato JJ, Haney AF, Weinberg JB. Sperm phagocytosis by human peritoneal macrophages: a possible cause of infertility in endometriosis. Am J Obstet Gynecol 1982;144:503-10.

Nasu K, Nishida M, Matsumoto H, Bing S, Inoue C, Kawano Y, Miyakawa I. Regulation of proliferation, motility and contractivity of cultured human endometrial stromal cells by transforming growth factor-beta isoforms. Fertil Steril 2005;84(Suppl. 2):1114-1123.

Neufeld G, Cohen T, Gengrinovitch S, and Poltorak Z (1999) Vascular endothelial growth factor (VEGF) and its receptors. *FASEB J* 13:9-22.

Nisolle, M., Casanas-Roux, F., Anaf, V. et al. (1993) Morphometric study of the stromal vascularization in peritoneal endometriosis. *Fertil. Steril.*, 59, 681-684.

Oosterlynck D, Meuleman M, Waer M, Koninckx P. Transforming growth factor-beta-activity is increased in peritoneal fluid from women with endometriosis. Obstet Gynecol 1994;83:287-92.

Orlando S, Sironi M, Bianchi G, Drummond AH, Boraschi D, Yabes D, et al. Role of metalloproteases in the release of the IL-1 type II decoy receptor. J Biol Chem 1997;272:31764-9.

Ortega N, Hutchings H, and Plouet J (1999) Signal relays in the VEGF system. *Front Biosci* 4:D141-D152.

Overton C, Fernandez-Shaw S, Hicks B, Barlow D, Starkey P. Peritoneal fluid cytokines and the relationship with endometriosis and pain. Hum Reprod 1996;11:380-386.

P.G Artini, M.Ruggiero, P. Monteleone, A. Carpi, F. Cristello, V. Cela, A.R. Genazzani (2008) Vascular endothelial growth factor and its soluble receptor in benign and malignant ovarian tumors. Biomedicine & Pharmacotherapy 62:373e377

Pizzo A, Salmeri F, Ardita F, Sofo V, Tripepi M, Marsico S. Behaviour of cytokine levels in serum and peritoneal fluid of women with endometriosis. Gynecol Obstet Invest 2002; 54: 82-87.

Punnonen J, Teisala K, Ranta H, Benneff B, Punnonen R. Increased level of interleukin-6 and interleukin-10 in peritoneal fluid of patients with endometriosis. Am J Obstet Gynecol 1996; 174: 1522-1526

Rana N, Gebel H, Braun DP, Rotman C, House R, Dmowski WP. Basal and stimulated secretion of cytokines by peritoneal macrophages in women with endometriosis. Fertil Steril 1996;65:925-30). role in the initiation of menstruation. Hum Reprod 11,134-143.

Ryan IP, Tseng JF, Schriock ED, Khoram O, Landers DV, Taylor RN. Interleukin-8 concentrations are elevated in the peritoneal fluid of women with endometriosis. Fertil Steril 1995; 63: 929-932.

Saare M, Lamp M, Kaart T, Karro H, Kadastik U, Metspalu A, Peters M, Salumets A. Polymorphisms in MMP-2 and MMP-9 promoter regions are associated with endometriosis. Fertil Steril. 2010 Sep;94(4):1560-3. Epub 2010 Jan 25.

Sakamoto Y, Harada T, Horie S, Iba Y, Taniguchi F, Yoshida S, Iwabe T, Terakawa N. Tumor necrosis factor-ainduced interleukin-8 (IL-8) expression in endometriotic stromal cells, probably through nuclear factor-kB activation: gonadotropin-releasing hormone agonist treatment reduced IL-8 expression. J Clin Endocrinol Metab 2003;88:730-735.

Salamonsen LA and Woolley DE (1996) Matrix metalloproteinases in normal menstruation. Hum Reprod 11,124 - 133.

Salata IM, Stojanovic N, Cajdler-Łuba A, Lewandowski KC, Lewiński A. Gelatinase A (MM-2), gelatinase B (MMP-9) and their inhibitors (TIMP 1, TIMP-2) in serum of women with endometriosis: Significant correlation between MMP-2, MMP-9 and their inhibitors without difference in levels of matrix metalloproteinases and tissue inhibitors of metalloproteinases in relation to the severity of endometriosis. Gynecol Endocrinol. 2008 Jun;24(6):326-30.

Sampson J (1927). Metastatic or Embolic Endometriosis, due to the Menstrual Dissemination of Endometrial Tissue into the Venous Circulation. Am J Pathology 3(2): 93–110.43.

Scott RB, Te Linde RW, Wharton LR Jr. Further studies on experimental endometriosis. Am J Obstet Gynecol 1953;60:1082–103.

Shan K, Lian-Fu Z, Hui D, Wei G, Na W, Xia J, Yan L. Polymorphisms in the promoter regions of the matrix metalloproteinases-7, -9 and the risk of endometriosis and adenomyosis in China. Mol Hum Reprod. 2006 Jan;12(1):35-9. Epub 2006 Feb 2.

Shull MM, Ormsby I, Kier AB, Pawlowski S, Diebold RJ, Yin M, Allen R, Sidman C, Proetzel G, Calvin D et al. Targeted disruption of the mouse transforming growth factor-b1 gene results in multifocal inflammatory disease. Nature 1992;359:693–699.

Sillem M, Prifti S, Monga B, Buvari P, Shamia U, Runnebaum B. Soluble urokinase-type plasminogen activator receptor is over-expressed in uterine endometrium from women with endometriosis. Mol Hum Reprod. 1997 Dec;3(12):1101-5.

Simpson JL,Bischoff FZ, Kamat A, et al. (2003). Genetics of endometriosis. *Obstet Gynecol Clin North Am.*30:21-40.

Smith RE, Hogaboam CM, Strieter RM, Lukas NW, Kunkel SL. Cell-to-cell and cell-to-matrix interactions mediate chemokine expression: an important component of the inflammatory lesion. J Leukoc Biol 1997;62:612–9.

Somigliana S, Vigano P, Rossi G, Carinelli S, Vignali M, Panina- Bordignon P. Endometrial ability to implant in ectopic sites can be prevented by interleukin-12 in a murine model of endometriosis Hum Reprod 1999;14:2944 –50.

Spuijbroek MDE, Dunselman GAJ, Menheere PPCA, Evers JLH. Early endometriosis invades the extracellular matrix. Fertil Steril 1992;58:929 –33

Subramaniam S, Stansberg C, Cunningham C. The interleukin 1 receptor family. Dev Comp Immunol 2004;28:415–28.

Sueldo CE, Kelly E, Montoro L, Subias E, Baccaro M, Swanson JA, et al. Effect of interleukin-1 on gamete interaction and mouse embryo development. J Reprod Med 1990;35:868–72.

Suginami H, Yano K. An ovum capture inhibitor (OCI) in endometriosis peritoneal fluid: an OCI-related membrane responsible for fimbrial failure of ovum capture. Fertil Steril 1988;50:648 –53.

Symons JA, Young PR, Duff GW. Soluble type II interleukin 1 (IL-1) receptor binds and blocks processing of IL-1 beta precursor and loses affinity for IL-1 receptor antagonist. Proc Natl Acad Sci USA 1995;92: 1714–8.

Syrop CH, Halme J. Peritoneal fluid environment and infertility. Fertil Steril 1987;48:1–9)

Tabibzadeh S, Mason JM, Shea W, Cai Y, Murray MJ, Lessey B Dysregulated expression of ebaf, a novel molecular defect in the endometria of patients with infertility. J Clin Endocrinol Metab 2000; 85:2526–2536.

Tabibzadeh S, Santhanam V, Sehgel PB, May LT. Cytokine-induced production of IFN-b2 by freshly explanted human endometrial stromal cells. Modulation by estradiol-17b. J Immunol 1989;142:3134 -9.

Tabibzadeh S. Homeostasis of extracellular matrix by TGF-beta and lefty. Front Biosci 2002;7:d1231–d1246.

Taketani Y, Kuo TM, Mizuno M. Comparison of cytokine levels and embryo toxicity in peritoneal fluid in infertile women with untreated or treated endometriosis. Am J Obstet Gynecol 1992;167:265–70.

Tamburro S, Canis M, Albuisson E, Dechelotte P, Darcha C, Mage G.Expression of transforming growth factorb1 in nerve fibers is related to dysmenorrhea and laparoscopic appearance of endometriotic implants. Fertil Steril 2003;80:1131–1136.

Tamura M, Fukaya T, Enomoto A, Murakami T, Uehara S, Yajima A Transforming growth factor-beta isoforms and receptors in endometriotic cysts of the human ovary. Am J Reprod Immunol 1999;42:160–167

Tokyol C, Aktepe F, Dilek FH, Sahin O, Arioz DT. Expression of cyclooxygenase-2 and matrix metalloproteinase-2 in adenomyosis and endometrial polyps and its correlation with angiogenesis. Int J Gynecol Pathol. 2009 Mar;28(2):148-56.

Tsudo T, Harada T, Iwabe T, Tanikawa M, Nagano Y, Ito M, Taniguchi F, Terakawa N. Altered gene expression and secretion of interleukin-6 in stromal cells derived from endometriotic tissues. Fertil Steril 2000;73:205–211

Ulloa L, Tabibzadeh S. Lefty inhibits receptor-regulated Smad phosphorylation induced by the transforming growth factor-beta receptor. J Biol Chem 2001;276:21397–21404.

Vinatier D, Dufour P, Oosterlynck D. Immunological aspects of endometriosis. Hum Reprod Update 1996;2:371- 84.

Wiegerick MAHM, Van Dop PA, Brosens IA. The staging of peritoneal endometriosis by the type active lesion in addition to the revised American Fertility Society classification. Fertil Steril 1993;60:461- 4

Wysocka M, Kubin M, Vieira LQ, Ozmen L, Garotta G, Scott P, et al. Interleukin-12 is required for IFN- production and lethality in lipopolysaccharide- induced shock in mice. Eur J Immunol 1995;25:672- 6.

Yanaihara A, Otsuka Y, Iwasaki S, Koide K, Aida T, Okai T. Comparison in gene expression of secretory human endometrium using laser microdissection. Reprod Biol Endocrinol. 2004;2:66. doi: 10.1186/1477-7827-2-66.

Ye S. Influence of matrix metalloproteinase genotype on cardiovascular disease susceptibility and outcome. Cardiovasc Res 2006;69: 636 - 645

Yilmaz B, Sucak A, Kilic S, Aksakal O, Aksoy Y, Lortlar N, Sut N, Gungor T. (2010) Metformin regresses endometriotic implants in rats by improving implant levels of superoxide dismutase, vascular endothelial growth factor, tissue inhibitor of metalloproteinase-2, and matrix metalloproteinase-9. Am J Obstet Gynecol.202(4):368.e1-8.

Yoshioka H, Harada T, Iwabe T, Nagano Y, Taniguchi F, Tanikawa M, et al. Menstrual cycle-specific inhibition of the proliferation of endometrial stromal cells by interleukin 6 and its soluble receptor. Am J Obstet Gynecol 1999;180:1088 -94

Zeyneloglu HB, Senturk LM, Seli E, Bahtiyar OM, Olive DL, Arici A. The peritoneal fluid levels of interleukin-12 in women with endometriosis.Am J Reprod Immunol. 1998;39:152- 6

Zhang X, Nothnick WB. The role and regulation of the uterine matrix metalloproteinase system in menstruating and non-menstruating species. Front Biosci. 2005;10:353–366. doi: 10.2741/1533.

Zhao Y, Nichols JE, Bulun SE, Mendelson CR, Simpson ER. Aromatase P450 gene expression in human adipose tissue: role of a Jak/STAT pathway in regulation of the adipose-specific promoter. J Biol Chem 1995;270:16449 –57.

Zhao Z, Nyholt DR, Thomas S, et al (2008) Polymorphisms in the vascular endothelial growth factor gene and the risk of familial endometriosis. *Molecular human reproduction* 14 (9):531-538.

11

The Local Immune Mechanisms Involved in the Formation of Endometriotic Lesions

Yulia Antsiferova and Natalya Sotnikova
Federal State Establishment Ivanovo's Research Institute of Maternity and Childhood Named V. N. Gorodkov, Russia

1. Introduction

According to common view, endometriosis is characterized by the presence and growth of the endometrium-like glandular tissue and stroma outside the uterus. So, endometriosis would represent an autotransplant in which tissue is transplanted to an ectopic location in an organism. It is well known that the immune system plays the main role in regulation of tissue homeostasis in an organism. Thus, immunologists have a special interest in this disease as insights in the pathogenesis of endometriosis would help not only to understand how ectopic lesions grow but also allow searching new approaches to the medical treatment of this disease.

Numerous theories have been proposed to explain the endometriosis pathogenesis till date. The most widely accepted Sampson's transplantation theory proposes that, during menstruation, there is reflux of endometrial tissue via fallopian tubes into abdominal cavity where endometrium could attach to peritoneal surfaces, proliferate, invade, and become the disease known as endometriosis. However, this theory does not account for the fact that most of women of reproductive age exhibit some degree of reflux of endometrial debris, but only some patients develop endometriosis (Harada et al., 2004; Vinatier et al., 2001). There are two main suggestions explaining this contradiction. The first explanation propose that there are some changes in the endometrium of women with endometriosis and these changes can promote the resistance of endometrial cells to normal peritoneal cleaning (Vinatier et al., 2001). The second theory suggests that impaired immune recognition in peritoneal cavity due to abnormalities of the cellular and humoral immunity can promote the endometriosis development (Kyama et al., 2003).

The suggestion that the primary defect in endometriosis is located in the eutopic endometrium, was proposed many years ago and supported now by many investigators (Vinatier et al., 2001; Kyama et al., 2003; Harada et al., 2004), though the eutopic endometrium of women with and without endometriosis is histologically similar. This hypothesis is confirmed by different studies revealing that there are many fundamental differences between these two tissues. Invasive properties, decreased apoptosis, and increased steroid hormones and cytokine production have been identified in eutopic endometrium of women with endometriosis compared to that in women without disease (Ulukus 2006). Impairment of some genes expression also was found in women with endometriosis. Aberrant expression of several genes such as matrix metalloproteinases, Hox genes, integrins, anti-apoptotic genes Bcl-2 was demonstrated in endometrium of women with endometriosis (Bondza et al., 2009). The significant increase of aromatase expression was shown in eutopic endometrium from endometriosis patients (Weiss et al., 2009). A constitutional or acquired anomaly in the nature of antigens, expressed by endometrium, such as transplantation antigens HLA-DR and HLA-A, B, C antigens, can explain the resistance of endometrium of women with endometriosis to the cytotoxicity of T-lymphocytes (Vinatier et al., 2001). Increased proliferative activity of endometrial cells due to altered expression of c-myc, TGF-β1 and bax genes was also found in patients with endometriosis (Jonson et al., 2005). Eutopic endometrium from endometriosis patients showed increased expression of midkine and pleiotropin mRNA expression compared with endometrium from normal women (Chung et al., 2002). It is known that midkine and pleiotropin function as tumor growth factors positively regulating tumor angiogenesis and metastasis of solid tumors. So these results evidence that eutopic endometrium from endometriosis patients may be more invasive and prone to implantation than that from women without endometriosis (Chung et al., 2002). All these findings let us to propose that cells and tissue elements derived from such an altered eutopic endometrium shed into peritoneal cavity would have a higher potential of implantation and growth on peritoneal surfaces. And many differences, observed between eutopic endometrium and ectopic tissue of patients with endometriosis, can be explained as the direct consequence of the specific environment of peritoneal fluid (Vinatier et al., 2001; Harada et al., 2004).

The local environment that surrounds the endometriotic implants in the peritoneal cavity is a dynamic one. Histologically, the peritoneum consists of a thin layer of loose connective tissue covered by a layer of mesothelium and is the most extensive serous membrane in the body, with a rich supply of subperitoneal blood vessels and lymphatics (Gazvani & Templeton, 2002). The peritoneal cavity is normally empty except for a thin film of fluid that keeps surfaces moist. The peritoneal fluid arises primarily from two sources: plasma transudate and ovarian exudate (Koninckx et al., 1998; Gazvani & Templeton, 2002). Peritoneal fluid contains a variety of free-floating immune cells, including macrophages, natural killer (NK) cells, lymphocytes, eosinophils and mast cells (Gazvani & Templeton, 2002). Macrophages are the most abundant cells among the peritoneal leukocytes. It is well known that macrophages are the main source of different cytokines, growth factors and other biologically active substances in the peritoneal fluid. Recent studies have also suggested that peritoneal fluid of women with endometriosis contain an increased number of activated macrophages and other immune cells and high amount of proinflammatory cytokines and growth factors, which exert a paracrine action on endometrial cells (Minici et al., 2007). So, endometriosis can be considered to be an inflammatory disease (Vigano et al., 2004). Possibly, this peritoneal inflammation might facilitate the implantation and growth of ectopic endometrial tissues. But we don't know exactly yet, whether endometriosis is caused by peritoneal inflammation? Or does endometriosis lead to inflammation caused by inappropriate immune response to endometrial debris? Can the inappropriate peritoneal environment directly influence lesions formation, or may be the intrinsic dysfunctions of endometrial cells play the main role in endometriosis development?

To concretize the role of cellular and humoral immune components of peritoneal fluid in their interaction with endometrial tissue in endometriosis and also to elucidate the local immune mechanisms participating in endometriotic lesions formation we attempted: a) to define the regulatory mechanisms of apoptosis and invasiveness of eutopic and ectopic endometrium in women with endometriosis, b) to elucidate the influence of autologous peritoneal macrophages and humoral factors of peritoneal fluid upon the parameters of eutopic endometrial tissue apoptosis and invasiveness in endometriosis women, c) to establish the changes in the functional state of peritoneal macrophages of women with endometriosis and d) to estimate the character of macrophages activity in response to autologous stimulation of endometrial cells.

2. Methods of investigation

2.1 Subjects

The study group consisted of 80 women of reproductive age undergoing diagnostic laparoscopies for infertility or pelvic pain. The presence and extent of the disease were determined laparoscopically and staging was performed according to the revised American Fertility Society classification (1985). Mild endometriosis (stage 1-2) was diagnosed in 51 women (64%), severe endometriosis (stage 3-4) was noted in 29 patients (36%). Laparoscopy was performed prior to the initiation of any treatment. Samples of peritoneal fluid and paired eutopic and ectopic endometrial biopsies were obtained from women with endometriosis. Endometrial tissue and peritoneal fluid from 30 control women without endometriosis, who underwent surgical sterilization were also collected. Informed consent was given by each woman participating in our study, according to local Ethical Committee protocol. Samples of peritoneal fluid from the Douglas pouch were aspirated into sterile tubes. Samples of ectopic and matched eutopic endometrium were collected into sterile flasks with isotonic saline solution and were immediately recruited into the study.

2.2 Co-cultivation of endometrial tissue and peritoneal macrophages

To evaluate the possible effect of peritoneal environment on the apoptosis and invasive capacity of endometrial tissue, the samples of eutopic endometrium of 10 women without endometriosis and 10 women with endometriosis were cultivated in the presence of autologous peritoneal fluid or autologous peritoneal macrophages. Samples of peritoneal fluid were centrifuged at 2000 g for 10 minutes to remove cellular component. Bloody samples of peritoneal fluid were excluded from our study. Enriched population of peritoneal macrophages was obtained from peritoneal fluid using standard Ficoll-Verografin gradient centrifugation (d-1.078) with subsequent removing of lymphocytes using standard procedure of macrophages adherence to plastic. The percentage of CD14+ macrophages in received fraction was 93-95% as it was established by flow cytometry analysis.

Endometrial tissue was minced by scissors into pieces of 1-2 mm in diameter. Approximately 40-50 mg of endometrial tissue were placed in 24 well plate, in 2 ml of whole RPMI 1640 medium with 2 mM of glutamine, 5% fetal calf serum and antibiotics supplemented with autologous peritoneal fluid or with peritoneal macrophages. Ratio of peritoneal fluid and whole RPMI 1640 in medium for cultivation was 1:1. The final concentration of macrophages in culture media was $2x10^6$ cell/ml. Endometrial explants were cultured at 37^0 C and 5% CO_2 for 24 hours. Samples of endometrium or peritoneal macrophages, cultured in the same conditions only in RPMI 1640, were used as controls. After termination of cultivation, endometrial tissue was washed up in phosphate-buffered saline (PBS) twice and was taken for subsequent RNA isolation or for enzymatic isolation of stromal endometrial cells. Peritoneal macrophages were collected from wells, filtered through 6 layers of gauze and analyzed using flow cytometry.

2.3 Quantitative real-time RT-PCR

The level of mRNAs expression of different factors, regulating apoptosis and invasiveness in endometrial tissue, was investigated using quantitative real time RT-PCR (reverse transcription- polymerase chain reaction). Total RNA was isolated from the whole endometrial tissue using the acid guanidinium thiocyanate-phenol-chloroform method. RNA was converted to complementary DNA (cDNA) using random hexamers and murine leukaemia virus reverse transcriptase (Promega, USA). Reverse transcription was performed at 70^0C for 3 min and 37^0C for 90 min. For real time quantitative RT-PCR, gene-specific primers and probes for human β2-microglobulin (housekeeper gene), XIAP, caspase-3, HSP27, MT-1, MMP-2, MMP-9, TIMP-2, TIMP-1 were designed and constructed in the Laboratory of Gene Engineering of National Research Center for Hematology (Moscow, Russia) using the Vector NTI Advance 10 design program (Invitrogen, USA). Commercial kit "Immunoscreen" (Gene Engineering of National Research Center for Hematology, Moscow, Russia) was used to perform real-time quantitative RT-PCR. For the thermocycle reactions and the detection of the fluorescence signals, iCycler iQ Multi-Color Real Time PCR Detection System (BIO-RAD Laboratories, California, USA) was used. To assess the number of cDNA copies in every sample, the standard curves for studied genes were constructed using control cDNA dilution series. As the controls sequences of cloned corresponding genes were used. For each endometrial sample, the amount of copies of housekeeper gene (β2-microglobulin) and specific genes were determined from the appropriate standard curve, generated by iCycler iQ software. The amount of specific gene was subsequently divided by the amount of housekeeper gene to obtain normalized specific gene value and results were presented as the ratio in a sample in the order of 10^3 per μl for MT-1, XIAP, caspase-3, MMP-2, TIMP-2, 10^4 per μl for HSP27 and 10^5 per μl for MMP-9 and TIMP-1.

2.4 Flow cytometry

The surface expression of the number of functional receptors and intracellular production of proinflammatory cytokines by peritoneal macrophages was estimated with monoclonal antibodies using flow cytometry method. The following monoclonal antibodies were used in this study: FITC-conjugated anti-human-CD45, CD36, CD204, IL-1beta, IL-8, Vimentin antibodies and PE-conjugated anti-human CD14, HLA-DR, CD49e, CD11b, CD95, CD95L, IL-6, IL-12, TNF alpha antibodies (BD Biosciences, USA). Intracellular staining procedure was carried out according to the manufacturer's instructions using the FIX & PERM cell permeabilization reagents (Invinrogen, Camarillo, CA, USA). The amount of apoptotic endometrial stromal cells after incubation with peritoneal fluid or with macrophages was assessed using commercial kit with Annexin V and propidium iodide (CALTAG

Laboratories, USA). Flow cytometry analyses were performed on FACScan (Becton Dickinson, USA) using CellQuest Pro software. Data from forward versus side scatter was obtained to analyze the CD45+CD14+ macrophage population and Vimentin+ endometrial stromal cell population.

2.5 ELISA

The content of IL-8, MCP-1 and calprotektin in the peritoneal fluid of women with and without endometriosis was assessed by ELISA (enzyme-linked immunosorbent assay) using commercial kits (Bender MedSystems, Austria).

2.6 Cell invasion assays

The influence of peritoneal fluid and culture media of 24-h cultures of peritoneal macrophages of women with endometriosis upon invasiveness of eutopic endometrial cells of women with endometriosis was estimated in the 2D Matrigel system using BD BioCoat Matrigel Invasion Chamber (BD Biosciences, USA). 50 μl of prepared endometrial stromal cells isolated from eutopic endometrium of women with endometriosis by enzymatic method were placed on top of porous membrane coated with Matrigel. Autologous peritoneal fluid or pooled culture media of 24-h cultures of peritoneal macrophages of women with endometriosis were added to the lower chamber and then incubated overnight. At the end of the incubation period the upper side of the membrane was cleaned with a cotton wool bud. For assessment of the number of invaded cells, the filters were stained with hematoxylin and eosin and mounted on glass microscope slides. Total number of cells that had invaded onto the underside of the filter was counted manually at 200x magnification.

2.7 Statistics

Results were presented as the mean ± standard error. All variables were checked for normal distribution with the Kolmogorov-Smirnov test. All the parameters studied showed a normal distribution. Student's t-test was used to compare results from different groups. Statistical significance was defined as $p < 0.05$.

3. Impairment of the apoptosis and invasiveness of endometrial tissue in endometriosis

The growing bodies of evidence indicate that the impairment of endometrial cell's apoptosis and the increase of tissue proteolysis supposedly are involved in the pathogenic mechanisms of endometriosis.

3.1 Regulation of apoptosis in the endometrium of women with endometriosis

Apoptosis is a fundamental process responsible for maintaining homeostasis in multicellular organisms (Mei et al., 2010). In contrast to necrotic cell death, which is usually a result of trauma, programmed cell death is a physiological process. The mechanisms of apoptosis are highly complex and sophisticated, involving an energy dependent cascade of molecular events. Two major apoptotic routes exist in mammalian cells: the intrinsic or mitochondrial pathway and extrinsic or death receptor pathway. The intrinsic pathway is characterized by the permeabilization of the outer mitochondrial membrane and the release of several pro-apoptotic factors into the cytosol. These include cytochrome c, Smac/Diablo, AIF (apoptosis-inducing factor), and serine protease HtrA2/Omi (Elmore 2007). These proteins activate the caspase dependent mitochondrial pathway. Cytochrome *c* binds and activates Apaf-1 (the apoptotic protease activating factor-1) as well as procaspase-9, forming an "apoptosome" (Hill et al., 2004). The clustering of procaspase-9 in this manner leads to caspase-9 activation. Different molecules from IAP family (inhibitors of apoptosis proteins) can inhibit activity of Smac/DIABLO and HtrA2/Omi on this stage of apoptosis (Schimmer et al., 2006). The control and regulation of these apoptotic mitochondrial events occurs through members of HSP (heat shock proteins) family, acting as inhibitors of apoptosis. Proteins from Bcl-2 family also regulate the mitochondrial stage of apoptosis and these factors can be either pro-apoptotic or antiapoptotic. Till date, a total of 25 genes have been identified in the Bcl-2 family. Some of the anti-apoptotic proteins include Bcl-2, Bcl-x, Bcl-XL, Bcl-XS, Bcl-w, BAG, and some of the pro-apoptotic proteins include Bcl-10, Bax, Bak, Bid, Bad, Bim, Bik, and Blk. These proteins have special significance since they can determine if the cell is committed to apoptosis or else abort the process. The tumor suppressor protein p53 has a critical role in regulation of the Bcl-2 family of proteins (Elmore 2007). The extrinsic pathway is activated by engaging death receptors such as Fas and Tumor Necrosis Factor Receptor (TNFR) with their cognate ligands. This leads to the formation of the membrane-bound death inducing signaling complex (DISC), which recruits the initiator procaspase-8 by the adaptor protein FADD. The intrinsic pathway responds to "intracellular" signals such as DNA damage, oncogene activation, nutrient deprivation, and lineage information (Elmore 2007). The final common end point of both pathways is initiation of execution stage of apoptosis and result in DNA fragmentation, degradation of cytoskeletal and nuclear proteins, crosslinking of proteins, formation of apoptotic bodies, expression of ligands for phagocytic cell receptors and finally uptake by phagocytic cells (Elmore 2007). Caspase-3 is considered to be the most important of the executioner caspases and is activated by any of the initiator caspases (caspase-8, caspase-9, or caspase-10). Caspase-3 specifically activates the endonuclease CAD and CAD then degrades chromosomal DNA within the nuclei and causes chromatin condensation. Caspase-3 also induces cytoskeletal reorganization and disintegration of the cell into apoptotic bodies (Elmore 2007). So, the apoptosis process is very complex and regulated numerous pro- and anti-apoptotic factors.

The role of apoptosis in endometriosis development is studied very intensively at last time. It was demonstrated that apoptosis aids in maintaining cellular homeostasis during the menstrual cycle by eliminating aging cells from the functional layer of the uterine endometrium (Agic et al., 2009). In the normal endometrium apoptosis was detected in the glandular epithelium of late secretory and menstruating endometrium, while very little apoptosis was detected during the proliferative or at the beginning of the secretory phase (Harada et al., 2004). Eutopic endometrium from women with endometriosis has some differences in apoptosis compared with normal endometrium. These differences could contribute to the survival of the regurgitating endometrial cells into the peritoneal cavity and the endometriosis development. It was found, that the percentage of apoptosis in sloughed endometrial cells was greatly reduced among women with endometriosis, implying that the number of surviving cells that enter the peritoneal cavity is greater in women who develop endometriosis (Harada et al., 2004). An increased expression of anti-apoptotic factor Bcl-2 and decrease expression of pro-apoptotic factor Bax were found in proliferative eutopic endometrium from women with endometriosis (Meresman et al., 2000). These differences could contribute to the survival of regurgitating endometrial cells into the peritoneal cavity and development of endometriosis (Taniguchi 2011). In ectopic endometrium of women with endometriosis the level of Bcl-2 expression was significantly increased in stromal cells (Harada et al., 2004). In endometriotic lesions the alterations in expression of different apoptosis-associated genes, such as PTEN, p52 and Bcl-2 were also demonstrated (Nezha et al., 2008). Authors thought that these changes are analogous in tumor tissue and evidence about possible malignant transformation of endometriotic tissue. At the same time there are some data about absence of significant changes of apoptotsis both in eutopic and in ectopic endometrium in women with endometriosis (Hassa et al., 2009). So, the study of the mechanisms, regulating apoptosis in endometriosis, need to be continued.

We also have checked out the expression of mRNA of some genes, possessed both pro- and anti-apoptotic action, in eutopic and ectopic endometrium of women with endometriosis. It was found that the expression of genes, regulating apoptosis, in endometrial tissue of women with endometriosis significantly differed from that in healthy women (Table 1).

Parameter, copies number/µl	Endometrium, control (n=7)	Eutopic endometrium, endometriosis (n=15)	Ectopic endometrium, endometriosis (n=15)
mRNA MT-1	361.89±124.74	46.56±23.76 *	42.36±17.42*
mRNA XIAP	0.38±0.18	22.51±9.62*	2.90 ± 1.59^{x}
mRNA caspase-3	0.72±0.33	0.38±0.09	$3.80\pm1.25^{*xx}$
mRNA HSP27	0.23±0.05	0.22±0.08	$1.75\pm0.55^{*x}$

Table 1. The level of the expression of mRNAs genes, regulating apoptosis, in the eutopic and ectopic endometrium of women with endometriosis (* - given in comparison to the endometrium of healthy women, *- $p<0.05$; ^{x} - given in comparison to the eutopic endometrium of women with endometriosis, ^{x} – $p<0.05$, ^{xx}- $p<0.01$)

In eutopic endometrium of women with endometriosis the expression of anti-apoptotic factor XIAP (X-linked inhibitor of apoptosis) mRNAs were statistically increased compared to that in the endometrium of women from the control group.

In ectopic endometrial tissue the high levels of caspase-3 and heat shock protein 27 (HSP27) mRNAs expression were seen. Both in eutopic and ectopic endometrium of endometriosis women the low level of metallothionein-1 (MT-1) mRNA expression was found compared to that in the endometrium of women without endometriosis.

Thus, the profile of genes, regulating apoptosis, was different in eutopic and ectopic endometrium in endometriosis except the expression of MT-1 mRNA which was decreased both in eutopic endometrium and in endometriotic lesions. It is known that metalloteoneins (MTs) are a group of ubiquitous low-molecular-weight proteins essential for the protection of cells against heavy metal ion toxicity. These molecules also are directly involved in regulation of cell growth, differentiation and apoptosis in different pathological conditions and in tumour as well (Inoue et al., 2009). Earlier the low level of MT-1 protein was demonstrated in ovarian endometriomas (Wicherek et al., 2006).

Likely, diminishment of the MT-1 synthesis in endometrium of women with endometriosis might lead to the impairment of apoptosis control during this pathology. Another important apoptosis regulator, XIAP, is one of the members of IAP (inhibitory apoptosis proteins) family (Mufti et al., 2007). IAPs proteins are selectively bind and inhibit caspases-3, -7 and -9. XIAP is the only member of this family able to directly inhibit both the initiation and execution phase of the caspase cascade. XIAP is frequently over-expressed in malignant cells and is associated with poor clinical outcome (Schimmer et al., 2006). According to our data XIAP synthesis was significantly increased in eutopic endometrium in endometriosis, but in endometriotic lesions the level of XIAP mRNA expression didn't differ from that in normal endometrium. The high level of XIAP mRNA expression in eutopic endometrium possibly can lead to the decrease of spontaneous apoptosis in endometrium of women with endometriosis and in menstrual endometrium as well. This phenomenon might be responsible for the elevation of viability of endometrial cells in peritoneal cavity and play an important role at the initial stages of endometriotic lesions formation. But the absence of the elevation of XIAP synthesis in ectopic endometrium evidence in favor of the benign character of endometriotic lesions growth. Likely, the growth of already formed endometriotic tissue isn't under the XIAP control. Evidently, mechanisms, regulating endometrial XIAP synthesis, are different in eutopic and ectopic endometrium. The same was noted for the caspase-3 and HSP27. Only in ectopic endometrium we have seen the high level of the caspase-3 and HSP27 synthesis compared to that in endometrium of healthy women. From one side, these results are controversial, because caspase-3 is one of the main proapoptotic factors, a central effector caspase involved in numerous apoptotic pathways (Voss et al., 2007). On the contrary, HSP27 is well known inhibitor of apoptosis because the most heat shock proteins and HSP27 as well have strong cytoprotective effects and behave as molecular chaperone for other cellular proteins (Schmitt et al., 2007). HSP27 can bind to pro-caspase-3 to prevent its cleavage and activation by caspase-9 (Pandey et al., 2000). It does so by directly sequestering cytochrome c when released from the mitochondria into the cytosol (Schmitt et al., 2007). But as it is known HSP27 can interact with different partners implicated in the apoptotic process. For example, under stress conditions HSP27 increases IκBα ubiquitination/degradation, which results in an increase in NFκ-B activity and increased survival (Parcellier et al., 2003). So, the high level of HSP27 synthesis in endometriotic lesions can protect cells form apoptosis in caspase-independent pathway. Possibly the thin balance between mechanisms inducing and inhibiting apoptosis exists in endometriosis tissue. The growth of the endometriotic tissue was accompanied by the high level of synthesis of anti-apoptotic molecules HSP27. These changes are similar to that in the cancer cells and might be responsible for the invasion of endometrium into the peritoneum in the process of lesions formation. But in contrast to tumor cells the high level of caspase-3 mRNA expression in endometriosis lesions might provide the benign character of its growth.

Thus, both literature data and our own results evidence the impairment of apoptosis regulation in endometriosis. It must be special noted, that mechanisms of regulation of apoptosis in eutopic and ectopic endometrium are different. In eutopic endometrium the expression profile of apoptosis-related genes possibly contribute to the increase of viability of endometrial cells. But in endometriotic lesions we found the simultaneously elevated expression of both pro- and anti-apoptotic genes. Likely, this phenomenon might be responsible for benign type of ectopic growth of endometrium in endometriosis.

3.2 Changes of the invasiveness of endometrium in endometriosis

It has been shown that early lesions formation is an invasion event that requires breakdown of the extracellular matrix (ECM) proteins (Nap et al., 2004). The ECM consists of collagens, proteoglycans and glycoproteins, including fibronectin and laminin (Curry & Osteen, 2003). The ECM has become recognized as a key regulatory component in cellular physiology, providing an environment for cell migration, division, differentiation, anchorage, and, in some cases, an ultimate fate between cell survival and cell death. Additionally, the ECM is important in metabolic processes, influencing cellular proliferation, differentiation and apoptosis and it serves as a repository for biologically active growth factors (Nap et al., 2004). The highly regulated control of ECM turnover and homeostasis occurs, in part, by the action of a specific class of proteolytic enzymes. Supposedly, enzymes which belong to the system of plasminogen and matrix metalloproteinase family play the important role in ECM remodeling during endometriotic lesions formation (Vinatier et al., 2001).

Plasminogen, a ubiquitous protein secreted by liver, is activated into a protease plasmin by two types of activators. These are tissue plasminogen activator (tPA) and urokinase plasminogen activator (uPA), which bind to a specific cellular receptor (uPA-R). uPA initiates pericellular proteolysis of the ECM. This system is perfectly controlled by powerful inhibitors, some at the level of the plasminogen activators (type 1 and type 2 Plasminogen Activator Inhibitor, PAI-1 and PAI-2, respectively), and others at the level of the plasmin. uPA plays an important role in uterine physiology and in menstruation (Vinatier et al., 2001). Some results evidence about involvement of plasminogen system in mechanisms of endometriosis development. It was found that concentrations of uPA and PAI-1 were strongly increased both in endometriotic lesions and in matched eutopic endometrium of women with endometriosis compared to that in healthy women (Bruse et al., 1998). But there are some works which didn't find any differences in the expression of the proteins from plasminogen system in endometrial tissue in endometriosis (Vinatier et al., 2001). So, the role of these enzymes in endometriosis is not clear yet.

In last years the role of proteases from matrix metalloproteinase (MMPs) family in mechanisms of endometriosis establishment is intensively investigated. It was found that the MMP system is actively involved in the control of different aspects of reproductive function. In the ovary and uterus, MMP system regulates the dynamic structural changes that occur throughout the menstrual cycle (Curry & Osteen, 2003). The MMPs family consists of several structurally related Zn^{2+}-dependent secreted endopeptidases. Currently, it is recognized more that 26 endopeptidases that include four broad classes: the collagenases, gelatinases, stromelysins, and membrane type enzymes (MT-MMPs). These proteinases exhibit numerous structural and functional similarities. All of them have conserved domain structures and specific domains related to substrate specificity and recognition of other proteins (Amalinie et al., 2010). Common features of the MMPs family include: 1) the presence of zinc in the active site of the catalytic domain, 2) synthesis of the MMPs as preproenzymes that are secreted in an inactive form, 3) activation of the latent zymogen in the extracellular space, 4) recognition and cleavage of the ECM by the catalytic domain of the enzyme, and 5) inhibition of enzyme action by both serum-borne and tissue-derived metalloproteinase inhibitors or TIMPs in the extracellular environment (Curry & Osteen, 2003). Although similarities exist in the structure of the MMPs, there are also distinct differences in the recognition and specificity for components of the ECM. For example, collagenases (MMP-1, MMP-8, and MMP-13) degrade native fibrillar collagen of types I, II, III, V, and XI. Gelatin, another important protein of ECM, is susceptible to a wide range of tissue proteinases, including the gelatinases MMP-2 and MMP-9. The stromelysin enzymes (MMP-3, MMP-7, MMP-10, and MMP-11) act on a broad and diverse array of ECM substrates. Both gelatinases and stromelysins are capable of degrading major constituents of basement membranes, including type IV collagen, laminin, and fibronectin. In addition to degrading the ECM, the MMPs exhibit activity toward other MMPs, growth factors, and cytokines such as IGF binding proteins, epidermal growth factor (EGF), TNF-α (Curry & Osteen, 2003).

Involvement of MMPs in endometriosis development was suspected after collagen breakdown products were found in the peritoneal fluid of patients with endometriosis (Spuijbroek et al., 1992) and since that time many studies have demonstrated that the pattern of MMPs expression in endometrium and peritoneal fluid of women with endometriosis significantly differ from that in healthy women (Nap et al, 2004). Increased levels of MMP-1, MMP-2, MMP-7 and MMP-9 were detected in peritoneal fluid of patients with endometriosis (Amalinie et al., 2010). At the same time the amount of the MMP-13 in peritoneal fluid of patients was significantly decreased in comparison to that in healthy women (Laudanski et al., 2005). In eutopic endometrium of women with endometriosis the elevation of the expression of MMP-1, MMP-2, MMP-3, MMP-9 was found (Di Carlo et al., 2009; Shaco-Levy et al., 2008). Diminishment of the expression of MMPs inhibitors TIMP-1 and TIMP-2 in endometrium of endometriosis patients was also noted (Colett et al., 2004; Uzan et al., 2004). The study of the character of MMPs production at the level of ectopic endometrium had shown that MMP-2 and MMP-3 overexpression were related to the infiltrative nature of endometriotic lesion (Uzan et al., 2004). It was also shown that circulating mRNA for MMP-3 was significantly higher in peripheral blood of patients with endometriosis than in control patients, regardless of the degree of endometriosis severity (De Sanctis et al., 2011). In a prospective, blinded, longitudinal study MMP-2 and MMP-9 were more likely to be detected in the urine of patients with endometriosis than in controls (Becker et al., 2010). Thus, practically all received data evidence about the increased production of MMPs both at the systemic and local level in endometriosis. But there are some reports that contradict these results. For example, Colett with coworkers didn't find any difference in the MMP-2 production in endometrial tissue of women with endometriosis in comparison with healthy women (Colett et al., 2004). Very low production of MMP-9 by endometrial cells was seen in endometriosis women (Sillme et al., 2001). So, the role of MMPs in endometriosis pathogenesis is still unclear.

The majority of works are only descriptive and functional involvement of MMPs in the development or progression of endometriosis has not been proven. It is very difficult to study the ectopic endometrium in humans as controlled experiments are limited, because it is not possible to monitor the disease progression without repeated laparoscopies which is difficult on many grounds. In such cases animal models are an extremely important tool in elucidating the pathogenesis of the disease. Animals with experimental endometriosis let us to evaluate the different stages of ectopic lesion formation. Both nonprimate and primate models have been used to study endometriosis for many years. Nonprimates, including rodents, do not undergo spontaneous disease, but it can be induced using either autologous uterine tissue or human endometrium (Story and Kennedy, 2004). Up to now the prominent changes of MMPs production in animals with experimental endometriosis have been demonstrated. The level of MMP-3 and MMP-9 was significantly higher in endometriotic lesions in rats with experimental endometriosis than in matched eutopic endometrium (Machado et al., 2010; Cox et al., 2001). Suppression of MMP-2 and MMP-9 activity in mice led to the inhibition of endometriosis progression in animals with the decrease of endometriotic lesions weight (Chen et al., 2010). Investigation of the role of MMPs in human endometrial explants in a chicken chorioallantoic membrane model (CAM) of endometriosis allowed to establish that endometrium both of healthy women and patients with endometriosis showed a statistically significant increase of MMP-1 mRNA expression 24, 48, 72, and 96 hours after transfer to the CAM and no statistically significant difference regarding the MMPs mRNA expression was shown for endometrium of healthy women and endometriosis patients (Juhasz-Boss et al., 2010). Earlier we have also studied the synthesis of mRNA of MMP-2 and TIMP-2 in rat ectopic endometrium at different stages of experimental endometriosis development. We found that the dynamic of MMP-2 mRNA expression in ectopic experimental lesions was characterized by its significant increase at 7th day after transplantation comparing to that in native uterine endometrium with subsequent declining to normal values at 14th and 21st days after surgery. The level of TIMP-2 mRNA expression on the contrary was sharply decreased at early and middle stages of endometriotic lesions formation and was elevated at the late stage of experimental endometriosis comparing to that in intact uterine endometrium (Sotnikova et al., 2010). So, during the first 7 days of experimental endometriosis lesions development, the balance of pro- and anti-proteolytic activity in endometrial tissue was shifted towards MMP-2 prevalence. It is known that during this period the maximal level of endometrial tissue invasion and cell proliferation are seen in rat endometriosis model. Our results evidence about the coincidence of high level of MMP-2 expression and high tissue's invasiveness in early experimental endometriosis lesions and allow us to suggest the direct involvement of MMP-2 in invasion of endometrial cells at the initial stage of endometriosis development.

The role of MMP-2 and MMP-9 in endometriosis development has a special interest. It was demonstrated that these two gelatinases actively participate in tumor invasion and progression (Amalinei et al., 2010). Initially, MMP-9 or gelatinase-B, was considered a key MMP in the invasion and metastasis, overexpressed by cancer cells and induced by several cytokines, growth factors and oncogene products (Okada et al., 2001), and its inhibition resulting in loss of metastatic potential. Subsequent studies demonstrated that the activation ratios of pro-MMP-2, not of pro-MMP-9, correlate with lymph node metastasis in breast, lung, thyroid and digestive tract carcinomas (Amalinei et al., 2010). MMP-2 has been shown to play a key role in promotion of invasiveness both of normal and neoplastic cells. Cellular localization in many tumor tissues indicates that MMP-2 mRNA appears to be localized to the stromal fibroblast adjacent to the sites of tumor invasion (Amalinei et al., 2010). It was also shown that MMP-2 and MMP-9 expression are closely associated with the parameters of tumor aggressiveness (Karahan et al., 2007) and tumor growth is reduced by the absence of MMP-2, and the metastatic processes is reduced by the lack of MMP-9 (Egeblad & Werb, 2002). But MMP-2 and MMP-9 are not tumor specific and are involved in ECM remodeling in a wide range of non-neoplastic processes, including embryonic development, trophoblastic invasion, angiogenesis, T-cell transmigration and wound healing (Amalinei et al., 2010).

Endometriosis often is defined as benign tumor. Taking into account literature data about action of MMP-2 and MMP-9 during tumor progression we checked out synthesis on these MMPs and its inhibitors TIMP-2 and TIMP-1 in eutopic and ectopic endometrium of healthy women and women with endometriosis. We found, that in eutopic endometrium of women with endometriosis the expression of MMP-2, TIMP-2 and TIMP-1 mRNAs were statistically increased compared to that in the endometrium of women from control group. In ectopic endometrial tissue the high levels of MMP-2, MMP-9 and TIMP-1 mRNAs expression were seen (Table 2). So, the distinct characteristic of endometriotic lesion is the high level of MMP-2 and MMP-9 synthesis which might provide invasive character of ectopic endometrium growth. But the eutopic endometrium doesn't posses such invasive activity. Evidently, some factors may influence upon MMPs synthesis in endometrial tissue of women with endometriosis elevating the mRNA expression of MMP-2 and MMP-9.

Parameter, copies number/μl	Endometrium, control (n=5)	Eutopic endometrium, endometriosis (n=17)	Ectopic endometrium, endometriosis (n=18)
mRNA MMP-2	0.89±0.27	2.40±0.63*	5.89±2.29*
mRNA TIMP-2	4.09±0.74	13.53±3.94*	6.44±1.59
mRNA MMP-9	0.27±0.16	1.37±0.62	13.78±5.04*x
mRNA TIMP-1	2.72±1.33	24.44±9.02*	87.73± 31.19*

Table 2. The level of the expression of mRNAs for genes, regulating invasiveness, in the eutopic and ectopic endometrium of women with endometriosis (* – given in comparison to the endometrium of healthy women, *- $p<0.05$; x – given in comparison to the eutopic endometrium of women with endometriosis, x – $p<0.05$)

It must be noted that the balance of pro- and anti-proteolytic enzymes synthesis was different in eutopic end ectopic endometrium (Fig.1). In eutopic endometrium we have seen the significant prevalence of the mRNA expression of specific inhibitors of MMPs - TIMP-2 and TIMP-1 upon the activity of MMP-2 and MMP-9, respectively. But in ectopic endometrium the level of mRNA expression of MMP-2 and TIMP-2 was practically the same (Fig.1). This situation allows us to compare the growth of ectopic endometrium with tumor growth. It is well known that in urothelial cancer patients the mean MMP-2/TIMP-2 ratio in patients with recurrence is significantly higher than that in patients without recurrence and the disease-free survival of patients with high MMP-2/TIMP-2 ratio is extremely poor compared with that of patients with lower ratios (Gohji et al., 1996). It was demonstrated also that evaluation of MMP-2: TIMP-2 mRNA balance may constitute an early prognostic indicator of human cancer (Onisto et al., 1995). Evidently, the elevation of the balance of MMP-2 and TIMP-2 in endometriotic tissue results in increase of invasive potential of ectopic endometrium. But mechanisms regulating such changes need to be further elucidated. It can be supposed that peritoneal fluid factors can directly influence upon endometrial invasiveness. But in our case we didn't observe such changes in the balance of MMP-9 and TIMP-1. Moreover, the synthesis of TIMP-1 in ectopic endometrium was very high. From one side these changes can be connected with the specific action of TIMP-1 during tumor progression. It was shown that in certain situations TIMP-1 can act as growth promoting factor and/or antiapoptotic factor to the cancer cells (Mannello & Gazzanelli, 2001). And high level of TIMP-1 synthesis might be attributive to enhance the invasive growth of ectopic lesion. But from another side, it was shown that excessive levels of TIMP-1 protein such as those secreted by endometriotic lesions into the peritoneal cavity negatively affects the reproduction function of rats with experimental endometriosis (Stilley et al., 2010). It was also shown that the rat embryo treated in vitro with endometriotic peritoneal fluid concentrations of TIMP-1 developed abnormally, and rats treated with a TIMP-1 function-blocking antibody had normal zygote, follicle and embryo quality (Stilley et al., 2010). Summarizing their results authors hypothesize that excessive TIMP-1 was deleterious to ovulation and embryo development because endometriotic lesion-secreted TIMP-1 can translocate to ovary/or oviduct and cause poor preimplantation embryo quality, developmental arrest and the subsequent embryo loss found in endometriosis (Stilley et al., 2010). Thus, the high level of TIMP-1 synthesis in ectopic endometrium might be associated with mechanisms of infertility development in women with endometriosis.

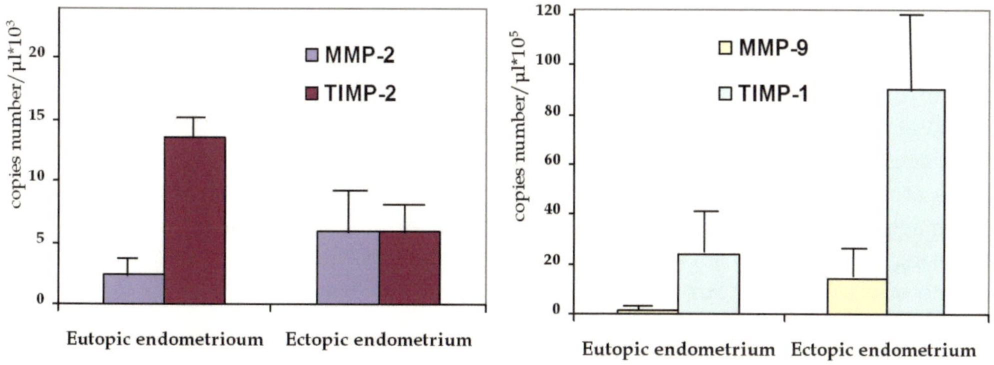

Fig. 1. Comparative characteristic of the synthesis of the enzymes with pro- and anti-proteolytic activity in eutopic and ectopic endometrium of women with endometriosis

Thus, endometriotic lesion establishment and growth are accompanied by the impairment of regulation of apoptosis and invasion in endometrial tissue. These changes at the level of eutopic endometrium possibly are associated with the increase of the viability of endometrial cells and participate in early lesions formation events. At the level of already formed ectopic endometrium we found the significant increase of invasive capacity and elevated synthesis of both pro- and anti-apoptotic factors which might be responsible for the benign type of ectopic lesions growth. Earlier it was suggested that many differences observed between eutopic and ectopic tissue of a patients with endometriosis can be explained as the direct consequence of the different environment of peritoneal fluid (Hara et al., 2004). So, the next step of our investigation was to study the possible peritoneal fluid factors influence upon apoptosis and invasiveness of endometrial cells.

4. Influence of peritoneal macrophages and peritoneal fluid upon mechanisms, regulating apoptosis and invasiveness of endometrium in endometriosis

The mechanisms by which regurgitated endometrial cells are cleared from the peritoneal cavity in the majority of women are poorly understood yet. However, it has been suggested that a peritoneal microenvironment might subserve this role (Vigano et al., 2004). There are two main factors which can contribute to the mechanisms regulating endometrial apoptosis and invasion - soluble biologically active factors of peritoneal fluid, including numerous cytokines, growth factors, metabolites of arachidonic acid, reactive oxygen species, etc. and peritoneal macrophages, the most abundant leukocytes population in peritoneal fluid. To estimate the possible influence both of humoral and cellular components of peritoneal fluid upon the apoptosis and invasiveness of endometrial cells which entered the peritoneal cavity due to the menstrual reflux, we had incubated explants of eutopic endometrial tissue in the presence of autologous peritoneal macrophages or in the presence of autologous peritoneal fluid. After termination of incubation we assessed the level of expression of genes regulating apoptosis and invasiveness in endometrial tissue.

4.1 Influence of peritoneal macrophages and peritoneal fluid upon apoptosis of eutopic endometrial tissue in healthy women and in women with endometriosis

Accumulation evidences suggest that apoptosis helps to maintain cellular homeostasis during the menstrual cycle through the elimination of senescent cells from the functional layer of the uterine endometrium during the late secretory and menstrual phases of the cycle (Vigano et al., 2004). It was proposed that in healthy women the majority of menstrual reflux cells undergo programmed cells death and do not survive in the peritoneal fluid (Gebel et al., 1998; Nasu et al., 2009). On the contrary in women with endometriosis the percentage of menstruated endometrial cells undergoing apoptosis is greatly reduced, increasing the number of surviving cells that could continue to exhibit physiological activity (Vigano et al., 2004). In our work we have checked out the influence of peritoneal fluid factors upon apoptosis endometrial cells both in healthy women and in women with endometriosis to elucidate the mechanisms responsible for elimination of menstrual endometrial cells from peritoneal cavity in women with and without endometriosis.

It was found that in women without endometriosis incubation of the endometrial explants with macrophages had led to the significant increase of the caspase-3 and MT-1 mRNAs expression in endometrial tissue (Table 3). Peritoneal fluid in this case didn't influence upon apoptosis-related gene expression in endometrial tissue.

Parameter, copies number/μl	Endometrium +RPMI 1640 (control) (n=10)	Endometrium+ autologous macrophages (n=10)	Endometrium + autologous peritoneal fluid (n=10)
mRNA MT-1	21.51±2.59	54.19±13.90*	68.79±21.68
mRNA XIAP	0.73±0.15	0.73±0.16	1.26±0.62
mRNA caspase-3	15.69±5.91	39.51±9.64*	131.21±73.54
mRNA HSP27	5.28±3.02	8.57±0.45	13.27±2.45

Table 3. The influence of peritoneal macrophages and peritoneal fluid upon the expression of mRNAs of genes, regulating apoptosis, in endometrium of healthy women (* – given in comparison to the control, *- $p<0.05$)

We also estimated the amount of apoptotic endometrial stromal cells in endometrium of healthy women after its incubation with macrophages or with peritoneal fluid in standard test with Annexin V and propidium iodide (Pi) staining. It was established that both macrophages and peritoneal fluid of healthy women increased the amount of apoptotic Annexin V+ endometrial cells (Table 4). The elevation of the amount of apoptotic cells was noted predominantly in population of endometrial stromal cells, entered in the late/irreversible apoptosis.

Parameter, %	Endometrium +RPMI 1640 (control) (n=5)	Endometrium+ autologous macrophages (n=5)	Endometrium + autologous Peritoneal fluid (n=4)
Annexin V+	63.36±2.86	78.14±4.21*	81.90±1.24***
Annexin V+Pi-	25.62±2.96	29.54±2.24	27.55±2.35
Annexin V+Pi+	37.74±4.12	53.23±4.25*	54.35±2.25**

Table 4. The influence of peritoneal macrophages and peritoneal fluid upon apoptosis of eutopic endometrium stromal cells in healthy women (* – given in comparison to the control, *- $p<0.05$, **- $p<0.01$, ***- $p<0.001$)

So, our results let us to conclude that in physiological conditions the endometrial cells are effectively eliminated from the peritoneal cavity due to induction of apoptosis by peritoneal macrophages. Peritoneal fluid, according to our data, is less important for induction of apoptosis in endometrium of healthy women. Only macrophages of women without endometriosis are capable to increase the synthesis one of the most important pro-apoptotic factor - caspase-3 in autologous endometrial tissue. Earlier it was shown that the control of tissue homeostasis by induction of apoptosis in aging and transformed cells is one of the important macrophages function (Gordon & Freedman, 2006). It is also known that apoptotic cells are rapidly engulfed by phagocytes in a process akin to macro pinocytosis. Normally, the uptake of apoptotic cells is accompanies by the induction of anti-inflammatory cytokine synthesis of phagocytes (Erwig & Henson, 2007). Our results have shown that MT-1 synthesis significant elevated in endometrium of healthy women after its incubation with peritoneal macrophages. It is known that metallothioneins demonstrated strong antioxidant properties and able to scavenge a wide range of reactive oxygen species thus serving as anti-inflammatory mediators (Inoue et al., 2009). So, the increase of MT-1 synthesis in endometrial cells, undergoing apoptosis, might be one of the factors, participating in the development of anti-inflammatory environment in the process of endometrial apoptotic cells uptake by phagocytes. Summarizing our data about the influence of peritoneal fluid factors upon apoptosis of endometrial cells in healthy women it can be concluded that the increase of the amount of endometrial stromal cells at the late stages of apoptosis after its incubation with autologous peritoneal macrophages or with peritoneal fluid is physiological process that prevent the survival and growth of menstrual endometrial cells in peritoneal cavity.

In women with endometriosis the response of endometrial cells upon the influence of peritoneal fluid factors significantly differed from that in healthy women. In vitro incubation of endometrial explants of women with endometriosis with the autologous peritoneal macrophages had led to the decrease of MT-1, XIAP, and caspase-3 mRNAs expression (Table 5). In these conditions the peritoneal fluid of endometriosis women significantly increased the level of HSP27 mRNA expression (Table 5) and diminished the amount of early apoptotic endometrial stromal cells (Table 6).

Parameter, copies number/µl	Endometrium +RPMI 1640 (control) (n=10)	Endometrium+ autologous macrophages (n=10)	Endometrium + autologous peritoneal fluid (n=10)
mRNA MT-1	43.95±7.88	13.02±4.03**	26.82±7.12
mRNA XIAP	0.47±0.19	0.04±0.01*	0.19±0.06
mRNA caspase 3	18.52±8.20	0.42±0.22*	2.81±1.09
mRNA HSP27	14.52±6.20	12.86±5.52	70.32±26.19*

Table 5. The influence of peritoneal macrophages and peritoneal fluid upon the expression of mRNAs of genes, regulating apoptosis, in eutopic endometrium of women with endometriosis (* – given in comparison to the control, *- p<0.05)

Parameter, %	Endometrium +RPMI 1640 (control) (n=8)	Endometrium+ autologous macrophages (n=8)	Endometrium + autologous peritoneal fluid (n=5)
Annexin V+	59.96±4.67	54.76±3.68	45.35±3.38*
Annexin V+Pi-	24.59±1.88	20.35±1.54	17.38±2.46*
Annexin V+Pi+	35.00±5.28	34.79±3.57	28.00±3.11

Table 6. The influence of peritoneal macrophages and peritoneal fluid upon apoptosis of eutopic endometrium stromal cells in women with endometriosis (* – given in comparison to the control, *- p<0.05).

Thus, the influence of both peritoneal macrophages and peritoneal fluid of women with endometriosis upon apoptosis of autologous eutopic endometrium was opposite to that in healthy women. Peritoneal macrophages decreased the expression of pro-apoptotic genes, and peritoneal fluid increased the synthesis of anti-apoptotic protein HSP27, diminishing the early apoptosis of endometrial stromal cells. We have seen only one exception from the anti-apoptotic action of peritoneal fluid factors in endometriosis. Peritoneal macrophages of women with endometriosis decreased the level of mRNA expression of apoptosis inhibitor factor XIAP. We thought that this effect might be responsible for the phenomenon of low expression of XIAP gene in ectopic endometrium in vivo. But in the general the action of peritoneal factors of women with endometriosis was directed to the inhibition of apoptosis of autologous endometrial cells. Evidently, this action of peritoneal fluid factors might serve as one of the fundamental mechanisms leading to survival of endometrial cells in peritoneal cavity and promotion of ectopic lesions formation and growth. Our results are in a good accordance to the literature data. Earlier it was shown that addition of plasma or peritoneal fluid of women with endometriosis to in vitro cultures of neutrophils from healthy donors reduced the percents of apoptotic cells (Kwak et al., 2002). Decrease of the sensitivity of endometrial cells of women with endometriosis to cytolysis by peritoneal macrophages was also noted (Dmowski et al., 1998). But all these works didn't light the mechanisms of apoptosis-inhibitory action of peritoneal fluid and peritoneal macrophages of women with endometriosis.

4.2 The influence of peritoneal macrophages and peritoneal fluid upon the invasiveness of eutopic endometrial tissue in endometriosis women

We also established that peritoneal fluid factors directly influenced upon invasive capacity of endometrial cells of women with endometriosis. In vitro incubation of endometrial explants of women with endometriosis with the autologous peritoneal macrophages had led to the decrease of TIMP-1 and TIMP-2 mRNAs expression and the peritoneal fluid of endometriosis women significantly increased the level of MMP-2 mRNA expression by eutopic endometrial cells (Table 7).

Parameter, copies number/µl	Endometrium +RPMI 1640 (control) (n=6)	Endometrium+ autologous macrophages (n=6)	Endometrium + autologous peritoneal fluid (n=6)
mRNA MMP-2	4.83±2.40	2.97±0.89	20.44±6.19*
mRNA TIMP-2	10.36±2.60	1.76±0.64*	8.25±2.57
mRNA MMP-9	0.18±0.09	0.17±0.13	0.98±0.68
mRNA TIMP-1	10.12±3.91	0.52±0.25*	15.00±6.98

Table 7. The influence of peritoneal macrophages and peritoneal fluid upon the expression of mRNAs of genes, regulating invasiveness, in eutopic endometrium of women with endometriosis (* - given in comparison to the control, *- $p<0.05$).

So, in endometriosis both soluble factors of peritoneal fluid and macrophages evidently increased the invasiveness of eutopic endometrial cells. The literature data about stimulatory action of peritoneal fluid from women with endometriosis upon uPA protein expression in endometrial cell culture from women with and without endometriosis are in a good accordance with our results (Cosin et al., 2010).

Results of our experiments, received after estimation of the invasiveness of endometrial stromal cells of women with endometriosis in matrigel system also have shown the prominent stimulatory effect of soluble factors of peritoneal fluid of women with endometriosis on endometrial cells invasiveness. We found the enhanced invasion of endometrial stromal cells in matrigel in the presence of autologous peritoneal fluid or in the presence of supernatants of 24-hours cultures of peritoneal macrophages of women with endometriosis (Fig.2). In every case we estimated the action of autologous peritoneal fluid, and the action of pooled supernatants of peritoneal macrophages cultures. When endometrial cells migrated through membrane pores with matrigel only in presence of culture media RPMI 1640 we have seen the only few migrated cells (coefficient of spontaneous invasion - 53.52±23.33%). In the cases of endometrial stromal cells invasion in the presence of autologous peritoneal fluid, coefficient of invasion was 71.85±2.15%, and addition of supernatants of peritoneal macrophages cultures in culture media elevated the coefficient of invasion to 76.07±1.43% ($p<0.001$ in both cases).

Thus, summarizing our results about the influence of peritoneal fluid factors on apoptosis and invasiveness of endometrial cells in endometriosis, it might be concluded that immunosurveillance in the peritoneal cavity of women with endometriosis promotes conditions favorable for apoptosis inhibition and invasiveness facilitation of endometrial cells. Incapability of macrophages of women with endometriosis to eliminate the ectopic cells from the peritoneal cavity and the stimulatory effect of humoral peritoneal factors on the synthesis of proteolytic enzymes by endometrial cells might be considered as the important pathogenetic mechanisms of endometriotic tissue formation and growth.

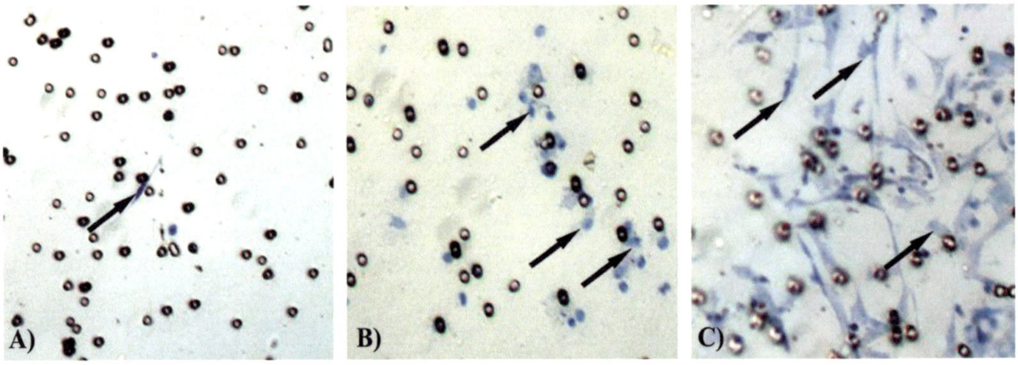

Fig. 2. Invasion of eutopic endometrium stromal cells of women with endometriosis. Holes represent the 8-µm pore in the filter. A- spontaneous invasion of endometrial stromal cells in RPMI 1640 medium; B - invasion of endometrial stromal cells in the presence of the supernatants of 24-h culture of macrophages; C - invasion of endometrial stromal cells in the presence of the autologous peritoneal fluid. Arrows indicate cells. (Original magnification x200)

5. Immune response in peritoneal cavity in endometriosis

As we can see from our results and from number of literature data, behavior of endometrial cells, floating in peritoneal fluid, is directly regulated by the peritoneal fluid microenvironment. Deficiency of immune response in peritoneal cavity supposedly might prevent clearance of the retrograde menstrual debris from the peritoneal environment and permits the implantation of misplaced endometrial cells that result in the development of endometriosis (Dmowski & Braun, 2004). To define more precisely the mechanisms attributing to the impairment of immune response in peritoneal fluid, we have studied the functional state of peritoneal macrophages and peritoneal fluid cytokine profile in endometriosis.

5.1 Peritoneal macrophages in endometriosis

Macrophages are key cellular constituents of the immune response in peritoneal cavity because macrophages comprise up to 90% of peritoneal fluid cells (Tariverdian et al., 2007). It is well known that macrophages are ubiquitous immune cells that play important role in both innate and acquired immunity (Wu et al., 2004). In addition to protection the body from foreign organisms and antigens, macrophages maintain homeostasis in many tissues and in peritoneal cavity as well through their cytokine production and remodeling capabilities. With regard to female reproduction macrophages contribute to the regulation of the pituitary-gonadal axis and are found throughout female reproductive tissues including the ovary, uterus, oviduct and mammary glands (Wu et al., 2004). Macrophages derive from bone-marrow precursors which when mature enter the bloodstream as monocytes and subsequent migrate into tissues and to various body cavities, where they function primarily as phagocytes when activated. Within tissues, differentiation of monocytes into macrophages occurs in response to the surrounding microenvironmental context, which directs the acquisition of tissue-specific phenotype. Within most organs macrophages are involved in tissue homeostasis via their ability to execute diverse functional activity, including (i) phagocytosis and degradation of foreign antigens, (ii) matrix dissolution and tissue remodeling, and (iii) production and secretion of growth factors, cytokines and chemokines (Wu et al., 2004). These effector functions allow macrophages to regulate local immune and inflammatory responses as well as influence normal tissue function.

Macrophages are identified in tissues by their expression of specific proteins markers which are predominantly cell surface receptors. The proteins considered most exclusively restricted to macrophages are CD68 molecules, class II MHC antigens, receptors, that are involved in phagocytosis, including Fc receptors, complement receptors, integrins, mannose receptor, sialoadhesin and scavenger receptors (Wu et al., 2004). Macrophages are considered "professional phagocytes" and can internalize particles much more rapidly and efficiently then other cells due to their expression of specific cell surface receptors, which initiates actin polymerization and internalization of the foreign molecule or organism into a phagosome. Macrophages phagocytose endogenous and exogenous substances, such as cell debris, bacteria and viruses. Macrophages in vivo recognize and internalize apoptotic and necrotic cells (Wu et al., 2004). Macrophages sequestered in the peritoneal cavity remove red blood cells, damaged tissue fragments, apoptotic cells, and probably endometrial cells that gain access to the peritoneal cavity through the fallopian tubes (Dmowski & Braun, 2004).

In endometriotic peritoneal fluid the concentration and number of peritoneal macrophages are significantly increased as compared to healthy controls (Tariverdian et al., 2007). These are large, activated macrophages that produce high levels of smooth-muscle-contracting prostaglandins, such as PGE2 and PGF2α (Gazvani & Templeton, 2002; Dmowski & Braun, 2004). Elevated PGE2 in the peritoneal fluid of endometriosis patients due to macrophages activation have been proposed to subsequently aggravate endometriosis-associated pain by altering uterine and tubal contractility and cause infertility due to a delayed ovum transport (Tariverdian et al., 2007). But despite of activated status macrophages evidently are not capable to effectively control the growth of endometrial tissue in peritoneal cavity of women with endometriosis. Molecular basis for this phenomenon isn't completely elucidated yet.

One of the mechanisms by which abnormally functioning macrophages could contribute to the growth of ectopic endometrial cells is through defective scavenging activity (Sidell et al., 2002). Important function of macrophages in the face of an invading "foreign" material or when encountering cellular debris and apoptotic cells is the scavenger function (Sidell et al., 2002). A family of specific scavenger receptors (SRs) is involved in this activity. This family was aptly named because these receptors have been found to bind and "scavenge" a broad array of modified self and nonself ligands, including apoptotic cells, anionic phospholipids and amyloid and pathogen components (Moore & Freeman, 2006). The SRs are believed to be members of the group of pattern recognition receptors (PRR) that mediate the innate immune host response through recognition of highly conserved pathogen-associated molecular patterns (PAMP). This evolutionarily ancient but highly effective system of host defense enables the immune system to discriminate between "noninfectious self" and "infectious nonself". However, there is a growing body of evidence to suggest that SRs may recognize endogenous neoantigens and apoptotic cells through molecular mimicry of microbial pathogen ligands (Moore & Freeman, 2006). In the last several years it was found that SRs initiate signaling cascades that regulate macrophages activation, lipid metabolism, and inflammatory programs. In addition, these receptors play role in the induction of apoptosis and apoptotic cell clearance. So, it is possible that SRs are directly involved in the clearance of endometrial debris from the peritoneal cavity. And it is also possible that peritoneal macrophages from women with endometriosis do not express fully functional scavenger receptors. But, now we know very little about the character of scavenger receptors expression by peritoneal macrophages of women with endometriosis. So, the study of the scavenger function of peritoneal macrophages in endometriosis has a special interest.

We have analyzed the expression of some surface functional receptors, such as integrin molecules CD11b and CD49e, HLA-DR molecules, CD95 and ligand for CD95 molecules (CD95L) and scavenger receptors SR-AI (CD204) and SR-B (CD36) as well by peritoneal macrophages of healthy women and women with endometriosis. It was found that peritoneal macrophages of women with endometriosis were characterized by the diminished level of the expression of scavenger receptors A and B type compared to that in healthy women (Table 8). More other, in women with endometriosis the amount of CD11b+, CD49e+, HLA-DR+ and CD95L+ macrophages in peritoneal fluid was also lower than that in healthy women (Table 8). We checked out the correlation between the character of receptors expression and the stage of endometriosis. All women with endometriosis were divided into two subgroups: women with mild and severe endometriosis. In subgroup with mild endometriosis the 1-2 stage of the disease was diagnosed during laparoscopy. Women with severe endometriosis have diagnosed of 3-4 stage of endometriosis during laparoscopic investigation.

Parameter,%	Control group (n=10)	Endometriosis (n=30)	1-2 stage of endometriosis (n=20)	3-4 stage of endometriosis (n=10)
CD204 (SR-AI)+	68.31±5.37	53.20±2.36*	50.88±3.20**	56.10±2.15*
CD36 (SR-B)+	70.86±9.22	57.20±2.36*	56.48±2.96*	59.53±2.00*
CD11b+	85.14±1.57	71.97±2.30***	71.58±2.91***	73.10±3.19**
CD49e+	87.91±2.19	80.16±2.34*	78.03±2.55**	87.6±4.12
HLA-DR+	87.35±2.28	78.35±2.43*	80.59±2.37*	71.97±6.23*
CD95+	48.12±3.16	51.39±2.54	47.46±4.32	54.02±3.05
CD95L+	60.62±2.42	46.37±2.65***	45.62±3.42***	48.50±3.41**

Table 8. Membrane expression of functional receptors by peritoneal macrophages of women with endometriosis (* - given in comparison to the control group, * - $p<0.05$, **- $p<-0.01$, ***- $p<0.001$)

Differential analysis of surface macrophages phenotype had shown that the expression of SRs, HLA-DR, CD11b and FasL molecules was significantly decreased both in mild and severe endometriosis compared to analogous parameters in control group (Table 8). The only association between the level of receptor expression and the stage of endometriosis was noted for CD49e molecules. The low expression of CD49e was seen only in women with 1-2 stage of the endometriosis, and in women with 3-4 stage of the disease the amount of CD49+ peritoneal macrophages was completely corresponded to that in healthy women. So, peritoneal macrophages in endometriosis independently from the stage of the disease are characterized by the low level of expression of functional receptors, such as integrins, scavenger receptors and apoptosis-inducing molecules.

This aberrant expression of the surface receptors might lead to the impairment of peritoneal macrophages function in endometriosis which in turn can contribute to the rescue of endometrial cells from immunosurveillance in peritoneal cavity. It is known that CD11b and CD49e molecules belong to the class of integrins, superfamily of cell adhesion receptors that bind to extracellular matrix ligands, cell-surface ligands and soluble ligands (Takakda et al., 2007). It is known that upon binding extracellular ligands, integrins generate an intracellular signal and, conversely, their functioning can be regulated by signals from within the cell. They serve as transmembrane links between extracellular contacts (other cells or the extracellular matrix) and the actin microfilaments of the cytoskeleton, whose behavior integrins also regulate and modulate. Extracellular ligation of integrins triggers a large variety of signal transduction events that modulate cell behaviors such as adhesion, proliferation survival or apoptosis, shape, polarity, motility and differentiation (Takakda et al., 2007). The low level expression of integrins by peritoneal macrophages might lead to the impairment of the interaction of macrophages with ECM and other cells, including the cells of reflux menstrual endometrium. More other, it is known, that if the peritoneal macrophages are not attached to extracellular matrix components, despite their differentiated status may not be competent scavengers (Sidell et al., 2002). Our results about the simultaneously diminishment of the expression of integrins and scavenger receptors A and B type by peritoneal macrophages of women with endometriosis completely confirmed the hypothesis that the defective scavenger function plays an important role in the immune mechanisms of endometriosis development.

Today the A class of SRs has grown to include 5 members that share common collagen-like domains and homotrimeric structure. SR-A receptors bind oxidized low-density lipoproteins, apoptotic cells, β-amyloid peptide, anionic phospholipids and advanced glycation end-products (Murphy et al., 2005). These receptors have also been implicated in both innate and adaptive immune responses through their recognition of pathogens and pathogen-associated molecules (Moore & Freeman, 2006). The B class of SRs was established with the identification of CD36 as a receptor for oxidized low-density lipoproteins. Unlike the SR-A family, CD36 is a type III (multiple transmembrane domains) receptor that traverses the membrane twice to form a heavily glycosylated extracellular loop with 2 short intracellular tails (Murphy et al., 2005). CD36 has a wider cellular distribution, including monocytes, macrophages, adipocytes, microvascular endothelium, platelets and erythroid precursors. CD36 bind several ligands common to SR-A (β-amyloid, anionic phospholipids, apoptotic cells, advanced glycation end-products), however, it is distinct from SR-A in its ability to bind native lipoproteins and very low-density lipoprotein as well as thrombospondin-I, collagen, fatty acids and pathogen-derived ligands (Moore & Freeman, 2006). As a result of its broad specificity, CD36 has been reported to contribute to a varied list of normal and pathologic processes such as apoptotic cell clearance, fatty acid transport, adhesion, angiogenesis and microbial defense (Murphy et al., 2005). Decrease of SR-AI and SR-B molecules on the surface of peritoneal macrophages of women with endometriosis likely might to contribute to the impairment of clearance of endometrial cells from peritoneal cavity and facilitate the implantation and growth of ectopic endometrium.

The low expression of FasL molecules by peritoneal macrophages might be attributed to the decrease of apoptosis-inducting function of macrophages in endometriosis. As we have demonstrated above macrophages of women with endometriosis were incapable to induce apoptosis in autologous eutopic endometrium. The observed low expression of FasL molecules on the macrophages surface likely is probably one of the possible mechanisms which impair the apoptosis-inducing function of macrophages in endometriosis. It is known that FasL or Fas ligand is one of the main transmembrane receptors initiating extrinsic pathway of apoptosis (Elmore 2007). The binding of FasL to its receptor Fas on the surface of cell-target results in the binding of the adapter protein FADD, activation of pro-caspase-8 and formation of death-inducing signaling complex (DISC) (Elmore 2007). So, the FasL-positive cells are powerful inducers of apoptosis and impairment of FasL expression on the surface of peritoneal macrophages might be an important factor contributing to inhibition of endometrial apoptosis.

We shown that the expression of HLA-DR molecules by peritoneal macrophages in endometriosis also was decreased comparing to that in healthy women. The same results were received Yamamoto et al. (2008), which observed low HLA expression and particularly reduced HLA-DR in the lipid raft. It is known that HLA-DR molecules are involved in antigen presentation by macrophages (Wu et al., 2004). So, impairment of HA-DR expression might compromise antigen presentation in women with endometriosis, limiting the immune response to peritoneal cavity antigens such as implanted or metaplastic endometrial cells.

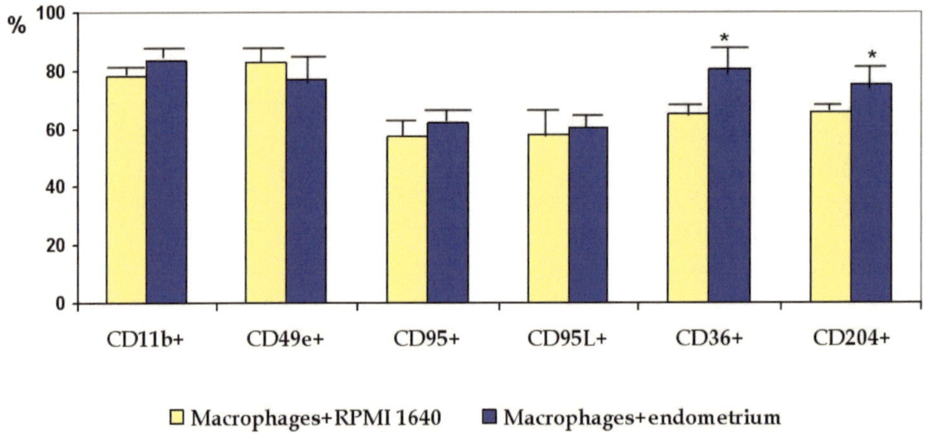

Fig. 3. Changes in the expression of functional molecules and scavenger receptors by peritoneal macrophages of healthy women after its incubation in vitro with autologous eutopic endometrium (* - given in comparison to macrophages incubating only in the presence of RPMI 1640, * - p<0.05).

Limited expression of the surface functional receptors by macrophages in endometriosis can lead to the incapability of macrophages to correctly response upon stimulation by autologous endometrial cells. We tried to prove this hypothesis and have done series of experiments in vitro for co-cultivation of peritoneal fluid macrophages with explants of autologous endometrial tissue with subsequent estimation of the surface membrane receptors by macrophages. We found that in healthy women the significant elevation of the scavenger receptors A and B type upon macrophages after their incubation with endometrial explants was seen (Fig.3). These results confirmed the suggestion about the direct involvement of SRs in normal response of peritoneal macrophages on the ectopic misplaced endometrium.

On the contrary, in endometriosis women the stimulation of peritoneal macrophages by autologous endometrial cells didn't change the expression of scavenger receptors by macrophages (Fig.4). Moreover, after co-cultivation of macrophages from endometriosis women with eutopic endometrial the significant diminishment of the number of FasL+, CD11b+ and CD49e+ macrophages was seen (Fig.4).

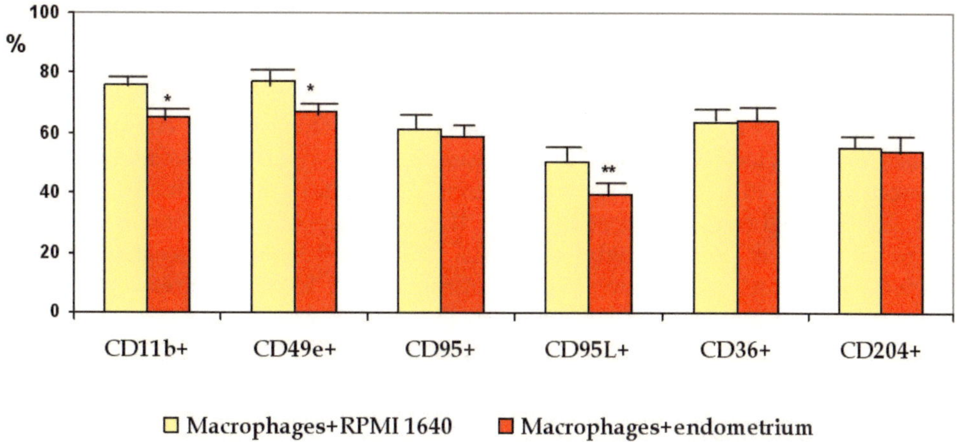

Fig. 4. Changes in the expression of functional molecules and scavenger receptors by peritoneal macrophages of women with endometriosis after its incubation in vitro with autologous eutopic endometrium (* - given in comparison to macrophages incubating only in the presence of RPMI 1640, * - $p<0.05$).

Supposedly, the initial aberrant expression of functional receptors by peritoneal macrophages results in inadequate response of macrophages to stimulation of self endometrial cells which, in turn escape the immunosurveillance in peritoneal cavity.

5.2 Peritoneal fluid cytokine production in endometriosis

The majority of studies up to now have shown significantly increase of the content of cytokines and growth factors in peritoneal fluid of women with endometriosis (Dmowski & Braun, 2004). It is known that cytokines and growth factors are proteins or glycoproteins produced by leukocytes or other cells, and secreted to the extracellular environment. These molecules exert their effects on the same (autocrine) or nearby cells (paracrine activity). They are key mediators of intercellular communication within immune system. Cytokines may have proliferative, cytostatic, chemo atractant or differetiative effects (Berkkanoglu & Arici, 2003). Cytokines possess pleiotropic function and act in cascade manner. The involvements of cytokines in the pathogenesis of many diseases, connected with inflammation and cells proliferation, such as autoimmune pathology, rheumatoid arthritis, cancer etc, have been proved. The role of cytokines system in pathogenesis of endometriosis was studied very intensively. The increased leukocyte number found in peritoneal fluid of women with endometriosis is likely to be attributable to the enhanced synthesis of various cytokines and growth factors (Dmowski & Braun, 2004). Cytokines also might be produced by endothelial cells, misplaced endometrial cells and ectopic tissue cells. The detailed analysis of the cytokines profile of peritoneal fluid of endometriosis women is above scope of this paper. To receive more information we recommend to direct reader's attention to some detailed reviews (Harada et al., 2001; Gazvani & Templeton, 2002; Kyama et al., 2003; Wu & Ho, 2003; Dmowski & Braun, 2004). Briefly, significantly elevated concentration of numerous proinflammatory cytokines such as IL-1β, TNFα, IL-6, IL-8, IL-12, IL-16, RANTES, EGF, TGF β, CSG, IFG, HGF was found in peritoneal fluid of endometriosis women and practically in all cases investigators conclude that this local sterile inflammation possibly "plays a decisive role in the pathogenesis if the endometriosis". This conclusion is based on the experimental data, showing capability of several proinflammatory cytokines increase the proliferation and growth endometrial cells. For example, experiments in vitro demonstrated that TNFα and IL-8 collaborate in the proliferation of stromal cells from ectopic endometrium and endometriomata (Harada et al., 2001). It was also shown that TNFα as the factor of peritoneal fluid from women with endometriosis promotes proliferation of eutopic and ectopic endometrial cells (Braun et al., 2002). IL-8 stimulates the adhesion of endometrial cells to fibronectin (Berkkanoglu & Arici, 2003). IL-1β promotes angiogenesis in endometriotic lesions by inducing the angiogenic factors in endometriotic stromal cells but not in normal endometrial stromal cells (Lebovis et al., 2000). But the majority of works are only descriptive and the functional involvement of cytokines in the development or progression of endometriosis has not been proven. Up to now we don't know exactly: is this peritoneal inflammation cause or consequence of the disease. From one side high concentration of growth factors and some cytokines, influencing upon cells proliferation, evidently might promote of endometrium implantation and growth in peritoneal cavity. Bur from another side, as ectopic endometrial lesions are a valuable source of cytokines itself, so peritoneal inflammation may be only the consequence of the presence of endometrial lesions in peritoneal cavity. Solutions of this problem evidently will be very helpful as to the endometriosis pathogenesis comprehension and search of new approaches to the medical treatment of endometriosis as well.

We attempted to trace the connection between cytokine profile of peritoneal fluid of women with endometriosis and possible mechanisms of peritoneal fluid action upon invasiveness of endometrial cells. To this purpose we estimated the concentration of few cytokines with possible action upon cells invasiveness, such as chemokines IL-8 and MCP and protein calprotektin, belonging to the family S100 proteins. We found the significant elevation all above mentioned cytokines in the peritoneal fluid of patients with endometriosis (Table 9). When we analyzed these cytokines content in subgroups of women with mild and severe endometriosis we found, that concentration of these cytokines correlated with the degree of endometriosis: maximal levels of IL-8, MCP-1 and calprotektin were seen in women with severe endometriosis (Table 9).

All of these cytokines are powerful stimulators of cells invasiveness. Earlier it was found that IL-8 directly increases the MMPs activity and invasive potential of endometrial cells in culture (Mulayim et al., 2004). Calprotektin, comprise the heterodimeric complex from C2a+-binding proteins S100A8 and S100 A9, also participates in cells invasiveness regulation. It was found that enhanced expression of S100A8/A9 gene is the marker of metastatic potential of epithelial tumor cells (Moon et al., 2008). It was also demonstrated that calprotektin is involved in the activation of gene MMP-2 transcription in tumor cell line SNU484 (Yong & Moon, 2007). Chemokine MCP-1 acts as paracrine and autocrine regulator of growth and invasion of prostate tumor (Lu et al., 2009). So, all these cytokines can be stimulators of the eutopic endometrial cells invasiveness in peritoneal fluid. But, the significant elevation of studied cytokines content was noted only in women with severe endometriosis. In cases of mild endometriosis the cytokines concentrations didn't differ from that in healthy women.

Parameter	Control group (n=10)	Endometriosis (n=35)	1-2 stage of endometriosis (n=18)	3-4 stage of endometriosis (n=17)
Calprotektin, µg/ml	0.44±0.17	1.28±0.38*	0.62±0.26	1.86±0.65*
IL-8, pg/ml	6.19±3.41	19.09±5.00*	10.83±4.18	27.73±9.12*
MCP-1, pg/ml	308.12±29.87	528.40±51.45**	376.56±50.32	689.18±74.79***xxx

Table 9. Cytokine content in peritoneal fluid of women with endometriosis (* - given in comparison to the control group, * - $p<0.05$, **- p<-0.01, ***- $p<0.001$; x - given in comparison to the group of women with 1-2 stage of endometriosis, xxx- $p<0.001$)

It is known, that peritoneal macrophages are the major producers of cytokines in peritoneal fluid (Wu & Ho, 2003). We assessed the production of several proinflammatory cytokines (IL-1β, IL-8, TNFα, IL-6, and IL-12) by peritoneal macrophages in endometriosis. It was found that that character of intracellular production of proinflammatory cytokines by macrophage was correspondent to cytokines content in peritoneal fluid (Table 10). The level of cytokines production directly correlated with the severity of endometriosis and significantly increased only in group of women with 3-4 stages of endometriosis. The only exception we noted for TNFα. We found that that the intracellular production of TNFα by peritoneal macrophages was significantly elevated both in women with mild and severe endometriosis (Table 10).

Parameter,%	Control group (n=10)	Endometriosis (n=28)	1-2 stage of endometriosis (n=18)	3-4 stage of endometriosis (n=10)
IL-1β+	64.51±3.40	74.69±2.90*	73.47±3.09	80.53±3.46***
IL-8+	67.10±2.96	75.13±2.03*	68.42±4.14	78.17±1.70**
TNFα+	63.11±3.37	74.77±1.95**	74.72±2.96**	76.24±2.38*
IL-6+	52.74±4.18	66.63±2.87	58.41±3.36	66.25±2.70*
IL-12+	67.35±3.39	63.64±2.56	63.268±3.32	65.53±0.95

Table 10. Intracellular production of cytokines by peritoneal macrophages of women with endometriosis (* - given in comparison to the control group, * - $p<0.05$, **- p<-0.01, ***- $p<0.001$)

TNFα or tumor necrosis factor α initially was identified for its ability to kill certain cell lines, but now it is known that TNFα have the ability to initiate the cascade of other cytokines and factors associated with inflammatory responses. Earlier it was shown that TNFα increased the adherence of cultured endometrial stromal cells to mesothelial cells (Zang et al., 1993). This finding suggests that the presence of TNFα in peritoneal fluid may facilitate the adherence of ectopic endometrial tissue to the peritoneum and allow implants to develop. There are some experimental data, also evidenced about implication of TNFα in the pathogenesis of endometriosis (Agic et al., 2006). In baboons with laparoscopically confirmed endometriosis, TNFα blockade with p55 soluble TNFα-receptors results in inhibition of the development and growth of endometriotic implants (D'Hooghe et al., 2006). In rats with ectopically transplanted endometrial tissue, the administration of recombinant human TNFα- binding protein-1 (r-hTBP-1) resulted in defective development of implants compared with controls (D'Antonio et al., 2000). All these data and our own results let us to suggest the possible involvement of TNFα in initial mechanisms of ectopic endometrium implantation and growth. But it must be special noted that the macrophage's production and peritoneal fluid content of the majority of proinflammatory cytokines significantly elevated only at advantage stages of endometriosis.

Thus, we must very careful to speculate about possible involvement of cytokines in the peritoneal fluid in regulation of the behavior of endometrial cells in peritoneal cavity, because the prominent action of peritoneal fluid cytokines generally is seen only in advantage stages of endometriosis. We thought that the impairment of peritoneal macrophages function plays the decisive role in immune mechanisms participating in implantation and growth of ectopic endometrium. Incapability of peritoneal macrophages to act as effective scavengers and adequately to eliminate the misplaced endometrial cells from peritoneal cavity possibly is one of the primary immunological disorders participating in endometriosis pathogenesis. Elevation of proinflammatory cytokines production in peritoneal cavity likely depends on the presence of ectopic lesions and can be stimulated by viable endometrial cells proliferating and growing in peritoneal cavity. Invasion of already implanted ectopic endometrial cells is evidently under the control of proinflammatory cytokines of peritoneal fluid.

6. Conclusions

Thus, it is very difficult to distinguish between the participation of endometrial abnormalities and immune impairments in peritoneal fluid in endometriosis pathogenesis. The frontiers between the two mechanisms are not clear-cut and evidently both mechanisms are responsible for endometriotic disease development. From one side, the development and growth of endometriosis lesions are associated with the significant changes in endometrium which are characterized by the high level of the expression of genes, stimulating invasiveness, and imbalanced production of anti- and pro-apoptotic factors in endometrial tissue. There are some differences in eutopic and ectopic endometrium in endometriosis. High level of anti-apoptotic factors XIAP synthesis is the characteristic feature of eutopic endometrium, which can provide high viability of menstrual endometrial cells in peritoneal cavity. But in endometriotic lesions the simultaneously elevated expression of both pro- and anti-apoptotic genes was seen. Likely, this phenomenon might provide the ectopic but not malignant growth of endometrium in endometriosis. The development and growth of already formed ectopic lesions but not the eutopic endometrium of women with endometriosis is under the control of proteolytic enzymes from metalloproteinases family. We found that some of these differences between eutopic and ectopic endometrium might be due to the impairment of immunosurveillance in peritoneal cavity. Both peritoneal macrophages and humoral factors of peritoneal fluid directly influenced upon apoptosis and invasiveness of endometrial cells. This action might be connected with the changes of functional activity of peritoneal macrophages and local cytokine production. The impairment of the scavenger function of peritoneal macrophages due to the decreased level of membrane expression of integrins, scavenger receptors and apoptosis-inducing molecules FasL is possibly one of the fundamental defects of immune response in peritoneal cavity, which allow endometrial cell to live, proliferate and be implanted. Altered cytokine profile of peritoneal fluid in endometriosis likely can promote the invasiveness of ectopic lesions. Though it can be said that now we don't fully understand the fine immune mechanisms providing the development of endometriosis. More studies into the macrophage functioning and cytokines production as well as clinical experiments on the animal model may improve our understanding of endometriosis pathogenesis and results in the novel therapeutic modalities for endometriosis.

7. References

Agi,c A,. Xu, H., Finas, D., Banz, C., Diedrich, K. & Hornung, D. Is endometriosis associated with systemic subclinical inflammation? *Gynecologic and Obstetric Investigation*, Vol.62, No.3, (April 2006), pp.139–147, ISSN 0378-7346

Agic, A., Djalali, S., Diedrich, K. & Hornung, D. Apoptosis in endometriosis. *Gynecology and Obstetrics Investigation*, Vol.68, No.4, (September 2009), pp.217-223, ISSN 0378-7346

Amalinei, C., Caruntu, I.D., Giusca, S.E. & Balan, R.A. Matrix metalloproteinases involvement in pathologic conditions. *Romanian Journal of Morphology and Embryology*, Vol.51, No.2, (June 2010), pp. 215-228. ISSN 1220-0522

Becker, C.M., Louis, G., Exarhopoulos, A., Machsner, A., Ebert, A.D., Zurakowski, D. & Moses M.A. Matrix metalloproteinases are elevated in the urine of patients with endometriosis. *Fertility and Sterility*, Vol.94, No.6, (November 2010), pp.2343-2346, ISSN 0015-0282

Berkkanoglu, M, & Arici, A. Immunology and endometriosis. *American Journal of Reproductive Immunology*, Vol.50, No.1, (July 2003), pp.48-59, ISSN 8755-8920

Bondza, P.K., Maheux, R. & Akoum, A. Insights into endometriosis-associated endometrial dysfunctions: a review. *Frontiers in Bioscience (Elite Edition)*, Vol.1, No.1, (June 2009), pp.415-438, ISSN 1945-0494

Braun, D.P., Ding, J & Dmowski, W.P. Peritoneal fluid-mediated enhancement of eutopic and ectopic endometrial cell proliferation is dependent on TNF-alpha in women with endometriosis. *Ferility and Sterility*, Vol.78, No.4, (October 2002), pp.727-732, ISSN 0015-0282

Bruse, C., Bergqvist, A., Calstrom, K., Fiaru-Jonasson, A., Lecander, I. & Astedt, B. Fibrinolytic factors in endometriotic tissue, endometrium, peritoneal fluid, and plasma from women with endometriosis and in endometrium and peritoneal fluid from healthy women. *Fertility and Sterility*, Vol.70, No.5, (November 1998), pp.821-826, ISSN 0015-0282

Chen, Q.H., Zhou, W.D., Pu, D.M., Huang, Q.S., Li, T. & Chen, O.X. 15-Epi-lipoxin A(4) inhibits the progression of endometriosis in a murine model. *Fertility and Sterility*, Vol.93, No.5, (March 2010), pp.1440-1447, ISSN 0015-0282

Colette, T., Bellehumeur, C., Kats, R., Maheux, R., Mailloux, J., Villeneuve, M , & Akoum, A. Evidence for an increased release of proteolytic activity by the eutopic endometrial tissue in women with endometriosis and for involvement of matrix metalloproteinase-9. *Humam Reproduction*, Vol.19, No.6, (June 2004), pp.1257-1264, ISSN 0268-1161

Cosin, R., Gilabert-Estelles, J., Ramon, L.A., Gomez-Lechon, M.J., Gialbert, J., Chirivella, M., Braza-Boils, A., Espana, F. & Estelles, A. Influence of peritoneal fluid on the expression of angiogenic and proteolytic factors in cultures of endometrial cells from women with endoemtriosis. *Human Reproduction*, Vol.25, No.2, (February 2010), pp.398-405, ISSN 0268-1161

Cox, K., Piva, M. & Sharpe-Timms, K.L. Differential regulation of matrix metalloproteinase-3 gene expression in endometriotic lesions compared with endometrium. *Biology of Reproduction*, Vol.65, No.4, (October 2001), pp.1297-1303, ISSN: 0006-3363

Curry, T.E. & Osteen, K.G. The matrix metalloproteinase system: changes, regulation, and impact throughout the ovarian and uterine reproductive cycle. *Endocrine Reviews*, Vol.24, No.4., (August 2003), pp. 428-465, ISSN 0163-769X

D'Antonio, M., Martelli, F., Peano, S., Papoian, R. & Borrelli, F. Ability of recombinant human TNF binding protein-1 (r-hTBP-1) to inhibit the development of experimentally-induced endometriosis in rats. *Journal of Reproductive Immunology*, Vol.48, No.2, (October-November 2000), pp.81–98, ISSN 0165-0378

De Sanctis, P., Elmakky, A., Farina, A., Caeamelli, E., Seracchioli, R., Mabrouk, M., Mignemi, G., Venturoli, S., Villa, G., Guerrini, M., Manuzzi, L., Montanari, G., Valvassori, L. & Zucchini, C. Matrix metalloproteinase-3 mRNA: a promising peripheral blood marker for diagnosis of endometriosis. *Gynecology and Obstetrics Investigation*, Vol. 71, No.2, (March 2011), pp.118-123, ISSN 0378-7346

Di Carlo, C., Bonifacio, M., Tommaselli, G.A., Bifulco, G., Guerra, G. & Nappi, C. Metalloproteinases, vascular endothelial growth factor, and angiopoietin 1 and 2 in eutopic and ectopic endometrium. *Fertility and Sterility*, Vol.91, No.6, (June 2009), pp. 2315-2323, ISSN 0015-0282

D'Hooghe, T.M., Nugent, N.P., Cuneo, S., Chai, D.C., Deer, F., Debrock, S., Kyama, C.M., Mihalyi, A. & Mwenda, J.M. Recombinant human TNFRSF1A (r-hTBP1) inhibits the development of endometriosis in baboons: a prospective, randomized, placebo-and drug-controlled study. *Biology of Reproduction*, Vol.74, No.1, (January 2006), pp.131–136, ISSN 0006-3363

Dmowski, W.P. & Braun, D.P. Immunology of endometriosis. *Best Practice & Research: Clinical Obstetrics & Gynaecology*, Vol.18, No.2, (April 2004), pp.245-263, ISSN 1521-6934

Dmowski, W.P., Gebel, H. & Braun, D.P. Decreased apoptosis and sensitivity to macrophage mediated cytolysis of endometrial cells in endometriosis. *Human Reproduction*, vol.4, No.5, (May 1998), pp.696-701, ISSN 0268-1161

Egeblad, M. & Werb, Z. New functions for the matrix metalloproteinases in cancer progression. *Nature Reviews Cancer*, Vol.2, No.3, (March 2002), pp.161-174, ISSN 1474-175X

Elmore, S. Apoptosis: a review of programmed cell death. *Toxicologic Pathology*, Vol.35, No.4, (June 2007), pp.495-516, ISSN 0192-6233

Erwig L.-P., Henson P.M. Immunological consequences of apoptotic cell phagocytosis. *The American Journal of Pathology*, Vol.171, No.1, (July 2007), pp.2-8, ISSN 0002-9440

Gazvani, R. & Templeton, A. Peritoneal environment, cytokines and angiogenesis in the pathophysyology of endometriosis. *Reproduction*, Vol 123, No.2, (February2002), pp.217-226, ISSN 1470-1626

Gebel, H.M., Braun, D.P., Tambur, A., Frame, D., Rana, N. & Dmowski W.P. Spontaneous apoptosis of endometrial tissue is impaired in women with endometriosis. *Fertility and Sterility*, Vol.69, No.6, (June 1998), pp.1042-1047, ISSN 0015-0282.

Gohji, K., Fujimoto, N., Fuji, A., Komiyama, T., Okawa, J & Nakajima, M. Prognostic significance of circulating matrix metalloproteinase-2 to tissue inhibitor of metalloproteinases-2 ratio in recurrence of urothelial cancer after complete resection. *Cancer Research*, Vol.56, No.14, (July 1996), pp.3196-3198, ISSN 0008-5472

Gordon, I.O. & Freedman, R.S. Defective antitumor function of monocyte-derived macrophages from epithelial ovarian cancer patients. *Clin.Cancer. Res.*, Vol.12, No.5, (March 2006), pp. 1515-1524, ISSN 1078-0432

Harada, T., Iwabe, T. & Terakawa, N. Role of cytokines in endometriosis. *Fertility and Sterility*, Vol 76, No.1, (July 2001), pp.1-10, ISSN 0015-0282.

Harada, T., Kaponis, A., Iwabe, T., Taniguchi, F., Makrydimas, G., Sofikitis, N., Paschopolous, M., Paraskevaidis, E. & Terakawa, N. Apoptosis in human endometrium and endometriosis. *Human Reproduction Update*, Vol.10, No.1, (January/February 2004), pp.29-38, ISSN 1355-4786

Hassa, H., Tanir, H.M., Tekin, B., Artan, S., Dundar, E., Kirilmaz, S.D. & Sahin Mutlu F. Apoptosis patterns in eutopic and ectopic endometrium, adhesions and normal-looking peritoneum from women with or without endometriosis. *Archives of Gynecology and Obstetrics*, Vol.280, No.2, (August 2009), pp.195-199, ISSN 0932-0067

Hill, M.M., Adrain, C., Duriez, P.J., Creagh, E.M. & Martin, S,J. Analysis of the composition, assembly kineticsand activity of native Apaf-1 apoptosomes. *The Embo Journal*, Vol.23, No.10, (May 2004), pp.2134–2145, ISSN 0261-4189

Inoue, K.-I., Takano, H., Shimada, A. & Satoh, M. Metallothionein as an anti-inflammatory mediator. Hindawi Publishing Corporation. *Mediators of inflammation*, 2009: 101659, (May 2009), ISSN 0962-9351

Jonson, M.S., Torres, M., Alves, A., Bacallao, K., Fuentes, A., Vega, M. & Boric, A. Augmented cell survival in eutopic endometrium from women with endometriosis: Expression of c-myc, TGF-bets1 and bax genes. *Reproductive Biology and Endocrinology*, Vol.3, No.1, (September 2005), pp.45, ISSN 1477-7827

Juhasz-Boss, I., Hofele, A., Lattrich, C., Buchholz, S., Ortmann, O. & Malik, E. Matrix metalloproteinase messenger RNA expression in human endometriosis grafts cultured on a chicken chorioallantoic membrane. *Fertility and Sterility*, Vol.94, No.1, (January 2010), pp.40-45, ISSN 0015-0282.

Karahan, N., Güney, M., Baspinar, S., Oral, B., Kapucuoglu, N. & Mungan, T. Expression of gelatinase (MMP-2 and MMP-9) and cyclooxygenase-2 (COX-2) in endometrial carcinoma. *European Journal of Gynaecological Oncology*, Vol. 28, No.3, (May 2007) 184-188, ISSN 0392-2936

Koninckx, P.R., Kennedy, S.H. & Barlow, D.H. Endometriotic disease: the role of peritoneal fluid. *Human Reproduction Update*, Vol.4, No.5, (September/October 1998), pp.741-751, ISSN1355-4786

Kwa, J.Y., Park, S.W., Kim, K.H., Na, Y.J. & Lee K.S. Modulation of neutrophils apoptosis by plasma and peritoneal fluid from patients with advance endometriosis. *Human Reproduction*, Vol.17, No.3, (March 2002), pp.595-600, ISSN 0268-1161

Kyama, C.M., Dabrock, S., Mwenda, J. & D'Hoogle, T. Potential involvement of the immune system in the development of endometriosis. *Reproductive Biology and Endocrinilogy,*Vol.1. No.1, (December 2003), pp.123, ISSN 1477-7827

Laudanski, P., Szamatowicz, J. & Ramel, P. Matrix metalloproteinase-13 and membrane typr-1 matrix metalloproteinase in peritoneal fluid of women with endometriosis. *Gynecological Endocrinology*, Vol. 21, No.2, (August, 2005), pp. 106-110, ISSN 0951-3590

Lebovic, D.I., Bentzien, I., Chao, V.A., Garett, E.N., Meng, Y.G. & Taylor, R.N. Induction of an angiogenec phenotype in endometriotic stromal cell cultures by interleukine-1β. *Molecular Human Reproduction*, Vol.6, No.3, (March 2000), pp.269-275, ISSN 1360-9947

Lu, Y., Chen, Q., Corey, E., Xie, W., Fan, J., Mizokami, A. & Zhang, J. Activation of MCP-1/CCR2 axis promotes prostate cancer growth in bone. *Clinical and Experimental Metastasis*, Vol. 26, No.2, (February 2009), pp.161-169, ISSN 0262-0898

Machado, D.E., Berardo, P.T., Palmero C.Y. & Nasciutti, L.E. Higher expression of vascular endothelial growth factor (VEGF) and its receptor VEGFR-2 (Flk-1) and metalloproteinase-9 (MMP-9) in a rat model of peritoneal endometriosis is similar to cancer diseases. *Journal of Experimental &Clinical Cancer Research*, Vol.29, No.1, (January 2010), pp.4, ISSN 0392-9078

Mannello, F. & Gazzanelli, G. Tissue inhibitors of metalloproteinases and programmed cell death: conundrums, controversies and potential implications. *Apoptosis*, Vol.6, No.6, (December 2001), pp.479-482, ISSN 1360-8185

Mei, Y., Stonestrom, A., Hou, Y.-M. & Yang, X. Apoptotic regulation and transfer RNA. *Protein & Cell*, Vol.1, No.9, (April 2010), pp.795-801, ISSN 1674-800X

Meresman, G.F., Vighi, S., Buquet, R.A., Contreras-Ortiz, O., Tesone, M. & Rumi, L.S. Apoptosis and expression of Bcl-2, Bax in eutopic endometrium from women with endometriosis. *Fertility and Sterility*, Vol.74., No.4, (October 2000), pp.760-766, ISSN 0015-0282.

Minici, F., Tiberi, F., Tropea, A., Miceli, F., Orlando, M., Gangale, M.F., Romani, F., Catino, S., Campo, S., Lanzone, A., & Apa, R. Paracrine regulation of endometriotic tissue.

Gynecological Endocrinology, Vol.23, No.10, (October 2007), pp.574-580, ISSN 0951-3590

Mulayim, N., Savlu, A., Guzeloglu-Kayisli, O., Kayisli, U.A. & Arici, A. Regulation of endometrial stromal cell matrix metalloproteinase activity and invasiveness by interleukin-8. *Fertility and Sterility*, Vol.81, Suppl 1, (March 2004), pp.904-911, ISSN 0015-0282

Moon, A., Yong, H.Y., Song, J.I., Cukovic, D., Salagrama, S., Kaplan, D., Kim, H., Dombkowski, A. & Kim, H.R. Global gene expression profiling unveils S100A8/A9 as candidate markers in H-ras-mediated human breast epithelial cell invasion. *Molecular Cancer Research*, Vol.6, No.10, (October 2008), pp.1544-1553, ISSN 1538-7445

Moore, K.J & Freeman, M.W. Scavenger receptors in atherosclerosis: beyond lipid uptake. *Arteriosclerosis, thrombosis and vascular biology*, Vol.26, No.8, (August 2006), pp.1702-1711, ISSN 1079-5642.

Mufti, A.R., Burstein, E. & Duckett, C.S. XIAP: cell death regulation meets copper homeostasis. *Archives of Biochemistry and Biophysics*, Vol.463, No.2, (July 2007), pp.168-174, ISSN 0003-9861

Murphy, J.E., Tedbury, P.R., Homer-Vanniasinkam, S., Walker, J.H. & Ponnambalam, S. Biochemistry and cell biology of mammalian scavenger receptors. *Atherosclerosis*, Vol.182, No.1, (September 2005), pp.1-15, ISSN 0021-9150

Nap, A.W., Groothuis, P.G., Demir, A.Y., Evers, J.L.H. & Dunselman, G.A.J. Pathogenesis of endometriosis. *Best Practice & Research: Clinical Obstetrics & Gynecology*, Vol.18, No.2, (April 2004), pp.233-244, ISSN 1521-6934

Nasu, K., Yuge, A., Tsuno, A., Nishida, M. & Narahara, H. Involvement of resistance to apoptosis in the pathogenesis of endometriosis. *Histology and Histopathology*, Vol.24, No.9, (September 2009), pp.1181-1192, ISSN, 1699-5848

Nezhat, F., Datta, M.S., Hanson, V., Pejovic, T., Nezhat, C. & Nezhat C. The relationship of endometriosis and ovarian malignancy: a review. *Fertility and Sterility*, Vol.90, No5, (November 2008), pp.1559-1570, ISSN 0015-0282

Okada, N., Ishida, H., Murata, N., Hashimoto, D., Seyama, Y. & Kubota, S. Matrix metalloproteinase-2 and -9 in bile as a marker of liver metastasis in colorectal cancer. *Biochemical and Biophysical Research* Communications, Vol.288, No.1, (January 2001), pp.212-216, ISSN 0006-291X

Onisto, M., Riccio, M.P., Scannapieco, P., Caenazzo, C., Groggio, L., Spina, M., Stetler-Stevenson, W.G. & Garbisa, S. Gelatinase A/TIMP-2 imbalance in lymph-node-positive breast carcinomas, as measured by RT-PCR. *International Journal of Cancer*, Vol.63, No.5, (November 1995), pp.621-626, ISSN 0020-7136

Pandey, P., Farber, R., Nakazawa, A., Kumar, S., Bharti, A., Nalin, C., Weichselbaum, R., Kufe, D. & Kharbanda S. Hsp27 functions as a negative regulator of cytochrome c-dependent activation of procaspase-3. *Oncogene*, Vol.19, No.16, (April 2000), pp. 1975-1981, ISSN 0950-9232

Parcellier, A., Schmitt, E., Gurbuxani, S., Seigneurin-Berny, D., Pance, A., Chantome, A., Plenchette, S., Khochbin, S., Solary, E. & Garrido C. Hsp27 is a ubiquitin-binding protein involved in IκBα proteasomal degradation. *Molecular and Cellular Biology,* Vol. 23, No.16, (August 2003), pp. 5790–5802, ISSN 0270-7306

Schimmer, A.D., Dalili, S., Batey, R.A. & Riedl, S.J. Targeting XIAP for the treatment of malignancy. Cell Death & Differentiation,-Vol.13, No.2, (February 2006), pp.179-188, ISSN 1350-9047

Schmitt, E., Gahrmann, M., Brunet, M., Multhoff, G. & Garrido, C. Intracellular and extracellular functions of heat shock proteins: repercussions in cancer therapy. *Journal of Leukocyte Biology,* Vol.81, No.1, (January 2007), pp.15-27, ISSN 0741-5400

Shaco-Levy, R., Sharabi, S., Benharroch, D., Piura, B. & Sion-Vardy, N. Matrix metalloproteinases 2 and 9, E-cadherin, and beta-catenin expression in endometriosis, low-grade endometrial carcinoma and non-neoplastic eutopic endometrium. *European Journal of Obstetrics &Gynecology and Reproductive Biology,* Vol.139, No.2, (August 2008), pp.226-232, ISSN 0301-2115

Sidell, N., Han, S.W. & Parthasarathy S. Regulation and modulation od abnormal immune responses in endometriosis. *Annals of the New York Academy of Sciences,* Vol.955, (March 2002), pp.159-173, ISSN 0077-8923

Sillme, M., Prifti, S., Koch, A., Neher, M., Jauckus, J. & Runnebaum, B. Regulation of matrix metalloproteinases and their inhibitors in uterine endometrial cells of patients with and without endometriosis. *European Journal of Obstetrics &Gynecology and Reproductive Biology,* Vol.95, No.2, (April 2001), pp.167-174., ISSN 0301-2115

Sotnikova, N.Y., Antsiferova, Y.S., Posiseeva, L.V., Shishkov, D.N., Posiseev D.V. & Filippova E.S. Mechanisms regulating invasiveness and growth of endometriosis lesions in rat experimental model and in humans. *Fertility and Sterility,* Vol.93, No.8, (May 2010), pp.2701-2705, ISSN 0015-0282.

Spuijbroek, M.D.E.H., Dunselman, G.A.J., Menheere, P.P.C.A. & Evers J.L.H. Early endometriosis invades the extracellular matrix. *Fertility and Sterility,* Vol.58, No.5, (November 1992), pp.929-933, ISSN 0015-0282.

Stilley, J.A.W., Birt, J., Nagel, S., Sutovsky, M., Sutovsky, P, & Sharpe-Timmps, K. Neutralizing TIMP1 restores fecundity in a rat model of endometriosis and treating control rats with TIMP1 causes anomalies in ovarian function. *Biology of reproduction,* Vol.83, No.2, (August 2010), pp.185-194, ISSN 0006-3363

Story, L. & Kennedy, S. Animal studies in endometriosis: a review. *ILAR Journal,* Vol.45, No.2, (February 2004). pp.132-138, ISSN 1084-2020

Takada, Y., Ye, X. & Simon, S. The integrins. *Genome Biology,* Vol.8, No.5, (June 2007), article 215, ISSN 1465-6906

Taniguchi, F., Kaponis, A., Izawa, M., Kiyama, T., Deura, I., Ito, M., Iwabe, T., Adonakis, G., Tarakawa, N. & Harada, T. Apoptosis and endometriosis. *Frontiers in Bioscience (Elite Edition),* Vol.3, No.1, (January 2011), pp.648-662, ISSN 1945-0494

Tariverdian, N., Theoharides, C., Siedentopf, F., Gutierrez, G., Jeschke, U., Rabinovich, G.A., Blois, S & Arck, P.C. Neuroendocrine-immune disequilibrium and endometriosis: an interdisciplinary approach. *Seminars in Immunopathology,* Vol.29, No.2, (June 2007), pp.193-210, ISSN 1863-2297

Ulukus, M., Cakmak, H. & Arici, A. The role of endometrium in endometriosis. *Journal of the Society for Gynecologic Investigation,* Vol.13, No.7. (October 2006), pp.467-476, ISSN 1071-5576

Uzan, C., Cortez, A., Dufournet, C., Fauvet, R., Siffroi, J.P. & Daraï E. Eutopic endometrium and peritoneal, ovarian and bowel endometriotic tissues express a different profile of matrix metalloproteinases-2, -3 and -11, and of tissue inhibitor metalloproteinases-1 and -2. *Virchows Archiv,* Vol.445, No.6, (December 2004), pp.603-609, ISSN 1432-2307

Vigano, P., Parazzini, F., Somogliana, E. & Vercellini, P. Endometriosis: epidemiology and aetiological factors. *Best Practice & Research: Clinical Obstetrics & Gynaecology,* Vol.18, No.2, (April 2004), pp.117-200, ISSN 1521-6934

Vinatier, D., Orazi, G., Cosson M. & Dufour, P. Theories of endometriosis. *European Journal of Obstetrics &Gynecology and Reproductive Biology,* Vol.96, No.1, (May 2001), pp.21-34, ISSN 0301-2115

Voss, O.H., Batrs, S., Kolattukudy, J., Gonzales-Mejia, M.E., Smith, J.B. & Doseff, A.I. Binding of caspase-3 prodomain to Heat Shock protein 27 regulates monocyte apoptosis by inhibiting caspase-3 proteolytic activation. *The Journal of Biological Chemistry,* Vol.282, No.34, (August 2007), pp.25088-25099, ISSN 0021-9258

Weiss, G., Goldsmith, L.T., Taylor, R., Bellet, D. & Taylor, H.S. Inflammation in reproductive disorders. *Reproductive Sciences,* Vol.16, No.2, (February 2009), pp.216-229, ISSN 1933-7191

Wicherek, L., Dutsch-Wicherek, M., Galazka, K., Banas, T., Popiela, T., Lazar, A. & Kleinrok-Podsiadlo, B. Comparison of RCAS 1 and metallothionein expression and the presence and activity of immune cells in human ovarian and abdominal wall endometriomas. *Reproductive Biology and Endocrinology,* Vol.4, No.41, (August 2006), pp.1-9, ISSN 14-77-7827

Wu, M.Y.& Ho, H.N. The role of cytokines in endometriosis. *American Journal of Reproductive Immunology,* Vol.49, No.5, (May 2003), pp.285-296, ISSN 8755-8920.

Wu, R., Van der Hock, K.H., Ryan, N.K., Norman, R.J. & Robker, R. Macrophages contribution to ovarian function. *Human Reproduction Update,* Vol.10, No.2, (March/April 2004), pp.119-133, ISSN 1355-4786

Yamamoto, Y., Maeda, N., Izumiya, C., Kusume, T., Oguri, H., Kawashima, M., Hayashi, K., Nomura, A., Yamashita, C. & Fukaya, T. Decreased human leukocyte antigen-DR expression in the lipid raft by peritoneal macrophages from women with endometriosis. *Fertility and Sterility,* Vol.89, No.1, (May 2007), pp.52-59, ISSN 0015-0282

Yong, H.Y. & Moon A. Roles of calcium-binding proteins, S100A8 and S100A9, in invasive phenotype of human gastric cancer cells. *Archives of Pharmacal Research,* Vol.30, No.1, (January 2007), pp.75-81, ISSN 0253-6269

Zang, R.J., Wild, R.A. & Ojago, J. Effect of tumor necrosis factor alpha on adhesion of human endometrial stromal cells to peritoneal mesothelial cells: an in vitro system. *Fertility and Sterility,* Vol.56, No.6, (June 1993), pp.1196-1201, ISSN 0015-0282

Zhou, H.E. & Nothnick, W.B. The relevancy of the matrix metalloproteinase system to the pathophysiology of endometriosis. *Frontiers in Bioscience (Elite Edition)*,Vol. 10, No.1, (January 2005), pp.569-575, ISSN 1945-0494

12

Virus Infection and Type I Interferon in Endometriosis

Pia M. Martensen[1], Anna L. Vestergaard[1,3] and Ulla B. Knudsen[2]
[1]Department of Molecular Biology, Aarhus University,
[2]Department of Gynecology and Obstetrics, Aarhus University Hospital, Skejby,
[3]Department of Biomedicine, Aarhus University,
Denmark

1. Introduction

Endometriosis is a chronic disease in which endometrium-like lesions are located ectopically, frequently in the pelvic cavity but also in more distant regions. It has been estimated that 5 to 10% of fertile women are suffering from the disease, and in a population of women with dysmenorrhoea (painful periods), around 50% have endometriosis (Faquhar, 2007). The symptoms include chronic pelvic pain, dysmenorrhoea, dyspareunia (pain during intercourse), and subfertility. The pathogenesis of endometriosis is unclear. Endometriosis is hormonal-dependent and therefore mainly found in women in the fertile age, although rare cases have been found in men and postmenopausal women. The risk is increased seven- to nine-fold for women who have a close relative (mother and/or sister) with endometriosis, indicating some genetic involvement (Simpson et al., 1980). Endometriosis displays malignant-like features, such as invasiveness and metastasis, and DNA viruses might play a role in endometriosis, like human papillomavirus (HPV) is part of the pathogenesis of cervix cancer (zur Hausen, 2009). Signs of inflammation are the key findings in endometriosis. From the above, some evidence points towards a possible involvement of the type I interferons (IFNs). This chapter will discuss whether DNA-viruses and the innate immune system might be involved in the pathogenesis of endometriosis.

1.1 Immunology and inflammation in endometriosis

Inflammation, characterized by activated lymphocytes, neutrophils, and macrophages, is a key feature of endometriosis tissue, associated with the overproduction of prostaglandins, metalloproteinases, cytokines, and chemokines (Bulun, 2009). It is debated whether the peritoneal inflammation is a consequence or a cause of endometriosis, or both. The immune system is involved in the pathogenesis of endometriosis on multiple levels, of which important features will be presented in this section.

It is believed that defective immunosurveillance in women with endometriosis contributes to the attachment, persistence and progression of the endometriosis tissue (Kyama et al., 2003; Osuga et al., 2011). Following retrograde menstruation, endometrial cells in the peritoneal cavity should be cleared by the immune system, and a number of mechanisms contribute to the failure of this in endometriosis. These mechanisms are summarized in figure 1 and will be addressed here in the order of disease progression.

1.1.1 Viable endometrial cells in the peritoneal cavity

The persistent endometriosis-associated presence of viable peritoneal endometrial cells is partially ascribed to augmented retrograde menstruation, which can directly induce endometriosis, probably by overcoming the immune systems by simple outnumbering (Kyama et al., 2003). Endometrial cell clearance is presumably also reduced by altered phagocytotic properties of peritoneal macrophages. Moreover, decreased cytotoxicity towards autologous endometrial cells by decreased natural killer (NK) cell activity is thought to be an immune defect in endometriosis and is correlated with disease severity (Osuga et al., 2011). The tightly regulated balance between T helper cells type 1 (Th1) and 2 (Th2) is altered towards higher Th2 activity in women with endometriosis. These cells secrete interleukin 4 (IL-4) and IL-10, which are speculated to reduce NK and T-cell cytotoxicity, and thus further reducing immune surveillance.

The endometrial cells themselves also contribute to their own enhanced survival. The transcriptional expression of intercellular adhesion molecule 1 (ICAM-1) is up-regulated in endometriosis lesions, a fact that might contribute to early implantation of peritoneal endometriosis (Wu et al., 2004). The inflammatory cytokines interferon γ (IFNγ) and IL-1β induce ICAM-1 protein expression and the secretion of the soluble form of ICAM-1, which competitively inhibits ICAM-mediated cytotoxicity thus increasing survival. Furthermore, the peritoneal endometrial cells also have a decreased ability to undergo apoptosis.

1.1.2 Endometrial-peritoneal adhesion

The immune system is believed to assist the adhesion of the viable endometrial cells (figure 1). Increased peritoneal infiltration of leukocytes, especially macrophages, and an increased proportion of activated macrophages, is found in endometriosis patients (Haider & Knöfler, 2009). Peritoneal macrophage depletion has been shown to effectively inhibit the initiation and growth of endometriosis implants in rats (Haber et al., 2009), pointing towards a pathogenic effect of macrophages. This inflammation is associated with elevated levels of inflammatory cytokines, growth factors and chemokines.

The pleiotropic pro-inflammatory cytokine tumor necrosis factor α (TNFα) is mainly produced by monocytes and macrophages and stimulates the secretion of the interleukins IL-1, IL-6 and IL-8 by endometriotic cells (Haider & Knöfler, 2009). TNFα can either promote cell regeneration (through the Nuclear Factor kB (NF-κB) pathway) or cell destruction (by initiating the caspase cascade), depending on its local concentration, expression pattern of receptors, and abundance of inhibitors. Macrophages in the peritoneal fluid from women with endometriosis secrete higher levels of TNFα than those from healthy women, and elevated peritoneal fluid levels of TNFα has been detected in women with endometriosis. The adherence of endometrial stromal cells to mesothelial cells is significantly increased by pretreatment of mesothelial cells with TNF-α *in vitro*, suggesting a role in facilitating pelvic adhesion.

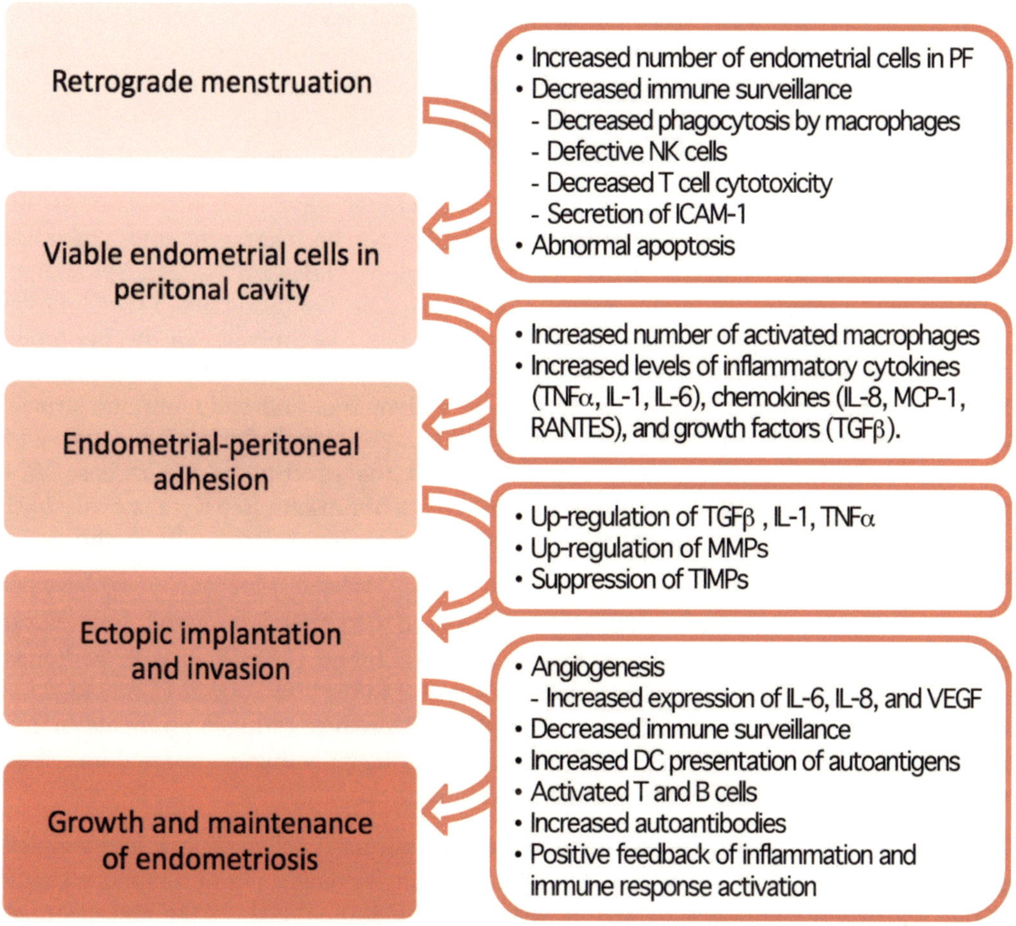

Fig. 1. The role of the immune system in the development and maintenance of endometriosis. Following retrograde menstruation, multiple altered actions of the immune system influence step-wise disease progression. PF, peritoneal fluid; NK cells, natural killer cells; ICAM, Intercellular Adhesion Molecule; TNF, Tumour Necrosis Factor; IL, interleukin; MCP, Monocyte Chemotactic protein; RANTES, Regulated upon Activation, Normal T-cell Expressed and Secreted; TGF, Transforming Growth Factor; MMP, Matrix Metalloproteinase; TIMPs, Tissue Inhibitor of Matrix Metalloproteinases; VEGF, Vascular Endothelial Growth Factor; DC, dendritic cells. Simplified overview inspired by (Kyama et al., 2003).

TNFα also stimulates the growth of both endometrial and endometriotic stromal cells from women with endometriosis, whereas it inhibits the growth of endometrial cells from healthy women (Haider & Knöfler, 2009). The peritoneal fluid level of TNFα is correlated with disease severity. In addition, anti-TNFα therapy effectively reduces endometriosis lesions in rats and baboons (Zulfikaroglu et al., 2010) revealing a potential future medical treatment for endometriosis. However, a placebo-controlled clinical trial of anti-TNFα treatment failed to demonstrate a significant decrease of pain associated with deep endometriosis (see Haider & Knöfler, 2009).

IL-1β and IL-6 are also a pro-inflammatory cytokine found elevated in the peritoneal fluid of women with endometriosis, and macrophages in the peritoneal fluid produce IL-1β *in vitro* in the absence of stimulants (Bondza et al., 2009). Both IL-1α and IL-1β as well as IL-6 are involved in the activation of T-lymphocytes and the differentiation of B-lymphocytes, thereby contributing to the increased peritoneal active immune state in endometriosis.

In addition to these cytokines, a number of chemokines have been implicated in the pathogenesis of endometriosis, believed to contribute by recruiting and activating leukocytes to the inflammatory sites, thereby assisting the adhesion process. Yet another member of the interleukin family, namely the chemokine IL-8 (also named CXCL-8) has been implicated in endometriosis (Bondza et al., 2009). Macrophages in the peritoneal fluid from women with endometriosis secrete higher levels of IL-8 than those from healthy women, which stimulate the growth of endometrial and endometriotic stromal cells. Elevated levels of IL-8 were found in the peritoneal fluid of women with endometriosis, and concentrations correlated with the severity of the disease. IL-8 stimulates the adhesion of endometrial stromal cells to fibronectin (see Kyama et al., 2003) and is therefore likely to contribute to the adhesion of endometrial cells in the pelvic cavity.

Monocyte chemotactic protein-1 (MCP-1, also named CCL2) is one of the most potent chemokines in attracting monocytes. MCP-1 has been found elevated in both peritoneal fluid and serum from women with endometriosis, and in the endometrial glands the level varies according to disease stage (Bondza et al., 2009). Moreover, estrogen up-regulates IL-1-induced MCP-1 expression, which may occur locally in the inflammatory site and contribute to peritoneal macrophage recruitment and activation.

The chemokine RANTES (regulated upon activation, normal T cell expressed and secreted, also named CCL5) plays an important role in recruiting several types of lymphocytes into the endometrium (Fang et al., 2009). It is secreted by stromal cells at the endometriosis lesions upon stimulation with TNFα, IFNγ, or IL-1β. IL-1β treatment yields a higher level of RANTES in endometriotic compared with endometrial cells from endometriosis patients, which in turn display higher levels than normal endometrial cells, entailing increased monocyte chemotactic activity. This is presumed to be a major contributor to leukocyte recruitment and inflammation in the pathogenesis of endometriosis.

It should be noted that the results on whether cytokines and chemokines are involved are equivocal. However, accumulating evidence predominantly reports that both cytokines and chemokines through enhanced local inflammation and cellular adhesion contribute to the pathogenesis of endometriosis.

Transforming growth factor β (TGFβ) peritoneal fluid levels are significantly higher in women with endometriosis compared with healthy control women, and the TGFβ level increases with the severity of the disease (Liu et al., 2009). The adhesion of human endometrial cells to murine peritoneum is increased by treatment with TGFβ (as well as with IL-1β, IL-6, and TNFα) (Omwandho et al., 2009). The same could not be shown for human peritoneal mesothelial cells, but TGFβ enhances trans-mesothelial invasion by primary and immortalized endometrial epithelial cell lines *in vitro* (Liu et al., 2009).

1.1.3 Ectopic implantation and invasion

TGF-β might not only facilitate adhesion but also implantation in endometriosis (figure 1). Its expression in the endometrium varies with the menstrual cycle, peaking at the time of menstruation (Omwandho et al., 2009). This expression pattern is roughly opposite to that of TNFα, and co-expression with progesterone occurs in the secretory phase (figure 2). TGFβ has been shown to mediate progesterone-associated suppression of matrix metalloproteinase (MMP) expression in endometrial tissue, and it is required for progesterone action in the prevention of experimental endometriosis (Bondza et al., 2009).

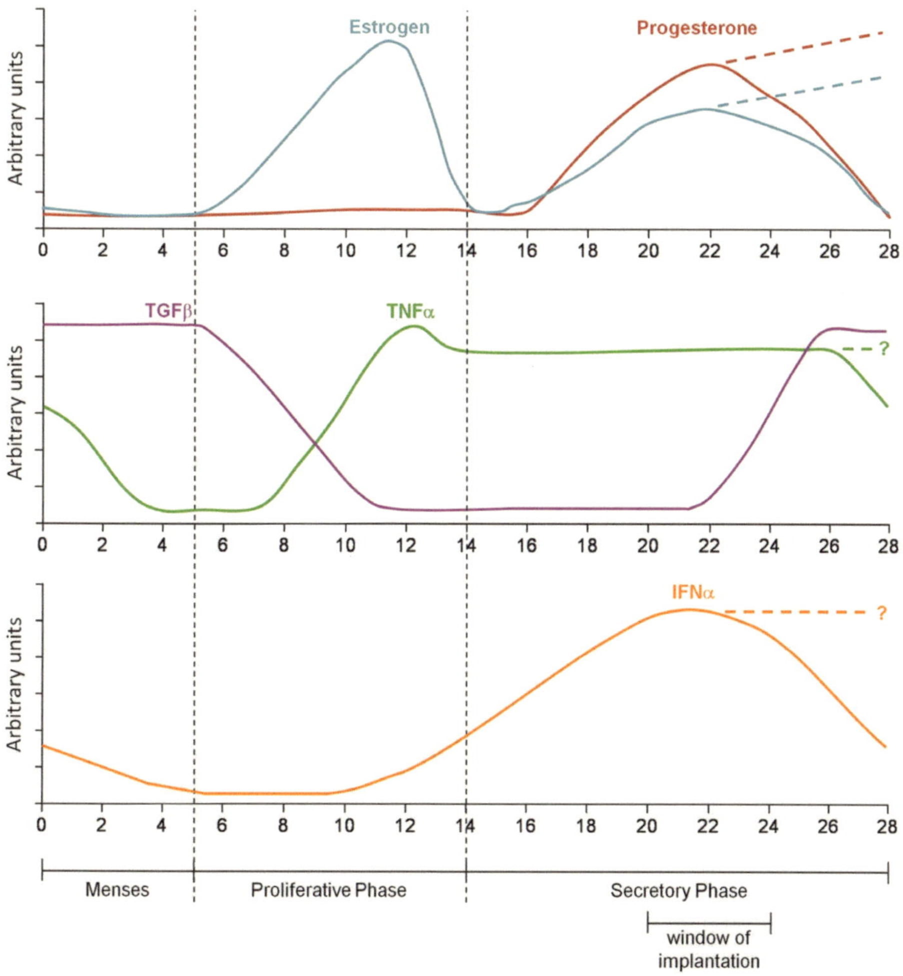

Fig. 2. Levels of estrogen, progesterone, TGFβ, TNFα, and IFNα in the human endometrium during menstrual cycling. Numbers denote days after the first menstrual day. Dashed lines show levels following implantation. There are indications that TNFα and IFNα levels are up-regulated in early pregnancy. TGF, Transforming Growth Factor; TNF, Tumour Necrosis Factor; IFN, interferon. Schematic representation based on (Li et al., 2001; Haider & Knöfler, 2009; Omwandho et al., 2009).

MMPs are important for the control of extracellular matrix turnover, and they are believed to influence the implantation of adhered endometriotic cells in endometriosis (Kyama et al., 2003). The level of MMPs is in up-regulated and tissue inhibitors of matrix metalloproteinases (TIMPs) down-regulated in the peritoneal fluid from women with endometriosis compared with controls (Bondza et al., 2009). MMPs are upregulated in response to the inflammatory cytokines TNFα and IL-1 and are expressed during the proliferative and menstrual phases but suppressed by progesterone in the secretory phase. In the absence of a normal progesterone response of the endometriosis lesions, sensitivity to TGFβ may be altered, and this may result in a failure to down-regulate MMPs, thus contributing to the implantation failure.

1.1.4 Growth and maintenance of endometriosis

Following implantation, the growth and maintenance of endometriosis lesions is influenced by a number of factors (figure 1). First of all, the implanted tissue is in need of vascularization and an increase in the concentration of several angiogenic factors has been reported. IL-6 and IL-8, which as stated above are up-regulated in endometriosis, both promote angiogenesis (Bondza et al., 2009). IL-1β, which is also elevated in the peritoneal fluid of endometriosis patients, induces IL-6, the vascular endothelial growth factor (VEGF), and an angiogenic phenotype in endometriotic but not endometrial stromal cells. Women with moderate and severe endometriosis have elevated levels of both IL-6 and VEGF in the peritoneal fluid compared with healthy controls (Kyama et al., 2003), underlining that angiogenesis is a feature of disease exacerbation. Furthermore, high proliferative activity of endometriosis lesions is associated with increased levels of VEGF and its receptor as well as increased microvessel density (Bondza et al., 2009).

A positive feedback of activated immune response contributes further to the maintenance of endometriosis. The reduced NK cell activity has been suggested to result in less effective killing of autologous dendritic cells (DCs) loaded with endometrial self-antigens. This would facilitate self-antigen presentation to autoreactive T cells and the subsequent production of autoantibodies (Kyama et al., 2003), pointing towards a pathogenic contribution by an autoimmune disease mechanism. Indeed, the frequency of autoantibodies towards endometrial antigens is elevated in both serum and peritoneal fluid of women with endometriosis compared with healthy women (Osuga et al., 2011). Activation of Th2 immune response in endometriosis and elevated B cell levels has been reported both systemically and locally in the endometriosis lesions, supposedly causing sustained autoantibody production and continuous infiltration of immune cells, thus maintaining the immunological contribution to the pathogenesis of endometriosis.

2. Virus and endometriosis

Pathogenic DNA virus infection has been associated with the aetiology of several human diseases. The double-stranded (ds) DNA viruses include herpesviruses, polyomaviruses, papillomaviruses, hepadnaviruses (e.g. hepatitis B virus (HBV)), adenoviruses and poxviruses. With the exception of poxviruses, these viruses often establish persistent or latent infections and can be reactivated in both healthy and immunosuppressed persons.

Only a few studies have addressed the possible involvement of a pathogenic virus in the aetiology of endometriosis (Oppelt et al., 2010; Vestergaard et al., 2010). The presence of specific human herpes viruses, human polyomaviruses, and human papillomaviruses was analysed. Also, the presence of human endogenous retroviruses have been investigated in endometriosis lesions (Hu et al., 2006; Oppelt et al., 2009), and these studies will be discussed in the following section.

2.1 Herpes viruses

The *Herpesviridae* are a large, diverse family of double-stranded, enveloped viruses. Eight human herpesviruses (HHVs) have been identified: Epstein-Barr virus (EBV, of the subfamily *Gammaherpesvirinae*), cytomegalovirus (CMV or HHV5 of the subfamily *Betaherpesvirinae*), herpes simplex virus type 1 and 2 (HSV-1 and HSV-2 of the subfamily *Alphaherpesvirinae*), varicella zoster (VZV), HHV6, HHV7, and the Karposi's sarcoma herpes virus (KHSV or HHV8). The seroprevalence of each of these herpes viruses varies according to a number of demographic factors (Prober, 2011). For EBV, CMV, and HSV-1 the prevalences range from 50 to 75%, whereas the prevalence for HSV-2 is about 25%. For VZV, HHV6 and HHV7 the seroprevalence is almost 100%, whereas the prevalence for HHV8 is less than 10%. The *Herpesviridae* family are found in many human tissue types, including the fallopian tubes (salpingitis) and the endometrium (see Vestergaard et al., 2010). These viruses are commonly distributed as asymptomatic infectious agents but are also all associated with diseases, such as genital sores or a variety of malignancies. EBV can cause infectious mononucleosis and has been associated with lymphomas of B, T and NK cell origin, but also cancers of epithelial origin like nasopharyngeal carcinomas and gastric adenocarcinomas (Dolcetti & Masucci, 2003). EBV maintains latency in B cells. CMV can cause pneumonitis and delayed neurological complications like sensory neural hearing deficits and learning disabilities (Brown & Abernathy, 1998). CMV maintains latency in monocytes and macrophages. HSV-1 and HSV-2 can cause encephalitis and genital ulcerative disease (Wilson et al., 2009). The HSVs maintain latency in neuronal cells. VSV cause chickenpox (varicella) as primary infection following which it becomes latent in neuronal cells (Kennedy & Cohrs, 2010). VZV can be reactivated and thus cause herpes zoster (shingles) and extremely painful vesicular eruption. HHV6 cause roseola during the primary infection (Prober, 2011). HHV6 becomes latent in salivary glands, the brain and in mononuclear cells or macrophages. Most reactived HHV6 infections are asymptomatic.

The presence of most of the herpes viruses in endometriosis has been analysed., Endometriosis samples from 32 patients were analysed for the presence of EBV, CMV, HSV-1 and HSV-2 by multiplex PCRs (Vestergaard et al., 2010). None of the clinical samples were positive for any of these four herpes viruses. In another study, 66 endometriosis samples from 56 patients were tested for the presence of EBV, CMV, HSV-1, HSV-2, VZV, and HHV6 by a PCR based analysis (Oppelt et al., 2010). Also this study failed to detect the presence of any of these six herpes viruses. Apart from HHV7 and HHV8, which has not yet been analysed, the six herpes viruses EBV, CMV, HSV-1, HSV-2, VZV, and HHV6 do not seem to be involved in the pathology of endometriosis.

2.2 Polyomaviruses

The well-described human polyomaviruses of the *Polyomaviridae* family, JC (JCV), BK (BKV) and simian virus 40 (SV40) are widely distributed in the general population (Moens & Johannessen, 2008). Thus antibodies against JCV and BKV have been found in more than 75% of the human adult population, and up to 15% of healthy humans are seropositive for SV40. These three polyomaviruses have been found in many different tissues (see Vestergaard et al., 2010). BKV has been found in the kidney tubule epithelium, urethral epithelium, the uterine cervix, and in the spleen. JCV has been found in tongue squamous cell epithelium, urethral epithelium, and in the spleen, whereas SV40 has been found in the liver and the mesothelium. Furthermore, these three polyomaviruses induce tumours in animal models and are able to transform cultured human cells (Moens & Johannessen, 2008). In 2007, two new human polyomaviruses, WU polyomavirus (WUV) and KI polyomavirus (KIV) were discovered in respiratory tract secretions and have subsequently been detected in faeces, blood, and lymphoid tissue (see Vestergaard et al., 2010). The full spectrum of their tissue tropism and their role in disease has yet to be elucidated. More recently, yet another human member of the *Polyomaviridae* family, the Merkel cell polyomavirus (MCV) was described in apparent association with Merkel cell carcinoma, an aggressive form of skin cancer (Moens & Johannessen, 2008). When analysed, none of these polyomaviruses were detected either in the endometrium or in endometriosis, suggesting an infrequent presence of polyomaviruses in the endometrium (Vestergaard et al., 2010).

2.3 Human papillomaviruses

Closely related to the polyomavirus family, the papillomavirus family is a very significant example of the large impact of a broad spectrum of pathogenic DNA viruses, which have emerged during the last two decades. More than 118 papillomaviruses have been fully described, and new virus types are constantly emerging (zur Hausen, 2009). The prevalence of human papillomavirus (HPV, of the family *Papillomaviridae*) in cervical carcinomas is 99.7%. Specific high-risk HPV types have been shown to cause the vast majority of cervical cancers as well as a substantial proportion of other anogenital and head and neck cancers as well as certain cutaneous cancers. HPV has not yet been detected in intraperitoneal tissues, but HPV has been detected in blood, including on the surface of peripheral blood mononuclear cells, suggesting a potential alternative route of transmission (see Vestergaard et al., 2010).

The prevalence of HPV in endometriosis has been analysed (Oppelt et al., 2010; Vestergaard et al., 2010). In one study, no HPV DNA was found in the endometriosis samples from 32 patients (Vestergaard et al., 2010). In another study, certain high-risk HPV types was found in endometriosis lesions (Oppelt et al., 2010). However, due to previous cervical HPV infections in the analysed patients, it was concluded that the detected HPV in the endometriosis samples possibly originated from these associated malignant transformations and might not have any association with the endometriosis *per se*.

In the endometrium, a HPV prevalence of less than 10% was found in samples from both women with endometriosis as well as controls, which is remarkably low compared with the well-known high frequencies of infection with these viruses (Vestergaard et al., 2010). It is estimated that 75% to 80% of sexually active individuals are infected with HPV during their lifetime, with the highest rates in women younger than 25 years of age. However, as the mean age of the women enrolled in this particular study were between 32 and 36 years of age, most HPV infections would have been cleared by the immune system, correlating well with the fact that none of these women had genital HPV infection in their cervical smears at the time of analysis. However, it is possible that transient HPV infections could cause the initiation of malignant-like processes by a "hit-and-run" mechanism and in this way contribute to the initiation of endometriosis. This theory is yet to be investigated further.

2.4 Endogenous retroviruses

Retroviruses are RNA viruses, which integrate into the genome of the host cell in the form of a DNA copy, which is denominated the provirus. Endogenous retroviruses refer to proviruses integrated into germ line cells, which are transmitted from one generation to the next. Approximately 5% of the human genome consists of complete and partial sequences from human endogenous retroviruses (HERVs) (Muir et al., 2004). The significance and consequences of the presence of HERVs in the human genome have been the subject of intensive investigation. HERVs have been implicated in autoimmune diseases and neoplasia as well as in placental function and protection from exogenous retroviral infection. Considering the placental function, it is now believed that syncytin, a retroviral envelope protein encoded by the endogenous retrovirus HERV-W, is involved in the fusion of the cytotrophoblast cells to form the syncytial layer of the placenta, and the envelope protein encoded by ERV3 has been associated with cytotrophoblast differentiation. Other endogenous retroviruses like HERV-E also seem to be involved in placental function (reviewed in Muir et al., 2004).

Expression of HERVs in endometriotic tissues has been detected, indicating that endogenous retrovirus expression might be involved in endometriosis (Hu et al., 2006; Oppelt et al., 2009). Endometriosis samples from 14 women were analysed for the presence of HERV-E HERV-W, HERV-I/T, and HERV-H mRNA by PCR analysis (Hu et al., 2006). It was found that HERV-E was expressed at higher levels in the endometriosis samples than in normal endometrium control samples. In another study, 15 endometriosis samples showed low levels of RNA encoding the HERV-W encoded envelope protein syncytin, as analysed by reverse transcriptase PCR (Oppelt et al., 2009). It was also found in this study that the endometriosis samples did not show an elevated expression of the HERV-W encoded envelope protein syncytin. Interestingly though, samples from the endometrium of women with endometriosis showed an increased expression of syncytin RNA compared with endometrial samples from controls, suggesting that this protein might be involved in the pathology of endometriosis. At this point, the involvement of endogenous virus expression in the pathology of endometriosis is not clarified. Further studies are required, analysing larger groups of endometriosis samples and including tissue samples from the endometrium of women with and without endometriosis.

3. Type I interferon and endometriosis

We will now focus on the putative implication of the important immune modulating cytokine family type I interferons in endometriosis, as a line of circumstantial evidence indicates that these cytokines could be involved. A key constituent of the immune system that has been only slightly investigated in relation to endometriosis is the family of interferons (IFNs). IFNs are cytokines secreted from cells in response to viral challenge and various other stimuli. The human interferons are by structural homology classified into type I, which consists of IFNα (counting 13 subtypes), IFNβ, IFNε, IFNκ, and IFNω, type II, which is only IFNγ, and type III, the more recently discovered IFNλ (comprising 3 subtypes) (Platanias, 2005; Hall & Rosen, 2010). Secreted IFNs bind to specific plasma membrane receptors, which initiate intracellular pathways leading to the transcription of hundreds of interferon stimulated genes (ISGs) (Platanias, 2005; Hall & Rosen, 2010). In spite of their common signaling pathway, IFNα and IFNβ display specific activity profiles.

Main biological activities resulting from IFN signaling are primarily antiviral but also anti-proliferative, anti-angiogenic, and antigen-presenting effects as well as regulation of pro- and anti-apoptotic genes and proteins (Platanias, 2005). The current state of the cells and complex balances of feedback mechanisms determine the overall outcome of the IFN response, *e.g.* survival vs. apoptosis. Recombinant human IFNs (mainly IFNα and IFNβ) are used as therapeutic agents against a variety of cancers, multiple sclerosis, and viral diseases, such as hepatitis B and C.

Type II IFN is produced only by activated T or NK cells and its primary role is to modulate the adaptive immune response, *e.g.* by contributing to the activation of macrophages and T cell development (Hall & Rosen, 2010). Expression of the receptors of type III IFN is primarily limited to epithelial and DCs, thus restricting their scope of action. We will only focus on type I IFNs and their possible role in endometriosis.

High levels of type I IFNs are secreted rapidly by most cell types upon stimuli (Hall & Rosen, 2010). Type 1 IFNs have immunostimulatory effects on NK cells, macrophages and DCs, which all are essential effector cells in the innate immune system. Among the downstream targets of type I IFN signaling are the IFNs themselves as well as associated receptors, signal transducers and transcription factors enabling a strong feed-forward mechanism. It is strongly believed that type I IFNs are directly involved in the pathogenesis of autoimmune disease by enhancing the self-amplification of systemic autoimmunity (Hall & Rosen, 2010). The aberrant antigen-presentation of debris from apoptotic cells and the resulting production of autoantibodies in endometriosis could be speculated to give rise to a type I IFN-amplified autoimmune pathogenic mechanism. In autoimmunity, self antigens elicit an immune response that includes substantial production of type I IFNs. Upon DC presentation of endometrial autoantigens, type I IFN may then promote monocyte differentiation, DC survival and cytotoxic T cell activity, which may enhance killing of endometrial cells presenting autoantigens. Debris from dying cells is then taken up by DCs and presented for recognition by T cells in a self-amplifying loop. Type I IFNs also induce the differentiation of B cells, which would promote autoantibody production. Immune complexes of endometrial self antigens and autoantibodies would further amplify the IFN production, constituting yet another positive feedback loop.

The approved drug Intron A (human recombinant IFNα-2b) has been proposed as a possible immunomodulatory therapeutic against reoccurrence of endometriosis cysts after surgery. The hypothesis was that this could enhance the cytotoxic activity of macrophages and natural killer cells and thus reduce the growth of endometriosis tissue (Acién et al., 2002). Rats with surgically induced endometriosis showed persistent significant reductions in the implant sizes upon intraperitoneal or subcutaneous administration of human IFNα-2b. However, a clinical study showed that intraperitoneal administration of IFNα-2b following surgical treatment for endometriosis increased the cyst reoccurrence rate significantly after 21 months. Hence, the normal anti-proliferative effects of type I IFNs appear to be challenged in endometriosis.

The endometrial level of IFNα mRNA is increased in the mid-secretory phase of the human menstrual cycle (Li et al., 2001), which is the putative window of implantation (figure 2). It has been found that the transcription of IFNα and the interferon α receptor 2 (IFNAR2) is highly up-regulated in the endometrium of women suffering from endometriosis compared with healthy women (Kao et al., 2003). Moreover, *JAK1*, which has an important function in type I IFN signaling, is up-regulated in endometriosis stromal cells compared with the endometrial cells from endometriosis patients (Matsuzaki et al., 2006). The sum of these findings suggests a role of type I IFN in the human endometrium and a possible dysregulation in endometriosis.

The possible involvement of type I IFNs in endometriosis has recently been investigated directly (Vestergaard et al., 2011). A type I interferon-specific PCR Array indicated significantly down-regulated transcription of the genes *HOXB2* and *ISG20* in endometriosis lesions compared with endometrium from endometriosis patients and healthy controls, but no difference in the expression of any other interferon stimulated genes were observed. These results were independent of the menstrual phase. As only two out of 84 genes of the type I IFN response was significantly dysregulated in endometriosis, the type I IFNs do not appear to be generally involved in the pathogenesis of endometriosis. Yet, specific gene regulation involving type I IFNs could still play distinct roles in endometriosis. The putative involvement of *ISG20, HOXB2* and *HOXA10* in the pathogenesis will now be discussed.

3.1 The ISG20 protein

The transcriptional expression of *ISG20* (interferon-stimulated gene product of 20 kDa, also called *HEM45*) was shown by validated qRT-PCR to be highly down-regulated in endometriosis lesions (Vestergaard et al., 2011). *ISG20* transcription is induced synergistically by type I and II IFNs, induced by estrogen, and regulated in a progesterone-dependent manner in mice, especially in the mouse endometrium. This gene encodes a 3′ to 5′ exonuclease with specificity for single-stranded RNA (and to a lesser extent for DNA), which is localized in the nucleus and is associated with promyelocytic leukemia (PML) protein nuclear bodies. The exonuclease has been proposed to down-regulate the estrogen-dependent transcriptional response by degrading estrogen-induced mRNAs within PML oncogenic domains (PODs). The subcellular localization of ISG20 in the nucleus argues for its involvement in the maturation rather than in the degradation of mRNAs.

ISG20 has also been implicated in the anti-angiogenic properties of interferon (Taylor et al., 2008). In an *in vitro* angiogenic assay system, ISG20 was found to be up-regulated in endothelial cells treated with interferon, however, overexpression of ISG20 did not lead to reduced angiogenesis *per se*. However, overexpression of the enzymatically inactive, dominant-negative ISG20 mutant inhibited angiogenesis in this system and potentiated the anti-angiogenic properties of interferon. How ISG20 might be involved in angiogenesis is currently not clear.

The ISG20 protein mediates antiviral effects of interferons by inhibiting the replication of several RNA viruses, like vesicular stomatitis virus, influenza virus, encephalomyocarditis virus, West Nile virus, Dengue virus, hepatitis A and C viruses, yellow fever virus, and bovine viral diarrhea virus (Zhou et al., 2011). The antiviral activity of ISG20 is only observed with enzymatically active ISG20 expression, since expression of an ISG20 mutant without enzymatic activity, did not possess the same antiviral activities.

Importantly, ISG20 mRNA was found to be up-regulated in the uterine epithelium during the implantation window in mouse (Pan et al., 2006). Whether abolished ISG20 enzyme activity is implicated in the pathogenesis of endometriosis or a marker of altered hormonal expression, or both, needs to be further investigated.

3.2 The HOX proteins

The HOX proteins encoded by the homeobox genes are DNA binding transcription factors known to regulate embryonic development. In addition, the *HOX* genes are dynamically expressed in the endometrium during the menstrual cycle, where they are necessary for endometrial growth, differentiation, and implantation (Cakmak & Taylor, 2010; Zanatta et al., 2010). Furthermore, HOX proteins are molecular mediators of the steroid hormones during endometrial cell development.

It has been suggested that a HOX gene-related defect in endometrial development exists in patients with endometriosis (Zanatta et al., 2010). According to this theory, endometriosis might originate from estrogen stimulated metaplasia of mesenchymal embryonic cells distributed in the pelvis during organogenesis. However, transcriptional dysregulation of the HOX genes in the adult endometrium compatible with the more well-supported retrograde menstruation pathogenesis model is also well substantiated. Recently, a systematic dysregulation of *HOX* genes in the endometrium from healthy women compared with the endometrium in women with endometriosis has been demonstrated (Borghese et al., 2008). A down-regulation of *HOXA* and *HOXB* genes and an up-regulation of HOXC genes were found in endometrium from women with endometriosis compared with endometrium from healthy women.

The HOXA10 protein is up-regulated in response to circulating estrogen and progesterone in the healthy endometrium, thus indicating a role in endometrial maturation, implantation and maintenance of pregnancy implantation (Cakmak & Taylor, 2010; Zanatta et al., 2010). *HOXA10* transcription is normally up-regulated in the endometrium during the window of implantation but this up-regulation is abolished in women with endometriosis. Low levels of HOXA10 could explain the lower fertility of women with endometriosis, and this is further supported by studies of the HOXA10 knock-out mice, in which the targeted disruption of the *HOXA10* gene generated uterine factor infertility. Also in the endometriotic tissue, the HOXA10 transcriptional levels were found to be low

(Langendonckt et al., 2010). The endometrial down-regulation of HOXA10 protein in women with endometriosis seems to be due to increased methylation of the *HOXA10* genomic enhancer region in the endometrium leading to epigenetic silencing of this gene (reviewed in Cakmak & Taylor, 2010). In conclusion, low levels of HOXA10 may result in resistance to progesterone action in the endometriotic tissue.

HOXB2 is part of the *HOX* gene family involved mainly in embryonic development. A very solid down-regulation of *HOXB2* in endometriotic lesions compared with endometrium from both endometriosis and healthy women has been observed (Vestergaard et al., 2011). Little is known about *HOXB2* expression in the endometrium, but several studies have demonstrated that *HOXB2* expression is altered in tumours. In a xenograft breast tumour mouse model, HOXB2 acts as a negative tumour growth regulator, since *HOXB2* expression decreases proliferation of tumour cells (Boimel et al., 2011). Other results have shown that overexpression of HOXB2 in pancreatic, lung and cervical cancer was associated with malignancy. However, a more in-depth analysis correlated lower HOXB2 expression with higher grades of tumours. Finally, it has been reported that the HOXB2 protein binds the interferon-induced protein p205, involved in the growth inhibitory activities of interferon (see Vestergaard et al., 2011). Whether HOXB2 interaction with p205 modifies the growth inhibitory activities of p205 has not yet been investigated. Further studies are needed to determine the mechanism and implications of the abolished *HOXB2* expression in endometriosis lesions.

4. Conclusion

The pathogenesis and the similarity to cancer invasiveness suggested that a viral background could be part of the pathogenesis of endometriosis, but so far no investigations have demonstrated this connection in the aetiology. The prevalence of pathogenic dsDNA viruses in the human endometrium was found to be generally low (0-10%), and nothing points towards any evidence that endometriosis is caused by currently known DNA viruses (Oppelt et al., 2010; Vestergaard et al., 2010). It can be speculated that the endometrium and endometriotic tissue is difficult to access or simply an unfavorable environment for virus progression, leading to a generally low prevalence in these deeper tissues. It is possible that viruses can infect the endometrium transiently but subsequently be either shed with the endometrial tissue during menstruation or be rapidly cleared by an efficient immune response. Thus stable infections of the endometrium would not be frequent. However, a pathogenic virus could theoretically initiate a malignant cell process during a shorter infectious period and then flee the scene. This "hit-and-run" strategy has been previously shown *e.g.* for CMV *in vitro* and indicated in clinical studies of both polyomaviruses and papillomaviruses (see Vestergaard et al., 2010). This could explain why no virus DNA so far has been found associated with endometriosis lesions.

To address the viral "hit-and-run" strategy hypothesis, one could analyse for an elevated level of serum antibodies against the viruses, which would then show previous viral infections. Even though a broad selection of the most common pathogenic DNA viruses have been tested for, other more rare or even undiscovered viruses or bacteria might still be involved. Conclusively, the prevalence of pathogenic DNA viruses in the endometrium and endometriosis lesions is very low and does not indicate a virological cause of endometriosis. However, the existence of a causative infectious agent can still not be ruled out at this point.

The altered expression of a large number of genes has been reported in endometriosis (Kao et al., 2003; Matsuzaki et al., 2006), an imbalance mediated by altered levels of a number of signaling molecules as well as by epigenetic alterations. Dysregulation of a large number of hormones, cytokines, chemokines, and growth factors is a feature of endometriosis. The abolished expression of *HOXA10*, *HOXB2* and *ISG20* in the endometriosis tissue seems to be influenced by a number of these factors, which regulate gene transcription via complex, overlapping mechanisms, possibly in combination with the action of estrogen and progesterone. The observed abolishment of *ISG20* and *HOXB2* expression in endometriosis lesions indicates that they fail to be induced by estrogen. The altered ERα/ERβ ratio in endometriosis could be important in this mechanism. The lack of *HOXA10* expression in the endometrium as well as in endometriotic lesions is probably due to epigenetic changes in the gene promoter, resulting in abolished response to estrogen and progesterone. Moreover, the expression of other *HOX* genes in endometriosis might shed a light on the function of this family of proteins in the development of this disease.

As the aetiology of endometriosis is unknown, and as several factors are thought to influence the course of the disease, the pathogenesis of endometriosis is still a challenge. One of the main problems is the lack of a non-invasive test to diagnose endometriosis. Several markers have been investigated. The best known is CA125, which is not specific to endometriosis but frequently also elevated in cancer. CA125 is often elevated in endometriosis, and the level is to some extend related to the degree of the infiltration in active endometriosis. However, the CA125 levels are individual, and change in intensity of pain or other symptoms related to endometriosis are not automatically reflected in the level. Therefore, the identification of a non-invasive marker able to diagnose endometriosis would be of great importance. Furthermore, if this marker could indicate changes in disease intensity this would be a great help both for the patient and the doctor. The success of different treatments could also be measured more objectively e.g. by an independent marker. So far hormonal treatment is the first line of treatment, and if pain cannot be resolved by medication, surgery may be performed. However, the endometriosis often reoccurs and more operations are needed, thus bringing the risk of complications.

As clarified in this chapter, many possibilities for causative or aetiological mechanism for the pathogenesis of endometriosis are in focus. If the aetiology of endometriosis is to be found related to virus, we can probably in the future prevent the disease or at least weaken the intensity. A marker for the disease based on virus aetiology would most likely be possible to develop, and the development of a specific treatment could be feasible. If HOX genes and/or ISG20 are involved in the aetiology of endometriosis, this would also give possibilities for new diagnostic tools and medical treatments.

In conclusion, the possible involvement of viruses, type I IFNs, and the innate immune system in the pathogenesis of endometriosis is yet unclear. More investigations are needed in order to resolve the riddle of endometriosis.

5. References

Acién, P., Quereda, F., Campos, A., Gomez-Torres, M.-J., Velasco, I., & Gutierrez, M. (2002). Use of intraperitoneal interferon α-2b therapy after conservative surgery for endometriosis and postoperative medical treatment with depot gonadotropin-releasing hormone analog: a randomized clinical trial. *Fertil Steril*, Vol. 78, No. 4, (October 2002), pp. 705-711, 0015-0282

Boimel, P. J., Cruz, C., & Segall, J. E. (2011). A functional in vivo screen for regulators of tumor progression identifies HOXB2 as a regulator of tumor growth in breast cancer. *Genomics*, Vol. 98, No. 3, (September 2011), pp. 164-172, 0888-7543

Bondza, P. K., Maheux, R., & Akuom, A. (2009). Insights into endometriosis-associated endometrial dysfunction: a review. *Frontiers in Bioscience*, Vol. 1, No. -, (June 2009), pp. 415-428, 1093-0046

Borghese, B., Mondon, F., Noel, J.-C., Fayt, I., Mignot, T.-M., Vaiman, D., & Chapron, C. (2008). Gene Expression Profile for Ectopic Versus Eutopic Endometrium Provides New Insights into Endometriosis Oncogenic Potential. *Mol Endocrinol*, Vol. 22, No. 11, (November 2008), pp. 2557-2562, 0888-8809

Brown, H. L., & Abernathy, M. P. (1998). Cytomegalovirus infection. *Semin Perinatol*, Vol. 22, No. 4, (August 1997), pp. 260-6, 0146-0005

Bulun, S. E. (2009). Endometriosis. *N Engl J Med*, Vol. 360, No. 3, (January 2009), pp. 268-279, 0028-4793

Cakmak, H., & Taylor, H. S. (2010). Molecular Mechanisms of Treatment Resistance in Endometriosis: The Role of Progesterone-Hox Gene Interactions. *Semin Reprod Med*, Vol. 28, No. 1, (January 2010), pp. 69-74, 1526-8004

Dolcetti, R., & Masucci, M. G. (2003). Epstein-Barr virus: induction and control of cell transformation. *J Cell Physiol*, Vol. 196, No. 2, (August 2003), pp. 207-18, 0021-9541

Fang, C.-L., Han, S.-P., Fu, S.-L., Wang, W., Kong, N., & Wang, X.-L. (2009). Ectopic, autologous eutopic and normal endometrial stromal cells have altered expression and chemotactic activity of RANTES. *Eur J Obstet Gynecol Reprod Biol*, Vol. 143, No. 1, (March 2009), pp. 55-60, 0301-2115

Faquhar, C. (2007). Endometriosis. *BMJ*, Vol. 334, No. 7587, (February 2007), pp. 249-253, 0959-8138

Haber, E., Danenberg, H. D., Koroukhov, N., Ron-El, R., Golomb, G., & Schachter, M. (2009). Peritoneal macrophage depletion by liposomal bisphosphonate attenuates endometriosis in the rat model. *Hum Reprod*, Vol. 24, No. 2, (February 2009), pp. 398-407, 0268-1161

Haider, S., & Knöfler, M. (2009). Human Tumour Necrosis Factor: Physiological and Pathological Roles in Placenta and Endometrium. *Placenta*, Vol. 30, No. 2, (February 2009), pp. 111-123, 0143-4004

Hall, J. C., & Rosen, A. (2010). Type I interferons: crucial participants in disease amplification in autoimmunity. *Nat Rev Rheumatol*, Vol. 6, No. 1, (January 2010), pp. 40-49, 1759-4790

Hu, L., Hornung, D., Kurek, R., Ostman, H., Blomberg, J., & Bergqvist, A. (2006). Expression of Human Endogenous Gammaretroviral Sequences in Endometriosis and Ovarian

Cancer. *AIDS Research and Human Retroviruses*, Vol. 22, No. 6, (November 2006), pp. 551-557, 0889-2229

Kao, L. C., Germeyer, A., Tulac, S., Lobo, S., Yang, J. P., Taylor, R. N., Osteen, K., Lessey, B. A., & Giudice, L. C. (2003). Expression profiling of endometrium from women with endometriosis reveals candidate genes for disease-based implantation failure and infertility. *Endocrinology*, Vol. 144, No. 7, (July 2003), pp. 2870-81, 0013-7227

Kennedy, P. G. E., & Cohrs, R. J. (2010). Varicella-zoster virus human ganglionic latency: a current summary. *J NeuroVirol*, Vol. 16, No. 6, (November 2010), pp. 411-418, 1355-0284

Kyama, C. M., Debrock, S., Mwenda, J. M., & D'Hooghe, T. M. (2003). Potential involvement of the immune system in the development of endometriosis. *Reprod Biol Endocrinol*, Vol. 1, No. -, (December 2003), pp. 123, 1477-7827

Langendonckt, A. V., Lyuckx, M., Gonzalez, M.-D., Defrère, S., Donnez, J., & Squifflet, J. (2010). Differential expression of genes from the homeobox A cluster in deep endometriotic nodules and peritoneal lesions. *Fertil Steril*, Vol. 94, No. 6, (November 2010), pp. 1995-2000, 0015-0282

Li, Q., Zhang, M., Kumar, S., Zhu, L. J., Chen, D., Bagchi, M. K., & Bagchi, I. C. (2001). Identification and implantation stage-specific expression of an interferon-α-regulated gene in human and rat endometrium. *Endocrinology*, Vol. 142, No. 6, (June 2001), pp. 2390-400, 0013-7227

Liu, Y.-g., Tekmal, R. R., Binkley, P. A., Nair, H. B., Schenken, R. S., & Kirma, N. B. (2009). Induction of endometrial epithelial cell invasion and c-fms expression by transforming growth factor β. *Mol Hum Reprod*, Vol. 15, No. 10, (October 2009), pp. 665-673, 1360-9947

Matsuzaki, S., Canis, M., Pouly, J.-L., Botchorishvili, R., Déchelotte, P. J., & Mage, G. (2006). Differential expression of genes in eutopic and ectopic endometrium from patients with ovarian endometriosis. *Fertil Steril*, Vol. 86, No. 3, (September 2006), pp. 548-553, 0015-0282

Moens, U., & Johannessen, M. (2008). Human polyomaviruses and cancer: expanding repertoire. *Journal der Deutschen Dermatologischen Gesellschaft*, Vol. 6, No. 9, (September 2008), pp. 704-708, 1610-0387

Muir, A., Lever, A., & Moffett, A. (2004). Expression and function of human endogenous retroviruses in the placenta: An update. *Placenta*, Vol. 25, No. suppl. 1, (April 2004), pp. S16-S25, 0143-4004

Omwandho, C. O. A., Konrad, L., Halis, G., Oehmke, F., & Tinneberg, H.-R. (2009). Role of TGF-βs in normal human endometrium and endometriosis. *Hum Reprod*, Vol. 25, No. 1, (November 2009), pp. 101-109, 0268-1161

Oppelt, P., Strick, R., Strissel, P. L., Winzierl, K., Beckmann, M. W., & Renner, S. P. (2009). Expression of the human endogenous retrovirus-W envelope gene syncytin in endometriosis lesion. *Gynecol Endocrinol*, Vol. 25, No. 11, (November 2007), pp. 741-747, 0951-3590

Oppelt, P., Renner, S. P., Strick, R., Valletta, D., Mehlhorn, G., Fasching, P. A., Beckmann, M. W., & Strissel, P. L. (2010). Correlation of high-risk human papilloma viruses but not of herpes viruses or Chlamydia trachomatis with endometriosis lesions. *Fertility and Sterility*, Vol. 93, No. 6, (April 2010), pp. 1778-1786, 0015-0282

Osuga, Y., Koga, K., Hirota, Y., Hirata, T., Yaoshino, O., & Taketani, Y. (2011). Lymphocytes in endometriosis. *Am. J. Reprod. Immunol.*, Vol. 65, No. 1, (January 2011), pp. 1-10, 1046-7408

Pan, H., Zhu, L., Deng, Y., & Pollard, J. (2006). Microarray analysis of uterine epithelial gene expression during the implantation window in the mouse. *Endocrinology*, Vol. 147, No.(October 2006), pp. 4904-4916, 0013-7227

Platanias, L. C. (2005). Mechanisms of type-I- and type-II-interferon-mediated signalling. Nat Rev Immunol, Vol. 5, No. 5, (May 2005), pp. 375-386, 1474-1733

Prober, C. G. (2011). Human Herpesvirus 6, In *Hot Topics in Infection and Immunity in Children VII, Curtis*, N., Finn, A. & Pollard, A., pp. 87-90, Springer, 978-1-4419-7184-5, New York, USA

Simpson, J. L., Eklias, S., Malinak, L. R., & Buttram, V. C., Jr. (1980). Heritable aspects of endometriosis. I. Genetic studies. *Am J Obstet Gynecol* Vol. 137, No. 3, (June 1980), pp. 327-331, 0002-9378

Taylor, K. L., Leaman, D. W., Grane, R., Mechti, N., Borden, E. C., & Lindner, D. J. (2008). Identification of interferon-β-stimulated genes that inhibit angiogenesis in vitro. *J Interferon Cytokine Res*, Vol. 28, No. 12, (December 2008), pp. 733-740, 1079-9907

Vestergaard, A. L., Knudsen, U. B., Munk, T., Rosbach, H., Bialasiewicz, S., Sloots, T. P., Martensen, P. M., & Antonsson, A. (2010). Low prevalence of DNA viruses in the human endometrium and endometriosis. *Arch Virol*, Vol. 155, No. 5, (May 2010), pp. 695-703, 0304-8608

Vestergaard, A. L., Knudsen, U. B., Munk, T., Rosbach, H., & Martensen, P. M. (2011). Transcriptional expression of type-I interferon response genes and stability of housekeeping genes in the human endometrium and endometriosis. *Mol Hum Reprod*, Vol. 17, No. 4, (April 2011), pp. 243-254, 1360-9947

Wilson, S. S., Fakioglu, E., & Herold, B. C. (2009). Novel approaches in fighting herpes simplex virus infections. *Expert Rev Anti Infect Ther*, Vol. 7, No. 5, (June 2009), pp. 559-68, 1744-8336

Wu, M.-H., Yang, B.-C., Lee, Y.-C., Wu, P.-L., & Hsu, C.-C. (2004). The Differential Expression of Intercellular Adhesion Molecule-1 (ICAM-1) and Regulation by Interferon-Gamma during the Pathogenesis of Endometriosis. *Am J Reprod Immunol*, Vol. 51, No. 5, (May 2004), pp. 373-380, 1600-0897

Zanatta, A., Rocha, A. M., Carvalho, F. M., Pereira, R. M. A., Taylor, H. S., Motta, E., Baracat, E. C., & Serafini, P. C. (2010). The role of *Hoxa10/HOXA10* gene in the etiology of endometriosis and its related infertility: a review. *J. Assist Reprod. Genet.*, Vol. 27, No. 12, (December 2010), pp. 701-710, 1058-0468

Zhou, Z., Wang, N., Woodson, S. E., Dong, Q., Wang, J., Liang, Y., Rijnbrand, R., Wei, L., Nichols, J. E., Guo, J.-T., Holbrook, M. R., Lemon, S. M., & Li, K. (2011). Antiviral activities of ISG20 in positive-strand RNA virus infection. *Virology*, Vol. 409, No. 2, (January 2011), pp. 175-188, 0042-6822

Zulfikaroglu, E., Kılıc, S., Islimye, M., Aydin, M., Zergeroglu, S., & Batioglu, S. (2010). Efficacy of anti-tumor necrosis factor therapy on endometriosis in an experimental rat model. *Arch Gynecol Obstet*, Vol. 283, No. 4, (March 2010), pp. 799-804, 0932-0067

zur Hausen, H. (2009). Papillomaviruses in the causation of human cancers - a brief historical account. *Virology*, Vol. 384, No. 2, (February 2009), pp. 260-265, 0042-6822

13

Stem Cell as the Novel Pathogenesis of Endometriosis

Eing-Mei Tsai
Kaohsiung Medical University,
Taiwan

1. Introduction

Endometriosis is a common gynecological disease. It is unique to have benign histology but with malignant characteristics. Easy recurrence, multiple organ involvement and malignant transformation potential make endometriosis a complex disease. Multi-factors contribute to the pathophysiology. Recently, endometriosis has been regarded as a stem cell disease (Sasson & Taylor, 2008). Some studies have provided evidence of the possible existence of stem cells in endometrial tissue (Gargett et al., 2004, 2007). We successfully isolated eutopic and ectopic endometrial mesenchymal stem cells (EN-MSCs) derived from one donor to examine the genetic difference analysis that provided a powerful tool for investigating the disease origin (Kao et al., 2011). Our results are consistent with the concept that endometriosis is a stem cell disease. We identified and characterized the MSCs from ectopic and eutopic endometrium by *in vitro* cell characteristics, including serpiginous morphology, surface biomarkers, a lack of gap junctional intercellular communication and the ability of differentiation and transdifferentiation into adipocytes, osteocytes, chondrocytes, neural cell and cardiomyocytes. In an *in vivo* animal study, we found the ability of invasion in eutopic and ectopic MSC.

The origins of endometrium stem cells are still under debate. Bone marrow is one of the origins. Bone marrow MSC circulates to the endometrium and reprograms into the endometrial MSC.

Aims of the chapter are to discuss about the endometrial stem cell identification and characterization and the stem cell theory of endometriosis will be discussed by search from the PubMed publications. The results will update our knowledge of the novel theory --- stem cell as the root of endometriosis.

2. Stem cells as the novel pathophysiology of endometriosis

2.1 Evidence of stem cell in the endometrium

The presence of endometrium stem cells can be identified by the property of clonogenicity, side population cells, stem cell markers, multipotent cells, xeno-transplantation. Expression of pluripotent marker such as Oct-4, and the stem cell factor in ectopic endometrium suggest that endometriosis has a stem cell origin (Pacchiarottic et al., 2011). There are two types of endometrium mesenchymal stem cells, one derived from the epitheilium and the other one from the stromal cells. The locations of these putative stem cells are supposed to be in the basalis of the endometrium (Figure 1). Some stem cell markers, for example, the RNA-binding protein Musashi-1 in colocalization with Notch-1 and telomerase increased in the basalis (Gotte et al., 2008). Recent study showed the endothelial progenitor/stem cells might reside in the endothelial cells (Maruyama et al., 2010). Some report showed the stem cell activity in endometrium through a stem cell niche with numbers of stem cells instead of a single stem cell (Kim et al., 2005). The function of endometrial stem cell/progenitor cell has be demonstrated to repair the damaged uterine surface in mouse model (Kaitu'u-Lino et al., 2010).

2.1.1 Cell cloning studies

The classic adult stem cell property, namely clonogenicity, is defined as a single cell to initiate a colony of cells when cultured at a single cell dilution condition. Both epithelium and stroma cells were reported to show clonogenicity (Gargett et al., 2007). The stromal cells display more clonogenicity than the epithelium cells. Both epithelium and stromal cells can develop large and small colonies. The large colonies were supposed to be initiated by stem cells while the small colonies by more mature transit amplifying cells (Figure 2).

2.1.2 Side population cells

Side population (SP) cells with the expression of ABCG2, which is a plasma membrane transporter, can extrude the DNA binding dye from cells. The cells in the side population are clonogenic and appear to be a universal marker of endometrial stem cell activity. SP cells are detected as a small fraction of cells within the endometrium after incubation with the Hoechst 33342 DNA binding dye. Recent study (Cervell et al., 2011) confirms the SP cells displays endometrial stem cell characteristics in molecular markers of undifferentiated cells (Oct-4, GDF3, Nanog, DNMT3betta, GABR3). Phenotype analysis verifies epithelial (CD9+), or stromal (vimentin+) cell origin. The mesenchymal markers (CD90+, CD73+, CD45-) are expressed in SP. All these data imply SP containing the endometrial stem cells.

2.1.3 Stem cell marker and expression of stemness-related genes

Since the lack of universal stem cell-specific markers, adult stem cells are difficult to purify. This is the same in the case of endometrial stem cells. Various markers or combinations of markers have been reported to purify endometrium MSC (Table 1).

The stem cell markers in endometrium are not fully recognized. Some studied have examined the expression of stem cell markers in the endometrium. Oct-4, bcl-2, c-kit (CD117), CD 34, CD45, CD7, CD56 are reported (Mattai C et al., 2006; Cho et al., 2004; Lnych et al., 2007). Forte et al (Forte et al., 2009) studied the expression a panel of stemness related genes in the human endometriotic and endometrial samples. They found genes *UTF1, TCL1,* and *ZFP42* showed higher frequency of expression in endometriosis than in endometrium.

The presence of the stem cell markers in the endometrium and endometriotic samples suggest stem cell contributes to the pathogenesis of endometriosis.

2.1.4 Multipotent cells identified in human endometrium

Schwab & Gargett isolated mesenchymal stem-like cells from human endometrium in 2007 (Schwab & Gargett, 2007). They identified the endometrial stromal cells with the capacity of differentiated into cells of adipogenic, myogenic, osteogenic, and chondrogenic cell lineages. In the same year, the other research group (Wolff et al., 2007) also identified the chondrocytes from the human endometrium. These reports demonstrated the multipotent stem cells in the human endometrium. These multipotent endometrial stem/progenitor cells have reported to differentiate into 9 lineages: cardiomyocytic, respiratory epithelial, neurocytic, myocytic, endothelial, pancreatic, hepatic, adipocytic and osteogenic (Meng et al., 2007).

2.1.5 Xenotransplantation

Some studies have demonstrated the formation of endometriotic lesion formation after transplantation of human endometrium into the immunodeficient mice such as severe combined immunodeficiency (SCID) and nude mice. Singly dispersed human endometrial cells were transplanted under the kidney capsules of non-obese diabetic (NOD)/SCID mice. They unveiled the reconstruction of endometrium by showing the formation of chimeric vessels, tortuous endometrial glands, tissue breakdown and bleeding (Masuda et al., PNAS 2007). Our previous investigation revealed the invasion and angiogenesis character after implanting with scaffolds seeded with eutopic or ectopic endometrial MSCs (Kao et al., 2011).

2.2 Source of the endometrium stem cells

Endometrium from the eutopic (inside the uterine cavity) or ectopic (outside of the uterine cavity), from the menstrual blood and bone marrow are the origin of the putative endometrial stem cells.

2.2.1 Isolation and culture of putative eutopic and ectopic endometrial mesenchymal stem cells

Endometrial stem cells can be cultivated from the endometrium epithelium and stroma. We isolated the putative eutopic and ectopic endometrial mesenchymal stem cells from the cases of endometriosis. According to our previous report (Kao et al., 2011), endometrial stromal cells were cultured from the tissue of eutopic and ectopic endometrium (from the endometrioma). At early passage (passage 5), endometrial stromal cells were seeded in triplicate at very low density (200 cells per 100 mm dish) in Dulbecco's modified Eagles's medium-Ham's F12 medium. After 21 days of incubation, large colonies were isolated and trypsinized into single cells. The diluted single cells were seeded in 96-well plates, clonally derived proliferating colonies were individually trypsinized and culture in a 100-mm dish after culture for 14 days. These isolated stem/progenitor cells illustrated the differentiation into mesoderm (adipogenesis, chondrogenesis, osteogenesis and cardiogenesis) and ectoderm (neurogenesis) (Figure 2).

2.2.2 Menstrual blood plays a role in the endometrial stem cells

Musina et al. isolated endometrium stem cells from the menstrual blood (Musina et al., 2008). The morphology resembled mesenchymal stem cells. The stem cells express CD44, CD90, CD 34, CD45, CD105/Endoglin. Cell differentiation revealed adipocytes, osteoblasts.

2.2.3 Bone marrow contributes to the sources of endometrial stem cells and pathogenesis of endometriosis

Currently, the ultimate source of endometrial stem cells is uncertain. Bone marrow derived stem cells (BMDCs) include hematopoietic stem cells (HSC) and MSC. BMDCs have been reported to be capable of transdifferentiation into hepatocytes, endothelial cells, neurons, cardiomyocyte, skin, gastrointestinal epithelium and endometrium (Taylor et al., 2004; Alison et al., 2000; Mezey et al., 2003; Quanini et al., 2002). Taylor et al. first provided the evidence of BMDCs as the sources of endometrial stem cells (Taylor et al., 2004). After bone marrow transplantation, they detected the endometrial epithelial cells and stromal cells with the donor human leukocyte antigen (HLA) in the recipient's endometrial samples. Another study observed the BMDCs derived from male donor mice engrafted the murine recipient endometrium (Du & Taylor, 2007). Although the transplanted BMDCs present in a small fraction (less than 0.01%), they could differentiate into endometrial cells in the uterus. Some novel theory of BMDCs in endometriosis pathogenesis was recently arisen. Bone marrow-derived circulating endothelial progenitor cells are recruited and incorporated into the vasculature of endometriotic lesions, thus contributing to the development of endometriosis (Matthias et al., 2011). In human studies, the donor BMDCs could transdifferentiate into the endometrial endothelial cells in a bone marrow transplantation recipient (Mints et al., 2008). BMDCs from human male donors were reported to differentiate into endometrial glands in a female transplant recipient (Ikoma et al., 2009). These data provide the evidence BMDCs as possible sources of endometrial stem/progenitor cells and endothelial progenitor cells.

2.2.4 Circulating endothelial progenitor cells (EPCs) contribute to the vascularization of endometriotic lesions

Endometriosis represents an angiogenic disease, rapid vascularization is essential to foster the ectopic endometrium survival and growth. One canonical characteristic of endometiosis is the vascularized endometriotic lesions inside the peritoneal cavity. Recent study (Matthias et al., 2011) indicates for the first time the circulating EPCs from the bone marrow contribute a relative high fraction (about 15%) of the microvascular networks in the engrafting endometriotic lesions in mice model. The recruited EPCs may contribute to the process of vasculogenensis (de novo generation of endothelial cells) (Figure 5). These data provide that the EPCs involve in the integral mechanism in the pathogenesis of endometriosis.

2.3 Endometrial stem cells as the pathogenesis and therapeutic target for endometriosis

2.3.1 Stem cells as a novel pathogenesis of endometriosis

Endometriosis is a multifactorial disease, the pathogenesis includes retrograde of endometrial cells, immunological insufficiency, genetics (Juo et al, 2006; 2009), metaplasia, and environmental hormone disruptor (Huang et al., 2011). Endometrial stem cells were identified in the endometrioma cyst walls (Chan et al., 2011; Kao et al., 2011).

Some hypotheses suggest the theory of stem cell in the pathogenesis of endometriosis (Figueira et al., 2011; Kao et al., 2010). Endometrium stem cells reside in the basalis layer can flux through the tubes and establish endometriotic lesions in the peritoneum. The stimulatory factors consisting of genetic, immunological and inflammatory, angiogenesis factors (Figure 6) promote the growth. An alternative hypothesis explores the extrauterine stem/progenitor cells (for example, from reprogram of bone marrow MSCs and circulating EPCs) function in the pathogenesis of endometriosis.

2.3.2 Therapeutic potential of human endometrial stem cells

Therapeutic potential of human endometrial stem cells has attracted interest of the researchers. Endometrial stem cells were obtained from nine healthy women and were transformed into the dopaminergic nerve cells. These cells were transplanted into the Parkinson-mice model (Wolff et al., 2010) and restored function of brain cells damage by producing dopamine.

The stem cell theory of endometriosis makes the advancement of targeting stem cells as the novel treatment. Stem cells flux and fostered by the peritoneal environment. The stem cells grow into endometriosis with increased survival and proliferative capacity along with environmental factors that contribute to stem cell survival and propagation. The treatment target can focus on the inhibition of stem cell flux and initiation and progression of endometriosis. Recent report (Zhou et al., 2011) cigarette smoke inhibits recruitment of bone marrow derived stem cells to the uterus. This finding is compatible with the epidemiological data of low incidence of endometriosis cases in smokers. Further investigation on the individual components of tobacco may unveil useful treatment in endometriosis. Our recent study reveals interleukin-1 beta can upregulate cyclooxygenase-2 and enhance invasion of human MSC derived from the ectopic endometrium (Kao et al., 2011). These results imply the interleukin-1 betta could be the targeting signalling. Stem cell therapy has been used in the lupus through anti-inflammatory activity (Traynor et al., 2002). Based on the same concept, bone marrow derived mononuclear stem cells has been transplanted in the experimental Wistar rats (Kondo et al., 2011). The expression of the inflammatory cytokines tumor necrosis factor-alpha (TNF-alpha) and vascular endothelial growth factor (VEGF) in the endometriotic implant decreased without reducing the lesion surface area. This provides the evidence that stem cells home the ectopic tissue to reduce the inflammatory process. This conflicts with the stem cell theory, which may indicate when the stem cells derived from the bone marrow, when they engrafte the endometrium, they are modified in the gene expression, what will lead to the development of the endometriosis. The modified stem cells play different function as those original stem cells used for therapy. Other targeting of inhibition in signalling pathways by stem cells and the microenvironment, self- renew pathway blocking, cell recruitment, flux and adhesion prevention will represent novel potential strategies (Taylor et al., 2011).

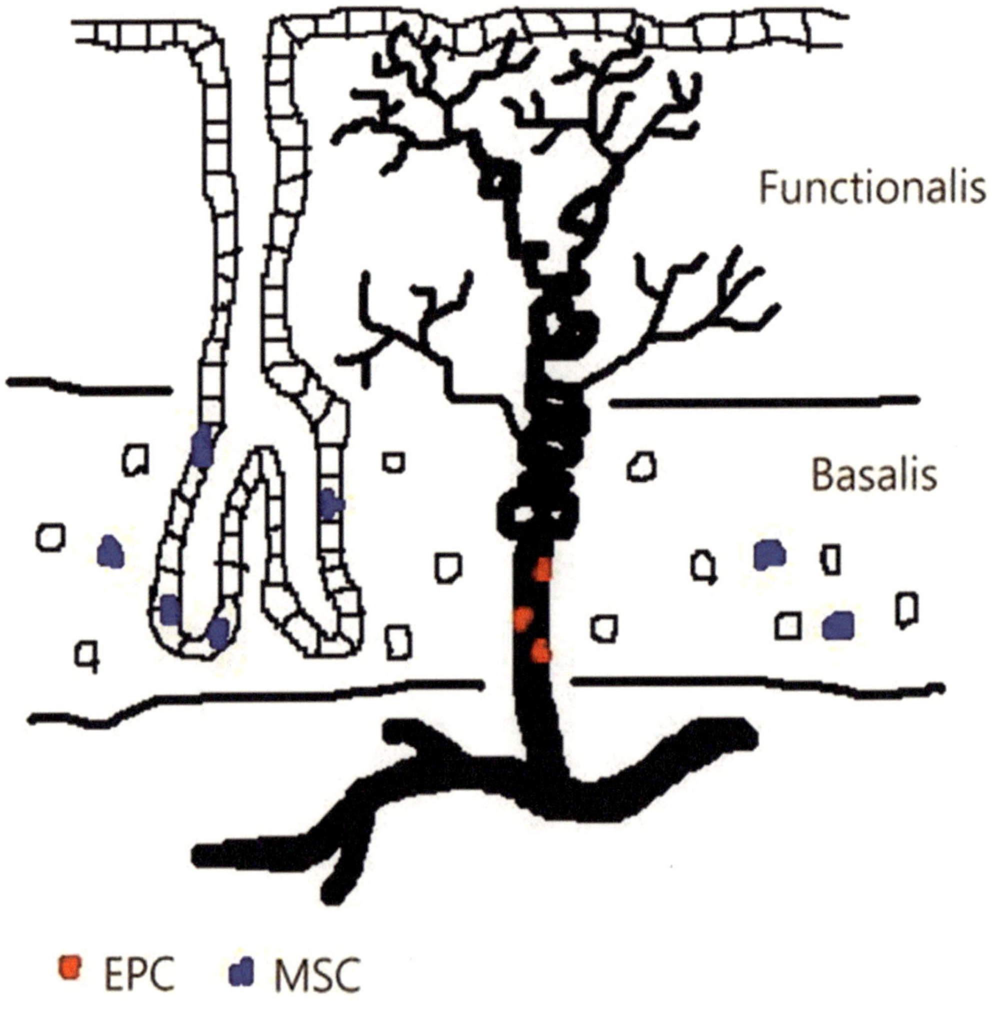

Fig. 1. The location of putative progenitor/stem cells is identified in the basalis of the endometrium. MSC denotes mesenchymal stem cells, and EPC indicates endothelial progenitor cells. (Modified from Maruyama et al., 2010)

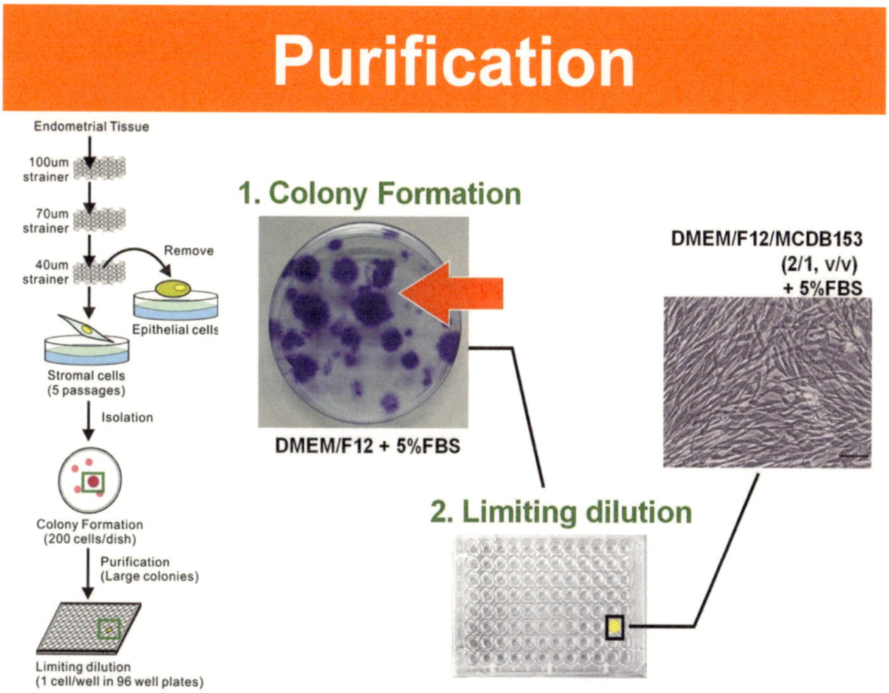

Fig. 2. Purification of stem cells from endometrial stromal cells. Large and small colonies develop after single cell limiting dilution. The large colonies are cultivated for stem cells identification.

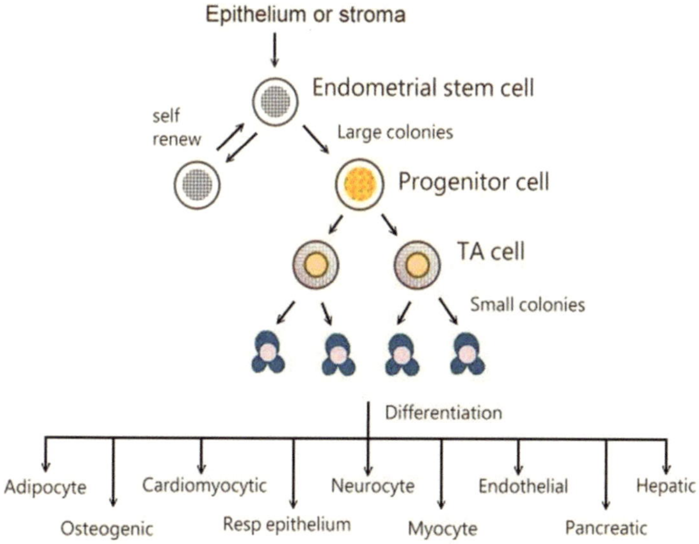

Fig. 3. Isolation and differentiation of endometrial stem/progenitor cells. Endometrial stem/progenitor cells can be isolated from endometrial epithelium and stromal cells. These cells can differentiated into 9 lineages, including adipocyte, myocyte, respiratory epithelium, neurocyte, osteogenic, cardiomyocytic, endothelial, pancreatic and hepatic cells.

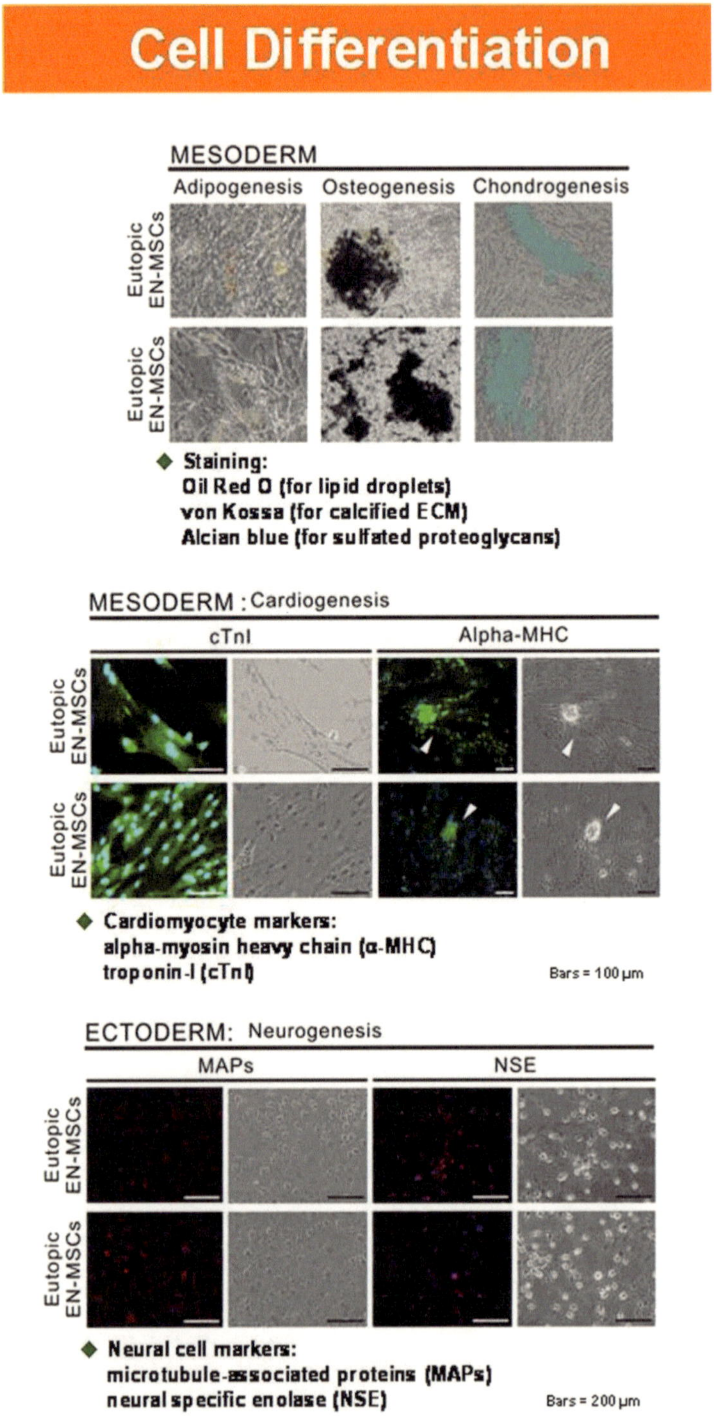

Fig. 4. Mesenchymal stem cells derived from eutopic and ectopic endometrial stromal cells differentiate into mesoderm and ectoderm lineages.

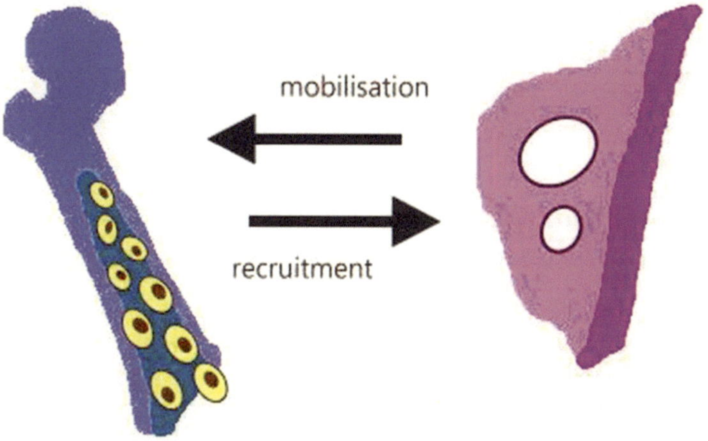

Fig. 5. Endothelial progenitor cells are mobilized and recruited to the endometriotic lesions, subsequently vasculogenensis (de novo generation of endothelial cells) occurs (modified from Laschke et al., 2011).

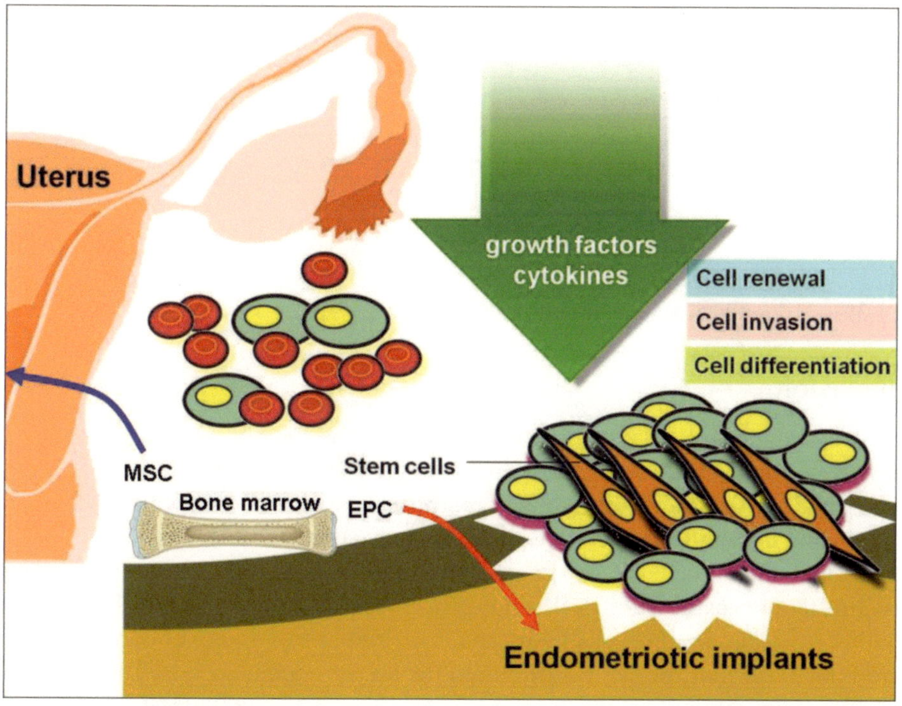

MSC indicates mesenchymal stem cell.
EPC means endothelial progenitor cell.

Fig. 6. The possible theory of endometrial stem/progenitor cells in the pathogenesis of endometriosis. The endometrial stem cells reflux to the peritoneum, and the microenvironmental factors such as growth factors, cytokines etc., stimulate the stem cells function (cell renew, invasion and cell differentiation). Bone marrow derived MSC and EPC may also contribute to the pathogenesis as described in the text.

Biomarker	Relevance/function	Expression
Oct-4	Stem cell	Positive
hTERT	Telomerase reverse transcriptase	Positive
CD9	MSC/angiogenesis	Positive
CD29	MSC/adhesion molecule	Positive
CD41a	MSC/fibrinogen receptor	Positive
CD44	MSC/hyaluronic acid receptor	Positive
CD73	MSC/migration	Positive
CD90	MSC/marker of T cells, hematopoietic and MSC	Positive
CD105	MSC	Positive
CD49f	MSC	Positive
Musashi-1	Endometrial stem cell	Positive
CD34	Hematopoietic stem cell	Negative
CD45	Leukocyte cell	Negative
SSEA-4	Embryonic stem cell	Negative
Nanog	Embryonic stem cell	Negative

MSC: mesenchymal stem cell
Modified from Meng et al., 2007

Table 1. Biomarkers of endometrial mesenchymal stem cells.

3. Conclusion

Since the retrograde implantation theory developed in the 1920s by Sympson, the etiology of endometriosis involves a complex interplay of genetic, immunologic, inflammatory and environmental factors. Nevertheless, endometriosis remains an enigmatic disease to cause pelvic pain and infertility. The characteristics of recurrence and wide spray make the disease malignant-like. Stem cell theory opens the latest advanced avenue for etiology of endometriosis. Increasing studies illustrate the presence of endometrial stem/progenitor cells, either from the residing cells in the endometrium or reprogram of bone marrow MSC. EPC from the bone marrow can contribute to the de novo angiogenesis. The EPC enhances endometriosis formation. Endometriosis is a recurrent disease, thus making the treatment costly and psychologically debilitating. Novel treatment modalities include selective ER modulators, tissue factor (the initiator of the hemostatic cascade) targets, statins and angiogenic blockers, immunoconjugate molecule and stem cells. Administration of endometrial stem cells to the disease model could suppress the immunological reaction, and was supposed to have potential in the treatment. Other therapy modalities to target the stem cells flux, adhesion and signalling control pathway are novel treatment strategies.

4. Acknowledgment

The author thanks sincerely to Dr. Yu-Chih Wang for his edition.

5. References

Alison M. R.; Poulsom R.; Jeffery R.; Dhillon A. P.; Quaglia A.; Jacob J.; Novelli M.; Prentice G.; Williamson J. & Wright N. A. (2000). *Nature,* Vol. 406, No. 6793, (July 2000), pp. 257, ISSN 0028-0836.

Bertolini F.; Pruneri G. (2002). Chimerism of the transplanted heart. *New England Journal of Medicine,* Vol. 346, No. 18, (January 2002), pp. 5-15, ISSN 1533-4406.

Cervello I.; Mas A.; Gil-Sanchis C.; Peris L.; Faus AS.; Saunder P.; Critchley H. & Simón H. (2011). Reconstruction of Endometrium from Human Endometrial Side Population Cell Lines. *PLoS one,* Vol. 6, No. 6, (June 2011), pp. e21221, ISSN 1932-6203.

Chan R. W.; Ng E. H. & Yeung W. S. (2011). Identification of Cells with Colony-Forming Activity, Self-Renewal Capacity, and Multipotency in Ovarian Endometriosis *The American Journal of Pathology,* Vol. 178, No. 6, (June 2011), pp. 2832-2844, ISSN 0002-9440.

Cho N. H.; Park Y. K.; Kim Y. T.; Yang H. & Kim S. K. (2004). Lifetime expression of stem cell markers in the uterine endometrium. *Fertility and Sterility,* Vol. 81, No. 2, (February 2004), pp. 403-407, ISSN 0015-0282.

Du, H. & Taylor H. S. (2007). Contribution of bone marrow-derived stem cells to endometrium and endometriosis. *Stem Cells,* Vol. 25, No. 8, (August 2007), pp. 2082-2086, ISSN 1066-5099.

Figueira P. G.; Abrão M. S.; Krikun G. & Taylor H. S. (2011). Stem cells in endometrium and their role in the pathogenesis of endometriosis. *Annals of The New York Academy of Sciences,* Vol. 1221, (March 2011), pp. 10-17, ISSN 1749-6632.

Forte A.; Schettino M. T.; Finicelli M.; Cipollaro M.; Colacurci N.; Cobellis L. & Galderisi U. (2009). Expression pattern of stemness-related genes in human endometrial and endometriotic tissues. *Molecular Medicine,* Vol. 15, No. 11-12, (November-Docember 2009),pp. 392-401, ISSN 1076-1551.

Gargett C. E. (2004). Stem cells in gynaecology. *Australian and New Zealand Journal of Obstetrics and Gynaecology,* Vol. 44, No. 5, (October 2004), pp. 380-386, ISSN 0004-8666.

Gargett C. E.; Chan R. W. & Schwab K. E. (2007). Endometrial stem cells. Current *Opinion in Obstetrics and Gynecology,* Vol. 19, No. 4, (August 2007), pp. 377-383, ISSN 1040-872X.

Götte M.; Wolf M.; Staebler A.; Buchweitz O.; Kelsch R.; Schüring A. N. & Kiesel L. (2008). Musashi-1 in endometriosis and endometrial carcinoma. *The Journal of Pathology,*Vol. 215, No. 3, (July 2008), pp. 317-329, ISSN 1096-9896.

Ikoma T.; Kyo S.; Maida Y.; Ozaki S.; Takakura M.; Nakao S. & Inoue M. (2009). Bone marrow-derived cells from male donors can compose endometrial glands in female transplant recipients. *American Journal of Obstetrics and Gynecology,* Vol. 21, No. 6, (December 2009), pp. 608. e1-8, ISSN 0002-9378.

Juo S. H.; Wang T. N.; Lee J. N.; Wu M. T.; Long C. Y. & Tsai E. M. (2006). CYP17, CYP1A1 and COMT polymorphisms and the risk of adenomyosis and endometriosis in Taiwanese women. *Human Reproduction,* Vol. 21, No. 6, (June 2006), pp. 1498-1502, ISSN 1460-2350.

Juo S. H.; Wu R.; Lin C. S.; Wu M. T.; Lee J. N. & Tsai E. M. (2009). A functional promoter polymorphism in interleukin-10 gene influences susceptibility to endometriosis. *Fertility and Sterility,* Vol. 92, No. 4, (October 2009), pp. 1228-1233, ISSN 0015-0282.

Kaitu'u-Lino T. J.; Ye L. & Gargett C. E. (2010). Reepithelialization of the uterine surface arises from endometrial glands: evidence from a functional mouse model of breakdown and repair. *Endocrinology,* Vol. 151, No. 7, (July 2010), pp. 3386-3395, ISSN 0013-7227.

Kao A. P.; Wang K. H.; Chang C. C.; Lee J. N.; Long C. Y.; Chen H. S.; Tsai C. F.; Hsieh T. H. & Tsai E. M. (2011). Comparative study of human eutopic and ectopic endometrial mesenchymal stem cells and the development of an in vivo endometriotic invasion model. *Fertility and Sterility,* Vol. 95, No. 4, (March 2011), pp. 1308-1315, ISSN 0015-0282.

Kao A. P.; Wang K. H.; Long C. Y.; Chai C. Y.; Tsai C. F.; Hsieh T. H.; Hsu C. Y.; Chang C. C.; Lee J. N. & Tsai E. M. (2011). Interleukin-1β induces cyclooxygenase-2 expression and promotes the invasive ability of human mesenchymal stem cells derived from ovarian endometrioma. , In 13. 07. 2011, *Fertility and Sterility* Available from
http://doi:10. 1016/j. fertnstert. 2011. 06. 041

Kim J. Y.; Tavaré S. & Shibata D. (2005). Counting human somatic cell replications: methylation mirrors endometrial stem cell divisions. *The Proceedings of the National Academy of Sciences USA,* Vol. 102, No. 49, (December 2005), pp. 17739-17744, ISSN 0027-8424.

Kondo W.; Dal Lago E. A.; Francisco J. C.; Simeoni R. B.; de Noronha L.; Martins A. P.; de Azevedo M. L.; Ferreira C. C.; Maestrelli P.; Olandoski M.; Guarita-Souza L. C. & do Amaral V. F. (2011). Effect of the bone marrow derived-mononuclear stem cells transplantation in the growth, VEGF-R and TNF-alpha expression of endometrial implants in Wistar rats, In 01. 06. 2011, *The European Journal of Obstetrics & Gynecology and Reproductive Biology* Available from
http://dx. doi. org/10. 1016/j. ejogrb. 2011. 05. 004.

Laschke M. W.; Giebels C.; Nickels R. M.; Scheuer C. & Menger M. D. (2011). Endothelial Progenitor Cells Contribute to the Vascularization of Endometriotic Lesions. *The American Journal of Pathology,* Vol. 178, No. 1, (January 2011), pp. 442-450, ISSN 0002-9440.

Lynch L.; Golden-Mason L.; Eogan M.; O'Herlihy C. & O'Farrelly C. (2007). Cells with haematopoietic stem cell phenotype in adult human endometrium: relevance to infertility? *Human Reproduction,* Vol. 22, No. 4, (April 2007), pp. 919-926, ISSN 0268-1161.

Maruyama T.; Masuda H.; Ono M.; Kajitani T. & Yoshimura Y. (2010). Human uterine stem/progenitor cells: their possible role in uterine physiology and pathology. *Reproduction,* Vol. 140, No. 1, (July 2010), pp. 11-22, ISSN 1470-1626.

Masuda H.; Maruyama T.; Hiratsu E.; Yamane J.; Iwanami A.; Nagashima T.; Ono M.; Miyoshi H.; Okano H. J.; Ito M.; Tamaoki N.; Nomura T.; Okano H.; Matsuzaki Y. & Yoshimura Y. (2007). Noninvasive and real-time assessment of reconstructed functional human endometrium in NOD/SCID/gamma c(null) immunodeficient mice. *The Proceedings of the National Academy of Sciences USA,* Vol. 104, No. 6, (February 2007), pp. 1925-1930, ISSN 0027-8424.

Meng X.; Ichim T. E.; Zhong J.; Rogers A.;, Yin Z.; Jackson J.; Wang H.; Ge W.; Bogin V.; Chan K. W.; Thébaud B. & Riordan N. H. (2007). Endometrial regenerative cells: a novel stem cell population. *Journal of Translational Medicine,* Vol. 5, (November 2007), pp. 57, ISSN 1479-5876.

Mints M.; Jansson M.; Sadeghi B.; Westgren M.; Uzunel M.; Hassan M. & Palmblad J. (2008). Endometrial endothelial cells are derived from donor stem cells in a bone marrow transplant recipient. *Human Reproduction,* Vol. 23, No. 1, (January 2008), pp. 139-143, ISSN 0268-1161.

Musina R. A.; Belyavski A. V.; Tarusova O. V.; Solovyova E. V. & Sukhikh G. T. (2008). Endometrial mesenchymal stem cells isolated from the menstrual blood. *Bulletin of experimental biology and medicine,* Vol. 145, No. 4, (April 2008), pp. 539-543, ISSN 0007-4888.

Pacchiarotti A.; Caserta D.; Sbracia M. & Moscarini M. (2011). Expression of oct-4 and c-kit antigens in endometriosis. *Fertility and Sterility,* Vol. 95, No. 3, (March 2011), pp. 1171-1173, ISSN 0015-0282.

Schwab K. E. & Gargett C. E. (2007). Co-expression of two perivascular cell markers isolates mesenchymal stem-like cells from human endometrium. *Human Reproduction,* Vol. 22, No. 11, (November 2007), pp. 2903-2911, ISSN 0268-1161.

Taylor H. S. (2004). Endometrial cells derived from donor stem cells in bone marrow transplant recipients. *Journal of the American Medical Association,* Vol. 292, No. 1, (July 2004), pp. 81-85, ISSN 0098-7484.

Taylor H. S.; Osteen K. G.; Bruner-Tran K. L.; Krikun G.; Sokalska A. & Duleba A. J. (2011). Novel Therapies Targeting Endometriosis. *Reproductive Sciences,* Vol. 18, No. 9, (September 2011), pp. 814-823, ISSN 1933-7191.

Traynor A. E.; Barr W. G.; Rosa R. M.; Rodriguez J.; Oyama Y.; Baker S.; Brush M. & Burt R. K. (2002). Hematopoietic stem cell transplantation for severe and refractory lupus. Analysis after five years and fifteen patients. *Arthritis and Rheumatism,* Vol. 46, No. 11, (November), pp. 2917-2923, ISSN 1529-0131.

Wolff E. F.; Wolff A. B.; Hongling D. & Taylor H. S. (2007). Demonstration of multipotent stem cells in the adult human endometrium by in vitro chondrogenesis. *Reproductive ciences,* Vol. 14No. 6, (September 2007), pp. 524-533, ISSN 1933-7191.

Wolff E. F.; Gao X. B.; Yao K. V.; Andrews Z. B.; Du H.; Elsworth J. D. & Taylor H. S. (2011). Endometrial stem cell transplantation restores dopamine production in a

Parkinson's disease model. *Journal of cellular and molecular medicine,* Vol. 15, No. 4, (April 2011), pp. 747-755, ISSN 1582-1838.

Zhou Y.; Gan Y. & Taylor H. S. (2011). Cigarette smoke inhibits recruitment of bone-marrow-derived stem cells to the uterus. *Reproductive Toxicology,* Vol. 31, No. 2, (February 2011), pp. 123-127, ISSN 0890-6238.

14

Green Tea for Endometriosis

Gene Chi Wai Man, Hui Xu and Chi Chiu Wang
Department of Obstetrics and Gynaecology, The Chinese University of Hong Kong, Prince of Wales Hospital, Shatin, New Territories, Hong Kong

1. Introduction

Endometriosis is a common gynaecological disease, defined by the presence of endometrial tissue outside the uterus, causing pain and infertility of women in reproductive age (Galle, 1989). It is estimated that it occurs in 10-15% for women in the reproductive age and more than 30% of all infertile women are affected (Cramer *et al.*, 2002). However, the actual figure on the total prevalence may even be higher, as the disease is often not diagnosed due to heterogenous clinical manifestations. These manifestations include dysmenorrhoea, dyspareunia, dysuria and chronic abdominal or pelvic pain as well as infertility, resulting in a severely limited quality of life (Davis *et al.*, 2003; Milingos *et al.*, 2006; Vercellini *et al.*, 2007). Thus, the aim on treating endometriosis should ideally target the endometriosis itself, i.e. relieves pain, promotes fertility and prevents reocurrence. Unfortunately, there is no current treatment being able to fulfill all these requirements. All conservative treatments, either medical or surgical, are still liable for disease reocurrence, and they do not address the cause and possible side effects brought upon to the disease mechanism and the patient outcomes.

In this chapter, we will analyze the rationale and limitations of the current therapy of endometriosis. Also, we will discuss on the latest therapies that hold a higher efficacy and sensitivity on treating the disease. Most importantly, we will highlight the effect of green tea on being a potential remedy toward tackling endometriosis.

1.1 Current and new treatment

In the past, the disease was best thought to be treated surgically. And with the advancement of operative laparoscopy, the treatment of endometriosis could be started as soon as it was diagnosis. However, different researches have shown surgical removal of endometriosis can bought upon many complications and chronicity. Likewise, without medical supplements, the patients would have a high chance for disease reocurrence. Hence, there is a great demand for medical treatments that can induce a suppression of this disease.

The type of treatments offer would depend on the extent or stage of the disease, the amount of pain suffered, and fertility wanted (Valle *et al.*, 2003) (Fig. 1). To perform the best therapy would require complete diagnosis and inspections of the lesion to determine the symptoms and staging of the patient's endometriosis (Olive *et al.*, 2001). The choices of present treatments include expectant management, medical therapy and surgical treatment (Table 1).

Traditional treatment
Expectant Management
Medical Therapy
- Analgesics
- Hormonal
- Selective progesterone receptor modulators
- Selective estrogen receptor beta agonists
- Gonadotropin releasing hormone antagonists
Surgical Treatment
- Conservative Surgery
- Definitive Surgery

New treatment
Angiogenesis inhibitors
Antioxidant therapy
Aromatase inhibitors
Tumor necrosis factor-alpha inhibitors
Matrix metalloproteinase inhibitors
Immunomodulators
Traditional Chinese medicines

Table 1. Treatment of Endometriosis

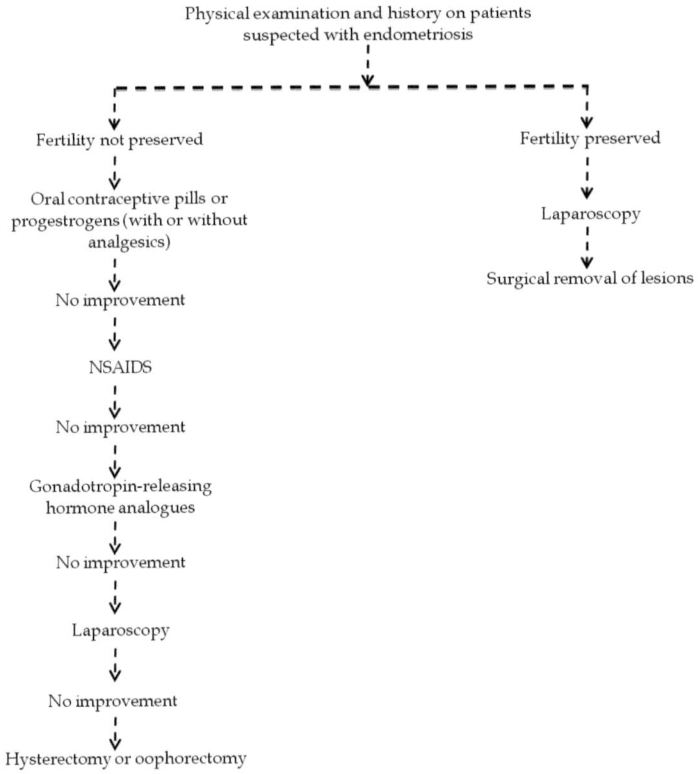

Fig. 1. Clinical evaluation on patients with endometriosis

1.1.1 Expectant management

In asymptomatic patients, those with mild symptoms or infertility with minimal endometriosis, expectant management may be prescribed. These women may opt for birth control pills because they can prevent endometriosis from progressing and protect against unwanted pregnancy (Bedaiwy *et al.*, 2009). While for women approaching the menopause, they may also be managed expectantly, because the growth of endometriosis is suppressed after the menopause.

1.1.2 Medical therapy

Medical therapies are typically used for patients with endometriosis that have minimal pelvic pain. The types of medical therapies can be divided into two main categories: analgesics and hormonal. However, medical therapy alone is not appropriate for women with more advanced stages of endometriosis or those desiring pregnancy. And unlike surgery, medical therapy does not enhance your chances of conception (Hansen *et al.*, 2006).

1.1.2.1 Analgesics

Analgesics treatments are often the first-line therapy in women with primary dysmenorrhea or pelvic pain and those with minimal pain symptoms associated with endometriosis. For mild cases of endometriosis, analgesic medications alone may be sufficient to relieve symptoms (Mahutte *et al.*, 2003). Commonly used analgesic medications include paracetamol and non-steroidal anti-inflammatory drugs (NSAID). Although the use of analgesic treatments for pain relief is regularly prescribed, lack of clinical studies have critically evaluated their effectiveness.

1.1.2.2 Hormonal

Hormonal treatments are aimed at decreasing the amount of estrogen in the body, which will inhibit the progression of the endometrial implants (Coutinho, 1982). The most common hormonal medications used are combined oral contraceptives, progestins, androgens, and gonadotropin-releasing hormone (GnRH) agonist analogs. Combined oral contraceptives has been used for women with endometriosis since the 1950s (Kistner, 1959). These pills consist of a low combination of synthetic estrogen and progesterone. They have been shown to be very effective for patients with mild symptoms of endometriosis (Vercellini *et al.*, 1993; Vessey *et al.*, 1993). The main advantages are that it is inexpensive and is usually reasonably well tolerated by women (Kennedy, 2004). It can also be taken safely for many years if necessary (Kennedy, 2004). However, it is not free of side effects. These include irregular vaginal bleeding, fluid retention, abdominal bloating, weight gain, increased appetite, nausea, headaches, breast tenderness and depression.

Progestins are a group of drugs that behave like the female hormone progesterone. Although the actual mechanism on how progestins relieve the symptoms of endometriosis remained unclear, a possible effect might be the growth of endometrial implants was suppressed by this hormone, causing them to gradually regress (Schweppe, 2001). Other reported that they may reduce endometriosis-induced inflammation in the pelvic cavity (Vercellini *et al.*, 2003). In clinical trials, it showed progestins being effective treatments for the symptoms of endometriosis (Kennedy *et al.*, 2005). When taken continuously daily, they have shown to relieve endometriosis-associated pain as effectively as the other hormonal drugs (Kennedy *et al.*, 2005). However, there are side effects, which include irregular menstrual cycle, sore breasts, headache, nausea, dizziness and bloating. These side effects are not usually serious and long-lasting (Winkel *et al.*, 2001), however many patients still feel unpleasant and difficult to cope with. Hence, most women could seldom complete this type of treatment.

Danazol is an effective androgen for treating endometriosis. It works by suppressing the growth and development of the endometriotic lesion temporarily, hence continuous medication is required. Clinical trials have shown that danazol is effective in relieving the pain symptoms of endometriosis (Kennedy *et al.*, 2005) for approximately 90% of women (Biberoglu *et al.*, 1981). However, common side effects from these treatments include acne, oily skin, increased hair growth, and weight gain. Its unpleasant side effects and its risk of developing cardiovascular disease mean it is not the first choice of treatment for endometriosis (Kennedy, 2004).

Gonadotropin releasing hormone (GnRH) agonists are a group of drugs that have been used to treat women with endometriosis for many years (Schweppe, 2005). They work by stopping the production of estrogen by a series of inhibition on the estrogen-related pathway mechanisms. Although this treatment can reduce 50% in symptoms, but in long-term, pain recurrence can be observed in up to 75% of the cases (Surrey *et al.*, 2002). Likewise, affecting the estrogen hormonal cycle can result in major side effects like bone thinning (Pierce *et al.*, 2000).

1.1.3 Surgical treatment

Typically surgery becomes a choice after expectant management and hormonal therapy failed to reduce the patient symptoms (Olive et al., 2001; Winkel et al., 2001). Likewise, when anatomic distortions due to endometrial growths are present, surgery would also be the primary choice for treatment (Surrey *et al.*, 2003). There are mainly two types of surgery associated with endometriosis: conservative and definitive.

1.1.3.1 Conservative surgery

This type of surgery is employed in cases of mild to moderate endometriosis, and for women who would like to retain fertility, as this surgery saves as much ovarian tissue and uterus as possible (Camanni *et al.*). The most common conservative surgical approach is the use of laparoscopy for treating endometriosis (Brosens *et al.*, 1981). The aim of this type of surgery is restoration of the normal anatomy of the pelvis. Clinically, it has been shown that most patients, who undergone conservative surgery, realize a relief of pain symptoms associated with endometriosis. Women who had their implants excised had fewer symptoms 12 months (Abbott *et al.*, 2004) and 18 months (Sutton *et al.*, 1994; Sutton *et al.*, 1997) after surgery compared with women who underwent a laparoscopy without excision of their implants, respectively. However, this type of surgery has a high reoccurrence rate of up to 40% at 10 years post surgery.

1.1.3.2 Definitive surgery

On the other hand, patients suffering from painful symptoms resulted from severe endometriosis, and when fertility does not need to be retained, may require definitive surgery. This can involves the removal of the uterus (hysterectomy), fallopian tubes (salpingectomy), deep endometrial implants (debulking) and scar tissue (fibrinolysis). The ovaries may also be removed (oophorectomy) to prevent fluctuation of estrogen levels, which may cause any remaining endometrial implants to continue to grow. In such cases, estrogen medication would be given to prevent menopausal symptoms to occur in the patients. Likewise, woman who underwent oophorectomy for endometriosis has greater pain relief and less likelihood of repeated surgery than those operated by hysterectomy with ovarian preservation (Namnoum *et al.*, 1995). In addition, the rate of recurrence in patients with definitive surgery is much lower than in those with conservative surgery.

1.1.4 Latest treatments developed against endometriosis

Recently, with the better understanding on the pathogenesis and progression toward endometriosis, novel medications on using molecular targets are developed for treatment of endometriosis. The advantages of such agents hold a higher efficacy and sensitivity on treating the disease, while minimizing evidence of side effects experienced by the patients.

1.1.4.1 Anti-angiogenesis inhibitors

One of the main etiologies of endometriosis is believe to be resulted from implantation of retrograde shed endometrium during menstruation (Sampson, 1927). The properties of the endometrium have the capacity to adhere, attach, and implant ectopically (Koks *et al.*, 1999; Maas *et al.*, 2001). Based on the anatomical surrounding, endometriotic lesions are found to be larger in size with the availability to rich blood supply. This suggesting that angiogenesis is prerequisite for the development of endometriosis.

The use of angiostatic agents may provide a new therapeutic option to inhibit this pathological process. The aim is to mainly control two processes involved in angiogenesis: endothelial cell growth and endothelial cell adhesion. Angiogenic cytokines are elevated in the peritoneal fluid in patients with endometriosis (Nisolle *et al.*, 1993). Anti-angiogenesis therapies have been shown effective in suppressing the development in endometriotic lesion in mice (Nap *et al.*, 2004). Common angiostatic compounds, such as anti-human vascular endothelial growth factor-A (anti-hVEGF), TNP-470, endostatin, and anginex, significantly decreased microvessel density and inhibited the established endometriosis lesions (Dabrosin *et al.*, 2002; Nap *et al.*, 2004; Yagyu *et al.*, 2005). By far, the only clinical trial conducted with an anti-angiogenesis therapy on treating endometriosis-associated pain was thalidomide (Scarpellini *et al.*, 2002). Although the result showed promising pain relief in the patients, however, thalidomide is a potential teratogen (Khoury *et al.*, 1987). Thus, women wanting pregnancy is prohibited.

1.1.4.2 Anti-oxidant therapy

Although the actual etiology of endometriosis remains unknown, it is widely accepted that retrograde menstruation is associated with endometriosis. However, it is unclear on why only a portion of women with retrograde menstruation develops endometriosis, while others do not. Studies proposed this might be due to the presence of elements such as macrophages, iron or environmental contaminants disrupting the balance between ROS and antioxidants in the peritoneal fluid of some women, leading to oxidative stress and endometriosis (Arumugam *et al.*, 1995; Donnez *et al.*, 2002; Murphy *et al.*, 1998). Likewise, the cyclical changes in the endometrium are accompanied by changes in the expression of various antioxidant enzymes in the endometrium (Gurdol *et al.*, 1997).

Patients with endometriosis have shown the increase in generation of ROS by peritoneal fluid macrophages, with increased lipid peroxidation (Halme *et al.*, 1983). The diminished peritoneal fluid antioxidants (Murphy *et al.*, 1998), elevated oxidized lipoproteins, lysophosphatidyl choline (Murphy *et al.*, 1998), and other markers of lipid peroxidation provide further evidence of oxidative stress in the peritoneal microenvironment of endometriosis (Ho *et al.*, 1997; Szczepanska *et al.*, 2003).

Currently, a study investigated whether there would be reduced total chemokines and inflammatory cytokines in women with endometriosis (Santanam *et al.*, 2003). As patients were given 1200 IU of vitamin E and 1 g of vitamin C for a period of 2 months, this resulted in a decrease in the inflammatory markers monocyte chemotactic protein-1, regulated on activation normal T cell expressed and secreted (RANTES), and interleukin-6 in peritoneal fluid. Similar study showed these antioxidant supplements can reduce pelvic pain in women with endometriosis (Kavtaradze *et al.*, 2003).

Recently, an inhibitory drug has been used in clinical trials to determine the effect of anti-oxidant therapy on endometriosis (Creus *et al.*, 2008). Pentoxifylline, a phosphodiesterase inhibitor, has the capability to maintain a higher pregnancy rates in patients suffering from endometriosis. RU 486 exerts an inhibitory effect on endometrial cell growth through its antioxidant properties *in vitro*. Although antioxidants have shown to have beneficial effects in patients with endometriosis, the limited number of trials conducted questions the actual efficacy.

1.1.4.3 Hormone inhibitors and modulators

As endometriosis is an estrogen-dependent disease, the estrogen-related pathways are often the treatment used to tackle the imbalanced of estrogen in these female patients. A way is to suppress the production of estrogen by inhibiting its synthetic and regulatory pathway. Another potential way is to influence estrogen receptors minimizing estrogen-dependent gene expressions.

Since aromatase, the key enzyme in estrogen synthesis in ovary, adipose tissue or endometriotic tissue, is encoded by a single gene, the inhibition of this gene or its production may cause an effective suppression of estrogen production (Simpson *et al.*, 2002). Preliminary evidence suggests that combined treatment with luteinizing-hormone-releasing hormone analogues and aromatase inhibitors may be superior to medical treatment with luteinizing-hormone-releasing hormone analogues (Shaw, 1988).

Another type of treatment is by using tumor necrosis factor alpha (TNF-α) inhibitor. This cytokine have been found to be overproduced in women with endometriosis, and partially responsible for the influx of peritoneal macrophages to occur in women with endometriosis (Montagna *et al.*, 2008; Richter *et al.*, 2005). A study was conducted to see the therapeutic effect on blocking this cytokine with recombinant human TNF binding protein-1 (TBP-1) in a baboon model (D'Hooghe *et al.*, 2005). The result demonstrated the inhibition in the baboon, suggesting the effective in treating the manifestations of endometriosis. However, there is currently no clinical study to determine the effect in human.

1.1.4.4 Proteases

Matrix metalloproteinases (MMPs) are a family of endopeptidases that play a role in the degradation and turnover of extracellular matrix proteins. Increased MMP activity has been described in endometriosis (Chung *et al.*, 2002; Gottschalk *et al.*, 2000). There function is believed to be integral in the ability of endometrium to invade tissue and implant successfully. Inhibition of these enzymes might be effective in inhibiting the development of endometriosis. Yet, there is no in-depth study being reported thus raising uncertainty on the value and practicality of this approach.

1.1.4.5 Traditional Chinese medicines

As surgical and hormonal treatment of endometriosis have unpleasant side effects and high rates of relapse, many patients began to explore more natural and traditional remedies. In China, treatment of endometriosis using Chinese herbal medicine is routine to alleviate pain, promote fertility, and prevent relapse. Study showed post-surgical administration of Chinese herbal medicine may have comparable benefits to western medicines but with fewer side effects (Flower *et al.*, 2009). In this study, it showed oral intake of traditional Chinese medicine have a better overall treatment effect than Danazol. Also, it is more effective in relieving dysmenorrheal and shrinking adnexal masses. Likewise, acupuncture is a new techniques employed to relieve the infertility associated with endometriosis in women (Mo *et al.*, 1993). However, due to the limited amount intervention studies reported, more rigorous researches are required to accurately assess the type, dose and potential role of Chinese herbal medicine in treating endometriosis.

2. Anti-angiogenesis therapy

2.1 Properties of anti-angiogenesis therapy

Angiogenesis is the physiological process involving the growth of new blood vessels from pre-existing vessels. It is a sequence of events that is fundamental to a broad array of physiological processes occurring in our body, including embryogenesis, development, the menstrual cycle and wound healing. Yet, it is also linked to many pathological situations such as cancer, chronic inflammation, ischemic diseases and endometriosis development (Griffioen *et al.*, 2000). In general, the turnover of capillary endothelial cells is extremely slow in physiological angiogenesis. However, in the normal endometrium and in tumors, the turnover rate is altered to a more rapid state in promoting angiogenesis. Angiogenesis involve activation of angiogenic factors, dissolution of basement membranes by proteases derived from vascular endothelial cells, migration and proliferation of the endothelial cells, and capillary tube formation. And various angiogenic factors are needed to regulate each step (Table 2).

Under normal physiological conditions, angiogenesis is well controlled by the local balance between endogenous angiogenesis stimulators and angiogenesis inhibitors, although the regulatory mechanism is still not clear. During wound healing, the expression of vascular endothelial growth factor (VEGF), one of the most potent angiogenic stimulators, is significantly upregulated to promote wound healing by restoring blood flow to the injured tissues. As wound healing resolves, the expression of VEGF is downregulated and most angiogenic capillaries regress, resulting in a residual normal vascularity (Tonnesen *et al.*, 2000). Other studies indicates that a number of endogenous angiogenic inhibitors are present in the normal retina to balance the stimulatory effect of VEGF in the regulation of angiogenesis and vascular permeability (Ma *et al.*, 2005). These studies suggest that endogenous angiogenic inhibitors can be used to balance the effect of angiogenic stimulators. Anti-angiogenic therapies have already been experimentally proven to be effective in preventing metastasis and shrinking the established experimental tumors to be formed (Camp-Sorrell, 2003). Angiogenesis therapeutic approaches can be divided into two major classes: (1) interference with the process of neovascularization and (2) directly destroying immature blood vessels.

Interleukin-1
Interleukin-6
Interleukin-8
Epidermal growth factor
Basic fibroblast growth factors
Insulin-like growth factors
Platelet-derived growth factor
Platelet-derived endothelial cell growth factor
Vascular endothelial growth factor
Endometriosis protein-I
Ovarian steroids
Estradiol
Angiogenin
Proliferin
Pleiotropin
Tumor necrosis factor-α
Hepatocyte growth factor
Transforming growth factor -α and -β
Placenta growth factor

Table 2. Angiogenic factors in endometriosis

Although they may not necessarily directly kill tumor cells, angiogenesis inhibitors significantly enhance the efficacy of standard chemotherapy and radiation therapy by inhibiting tumor growth and tumor metastasis. Therefore, this type of therapy may need to be administered over a long period of time. In the normal healthy body, the process of angiogenesis is dormant and the angiogenesis switch is kept "off" with inhibitors being dominant over stimulators. Since anti-angiogenesis therapy is a targeted therapy aimed specifically at the angiogenic stimulators and the angiogenic microvascular endothelial cells, anti-angiogenesis therapy usually produces only mild side effects and is less toxic to most healthy cells. But as physiological angiogenesis is important in wound healing and reproduction, bleeding, blood clotting, heart function, the immune system, and the reproductive system, the unknown consequences on long-term treatment with anti-angiogenic agents would still be a great concern (Board *et al.*, 2006; Cabebe *et al.*, 2007).

2.2 Anti-angiogenesis potentials for endometriosis

To date, endometriosis is often treated by hormonal medication, which aims at achieving a hypoestrogenic state. However, hormonal therapy would only suppress the symptoms associated with endometriosis, but not eradicating the ectopic implant. Moreover, significant side effects hinder the continuation of treatment (Saltiel *et al.*, 1991). Long-term hormonal therapy, therefore, is not an attractive option. Alternatively, endometriosis can also be treated surgically. Conservative surgery consists of ablation of endometriosis lesions, resulting in pain relief, but high symptoms recurrence has been reported in a majority of patients (Vercellini *et al.*, 2009). While definitive surgery includes removal of uterus, with or without ovaries, giving more permanent symptom relief, this therapy would result in the end of reproductive life. Therefore, an effective therapeutic agent for endometriosis would be a compound that not only prevents the development of endometriosis lesions, but would also be effective against the growth of established lesions. In cancer, endothelial cells have been shown to play a pivotal role in tumor cell survival and growth. In analogy with tumor growth, endometriosis is shown to be highly dependent on angiogenesis, which makes the achievements in the field of cancer research applicable to endometriosis.

Most of the studies on the role of angiogenesis in endometriosis have been performed in animal models so far. Still, more experiments are urgently needed to distinguish the effect of angiogenesis inhibitors on physiological and pathological angiogenesis. Like in a recently published study, the effect of angiogenesis inhibition was studied in nude mice. VEGF-A inhibitors were administered immediately after implantation of cultured human endometrium fragments (Hull *et al.*, 2003). The results showed impaired lesion formation, which concluded that angiostatic agents may be effective in the treatment of endometriosis. And recently, encouraging results have been achieved with the use of Avastin, a humanized anti-VEGF antibody, on cancer. This approach of neutralizing VEGF provided the first proof of concept that anti-angiogenesis is applicable in humans (Ferrara, 2002; McCarthy, 2003). Yet, it still needs clinical trial to make a more concrete result on the anti-angiogenesis effect. With prior to clinical testing to commence, the optimal mode of delivery and the best indication of anti-angiogenic therapy would still need to be determined. However, the encouraging results of some anti-angiogenic drugs and the pressing need for new therapeutic approaches make angiogenesis an attractive novel target for the treatment of patients with endometriosis.

2.3 Limitations

The limitation of anti-angiogenesis therapy is that the patient's immune system may be compromised (Calabrese *et al.*, 2000). This would make the patient more susceptible to infection and delay wounds healing. In addition, patients may experience reproductive problems and damage to the fetus, if the patient was pregnant while taking the anti-angiogenic drug. Other research has reported such therapy can enhance heart problems, elevating blood pressure and bleeding or blood clots could increase. Since angiogenesis inhibitor therapy is still under investigation, the definite possible complications and side effects are still unknown.

3. Green tea and its clinical values

3.1 Properties of green tea

Tea (*Camellia sinensis*) is an aromatic beverage prepared from boiling or simmering of cured leaves. Apart from water, tea is one of the most popular consumed beverages worldwide, with a consumption of 120mL/day/capita (Graham, 1992). Of the different varieties of tea, the most commonly found on the market are white, green, oolong and black tea. And over the last few decades, green tea has been subjected to many scientific and medical studies on its potential health beneficial effects (Table 3).

Anti-aging
Anti-bacterial
Anti-inflammatory
Anti-angiogenic
Anti-cancer
Lowering blood fat
Prevent tooth decay and clear bad breath
Enhanced skin whitening

Table 3. Benefits of green tea

Green tea contains polyphenols, particularly catechins, accounting for 30-40% of the dry weight (Balentine *et al.*, 1997; Graham, 1992). The main components of green tea consist of catechins, minor flavanols and polymeric flavonoids (de Mejia *et al.*, 2009). It contains more catechin concentrations than black tea or oolong tea, due to the minimal oxidation during processing. The compositions of green tea catechins are mainly comprised of (-)-epicathecin (EC), (-)-epigallocatechin (EGC), (-)-epigallocatechin gallate (EGCG), (-)-epicathecin gallatis (ECG), (-)-gallocatechin gallate (GCG), (-)-catechin gallate (CG) and (+)-cathecin (CT) (Miura *et al.*, 1994) (Fig. 2). Among the components of green tea, (-)-epigallocatechin gallate (EGCG) is the most abundant and the most extensively studied catechin, accounting to 50-80% of the total catechins in green tea (Yang *et al.*, 2002).

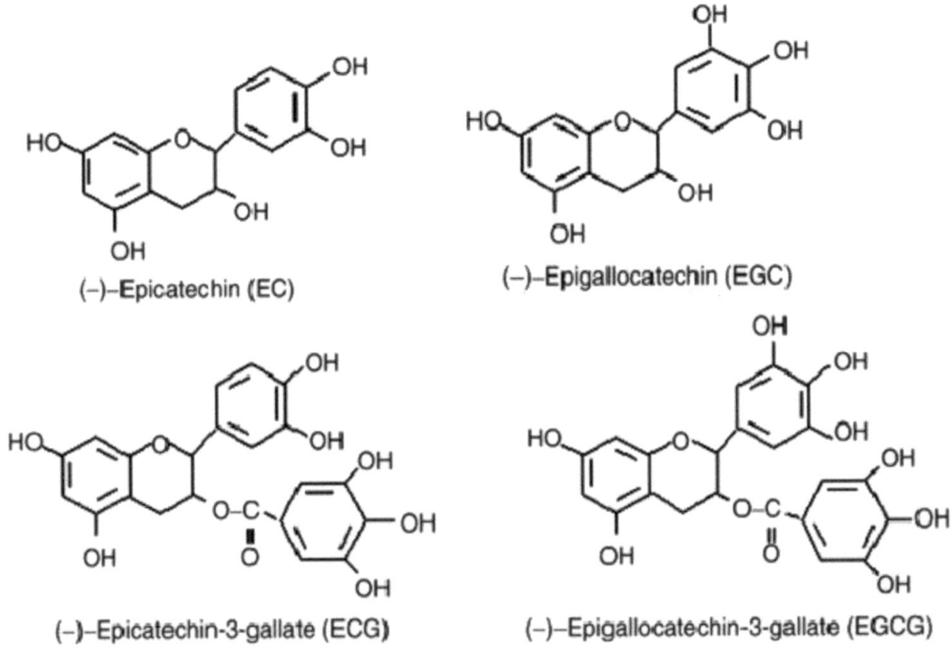

Fig. 2. The main catechins components found in green tea

3.2 Biological activities

3.2.1 Anti-oxidant activity

Free-radical damage has been postulated to contribute to the etiology of aging, and many chronic health problems such as cardiovascular, inflammatory diseases, and cancer (Rice-Evans *et al.*, 1993; Spiteller, 2001). The productions of free radicals, including reactive oxygen species (ROS), are capable of chemically altering many natural bio-molecules in our body, resulting in changes in their structure and function, leading to aging and the development of chronic diseases (McCall *et al.*, 1999).

Like most polyphenols, catechins and procyandins have an anti-oxidant activity. In a study conducted by Guo *et al*, ECG and EGCG displayed better antioxidant activity than EC and EGC on lipid peroxidation (Guo *et al.*, 1996). Also, green tea catechins have been shown to protect or regenerate α-tocopherol in human low-density lipo-protein (LDL), which functions as a major antioxidant in human LDL (Zhu *et al.*, 1999). Similarly, EGCG and EGC show potent inhibitory effects on LDL oxidation *in vitro*, with EC and ECG being even more effective on protective activity on the depletion of α-tocopherol in LDL. And a clinical study claimed the consumption of 300 mg of green tea polyphenol extract twice daily for 1week can delayed the oxidation of human LDL *ex vivo* (Miura *et al.*, 2000).

3.2.2 Anti-mitotic

Proliferation and migration of endothelial cells are major events in the angiogenic process for the formation of endometriosis. Matrix metalloproteinase-2 is expressed abundantly in lesions and has been suggested to play a key role in the degradation of the basement membrane, thereby promoting migration of endothelial cells (Zempo *et al.*, 1994). Green tea polyphenols can significantly reduced endothelial cells proliferation in a dose-dependent manner and caused the accumulation of cells in the G_1 phase without affecting cell viability (Kojima-Yuasa *et al.*, 2003). In addition, EGCG suppressed endothelial cells proliferation and migration by inducing apoptosis through mitochondrial depolarization, activation of caspase-3 and reduction of binding of VEGF to its receptors in human ECs (Kondo *et al.*, 2002; Yoo *et al.*, 2002).

3.2.3 Anti-inflammatory

Cytokines are a group of multifunctional proteins that mediate the regulation of inflammatory responses. These cytokines are expressed in a number of tissues, including macrophages, vascular endothelial cells, adipose tissue and neurons. In general, the role of cytokines can be further classified depending on the way they influence inflammation, such as pro- or anti-inflammatory (Kundu *et al.*, 2008). Factors such as tumor necrosis factor-α, IL-6, IL-1, GM-CSF, interferon-c, and IL-12 played a major role on the induction of the inflammatory response.

EGCG has been shown to possess anti-inflammatory properties *in vivo* and *in vitro* (Hamer *et al.*, 2007). The potent effects of tea polyphenols toward inflammation have also been known to cancer prevention (Beltz *et al.*, 2006). Tea polyphenols appear to modulate at different targets the anti-inflammatory activities related to arachidonic acid-dependent pathways, such as cyclooxygenase (COX) inhibition. Within the arachidonic acid-independent pathways, nitric-oxide synthase (NOS) and nuclear factor kappa-light-chain-enhancer of activated B cells (NF-κB) are targets of polyphenols (Miles *et al.*, 2005). The released phytochemicals inhibit cyclooxygenase-2 (COX-2) and inducible nitric-oxide synthase (iNOS) expression by blocking NF-κB activation. Particularly EGCG suppresses activation of NF-κB by repression of degradation of inhibitory unit, IκBκ, which hampers subsequent nuclear translocation of the functionally active subunit of NF-κB (Kundu *et al.*, 2008).

3.2.4 Anti-angiogenic

It has been widely shown that green tea have the ability to inhibit angiogenesis in *in vitro* proliferation studies (Laschke *et al.*, 2008; Park *et al.*, 2006; Slivova *et al.*, 2005) and in *in vivo* angiogenesis assays (Laschke *et al.*, 2008; Xu *et al.*, 2009). Anti-angiogenesis plays a crucial role accounting to the cancer-preventive effect made by green tea. As angiogenesis is a complex multi-step process that includes the proliferation, migration and differentiation of endothelial cells into tube-like structures. The initiation of each step involves multiple growth factors, proteases and adhesion molecule secreted by the endothelial cells, as well as supporting cells from the surrounding (Carmeliet *et al.*, 2000). Pathogenesis related to abnormal angiogenesis can be demonstrated in rheumatoid arthritis, diabetic retinopathy, and cancer growth and metastasis. Therefore, angiogenesis would be a crucial process that may account for part of the mechanisms of the cancer preventive effect of green tea. Studies have shown green tea's potential to decrease vital angiogenic factors in breast cancer (Sartippour *et al.*, 2002; Sartippour *et al.*, 2002). Similarly, other showed the mark decrease of IL-8 production by endothelial cells (Tang *et al.*, 2001). Likewise, tumor necrosis factor-α and matrix metalloprotinases were suppressed by the incorporation of EGCG (Annabi *et al.*, 2002; Yang *et al.*, 1998). The observation on the effect of green tea being anti-angiogenic is clinically very significant (Kabbinavar *et al.*, 2003). With the lack of information on clinical trials, work is still needed on promoting green tea as a possible medication on anti-angiogenesis therapy.

3.3 Side effects of green tea

The preliminary efficacy results of a phase I–II clinical study from a cohort of non-cancer patients demonstrated no uncomfortable side effects (Choan *et al.*, 2005). To date, the only side effect reported from drinking green tea is to cause insomnia, increase heart rate and nausea in selected individual, due to the presence of caffeine. An average cup of tea (10 g of tea leaves in 1 L water) contains around 300 mg of crude solids with 30–42% catechins and 3–6% caffeine (Khan *et al.*, 2007). However, the amount of caffeine is three times less than that of drinking coffee. Thus, this makes drinking green tea a prospective and very safe treatment for clinical use.

4. Green tea for endometriosis

As already proven, the catechins, notably EGCG, found in green tea are potential candidates to inhibit the growth of tumors (Jung *et al.*, 2001; Nakachi *et al.*, 1998; Uesato *et al.*, 2001). They act as a pleiotropic substance, which influencing multiple mechanisms that are involved in carcinogenesis (Beltz *et al.*, 2006; Khan *et al.*, 2006) through suppressing angiogenesis (Kondo *et al.*, 2002; Zhu *et al.*, 2007). With these basic finding, recent direction pointed out that the anti-angiogenic and anti-oxidation properties of ECGC may be a promising therapeutic agent in treating endometriosis.

So far, there are two major groups studying the use of EGCG to relate with the inhibition of endometriosis (Laschke *et al.*, 2008; Xu *et al.*, 2009). In the study conducted by Laschke *et al.*, the study showed that EGCG suppresses E2-stimulated activation, proliferation and VEGF expression of endometrial cells *in vitro*. While in the *in vivo* study using dorsal skinfold chamber model, EGCG selectively inhibited angiogenesis and blood perfusion of endometriotic lesions. Similarly, histology of the endometriotic lesion revealed induced regression when EGCG was prescribed. The author proposed the possible mechanism on the inhibition on the growth of the lesion may be due to attenuation of VEGF expression by EGCG in cultured endothelial cells, with the stimulation with estrogen. This indicates that EGCG specifically blocks the E2-induced activation in endometrial cells, which EGCG would compete with E2 for binding to estrogen receptors. In addition, the study found that EGCG treatment may not only induce regression of endometriotic lesions, but may also have a positive anti-angiogenic effect on the eutopic endometrium of endometriosis patients. This was shown by the decrease in VEGF expression in the eutopic endometrium.

Likewise, the possible toxicity by EGCG toward the reproductive organs was also investigated. The treatment marked by EGCG showed no adverse effect neither on angiogenesis and blood perfusion nor tissue integrity of ovarian follicles.

In another study conducted by our team, we demonstrated the anti-angiogenic effects of green tea catechin on a mouse model induced with endometriosis (Xu *et al.*, 2009). These immunosuppressent mice were induced with endometriosis by subcutaneously implanting human endometrial tissues from patients with endometriosis. Following the day of operation, endometriosis induced mice were treated daily with saline, Vitamin E or EGCG for two weeks. The result showed those treated with EGCG, but not Vitamin E, have the smallest size of lesion growth. Angiogenesis in lesions from the implant and adjacent tissues was under-developed, and microvessel size and density were lower. With regards to the lower expression of VEGF expression, EGCG significantly inhibits the development of experimental endometriosis can be through anti-angiogenic effects. Following on this study, we investigate the likely mechanism would involve the selective inhibition of angiogenic factors, mainly VEGF-C/VEGFR2 pathway by EGCG to suppress the growth of the endometriotic lesions (Xu *et al.*, 2011) (Fig 3). With these studies, the potential of green tea as an anti-angiogenic agent is high because of its low cost, wide availability, and apparent low toxicity.

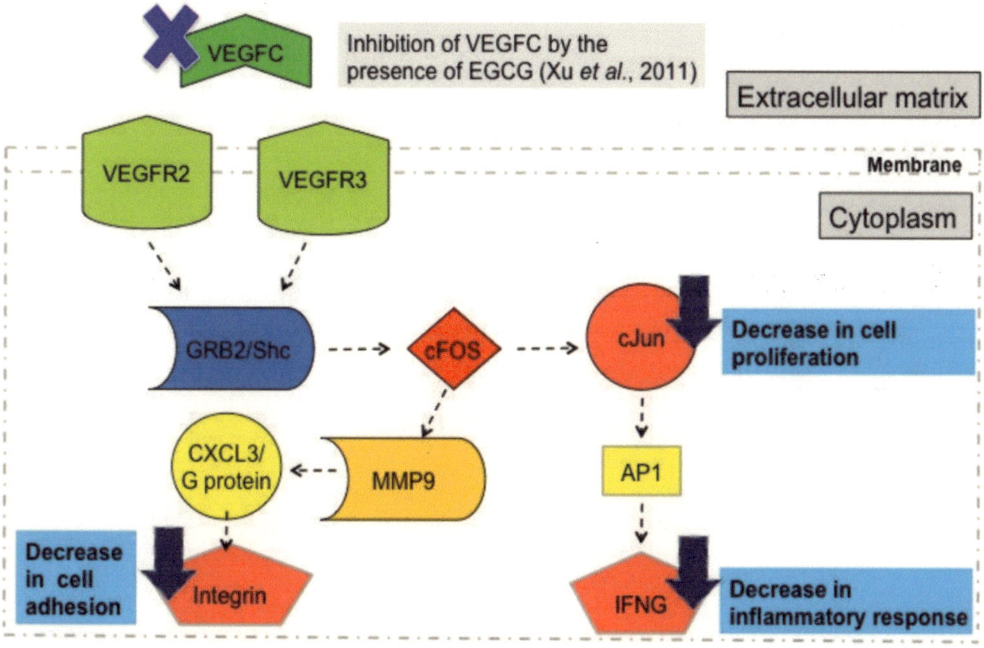

Fig. 3. Summary of the mechanism of green tea for endometriosis

5. Conclusion

Endometriosis is one of the most common benign gynaecological conditions. It affects an estimated 176 million worldwide regardless to their ethnics and social background. And it is estimated that 30-40% of women with endometriosis may not be able to have children. However, there is currently no single etiology that can explain the pathogenesis and pleomorphic manifestations of endometriosis.

Current treatments for endometriosis remain unsatisfactory, owing to their focus on treating the symptoms rather than curing the disease. In addition, each treatment proved to have many side effects (Rice, 2002). Hence, there is a need to derive a new therapy to provide a more efficient and specific therapeutic alternatives to eliminate the lesions, while preventing reoccurrence and retaining fertility.

To provide additional evidence to support the role of green tea in suppressing endometriosis, it would be an important future research goal. Several study areas should be emphasized. These areas include a more detailed molecular and cellular mechanism studies in animals and humans to verify the effects of green tea in humans, compared with those studied in animals. Next, the interactions between the green tea polyphenols and endometriosis have not been extensively investigated. This drawback can cause many important details being vague. Furthermore, the potential interactions of active compounds in green tea with other dietary active components and the roles of polymorphisms on the protective effects of tea need to be examined in future studies. Ultimately, clinical intervention trials should be conducted to verify the mechanisms of action of tea observed in animal studies in which tea does not show any unwanted side effect.

6. Acknowledgment

Hong Kong Obstetrical and Gynaecological Trust Fund 2010

7. References

Abbott, J, Hawe, J, Hunter, D, Holmes, M, Finn, P & Garry, R (2004). Laparoscopic excision of endometriosis: a randomized, placebo-controlled trial, *Fertil Steril* 82(4): 878-84.

Annabi, B, Lachambre, MP, Bousquet-Gagnon, N, Page, M, Gingras, D & Beliveau, R (2002). Green tea polyphenol (-)-epigallocatechin 3-gallate inhibits MMP-2 secretion and MT1-MMP-driven migration in glioblastoma cells, *Biochim Biophys Acta* 1542(1-3): 209-20.

Arumugam, K & Dip, YC (1995). Endometriosis and infertility: the role of exogenous lipid peroxides in the peritoneal fluid, *Fertil Steril* 63(1): 198-9.

Balentine, DA, Wiseman, SA & Bouwens, LC (1997). The chemistry of tea flavonoids, *Crit Rev Food Sci Nutr* 37(8): 693-704.

Bedaiwy, MA, Abdel-Aleem, MA, Miketa, A & Falcone, T (2009). Endometriosis: a critical appraisal of the advances and the controversies of a challenging health problem, *Minerva Ginecol* 61(4): 285-98.

Beltz, LA, Bayer, DK, Moss, AL & Simet, IM (2006). Mechanisms of cancer prevention by green and black tea polyphenols, *Anticancer Agents Med Chem* 6(5): 389-406.

Biberoglu, KO & Behrman, SJ (1981). Dosage aspects of danazol therapy in endometriosis: short-term and long-term effectiveness, *Am J Obstet Gynecol* 139(6): 645-54.

Board, RE, Thatcher, N & Lorigan, P (2006). Novel therapies for the treatment of small-cell lung cancer: a time for cautious optimism?, *Drugs* 66(15): 1919-31.

Brosens, I, Koninckx, P & Boeckx, W (1981). Endometriosis, *Clin Obstet Gynaecol* 8(3): 639-51.

Cabebe, E & Wakelee, H (2007). Role of anti-angiogenesis agents in treating NSCLC: focus on bevacizumab and VEGFR tyrosine kinase inhibitors, *Curr Treat Options Oncol* 8(1): 15-27.

Calabrese, L & Fleischer, AB (2000). Thalidomide: current and potential clinical applications, *Am J Med* 108(6): 487-95.

Camanni, M, Delpiano, EM, Bonino, L & Deltetto, F Laparoscopic conservative management of ureteral endometriosis, *Curr Opin Obstet Gynecol* 22(4): 309-14.

Camp-Sorrell, D (2003). Antiangiogenesis: the fifth cancer treatment modality?, *Oncol Nurs Forum* 30(6): 934-44.

Carmeliet, P & Jain, RK (2000). Angiogenesis in cancer and other diseases, *Nature* 407(6801): 249-57.

Choan, E, Segal, R, Jonker, D, Malone, S, Reaume, N, Eapen, L & Gallant, V (2005). A prospective clinical trial of green tea for hormone refractory prostate cancer: an evaluation of the complementary/alternative therapy approach, *Urol Oncol* 23(2): 108-13.

Chung, HW, Lee, JY, Moon, HS, Hur, SE, Park, MH, Wen, Y & Polan, ML (2002). Matrix metalloproteinase-2, membranous type 1 matrix metalloproteinase, and tissue inhibitor of metalloproteinase-2 expression in ectopic and eutopic endometrium, *Fertil Steril* 78(4): 787-95.

Coutinho, EM (1982). Treatment of endometriosis with gestrinone (R-2323), a synthetic antiestrogen, antiprogesterone, *Am J Obstet Gynecol* 144(8): 895-8.

Cramer, DW & Missmer, SA (2002). The epidemiology of endometriosis, *Ann N Y Acad Sci* 955: 11-22; discussion 34-6, 396-406.

Creus, M, Fabregues, F, Carmona, F, del Pino, M, Manau, D & Balasch, J (2008). Combined laparoscopic surgery and pentoxifylline therapy for treatment of endometriosis-associated infertility: a preliminary trial, *Hum Reprod* 23(8): 1910-6.

D'Hooghe, TM, Nugent, NP, Cuneo, S, Chai, DC, Deer, F, Debrock, S, Kyama, CM, Mihalyi, A & Mwenda, JM (2005). Recombinant human TNF binding protein-1 (r-hTBP-1) inhibits the development of endometriosis in baboons; a prospective, randomized, placebo and drug controlled study., *Biol Reprod* 74(131-6).

Dabrosin, C, Gyorffy, S, Margetts, P, Ross, C & Gauldie, J (2002). Therapeutic effect of angiostatin gene transfer in a murine model of endometriosis, *Am J Pathol* 161(3): 909-18.

Davis, CJ & McMillan, L (2003). Pain in endometriosis: effectiveness of medical and surgical management, *Curr Opin Obstet Gynecol* 15(6): 507-12.

de Mejia, EG, Ramirez-Mares, MV & Puangpraphant, S (2009). Bioactive components of tea: cancer, inflammation and behavior, *Brain Behav Immun* 23(6): 721-31.

Donnez, J, Van Langendonckt, A, Casanas-Roux, F, Van Gossum, JP, Pirard, C, Jadoul, P, Squifflet, J & Smets, M (2002). Current thinking on the pathogenesis of endometriosis, *Gynecol Obstet Invest* 54 Suppl 1: 52-8; discussion 59-62.

Ferrara, N (2002). VEGF and the quest for tumour angiogenesis factors, *Nat Rev Cancer* 2(10): 795-803.

Flower, A, Liu, JP, Chen, S, Lewith, G & Little, P (2009). Chinese herbal medicine for endometriosis, *Cochrane Database Syst Rev* (3): CD006568.

Galle, PC (1989). Clinical presentation and diagnosis of endometriosis, *Obstet Gynecol Clin North Am* 16(1): 29-42.

Gottschalk, C, Malberg, K, Arndt, M, Schmitt, J, Roessner, A, Schultze, D, Kleinstein, J & Ansorge, S (2000). Matrix metalloproteinases and TACE play a role in the pathogenesis of endometriosis, *Adv Exp Med Biol* 477: 483-6.

Graham, HN (1992). Green tea composition, consumption, and polyphenol chemistry, *Prev Med* 21(3): 334-50.

Griffioen, AW & Molema, G (2000). Angiogenesis: potentials for pharmacologic intervention in the treatment of cancer, cardiovascular diseases, and chronic inflammation, *Pharmacol Rev* 52(2): 237-68.

Guo, Q, Zhao, B, Li, M, Shen, S & Xin, W (1996). Studies on protective mechanisms of four components of green tea polyphenols against lipid peroxidation in synaptosomes, *Biochim Biophys Acta* 1304(3): 210-22.

Gurdol, F, Oner-Yyidothan, Y, Yalcyn, O, Genc, S & Buyru, F (1997). Changes in enzymatic antioxidant defense system in blood and endometrial tissues of women after menopause, *Res Commun Mol Pathol Pharmacol* 97(1): 38-46.

Halme, J, Becker, S, Hammond, MG, Raj, MH & Raj, S (1983). Increased activation of pelvic macrophages in infertile women with mild endometriosis, *Am J Obstet Gynecol* 145(3): 333-7.

Hamer, M & Steptoe, A (2007). Association between physical fitness, parasympathetic control, and proinflammatory responses to mental stress, *Psychosom Med* 69(7): 660-6.

Hansen, KA & Eyster, KM (2006). A review of current management of endometriosis in 2006: an evidence-based approach, *S D Med* 59(4): 153-9.

Ho, HN, Wu, MY, Chen, SU, Chao, KH, Chen, CD & Yang, YS (1997). Total antioxidant status and nitric oxide do not increase in peritoneal fluids from women with endometriosis, *Hum Reprod* 12(12): 2810-5.

Hull, ML, Charnock-Jones, DS, Chan, CL, Bruner-Tran, KL, Osteen, KG, Tom, BD, Fan, TP & Smith, SK (2003). Antiangiogenic agents are effective inhibitors of endometriosis, *J Clin Endocrinol Metab* 88(6): 2889-99.

Jung, YD & Ellis, LM (2001). Inhibition of tumour invasion and angiogenesis by epigallocatechin gallate (EGCG), a major component of green tea, *Int J Exp Pathol* 82(6): 309-16.

Kabbinavar, F, Hurwitz, HI, Fehrenbacher, L, Meropol, NJ, Novotny, WF, Lieberman, G, Griffing, S & Bergsland, E (2003). Phase II, randomized trial comparing bevacizumab plus fluorouracil (FU)/leucovorin (LV) with FU/LV alone in patients with metastatic colorectal cancer, *J Clin Oncol* 21(1): 60-5.

Kavtaradze, ND, Dominguez, CE, Rock, JA & Parthasarathy, S (2003). Vitamin E and C supplementation reduces endometriosis related pelvic pain, *Fertil Steril* 80: S221-222.

Kennedy, S (2004). *The Patient's Essential Guide to Endometriosis.*, Alden Press.

Kennedy, S, Bergqvist, A, Chapron, C, D'Hooghe, T, Dunselman, G, Greb, R, Hummelshoj, L, Prentice, A & Saridogan, E (2005). ESHRE guideline for the diagnosis and treatment of endometriosis, *Hum Reprod* 20(10): 2698-704.

Khan, N, Afaq, F, Saleem, M, Ahmad, N & Mukhtar, H (2006). Targeting multiple signaling pathways by green tea polyphenol (-)-epigallocatechin-3-gallate, *Cancer Res* 66(5): 2500-5.

Khan, N & Mukhtar, H (2007). Tea polyphenols for health promotion, *Life Sci* 81(7): 519-33.

Khoury, MJ, Adams, MM, Rhodes, P & Erickson, JD (1987). Monitoring for multiple malformations in the detection of epidemics of birth defects, *Teratology* 36(3): 345-53.

Kistner, RW (1959). Conservative management of endometriosis, *J Lancet* 79(5): 179-83.

Kojima-Yuasa, A, Hua, JJ, Kennedy, DO & Matsui-Yuasa, I (2003). Green tea extract inhibits angiogenesis of human umbilical vein endothelial cells through reduction of expression of VEGF receptors, *Life Sci* 73(10): 1299-313.

Koks, CA, Groothuis, PG, Dunselman, GA, de Goeij, AF & Evers, JL (1999). Adhesion of shed menstrual tissue in an in-vitro model using amnion and peritoneum: a light and electron microscopic study, *Hum Reprod* 14(3): 816-22.

Kondo, T, Ohta, T, Igura, K, Hara, Y & Kaji, K (2002). Tea catechins inhibit angiogenesis in vitro, measured by human endothelial cell growth, migration and tube formation, through inhibition of VEGF receptor binding, *Cancer Lett* 180(2): 139-44.

Kundu, JK & Surh, YJ (2008). Inflammation: gearing the journey to cancer, *Mutat Res* 659(1-2): 15-30.

Laschke, MW, Schwender, C, Scheuer, C, Vollmar, B & Menger, MD (2008). Epigallocatechin-3-gallate inhibits estrogen-induced activation of endometrial cells in vitro and causes regression of endometriotic lesions in vivo, *Hum Reprod* 23(10): 2308-18.

Ma, JX, Zhang, SX & Wang, JJ (2005). Down-regulation of angiogenic inhibitors: a potential pathogenic mechanism for diabetic complications, *Curr Diabetes Rev* 1(2): 183-96.

Maas, JW, Groothuis, PG, Dunselman, GA, de Goeij, AF, Struijker-Boudier, HA & Evers, JL (2001). Development of endometriosis-like lesions after transplantation of human endometrial fragments onto the chick embryo chorioallantoic membrane, *Hum Reprod* 16(4): 627-31.

Mahutte, NG & Arici, A (2003). Medical management of endometriosis-associated pain, *Obstet Gynecol Clin North Am* 30(1): 133-50.

McCall, MR & Frei, B (1999). Can antioxidant vitamins materially reduce oxidative damage in humans?, *Free Radic Biol Med* 26(7-8): 1034-53.

McCarthy, M (2003). Antiangiogenesis drug promising for metastatic colorectal cancer, *Lancet* 361(9373): 1959.

Miles, EA, Zoubouli, P & Calder, PC (2005). Effects of polyphenols on human Th1 and Th2 cytokine production, *Clin Nutr* 24(5): 780-4.

Milingos, S, Protopapas, A, Kallipolitis, G, Drakakis, P, Loutradis, D, Liapi, A & Antsaklis, A (2006). Endometriosis in patients with chronic pelvic pain: is staging predictive of the efficacy of laparoscopic surgery in pain relief?, *Gynecol Obstet Invest* 62(1): 48-54.

Miura, S, Watanabe, J, Tomita, T, Sano, M & Tomita, I (1994). The inhibitory effects of tea polyphenols (flavan-3-ol derivatives) on Cu2+ mediated oxidative modification of low density lipoprotein, *Biol Pharm Bull* 17(12): 1567-72.

Miura, Y, Chiba, T, Miura, S, Tomita, I, Umegaki, K, Ikeda, M & Tomita, T (2000). Green tea polyphenols (flavan 3-ols) prevent oxidative modification of low density lipoproteins: an ex vivo study in humans, *J Nutr Biochem* 11(4): 216-22.

Mo, X, Li, D, Pu, Y, Xi, G, Le, X & Fu, Z (1993). Clinical studies on the mechanism for acupuncture stimulation of ovulation, *J Tradit Chin Med* 13(2): 115-9.

Montagna, P, Capellino, S, Villaggio, B, Remorgida, V, Ragni, N, Cutolo, M & Ferrero, S (2008). Peritoneal fluid macrophages in endometriosis: correlation between the expression of estrogen receptors and inflammation, *Fertil Steril* 90(1): 156-64.

Murphy, AA, Palinski, W, Rankin, S, Morales, AJ & Parthasarathy, S (1998). Evidence for oxidatively modified lipid-protein complexes in endometrium and endometriosis, *Fertil Steril* 69(6): 1092-4.

Murphy, AA, Palinski, W, Rankin, S, Morales, AJ & Parthasarathy, S (1998). Macrophage scavenger receptor(s) and oxidatively modified proteins in endometriosis, *Fertil Steril* 69(6): 1085-91.

Murphy, AA, Santanam, N, Morales, AJ & Parthasarathy, S (1998). Lysophosphatidyl choline, a chemotactic factor for monocytes/T-lymphocytes is elevated in endometriosis, *J Clin Endocrinol Metab* 83(6): 2110-3.

Nakachi, K, Suemasu, K, Suga, K, Takeo, T, Imai, K & Higashi, Y (1998). Influence of drinking green tea on breast cancer malignancy among Japanese patients, *Jpn J Cancer Res* 89(3): 254-61.

Namnoum, AB, Hickman, TN, Goodman, SB, Gehlbach, DL & Rock, JA (1995). Incidence of symptom recurrence after hysterectomy for endometriosis, *Fertil Steril* 64(5): 898-902.

Nap, AW, Griffioen, AW, Dunselman, GA, Bouma-Ter Steege, JC, Thijssen, VL, Evers, JL & Groothuis, PG (2004). Antiangiogenesis therapy for endometriosis, *J Clin Endocrinol Metab* 89(3): 1089-95.

Nisolle, M, Casanas-Roux, F, Anaf, V, Mine, JM & Donnez, J (1993). Morphometric study of the stromal vascularization in peritoneal endometriosis, *Fertil Steril* 59(3): 681-4.

Olive, DL & Pritts, EA (2001). Treatment of endometriosis, *N Engl J Med* 345(4): 266-75.

Park, JS, Kim, MH, Chang, HJ, Kim, KM, Kim, SM, Shin, BA, Ahn, BW & Jung, YD (2006). Epigallocatechin-3-gallate inhibits the PDGF-induced VEGF expression in human vascular smooth muscle cells via blocking PDGF receptor and Erk-1/2, *Int J Oncol* 29(5): 1247-52.

Pierce, SJ, Gazvani, MR & Farquharson, RG (2000). Long-term use of gonadotropin-releasing hormone analogs and hormone replacement therapy in the management of endometriosis: a randomized trial with a 6-year follow-up, *Fertil Steril* 74(5): 964-8.

Rice-Evans, CA & Diplock, AT (1993). Current status of antioxidant therapy, *Free Radic Biol Med* 15(1): 77-96.

Rice, VM (2002). Conventional medical therapies for endometriosis, *Ann N Y Acad Sci* 955: 343-52; discussion 389-93, 396-406.

Richter, ON, Dorn, C, Rosing, B, Flaskamp, C & Ulrich, U (2005). Tumor necrosis factor alpha secretion by peritoneal macrophages in patients with endometriosis, *Arch Gynecol Obstet* 271(2): 143-7.

Saltiel, E & Garabedian-Ruffalo, SM (1991). Pharmacologic management of endometriosis, *Clin Pharm* 10(7): 518-31.

Sampson, JA (1927). Metastatic or Embolic Endometriosis, due to the Menstrual Dissemination of Endometrial Tissue into the Venous Circulation, *Am J Pathol* 3(2): 93-110 43.

Santanam, NK, Kavtaradze, N, Dominguez, C, Rock, JA, Parthasarathy, S & Murphy, AA (2003). Antioxidant supplementation reduces total chemokines and inflammatory cytokines in women with endometriosis., *Fertil Steril* 80: S32-33.

Sartippour, MR, Heber, D, Zhang, L, Beatty, P, Elashoff, D, Elashoff, R, Go, VL & Brooks, MN (2002). Inhibition of fibroblast growth factors by green tea, *Int J Oncol* 21(3): 487-91.

Sartippour, MR, Shao, ZM, Heber, D, Beatty, P, Zhang, L, Liu, C, Ellis, L, Liu, W, Go, VL & Brooks, MN (2002). Green tea inhibits vascular endothelial growth factor (VEGF) induction in human breast cancer cells, *J Nutr* 132(8): 2307-11.

Scarpellini, F, Sbracia, M, Lecchini, S & Scarpellini, L (2002). Anti-angiogenesis treatment with thalidomide in endometriosis: a pilot study., *Fertil Steril* 78: S87.

Schweppe, KW (2001). Current place of progestins in the treatment of endometriosis-related complaints, *Gynecol Endocrinol* 15 Suppl 6: 22-8.

Schweppe, KW (2005). [Guidelines for the use of GnRH-analogues in the treatment of endometriosis], *Zentralbl Gynakol* 127(5): 308-13.

Shaw, RW (1988). LHRH analogues in the treatment of endometriosis--comparative results with other treatments, *Baillieres Clin Obstet Gynaecol* 2(3): 659-75.

Simpson, ER, Clyne, C, Rubin, G, Boon, WC, Robertson, K, Britt, K, Speed, C & Jones, M (2002). Aromatase--a brief overview, *Annu Rev Physiol* 64: 93-127.

Slivova, V, Zaloga, G, DeMichele, SJ, Mukerji, P, Huang, YS, Siddiqui, R, Harvey, K, Valachovicova, T & Sliva, D (2005). Green tea polyphenols modulate secretion of urokinase plasminogen activator (uPA) and inhibit invasive behavior of breast cancer cells, *Nutr Cancer* 52(1): 66-73.

Spiteller, G (2001). Lipid peroxidation in aging and age-dependent diseases, *Exp Gerontol* 36(9): 1425-57.

Surrey, ES & Hornstein, MD (2002). Prolonged GnRH agonist and add-back therapy for symptomatic endometriosis: long-term follow-up, *Obstet Gynecol* 99(5 Pt 1): 709-19.

Surrey, ES & Schoolcraft, WB (2003). Management of endometriosis-associated infertility, *Obstet Gynecol Clin North Am* 30(1): 193-208.

Sutton, CJ, Ewen, SP, Whitelaw, N & Haines, P (1994). Prospective, randomized, double-blind, controlled trial of laser laparoscopy in the treatment of pelvic pain associated with minimal, mild, and moderate endometriosis, *Fertil Steril* 62(4): 696-700.

Sutton, CJ, Pooley, AS, Ewen, SP & Haines, P (1997). Follow-up report on a randomized controlled trial of laser laparoscopy in the treatment of pelvic pain associated with minimal to moderate endometriosis, *Fertil Steril* 68(6): 1070-4.

Szczepanska, M, Kozlik, J, Skrzypczak, J & Mikolajczyk, M (2003). Oxidative stress may be a piece in the endometriosis puzzle, *Fertil Steril* 79(6): 1288-93.

Tang, FY & Meydani, M (2001). Green tea catechins and vitamin E inhibit angiogenesis of human microvascular endothelial cells through suppression of IL-8 production, *Nutr Cancer* 41(1-2): 119-25.

Tonnesen, MG, Feng, X & Clark, RA (2000). Angiogenesis in wound healing, *J Investig Dermatol Symp Proc* 5(1): 40-6.

Uesato, S, Kitagawa, Y, Kamishimoto, M, Kumagai, A, Hori, H & Nagasawa, H (2001). Inhibition of green tea catechins against the growth of cancerous human colon and hepatic epithelial cells, *Cancer Lett* 170(1): 41-4.

Valle, RF & Sciarra, JJ (2003). Endometriosis: treatment strategies, *Ann N Y Acad Sci* 997: 229-39.

Vercellini, P, Trespidi, L, Colombo, A, Vendola, N, Marchini, M & Crosignani, PG (1993). A gonadotropin-releasing hormone agonist versus a low-dose oral contraceptive for pelvic pain associated with endometriosis, *Fertil Steril* 60(1): 75-9.

Vercellini, P, Fedele, L, Pietropaolo, G, Frontino, G, Somigliana, E & Crosignani, PG (2003). Progestogens for endometriosis: forward to the past, *Hum Reprod Update* 9(4): 387-96.

Vercellini, P, Fedele, L, Aimi, G, Pietropaolo, G, Consonni, D & Crosignani, PG (2007). Association between endometriosis stage, lesion type, patient characteristics and severity of pelvic pain symptoms: a multivariate analysis of over 1000 patients, *Hum Reprod* 22(1): 266-71.

Vercellini, P, Crosignani, PG, Abbiati, A, Somigliana, E, Vigano, P & Fedele, L (2009). The effect of surgery for symptomatic endometriosis: the other side of the story, *Hum Reprod Update* 15(2): 177-88.

Vessey, MP, Villard-Mackintosh, L & Painter, R (1993). Epidemiology of endometriosis in women attending family planning clinics, *Bmj* 306(6871): 182-4.

Winkel, CA & Scialli, AR (2001). Medical and surgical therapies for pain associated with endometriosis, *J Womens Health Gend Based Med* 10(2): 137-62.

Xu, H, Lui, WT, Chu, CY, Ng, PS, Wang, CC & Rogers, MS (2009). Anti-angiogenic effects of green tea catechin on an experimental endometriosis mouse model, *Hum Reprod* 24(3): 608-18.

Xu, H, Becker, CM, Lui, WT, Chu, CY, Davis, TN, Kung, AL, Birsner, AE, D'Amato, RJ, Man, CW & Wang, CC (2011). Green tea epigallocatchin-3-gallate inhibits angiogenesis and suppresses VEGFC/VEGFR2 expression and signaling in experimental endometriosis in vivo, *Fertil Steril* Oct; 96(4):1021-1028.e1.'

Yagyu, T, Kobayashi, H, Matsuzaki, H, Wakahara, K, Kondo, T, Kurita, N, Sekino, H, Inagaki, K, Suzuki, M, Kanayama, N & Terao, T (2005). Thalidomide inhibits tumor necrosis factor-alpha-induced interleukin-8 expression in endometriotic stromal cells, possibly through suppression of nuclear factor-kappaB activation, *J Clin Endocrinol Metab* 90(5): 3017-21.

Yang, CS, Yang, GY, Landau, JM, Kim, S & Liao, J (1998). Tea and tea polyphenols inhibit cell hyperproliferation, lung tumorigenesis, and tumor progression, *Exp Lung Res* 24(4): 629-39.

Yang, CS, Maliakal, P & Meng, X (2002). Inhibition of carcinogenesis by tea, *Annu Rev Pharmacol Toxicol* 42: 25-54.

Yoo, HG, Shin, BA, Park, JC, Kim, HS, Kim, WJ, Chay, KO, Ahn, BW, Park, RK, Ellis, LM & Jung, YD (2002). Induction of apoptosis by the green tea flavonol (-)-epigallocatechin-3-gallate in human endothelial ECV 304 cells, *Anticancer Res* 22(6A): 3373-8.

Zempo, N, Kenagy, RD, Au, YP, Bendeck, M, Clowes, MM, Reidy, MA & Clowes, AW (1994). Matrix metalloproteinases of vascular wall cells are increased in balloon-injured rat carotid artery, *J Vasc Surg* 20(2): 209-17.

Zhu, BH, Zhan, WH, Li, ZR, Wang, Z, He, YL, Peng, JS, Cai, SR, Ma, JP & Zhang, CH (2007). (-)-Epigallocatechin-3-gallate inhibits growth of gastric cancer by reducing VEGF production and angiogenesis, *World J Gastroenterol* 13(8): 1162-9.

Zhu, QY, Huang, Y, Tsang, D & Chen, ZY (1999). Regeneration of alpha-tocopherol in human low-density lipoprotein by green tea catechin, *J Agric Food Chem* 47(5): 2020-5.

15

Endometrial Stem Cells and Endometriosis

Jafar Ai and Esmaeil Sadroddiny
*Department of Tissue Engineering, School of Advanced Medical Technologies,
Tehran University of Medical Sciences, Tehran,
Iran*

1. Introduction

Stem cells (SCs) are undifferentiated cells which are able to remain at this state for several generations following cell proliferations. SCs are also able to take part in natural *in vivo* phenomena such as wound repair after physical damages or tissue regenerations.

On this basis, endometrial stem cells (EnSCs), characterized by higher abilities for proliferation, differentiation, fast angiogenesis during menstruation and immune tolerance for embryo during pregnancy, have been considered as a valuable source of stem cells (Gargett, Chan et al. 2007; Meng, Ichim et al. 2007). Several researches have demonstrated presence of highly pleuripotent mesenchymal stem cells in endometrium by differentiation potency to various cell types such as, insulin producer cells (Li, Chen et al. 2010), osteoblasts (Ai, Mehrabani. 2010) , odontoblasts (Ai, Tabatabaei et al. 2009), neurons (Wolff, Gao et al. 2011) (Ai, Tabatabaei et al. 2009) and Myoblast (Ai, Tabatabaei et al. 2009). These findings may open up new opportunities to use endometrial stem cells in tissue engineering and cell therapy (Ai , Mehrabani. 2009).

Additionally our previous studies demonstrated that EnSCs are able to participate at a phenomenon like angiogenesis in 3-D cultures which is similar to early stages of endometriosis (Esfandiari, Ai et al. 2007; Esfandiari, Khazaei et al. 2007; Esfandiari, Ai et al. 2008) which may propose a novel mechanism in pathogenesis of endometriosis compared to the traditional theory that emphasis on retrograde menstruation as a possible factor. These studies are supported by others who demonstrated recruitment of bone marrow-derived mesenchymal stem cells to the endometrium (Taylor 2004) and these all may point to the role of stem cells at the pathogenesis of endometriosis (Figueira, Abrão et al.; Sasson and Taylor 2008). Therefore, endometrial stem cells could be considered as binary role-player in natural function of endometrium and endometriosis and potentially could be used as a target in endometriosis therapy.

2. Histology of human uterus

The inner layer of uterus (Endometrium) comprises the mucosal lining which is highly regenerative tissue during menstrual cycle. The human endometrium undergoes more than 400 cycles of shedding and regeneration during a woman's reproductive years (McLennan and Rydell 1965). This layer is backed by a thick muscular myometrium which consists of muscular cells. There is no submucosal tissue to separate endometrial glandular tissue from underlying smooth muscle. The endometrium is composed of single columnar epithelial layer, resting on a layer of connective tissue, the stroma. Tubular glands reach through the endometrial surface to the base of stroma. In a woman of reproductive age, the endometrium itself is structurally and functionally divided into two relatively distinct layers of upper functionalis and lower basalis. The functionalis zone is adjacent to uterine cavity and contains glands and supportive stroma for optimal implantation and growth condition of embryo. Basalis (basal layer), adjacent to myometrium, provides basal region of glands, dense stroma and lymphoid aggregates and from it functional layer develops. During menstrual cycle only the functional layer is regenerated and the basal layer is not affected.

Both endometrium and subendometrial myometrium originate from the Müllerian ducts during embryonic life. However, outer myometrial layer is formed during fetal life and from non- Müllerian origin (Ferenczy and Bergeron 1991).

The cellular components of human endometrium can be primarily divided into two cell types; the epithelial cells (luminal and glandular) and the supporting mesenchymal cells (stromal cells) as well as vascular (endothelial) cells and leukocytes.

3. Endometriosis

It is acknowledged that about 11% of all women population during reproductive age is affected by endometriosis (Buck Louis, Hediger et al. 2011). Endometriosis is a chronic benign gynecological disease which is characterized by the ectopic formation of endometrial stroma and glands mostly seen in pelvic peritoneum. However, it might be seen outside the pelvic peritoneum such as, pelvic viscera(Vercellini, Meschia et al. 1996), rectovaginal septum (Nisolle and Donnez 1997), pleura, abdominal wall, and even sometime in brain (Thibodeau, Prioleau et al. 1987). Briefly, the underlay mechanism is attachment of endometrial cells to the pelvic peritoneum, invasion into the mesothelium, and survival and proliferation of the ectopic endometrial cells. Endometriosis is usually diagnosed after symptoms such as pelvic pain, which might correlate with menstrual cycle, or infertility.

4. Etiology and pathophysiology of endometriosis

The source of endometrial implants is not fully understood. However, there are evidences for competence of some women over others (Di and Guo 2007). The reasons for susceptibility of some patients for development of ectopic lesions are not clear. Comparative microarray analysis of gene expression in patients with ectopic endometrial cells and that of eutopic endometrium has demonstrated an alternative pattern of gene expression in two groups (Taylor, Lundeen et al. 2002; Giudice 2003; Giudice 2006). This is also seen between patient and non-affected women (Gogusev, de Joliniere et al. 1999; Taylor, Lundeen et al. 2002; Giudice 2003; Giudice 2006; Wu, Strawn et al. 2006).

Although etiology of disease has not been clearly understood, a number of theories have been proposed in correlation with the pathogenesis of endometriosis which includes: genetic and environmental factors, immune system, retrograde menstruation, coelomic metaplasia, embryonic rest theory, lymphovascular metastasis and stem cell-based theory. Clinical manifestation of endometriosis and ectopic formation of endometriotic lesions usually considered as end point result of several aberrant biological process.

5. Stem cell-based theory

5.1 Stem cells

Stem cells are undifferentiated cells which are defined by their functional properties such as; high proliferative potential, substantial self-renewal capacity and ability to differentiate to other organ/tissue-specific cell types. Cellular self- renewal is a capacity that parental stem cells are able to divide into two daughter cells which can happen through symmetrical or asymmetrical division. The symmetrical division produces two identical daughter stem cells or transit amplifying (TA) cells. TA cells undergo repetitive cell division cycles and progressively acquire differentiation marker and lose their self-renewal capacity. Asymmetrical division leads to an identical daughter cell as well as a more differentiated cell.

Although stem cells are potentially capable to proliferation, they remain mostly in a quiescent state until an inductive factor to induce them to proliferation.

Adult stem cells present in all organs and tissues and are responsible for tissue regeneration and repair after damage and trauma encountered during life time.

Rarity and lack of distinguishable morphological features and specific molecular markers of stem cells have hindered their isolation, purification and studies for several years.

Broadly they can be divided into two categories, embryonic and adult stem cells. Stem cells can also be divided into various groups according to their differentiation capacity. For example, the zygote can be considered as a totipotent stem cell, which means it is able to differentiate into all other cell types in embryo and extraembryonic tissue. Other stem cells with decreased levels of potency can be named as; pluripotent, which can differentiate into nearly all cell types (e.g., inner cell mass of the blastocyst), multipotent, which can differentiate into a number of cells that are closely related family of cell (e.g., Hematopoetic stem cells), oligopotent which differentiate into a few cell types (e.g., myeloid or lymphoid stem cells) and unipotent, which differentiate into only one cell type with self-renewal capacity(e.g., muscle stem cell).

Anatomic structure surrounding stem cells which have profound effect on cell function is called niche. Signaling elements and various cellular and molecular interactions inside the niche can determine the fate of cell to stay in undifferentiated state until tissue regeneration or repair to motivate stem cell differentiation.

5.2 Evidences for existence of endometrial stem cells

5.2.1 Indirect evidences

Adult stem cells present throughout whole body and responsible for replenishment and regeneration of damaged tissues and contribute to the structural and functional maintenance of tissues and organs. Human endometrium undergoes periodical process of regeneration during menstrual cycle. The growth rate may vary between 0.5 -7mm in thickness. Menstruation is a phenomenon consisted of various cellular and tissue functions from cell proliferation and differentiation to shedding and regeneration. During each menstrual cycle, the functionalis and a part of basalis layer of endometrium undergo shedding. After shedding, the endometrium regrows under the influence of estrogen.

Regeneration process is comprised of endometrial regrowth, angiogenesis and proliferation of endometrial stromal cells. Shedding and regeneration of the endometrial layer during menstruation and regeneration of functional layer may be considered as an indirect evidence for presence of progenitor/ stem cells. This concept was proposed in 1978 by Prianishnikov (Prianishnikov 1978), and then confirmed by following clinical observations (Wood and Rogers 1993), proliferation experiments and demonstration of gland monoclonality (Tanaka, Kyo et al. 2003; Chan, Schwab et al. 2004; Schwab, Chan et al. 2005). In some other species this process is carried out in the form of endometrial growth and apoptosis rather than menstrual cycle. Therefore, this is conceivable that endometrium consists of an active and regenerative population of cells which are known as endometrial progenitor/stem cells (EnSCs). Since endometrium consists of glands, surface epithelium and supportive stroma, the existence of both epithelial and stromal stem/progenitor cells are plausible.

5.3 Evidence from cell cloning studies

The first reports for the existence of EnSCs on human endometrium came from clonogenic studies which identified epithelial and stromal stem cells (Tanaka, Kyo et al. 2003). By study carried out later on purified single cell suspensions obtained from hysterectomy tissue, 0.22±0.07% of endometrial epithelial cells and 1.25±0.18% of stromal cells formed individual colonies within 15 days (Chan, Schwab et al. 2004). Although both were clonogenic, the stromal stem cells were significantly more clonogenic than epithelial stem cells, and small and large colonies were observed in two types. The number of large colonies was lower than the smaller (0.09% of epithelial cells and 0.02% of stromal cells) and it may be hypothesized that they belong to stem cells population which are rare among other more mature transit amplifying cells. These colonies displayed significantly greater self-renewal capacity compared with the small and loose colonies. This observation lead to the hypothesis that larger colonies belong to endometrial stem/progenitor cells, and the smaller belong to transit amplifying (TA) cells with greater extent of differentiation.

The presence of clonogenic stromal and epithelial cells are also reported in inactive, noncycling endometrium (Schwab, Chan et al. 2005). This study showed similar frequency of clonogenicity for epithelial and stromal cells in different phases of the menstrual cycle or in inactive endometrium. These data further point to the presence of endometrial stem/progenitor cells within basalis layer in higher number than the functionalis layer.

5.4 Side population cells

Side population (SP) cells are a small fraction of cells within tissues with dye-effluxing properties. They are detected by flowcytometric analysis of pre-incubated cells with DNA-binding dye, Hoechst 33342. This is due to the expression of ABCG2, a plasma membrane transporter. SP cells have been identified from various adult tissues, demonstrating that this phenotype may represent a common feature of adult stem cells. SP cells were identified in short-term culture of two fractions filtered from human endometrial cell suspension (Kato, Yoshimoto et al. 2007). Upper fraction comprised mainly of epithelial ($CD9^{+}$) cells and the lower fraction contained both epithelial and stromal ($CD13^{+}$) cells. Further differentiation studies on Matrigel demonstrated the capacity of epithelial side population to differentiate into gland-like structures expressing CD9 and E-cadherin. On the side, cell differentiation study of lower fraction showed the capacity to differentiate into $CD13^+$ stromal-like clusters. Additionally, to test whether endometrial SP cells reconstitute the endometrial tissue with stromal and glandular structure, they were xenotransplanted into NOG mice (Maruyama 2010). These studies not only demonstrated the presence of endometrial stem/progenitor cells, they have also provided an experimental animal model for endometriosis which is valuable in endometriosis studies.

5.5 Evidence from mouse

Mouse could be used as an experimental model for endometriosis and endometrial stem cell studies. However, the structure and physiology of mouse endometrium is not exactly similar to that of human. The mouse lacks an endometrial basalies layer, and the endometrium does not shed during menstruation but rather it is reabsorbed after the cycle. In spite of these dissimilarities, the murine estrous cycle has characteristics similar to those of human menstrual cycle and then mouse uterus can provide data on the molecular and cellular information for the pathogenesis of endometriosis and normal activity of endometrium tissue.

On this basis, several studies have been conducted to demonstrate the presence of endometrial stem cells in mouse endometrium (Cervello, Martinez-Conejero et al. 2006; Chan and Gargett 2006). For example, label-retaining cells (LRCs) have been shown in the mouse uterus. Label retaining is a technique to identify a stem cell population *in vivo* on the basis of quiescent state of stem/progenitor cells. The cells in this state are able to retain DNA strand incorporated stains such as, 5-bromo-2´-deoxyuridine (BrdU) for a longer period than the active dividing cells. A study conducted by Chan and Gargett showed that 3% of mouse endometrial epithelium after a 56-day chase period and 6% of endometrial stromal cells after an 84-day chase period are LRCs. Also, in another study Cevello et al demonstrated that 9% of stromal cells after 49 days were LRCs and this decreased to 1.7% after 112-day chase period. However, no epithelial LRCs were identified even after 21 days (Cervello, Martinez-Conejero et al. 2006). Presence of LRCs have also been demonstrated in myometrium (Szotek, Chang et al. 2007).

5.6 Endometrial regenerative cells (ERCs) from menstrual blood

Endometrial stem/progenitor cells have also been obtained from menstrual blood. These cells can be maintained in culture for more than 68 doubling and during this time they are able to retain their markers such as CD9, CD29, CD41a, CD44, CD59, CD73, CD90 and CD105 without karyotypic abnormalities (Musina, Belyavski et al. 2008). Proliferative rate of these cells are also significantly more than mesenchymal stem cells from the source of umbilical cord.

Endometrial regenerative cells (EnRCs) from menstrual blood are different from endometrial stem cells at expression of STRO-1. These cells are also negative for hematopoetic markers such as, CD34, CD45, CD133, but express embryonic stem cell marker, Oct4.

Ease of collection could be considered as an important characteristic of EnRCs which make them more attractive. Karyotypic stability of EnRCs suggests a large scale expansion capability.

5.7 Endometrial cancer stem cells

Presence of specific type of stem cells called cancer stem cells have been pointed at recent years (Bomken, Fišer et al. 2010). Cancer stem cell refers to a subset of tumour cells which are able to self-renew and generate the diverse cells in tumour cell mass. In fact, many features of carcinoma can be explained by the stem cell concept, including clonal origin and heterogeneity of tumors, the mesenchymal influence on cancer behavior, the local formation of precancerous lesions and the plasticity of tumor cells (Miller, Lavker et al. 2005).

A gold standard to evaluate the presence of cancer stem cells is to check their tumorogenicity on immunocompromised mice following serial transplantation. It is now postulated that cancer stem cells are responsible for cancer return after current cancer therapies e.g., radio- or chemotherapy. Recently, presence of endometrial cancer stem cells among endometrial carcinoma cells has been reported (Hubbard, Friel et al. 2009).

5.8 Signalling pathways involved in EnSCs' biology

Evidences from early studies of human EnSCs revealed the influences of three growth factors on clonogenisity of both epithelial and stromal cells. These are platelet-derived growth factor-BB (PDGF-BB), transforming growth factor-α (TGF-α) and epithelial growth factor (EGF). Basic fibroblast growth factor (b-FGF) was also able to induce clonogenicity on stromal stem cells but was not effective on epithelial cells. This could point to the difference of two cell types in expression of cognate receptor and this may propose two relatively distinct niches for them.

Also in serum-free culture condition, epithelial cells are relying on fibroblast feeder layer for clonogenicity. This may emphasis on the importance of epithelial-stromal interactions.

5.9 Endometrial stem cell markers

No specific marker has been identified for endometrial progenitor stem cells. This may hinder the isolation of EnSCs from surrounding cells utilizing the techniques such as FACS and MACS. Instead, a technique called label-retaining cell (LRC) have been successfully utilized to identify progenitor/stem cells among others in vivo.

Oct-4 is a transcription factor which is crucial for the maintenance of cell pluripotency and is known to be expressed in embryonic stem cells, germ cells, whole embryos at various stages of development and adult stem cells. It is also reported in almost half of the endometrial samples (Matthai, Horvat et al. 2006). Expression of Oct4 mRNA has been detected in all endometrial samples of 89 women in follicular or luteal phase of menstrual cycle (Bentz, Kenning et al. 2010).

Expression of other general stem cell markers such as bcl-2, c-kit (CD117) and CD34 have also been reported on endometrial stem cells (Cho, Park et al. 2004). Haematopoietic stem cell markers (CD34 and CD45) that co-express CD7 and CD56 have also been identified in human endometrial cell suspension that may belong to lymphoid progenitors.

Expression and localization of Musashi-1, a RNA-binding protein, have been evaluated in endometrial, endometriotic and endometrial carcinoma tissue specimens (Götte, Wolf et al. 2008). Musashi-1 is an epithelial progenitor cell marker. It is expressed on endometrial glandular and stromal cells and in proliferative endometrium. The proportion of Musashi-1-

positive cells in the basalis layer significantly increase in the stroma (1.5 fold) and in endometrial glands (three fold) compared to functionalis. Musashi-1 is also expressed in high levels in endometriosis and endometrial carcinoma (Götte, Wolf et al. 2008).

5.10 Differentiation ability of endometrial stem cells

Differentiation potency of endometrial stem cells has been demonstrated in several studies, suggesting their potency to be used as a useful source in cell therapy and tissue engineering. Kato et al used two markers of CD9 and CD13 to show that side population cells can differentiate into endometrial epithelial and stromal cells respectively(Kato, Yoshimoto et al. 2007).

Additionally, endometrial stromal cells have the potency to differentiate into chondrocytes when cultured in a defined chondrocyte medium. Also, large putative stromal stem/progenitor cell colonies consist of multipotency by differentiation into mesenchymal lineages-adipocytes, smooth muscle cells, chondrocytes and osteoblasts when cultured in an appropriate differentiation medium. By contrast, the small, loose colonies failed to demonstrate similar differentiation capacity that may suggest these cells are derived from TA cells.

Endometrial regenerative cells from menstrual blood are also able to differentiate to various cell lineages such as, insulin producer cells (Li, Chen et al. 2010), osteoblast (Ai, Mehrabani. 2010) , odontoblasts (Ai, Tabatabaei et al. 2009), and neurons (Wolff, Gao et al. 2011 and Ai, Esfandiari et al. 2009a).

EnSCs have been recently used to replace dopaminergic neurons in a murine model of Parkinson's disease (Wolff, Gao et al. 2011). Cardiogenic potential of EnSCs have also been high-lighted by several studies (Hida, Nishiyama et al. 2008).

5.11 Endometrial regeneration and angiogenesis

Endometrium is well known for its profound angiogenic potency which may point to the presence of a highly regenerative back-up layer (Esfandiari, Ai et al. 2007; Esfandiari, Khazaei et al. 2007; Esfandiari, Ai et al. 2008 and Ai, Esfandiari et al 2009a and 2009b). Angiogenesis plays a pivotal role in endometrium regeneration during menstrual cycle. It is also involved in establishment and development of endometriosis lesions (Donnez, Smoes et al. 1998; Fujishita, Hasuo et al. 2000).

5.12 Sources of endometrial stem/progenitor cells

5.12.1 Fetal stem cells

It is thought that some embryonic cells in the intermediate mesoderm undergo mesenchymal to epithelial transitions to form the coelomic epithelium that later invaginates to make the paramesonphric or Murrelian ducts (Kobayashi and Behringer 2003). Müllerian ducts comprise of surface epithelium and underlying urogenital ridge mesenchyme which are the source of endometrium and myometrium. A few epithelial and mesenchymal cells are thought to remain in the adult endometrium and contribute to tissue regeneration during menstrual cycle. This small population of stem cells might be subdivided into epithelial and stromal or even more committed sub-lineages or might exist in the form of ultimate uterine stem cells with a capacity to replace all endometrial and myometrial cells.

5.13 Bone marrow-derived stem cells as a possible source of endometrial progenitor/stem cells

Interestingly, regenerative turnover in endometrium is equivalent to that in bone marrow (Fuchs and Segre 2000). Bone marrow is commonly known as a source of hematopoetic and non-hematopoetic stem cells. Hematopoetic stem cells are mainly involved in the homeostasis of cellular part of blood. However, non-hematopoetic stem cells can differentiate into various cell types, e.g., endothelial cells, hepatocytes, neurons, skin, cardiomyocyte, gastrointestinal epithelium (Alison, Poulsom et al. 2000; Mezey, Key et al. 2003; Taylor 2004), suggesting their possible contribution to the maintenance of multiple tissues.

Apart from fetal source of stem cells resideing in adult endometrium which is speculated to account for the endometrium replacement after each menstrual cycle, new observations support the role of bone marrow-derived stem cells at endometrial regeneration.

Migration and presence of donor-derived bone marrow cell to/in endometrium and generation of experimental endometriosis have been reported after murine bone marrow transplantation (Taylor 2004; Du and Taylor 2007). Also, presence of chimerism in the endometrial glands and stroma of four women who received single-antigen HLA-mismatched bone marrow transplants can point to the contribution of bone marrow stem cells to the repopulation of the endometrium (Taylor 2004). Bone marrow-derived cells are indistinguishable from endogenous endometrial cells and express glandular and stromal differentiation markers.

Whether bone marrow-derived stem cells are involved in the normal function and regeneration of endometrium or pathogenesis of endometriosis is not clear. However, this theory is appropriately able to explain ectopic endometriosis.

5.14 Stem cell-based theory of endometriosis

Today, a combination theory is more acceptable for the pathogenesis of endometriosis. Evidences for existence of pluripotent endometrial stem cells, and contribution of bone marrow as an alternative source of EnSCs as well as the direct correlation of endometriosis and menstrual retrograde have convinced researchers to propose that stem/progenitor cells are present in the blood that reach the peritoneal cavity (Figueira, Abrão et al. 2011). Endometrial stem cells shed through fallopian tube during menstruation might be responsible for endometriotic implants. Also, this theory could account for the distant ectopic implants, as circulatory stem cells are able to reach peritoneal cavity as well as distant tissues and organs such as brain.

Several experiments have demonstrated that endometrium-derived cells are capable of establishing endometriotic implants (Te Linde and Scott 1950; Ridley and Edwards 1958; D'Hooghe, Bambra et al. 1995). Xenografts of human endometrial tissue or dissociated endometrial cells have been used in immunocompromised mouse to investigate pathogenesis of endometriosis (Grümmer 2006; Masuda, Maruyama et al. 2007). This model provides an appropriate in vivo system to test the possible role of EnSCs in endometriosis. This is further supported by the demonstration of clonogenic cells in a long-term culture derived from a sample of endometriosis tissue (Tanaka, Nakajima et al. 2003).

The monoclonality of some endometrial lesions (Jimbo, Hitomi et al. 1997; Tamura, Fukaya et al. 1998; Wu, Basir et al. 2003) is consistent with the concept that endometriosis could have a stem cell origin. Furthermore, polyclonal endometriotic lesions may point to repeated seeding of the lesions with cells from other sources such as bone marrow or from establishment of different fragments of shed endometrium containing several stem cells. Although stem cell-based pathogenesis of endometriosis is not fully established the previous studies have demonstrated the role of unfractionated endometrial stem cells to ectopic endometrial growth (Sasson and Taylor 2008). Endometriosis was also generated experimentally by ectopic wild-type endometrial implantation in the peritoneal cavity of hysterectomized LacZ transgenic mice (Du and Taylor 2007). LacZ-expressing stem cells of extrauterine origin were incorporated into the endometriosis implants. These cells were able to differentiate into epithelial and stromal cells at a frequency of 0.04% and 0.1%, respectively (Du and Taylor 2007).

In a study carried out by Leyendecker et al. expression pattern of estrogen receptor, two isoforms of progesterone receptor and P450 aromatase were compared on normal endometrium and ectopic endometriotic implants (Leyendecker, Herbertz et al. 2002). The expression pattern of the endometriotic implants was identical to that of basalis layer of eutopic endometrium and was out of phase with the functionalis layer. This study also demonstrated that more basalis layer was shed in women with endometriosis compared to the normal women. As basalis layer contain endometrial stem/progenitor cells and it is shed in larger extent in endometriosis that is in accordance with the larger volume of retrograde menstrual flow, this may suggest that endometriosis implants results from the retrograde menstruation of endometrial stem/progenitor cells.

Additionally, it has been postulated that some forms of endometriosis may arise from remnants of fetal müllerian cells which have characteristics of stem cells such as multipotency and self-renewal.

Thus, stem cell-based pathogenesis of endometriosis could be suggested and this theory could account for the observations that support the cellular origin of ectopic implants.

6. References

Ai, J. and D. Mehrabani (2010). "The Potential of Human Endometrial Stem Cells for Osteoblast Differentiation." Iranian Red Crescent Medical Journal 12(5): 585-587.

Ai, J., F. S. Tabatabaei, et al. (2009). "Human endometrial adult stem cells may differentiate into odontoblast cells." Hypothesis 7(1).

Alison, M. R., R. Poulsom, et al. (2000). "Cell differentiation: hepatocytes from non-hepatic adult stem cells." Nature 406: 257.

Bentz, E. K., M. Kenning, et al. (2010). "OCT-4 expression in follicular and luteal phase endometrium: a pilot study." Reproductive Biology and Endocrinology 8(1): 38-45.

Bomken, S., K. Fišer, et al. (2010). "Understanding the cancer stem cell." British journal of cancer 103:439-445.

Buck Louis, G. M., M. L. Hediger, et al. (2011). "Incidence of endometriosis by study population and diagnostic method: the ENDO study." Fertility and sterility. 96(2): 360-365

Cervello, I., J. A. Martinez-Conejero, et al. (2006). "Identification, characterization and co-localization of label-retaining cell population in mouse endometrium with typical undifferentiated markers." Human Reproduction 22(1): 45-51.

Chan, R. W. S. and C. E. Gargett (2006). "Identification of Label Retaining Cells in Mouse Endometrium." Stem Cells 24(6): 1529-1538.

Chan, R. W. S., K. E. Schwab, et al. (2004). "Clonogenicity of human endometrial epithelial and stromal cells." Biology of reproduction 70(6): 1738-1750.

Cho, N. H., Y. K. Park, et al. (2004). "Lifetime expression of stem cell markers in the uterine endometrium." Fertility and sterility 81(2): 403-407.

D'Hooghe, T. M., C. S. Bambra, et al. (1995). "Intrapelvic injection of menstrual endometrium causes endometriosis in baboons (Papio cynocephalus and Papio anubis)* 1." American journal of obstetrics and gynecology 173(1): 125-134.

Di, W. and S. W. Guo (2007). "The search for genetic variants predisposing women to endometriosis." Current Opinion in Obstetrics and Gynecology 19(4): 395-401.

Donnez, J., P. Smoes, et al. (1998). "Vascular endothelial growth factor (VEGF) in endometriosis." Human Reproduction 13(6): 1686-1690.

Du, H. and H. S. Taylor (2007). "Contribution of Bone Marrow Derived Stem Cells to Endometrium and Endometriosis." Stem Cells 25(8): 2082-2086.

Esfandiari, N., J. Ai, et al. (2007). "Expression of Glycodelin and Cyclooxygenase 2 in Human Endometrial Tissue Following Three dimensional Culture." American Journal of Reproductive Immunology 57(1): 49-54.

Esfandiari, N., M. Khazaei, et al. (2007). "Effect of a statin on an in vitro model of endometriosis." Fertility and sterility 87(2): 257-262.

Ferenczy, A. and C. Bergeron (1991). "Histology of the human endometrium: from birth to senescence." Annals of the New York Academy of Sciences 622(1): 6-27.

Figueira, P. G. M., M. S. Abrão, et al. "Stem cells in endometrium and their role in the pathogenesis of endometriosis." Annals of the New York Academy of Sciences 1221(1): 10-17.

Figueira, P. G. M., M. S. Abrão, et al. (2011). "Stem cells in endometrium and their role in the pathogenesis of endometriosis." Annals of the New York Academy of Sciences 1221(1): 10-17.

Fuchs, E. and J. A. Segre (2000). "Stem cells: a new lease on life." Cell (Cambridge) 100(1): 143-155.

Fujishita, A., A. Hasuo, et al. (2000). "Immunohistochemical study of angiogenic factors in endometrium and endometriosis." Gynecologic and obstetric investigation 48(1): 36-44.

Gargett, C. E., R. W. S. Chan, et al. (2007). "Endometrial stem cells." Current Opinion in Obstetrics and Gynecology 19(4): 377-383.

Giudice, L. C. (2003). Genomics' role in understanding the pathogenesis of endometriosis, 21(2): 119-124.

Giudice, L. C. (2006). "Application of functional genomics to primate endometrium: insights into biological processes." Reprod Biol Endocrinol 4(suppl 1): S4.

Gogusev, J., J. B. de Joliniere, et al. (1999). "Detection of DNA copy number changes in human endometriosis by comparative genomic hybridization." Human genetics 105(5): 444-451.

Götte, M., M. Wolf, et al. (2008). "Increased expression of the adult stem cell marker Musashi 1 in endometriosis and endometrial carcinoma." The Journal of Pathology 215(3): 317-329.

Grümmer, R. (2006). "Animal models in endometriosis research." Human reproduction update 12(5): 641-649.

Hida, N., N. Nishiyama, et al. (2008). "Novel Cardiac Precursor Like Cells from Human Menstrual Blood Derived Mesenchymal Cells." Stem Cells 26(7): 1695-1704.

Hubbard, S. A., A. M. Friel, et al. (2009). "Evidence for cancer stem cells in human endometrial carcinoma." Cancer research 69(21): 8241-8248.

Jimbo, H., Y. Hitomi, et al. (1997). "Evidence for monoclonal expansion of epithelial cells in ovarian endometrial cysts." The American Journal of Pathology 150(4): 1173-1178.

Kato, K., M. Yoshimoto, et al. (2007). "Characterization of side-population cells in human normal endometrium." Human Reproduction 22(5): 1214-1223.

Kobayashi, A. and R. R. Behringer (2003). "Developmental genetics of the female reproductive tract in mammals." Nature Reviews Genetics 4(12): 969-980.

Leyendecker, G., M. Herbertz, et al. (2002). "Endometriosis results from the dislocation of basal endometrium." Human Reproduction 17(10): 2725-2736.

Li, H. Y., Y. J. Chen, et al. "Induction of Insulin-Producing Cells Derived from Endometrial Mesenchymal Stem-like Cells." Journal of Pharmacology and Experimental Therapeutics 335(3): 817-829.

Maruyama, T. (2010). "Stem/progenitor cells and the regeneration potentials in the human uterus." Reproductive Medicine and Biology 9(1): 9-16.

Masuda, H., T. Maruyama, et al. (2007). "Noninvasive and real-time assessment of reconstructed functional human endometrium in NOD/SCID/ cnull immunodeficient mice." Proceedings of the National Academy of Sciences 104(6): 1925-1930.

Matthai, C., R. Horvat, et al. (2006). "Oct-4 expression in human endometrium." Molecular human reproduction 12(1): 7-10.

McLennan, C. E. and A. L. F. H. Rydell (1965). "Extent of endometrial shedding during normal menstruation." Obstetrics & Gynecology 26(5): 605-621.

Meng, X., T. E. Ichim, et al. (2007). "Endometrial regenerative cells: a novel stem cell population." Journal of Translational Medicine 5(1): 57-67.

Mezey, É., S. Key, et al. (2003). "Transplanted bone marrow generates new neurons in human brains." Proceedings of the National Academy of Sciences of the United States of America 100(3): 1364-1369.

Miller, S. J., R. M. Lavker, et al. (2005). "Interpreting epithelial cancer biology in the context of stem cells: tumor properties and therapeutic implications." Biochimica et Biophysica Acta (BBA)-Reviews on Cancer 1756(1): 25-52.

Musina, R. A., A. V. Belyavski, et al. (2008). "Endometrial mesenchymal stem cells isolated from the menstrual blood." Bulletin of experimental biology and medicine 145(4): 539-543.

Nazemian, Z., A. Jolly, et al. (2008). "Angiogenesis following three-dimensional culture of isolated human endometrial stromal cells." International Journal of Fertility and Sterility 2(1): 19-22.

Nisolle, M. and J. Donnez (1997). "Peritoneal endometriosis, ovarian endometriosis, and adenomyotic nodules of the rectovaginal septum are three different entities." Fertility and sterility 68(4): 585-596.

Prianishnikov, V. A. (1978). "On the concept of stem cell and a model of functional-morphological structure of the endometrium." Contraception 18(3): 213-223.

Ridley, J. H. and I. K. Edwards (1958). "Experimental endometriosis in the human." American journal of obstetrics and gynecology 76(4): 783.

Sasson, I. E. and H. S. Taylor (2008). "Stem cells and the pathogenesis of endometriosis." Annals of the New York Academy of Sciences 1127(1): 106-115.

Schwab, K. E., R. W. S. Chan, et al. (2005). "Putative stem cell activity of human endometrial epithelial and stromal cells during the menstrual cycle." Fertility and sterility 84: 1124-1130.

Szotek, P. P., H. L. Chang, et al. (2007). "Adult Mouse Myometrial Label Retaining Cells Divide in Response to Gonadotropin Stimulation." Stem Cells 25(5): 1317-1325.

Tamura, M., T. Fukaya, et al. (1998). "Analysis of clonality in human endometriotic cysts based on evaluation of X chromosome inactivation in archival formalin-fixed, paraffin-embedded tissue." Laboratory investigation 78(2): 213-218.

Tanaka, M., S. Kyo, et al. (2003). "Evidence of the monoclonal composition of human endometrial epithelial glands and mosaic pattern of clonal distribution in luminal epithelium." American Journal of Pathology 163(1): 295-301.

Tanaka, T., S. Nakajima, et al. (2003). "Cellular heterogeneity in long-term surviving cells isolated from eutopic endometrial, ovarian endometrioma and adenomyosis tissues." Oncology reports 10(5): 1155-1160.

Taylor, H. S. (2004). "Endometrial cells derived from donor stem cells in bone marrow transplant recipients." JAMA: the journal of the American Medical Association 292(1): 81-85.

Taylor, R. N., S. G. Lundeen, et al. (2002). "Emerging role of genomics in endometriosis research* 1." Fertility and sterility 78(4): 694-698.

Te Linde, R. W. and R. B. Scott (1950). "Experimental endometriosis." American journal of obstetrics and gynecology 60(5): 1147-1173.

Thibodeau, L. L., G. R. Prioleau, et al. (1987). "Cerebral endometriosis." Journal of neurosurgery 66(4): 609-610.

Vercellini, P., M. Meschia, et al. (1996). "Bladder detrusor endometriosis: clinical and pathogenetic implications." The Journal of urology 155(1): 84-86.

Wolff, E. F., X. B. Gao, et al. (2011). "Endometrial stem cell transplantation restores dopamine production in a Parkinson's disease model." Journal of Cellular and Molecular Medicine 15(4): 747-755.

Wood, C. and P. Rogers (1993). "A pregnancy after planned partial endometrial resection." Australian and New Zealand journal of obstetrics and gynaecology 33(3): 316-318.

Wu, Y., Z. Basir, et al. (2003). "Resolution of clonal origins for endometriotic lesions using laser capture microdissection and the human androgen receptor (HUMARA) assay* 1." Fertility and sterility 79: 710-717.

Wu, Y., E. Strawn, et al. (2006). "Genomic alterations in ectopic and eutopic endometria of women with endometriosis." Gynecologic and obstetric investigation 62(3): 148-159.

Section 3

Recent Research Trends

16

Endometriosis-Associated Ovarian Cancer: The Role of Oxidative Stress

Yoriko Yamashita and Shinya Toyokuni
Nagoya University Graduate School of Medicine, Japan

1. Introduction

Recent studies indicated that oxidative stress has a causal role in the carcinogenesis of mainly two histological subtypes of ovarian cancer, namely, clear cell carcinoma and endometrioid adenocarcinoma. Because of recurrent hemorrhage in endometrial cysts, excess of reactive oxygen species are produced due to iron deposition, which results in direct genomic mutation of the epithelial cells and exaggeration of oxidative stress by stromal cells such as macrophages. In endometriosis-associated ovarian cancer, genomic mutations in specific genes such as ARID1A, p53, K-ras, PTEN, PI3CA and Met have been reported. Mechanism of carcinogenesis, especially focusing on the precise role of oxidative stress, remains to be clarified. Development of novel drugs and methods for therapy or prevention of endometriosis-associated ovarian cancer is necessary.

2. Risk of cancer development in endometriosis

Endometriosis is a common disease affecting 10 to 15% of women of reproductive age (Irving, 2011). An association between endometriosis and cancer was reported as early as the 1920s in English publications. Sampson (Sampson, 1925) proposed that endometrial carcinoma of the ovary develops from endometrial tissue, based on classic microscopic observation using several strict criteria (i.e., the coexistence of benign and malignant tissue with a shared histologic relationship in the same organ and evidence against invasion from other sites or sources). Further studies were interrupted by World War II; however, in the late 1940s and 1950s, several groups published case reports that met Sampson's criteria (Scott, 1953; Postoloff & Rodenberg, 1955). Although none of the studies demonstrated any direct evidence, the consensus of the major researchers in the field at that time was that malignant transformation or transition occurred in ovarian endometriosis.

In 1990, Heaps et al. analyzed 195 cases that mostly fulfilled Sampson's criteria (Heaps, 1990). They found that the primary endometriosis site was most frequently the ovary (78.7%), followed by various other sites such as the pelvis, rectovaginal septum, colon or rectum, or the vagina. The most frequent histologic subtype was endometrioid adenocarcinoma in either of the primary sites, ovarian (69%) or extragonadal (66%), followed by clear cell carcinoma and sarcoma in 13.5% and 11.6% of ovarian tumors, respectively, and sarcomas in 25% of extragonadal tumors. More recently, an elevated risk of ovarian cancer development in endometriosis has been shown by statistical analyses. A direct prospective study of 20,686 Swedish patients hospitalized with endometriosis between 1969 and 1983 with a mean follow-up period of 11.4 years demonstrated a standardized incidence ratio (SIR) of 1.9 and a 95% confidence interval [CI] of 1.3 to 2.8 (Brinton, 1997). Similar results were reported in a case-control study analyzing patients from the United States, in which the relative risk for ovarian cancer development in endometriosis patients was 1.7 (Ness, 2000). A nationwide case-control study of Australian patients with ovarian cancer revealed that endometriosis increased the risks of both endometrioid adenocarcinoma and clear cell carcinoma, with odds ratios of 3.0 and 2.2, respectively (Nagle, 2008). A recent retrospective study from Canada also showed a significant increase in the relative risk (rate ratio [RR], 1.6; 95% CI, 1.12 to 2.09) of ovarian cancer in patients with endometriosis (Aris, 2010). In line with these reports, a recent prospective study from Japan showed a significant and much greater elevation in the relative risk (SIR, 8.95; CI, 4.12 to 115.3) of cancer development in Japanese patients with endometrioma, or endometrial cyst of the ovary (Kobayashi, 2007). The reason for this discrepancy is unclear, but one possibility is that the endometriosis patients in the Japanese study included only those with clinically detectable ovarian endometrial cysts. It is also important to note that Danazol (17-α-ethinltestosterone), a synthetic androgen that has been used to treat endometriosis, has been revealed to be an independent risk factor for the development of ovarian cancer. A negative correlation between oral contraceptive use and ovarian cancer, regardless of histologic type other than mucinous tumors, was recently shown by a collaboration of various groups worldwide (Cottreau, 2003). These factors may also influence the relative risk of ovarian cancer development.

In addition to an epidemiologic approach, the retrospective pathological analysis of samples from ovarian cancer patients is also useful to confirm the presence of endometriosis associated with ovarian cancers of various histological types. A comprehensive review of 2,807 ovarian cancer patients from 15 independent publications from western countries from the 1970s to 1990s, including 3 articles from Japan, revealed that endometriosis was incidentally found in 14.1% of ovarian cancer patients (39.2%, 21.2%, 3.3% and 3.0% of clear cell, endometrioid, serous and mucinous carcinoma patients, respectively), with a tendency toward a higher incidence of endometriosis in Japanese patients with clear cell carcinoma (Yoshikawa, 2000).

3. Pathogenesis of endometriosis-associated ovarian cancer; the role of iron overload-induced oxidative stress

Endometrial cysts, or so-called chocolate cysts, are well-known lesions in endometriosis that contain fluid with an excess of free iron because of recurring hemorrhage in the cyst. It is interesting to note that Sampson mentioned in his first report of endometriosis-associated cancer that old hemorrhages should be considered additional evidence that meets his criteria (Sampson, 1925). Hemosiderin, heme, or iron deposition in endometriotic lesions have been assumed to trigger oxidative damage and chronic inflammation (Van Langendonckt, 2002a; Van Langendonckt, 2002b; Van Langendonckt, 2004; Toyokuni, 2009). In particular, iron storage in macrophages is significantly increased in patients with endometriosis; and intracellular iron activates the nuclear factor-κB pathway and exaggerates chronic inflammation (Lousse, 2009; Lousse, 2008). As a result, prominent oxidative stress, or an excess of reactive oxygen species, is consistently produced. This process is thought to have a causative role in endometriosis development and progression, leading to carcinogenesis (Murphy, 1998; Ness & Cottreau, 1999; Ngo, 2009). Alternatively, the high concentration of free iron in endometrial cysts may directly provide oxidative stress that induces genomic mutation in epithelial cells (Yamaguchi, 2008), and whether the direct pathway or the indirect pathway involving macrophages has a major role in carcinogenesis remains to be resolved. Iron overload in experimental animals enhances epithelial cell proliferation (Defrere, 2006) and causes malignant tumors with genomic abnormalities (Hu, 2010), which suggests a similar mechanism leading to carcinogenesis in human endometriosis (Fig. 1). However, further studies are awaited to elucidate the precise role of iron-deposition induced oxidative stress in carcinogenesis of endometriosis-associated cancer.

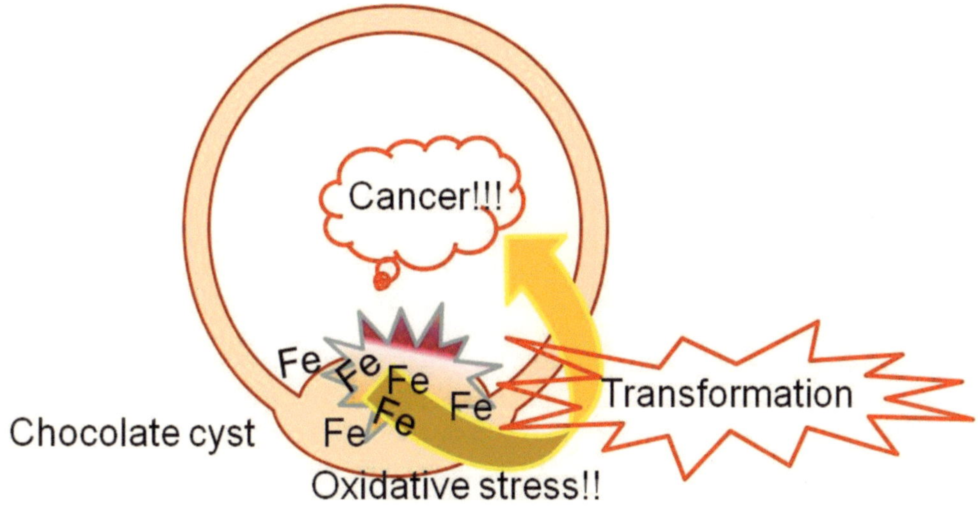

Fig. 1. A proposed mechanism of carcinogenesis in endometriotic (chocolate) cysts

4. Precancerous lesions in endometriosis

Endometriosis itself is generally considered a benign disease; however, endometriosis shares certain features with cancer, including the ability of cells from different lineages (i.e., epithelial cells, stromal cells, and the vasculature) to proliferate in ectopic sites. Thus, earlier studies have focused on the clonal or malignant potential of endometriosis by analyzing the loss of heterozygosity (LOH) at several candidate tumor suppressor gene loci. Positive results, such as the detection of LOH at the p53, p16 or PTEN gene, were observed in the majority of the endometriosis samples ((Jiang, 1996; Jiang, 1998; Sato, 2000), for review of other studies with similar results, see (Prowse, 2005)). Another approach, which assesses the clonality of endometriosis samples by analyzing methylation-related marker genes, also demonstrated the clonal nature of endometriosis (Jimbo, 1997). The findings, together with the LOH analysis, led to the conclusion that endometriosis was a neoplasm that may even have malignant potential. However, recent studies deny the malignant or neoplastic potential of endometriosis, demonstrating that most endometriosis tissues are not monoclonal (Mayr, 2003). Furthermore, neither LOH of tumor suppressor genes, promoter methylation of oncogenes, nor oncogenic mutations of known tumor-related genes was frequently observed in the majority of the cases, further denying the neoplastic theory (Prowse, 2005; Vestergaard AL, 2011). In contrast with these results, a third approach (fluorescent in situ hybridization [FISH]) used to investigate chromosomal aberrations in endometriosis samples revealed a significantly elevated proportion of aneusomic (monosomic > trisomic) cells in endometriosis in multiple groups (Koerner, 2006) (Bischoff, 2002). However, both endometriosis tissue and normal endometrium also contain a certain proportion of aneusomic cells (Koerner, 2006), and telomerase expression, telomere elongation, higher expression of DNA replication markers and lower expression of DNA damage response markers are all observed in endometriosis tissue, but not in normal endometrium (Hapangama, 2008; Hapangama, 2009). Thus, it may be reasonable to conclude that although endometriosis is generally considered non-neoplastic, the relative rates of abnormal cells are higher in endometriosis than in normal endometrium.

In this case, then, which cells are premalignant? Is there a focal area representing the precancerous state of endometriosis that is morphologically distinguishable from other, presumably benign, areas? "Atypical endometriosis" is the term used to describe this state, which has been found in cases of extraovarian and ovarian cancer as atypical epithelium showing hyperchromatism and stratification continuous with the malignant tumor (Brooks&Wheeler, 1977; Lagrenade&Silverberg, 1988). Fukunaga et al. found atypical endometriosis in 61% of endometriosis-associated ovarian cancers, in contrast with 1.7% of benign endometriosis samples (Fukunaga, 1997). Immunohistochemical markers distinguishing atypical endometriosis from benign endometriosis have not been fully established, but staining patterns of Ki67, Bcl-2, and p53 have been reported as useful markers (Nezhat, 2002; Ogawa, 2000). Extraovarian endometriosis may also show atypical changes. Hyperplastic changes, including atypical hyperplasia and malignant changes, were observed in more than half of the adenomyosis cases associated with endometrioid adenocarcinoma arising from the endometrium (Jacques&Lawrence, 1990; Kucera, 2011), and histologically atypical hyperplasia has been reported in some cases of gastrointestinal endometriosis (Yantiss, 2000).

5. Histological characteristics of endometriosis-associated malignancies

Clear cell carcinoma (Fig. 2) and endometrioid adenocarcinoma are well-known histological subtypes in ovarian cancer associated with endometriosis (Fukunaga, 1997; Heaps, 1990; Modesitt, 2002; Ogawa, 2000; Yoshikawa, 2000). Endometrioid adenocarcinoma is the most frequently observed phenotype in western countries (Heaps, 1990; Modesitt, 2002); however, clear cell carcinoma predominates in the Japanese cases (Ogawa, 2000; Yoshikawa, 2000). Veras et al. recently subdivided clear cell carcinoma into 3 groups (cystic, adenofibromatous, and indeterminate clear cell carcinoma) to further reveal the association between endometriosis and cystic clear cell carcinoma subtypes (Veras, 2009). Endometrioid adenocarcinomas arising in endometriotic lesions are often Grade 1 at presentation (Horiuchi, 2003), mostly showing typical morphology with various degrees of squamous differentiation (Heaps, 1990; Staats, 2007), similar to endometrioid adenocarcinoma without endometriosis. Sarcomas are the second and third most frequent endometriosis-associated extraovarian and ovarian tumors, respectively. Adenosarcoma and endometrial stromal sarcoma are the major histological types of sarcomas (Baiocchi, 1990; Heaps, 1990; Slavin, 2000). At least partially, differences in the incidences of tumor types (carcinoma versus sarcoma) depend on the tumor site, and further studies are needed to elucidate this mechanism. Other rare malignant tumors, such as squamous cell carcinoma, malignant mesodermal mixed tumor, and yolk sac tumor, are also reported to develop from endometriosis (Irving, 2011). Although its incidence is very low compared with endometrioid adenocarcinoma or clear cell carcinoma, serous adenocarcinoma has also been associated with endometriosis (Fukunaga, 1997; Modesitt, 2002; Yoshikawa, 2000). Much more rarely, mucinous carcinomas with unusual morphology resembling Mullerian mucinous borderline tumors have also been reported in association with endometriosis (Lee&Nucci, 2003).

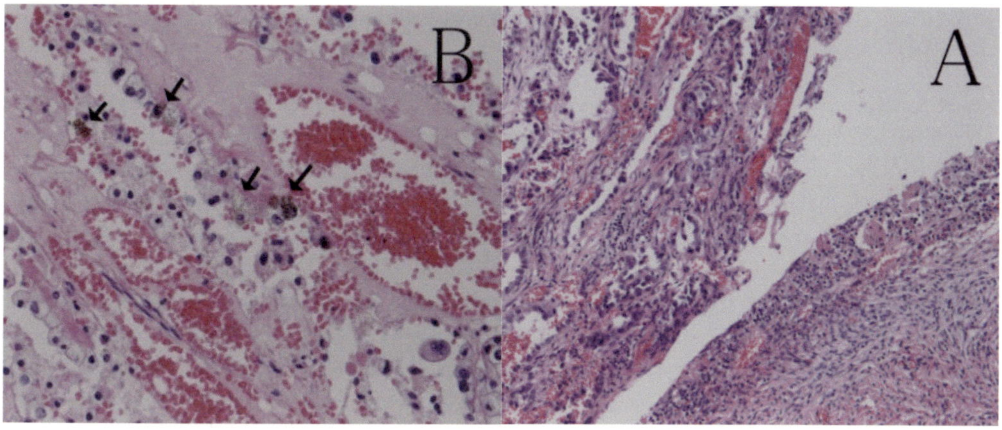

Fig. 2. A. Clear cell carcinoma (left) arising in a endometriotic cyst. B. Hemosiderin deposition (arrows) is observed in the stroma of clear cell carcinoma.

6. Genetic abnormalities and phenotypes of endometriosis-associated ovarian cancer

Genetic mutations specifically associated with ovarian cancer subtypes have been reported (reviewed by (Kurman&Shih, 2011)). Focusing on endometrioid adenocarcinomas, genetic mutations of K-ras, p53, PTEN, beta-catenin, and ATR have been reported (Mizuuchi, 1992; Milner, 1993; Palacios&Gamallo, 1998; Tashiro, 1997; Zighelboim, 2009). Mouse models of endometrioid adenocarcinoma have been reported, either with oncogenic K-ras and conditional PTEN deletion (Dinulescu, 2005) or dysfunction of both the Wnt/beta-catenin and PI3CA/PTEN pathways (Wu, 2007). However, specific genetic alterations of clear cell carcinoma were mostly unknown. Recently, a frequently activated mutation of the PI3CA gene was observed in clear cell carcinoma samples (Kuo, 2009). Most recently, several studies based on novel sequencing technology have elucidated that a significant proportion of clear cell carcinomas harbor a mutation of the ARID1A gene, which encodes the chromatin-remodeling complex protein BAF250A (Jones, 2010; Wiegand, 2010). ARID1A mutation and the consequent loss of BAF250A expression were found not only in clear cell carcinoma samples, but also in endometrioid adenocarcinomas, especially high-grade types

(Wiegand 2010; Wiegand, 2011). Whether ARID1A mutation is an early or late event in endometriosis-associated ovarian cancers related to atypical endometriosis remains to be elucidated. Alterations of other genes, such as p53, p16, and PTEN, have been detected in a low percentage of endometriotic lesions (Martini, 2002; Nezhat, 2008). hMLH, a DNA mismatch repair gene, is another candidate for the malignant transformation of endometriosis (Nyiraneza, 2010 ; Ren F, 2011). hMLH is the causal gene of Lynch syndrome, in which the risk of developing endometrial and ovarian cancers is significantly increased (Schmeler&Lu, 2008). K-ras may also be important because mutated K-ras promotes endometriosis in a mouse model, suggesting that K-ras mutation may be an early event in the carcinogenesis of endometriosis-associated cancers (Cheng, 2011). Finally, a single-nucleotide polymorphism in the intron of ANRIL, a non-coding RNA that regulates p16 expression, has been recently reported to have a strong association with endometriosis (Uno, 2010). The molecular steps from endometriosis development to carcinogenesis remain to be further clarified.

Recent studies have proposed classifying ovarian cancers into two categories: Type I tumors, which rarely harbor the p53 mutation and have an indolent clinical course, and Type II tumors, which feature the p53 mutation and are aggressive (Kurman&Shih, 2010). Within endometriosis-associated ovarian cancers, low-grade endometrioid adenocarcinoma and clear cell carcinomas are considered Type I, while high-grade endometrioid adenocarcinoma is included in the Type II category. However, p53 mutations are detected in both low- and high-grade endometriosis-associated ovarian endometrioid adenocarcinomas (Okuda, 2003), and PI3CA, PPP2R1A, and K-ras mutations are commonly detected in both endometrioid adenocarcinoma and clear cell carcinoma (Campbell, 2004; Jones, 2010 ; Kuo, 2009; McConechy, 2011 ; Mizuuchi, 1992). Recent evidence indicates that ovarian cancers arise from different cell lineages, such as preexisting cystadenomas, ectopic endometrium in endometriotic lesions, and epithelial cells of the Fallopian tubes (Bell, 2005; Kurman&Shih, 2011). Thus, it may be an oversimplification to divide all ovarian cancers into two groups. It may more accurate to categorize endometriosis-associated cancers into the same group, regardless of the histological subtype or tumor grade.

Numerous studies of expression microarray analyses have been published. Cytokines and chemokines, such as interleukin-1 and its downstream factor cyclooxygenase (COX)-2, interleukin-8, TNF-α and its downstream VEGF, TGF- α, and interleukin-6 have been reported to be involved in endometriosis and endometriosis-associated carcinoma (reviewed by (Nezhat, 2008)). An interesting study by Banz et al. revealed that SICA2, CCL14, and TDGF1 were specifically upregulated in both endometriosis samples and endometriosis-associated endometrioid adenocarcinomas, in contrast with serous adenocarcinomas or normal ovarian tissues (Banz, 2010). Another microarray study focusing on endometriosis-associated clear cell carcinoma showed upregulation of hepatocyte nuclear factor (HNF)-1β, versican, and other markers related to oxidative stress (Yamaguchi, 2010). HNF-1β is a transcription factor, involved in the regulation of glucose homeostasis and glycogen accumulation, normally expressed in the liver and other organs, which is assumed to have some role in the pathogenesis of clear cell carcinoma of the ovary (Kobayashi, 2009). Recently, a novel attempt to classify histological subtypes using a small number of biomarkers has been applied to ovarian cancers. A tissue microarray-based analysis selected 21 markers, including CA125, estrogen receptor (ER), insulin-like growth factor 2 (IGF2), Ki-67, p21, p53, progesterone receptor (PGR), and Wilms tumor 1 (WT1), to distinguish histological subtypes; however, only three of the 21 markers could predict outcomes in only high-grade serous carcinoma patients (Koebel, 2008). More recently, however, Kalloger et al. succeeded in reproductively diagnosing five major subtypes of ovarian cancers (high-grade serous, clear cell, endometrioid, mucinous, and low-grade serous) using only nine markers: p16, DKK1 (a Wnt antagonist), HNF-1β, MDM2, PGR, trefoil factor 3 (TFF3), p53, vimentin, and WT1 (Kalloger, 2011). Immunohistochemical analysis of 155 cases by De Lair et al demonstrated that 89% of clear cell carcinoma had HNF-1β positive, ER, PGR, and WT1 negative phenotype (DeLair, 2011).

7. Prognosis of endometriosis-associated ovarian cancer

Clear cell adenocarcinoma is known to be associated with chemoresistancy and a poor prognosis (Itamochi, 2008). However, most reports analyzing the prognosis of endometriosis-associated ovarian carcinomas (including mostly endometrioid adenocarcinoma and few clear cell carcinoma samples) have shown that endometriosis-associated ovarian carcinomas presented at younger ages, in lower grades and stages, and had significantly better overall survival compared with age-matched controls without endometriosis (Erzen, 2001; Kumar, 2011; Melin, 2011 ; Orezzoli, 2008). However, recent studies from various countries indicate that clear cell carcinomas consist of heterogenous tumors with gene alterations, such as HER2 or Met gene amplification (Tan, 2011 ; Yamamoto, 2011; Yamashita, 2011). Therefore, clear cell carcinomas as a subtype are considered to have a worse prognosis than endometrioid adenocarcinomas, especially in Asian cases (Lee, 2011). Recently, the first international symposium of ovarian clear cell carcinoma concluded that although patients with low-stage clear cell carcinoma had a better prognosis than matched controls with high-grade serous carcinoma, high-stage clear cell carcinoma cases had the worst prognosis (Anglesio, 2010). Thus, alternative therapy, such as molecular targeted therapy, should be applied to these aggressive tumors, and a further understanding of the basic biology of the endometriosis-cancer progression, especially the role of oxidative stress, is necessary to prevent carcinogenesis in endometriosis patients (Aris, 2010).

8. Conclusion

We have reviewed the literature on endometriosis-associated ovarian cancer. Further studies are awaited to clarify the exact role of oxidative stress in carcinogenesis.

9. References

Anglesio, M. S., Carey, M. S., Koebel, M., MacKay, H. and Huntsman, D. G. (2010). Clear cell carcinoma of the ovary: A report from the first Ovarian Clear Cell Symposium, June 24th, 2010. *Gynecologic Oncology* 121, 407-415.

Aris, A. (2010). Endometriosis-associated ovarian cancer: A ten-year cohort study of women living in the Estrie Region of Quebec, Canada. *Journal of Ovarian Research* 3, 2.

Baiocchi, G., Kavanagh, J. J. and Wharton, J. T. (1990). Endometrioid Stromal Sarcomas Arising from Ovarian and Extraovarian Endometriosis - Report of 2 Cases and Review of the Literature. *Gynecologic Oncology* 36, 147-151.

Banz, C., Ungethuem, U., Kuban, R.-J., Diedrich, K., Lengyel, E. and Hornung, D. (2010). The molecular signature of endometriosis-associated endometrioid ovarian cancer differs significantly from endometriosis-independent endometrioid ovarian cancer. *Fertility and Sterility* 94, 1212-1217.

Bell, D. A. (2005). Origins and molecular pathology of ovarian cancer. *Modern Pathology* 18, S19-S32.

Bischoff, F. Z., Heard, M. and Simpson, J. L. (2002). Somatic DNA alterations in endometriosis: high frequency of chromosome 17 and p53 loss in late-stage endometriosis. *Journal of Reproductive Immunology* 55, 49-64.

Brinton, L. A., Gridley, G., Persson, I., Baron, J. and Bergqvist, A. (1997). Cancer risk after a hospital discharge diagnosis of endometriosis. *American Journal of Obstetrics and Gynecology* 176, 572-579.

Brooks, J. J. and Wheeler, J. E. (1977). Malignancy Arising in Extra-Gonadal Endometriosis - Case-Report and Summary of World Literature. *Cancer* 40, 3065-3073.

Campbell, I. G., Russell, S. E., Choong, D. Y. H., Montgomery, K. G., Ciavarella, M. L., Hooi, C. S. F., Cristiano, B. E., Pearson, R. B. and Phillips, W. A. (2004). Mutation of the PIK3CA gene in ovarian and breast cancer. *Cancer Research* 64, 7678-7681.

Cheng, C.-w., Licence, D., Cook, E., Luo, F., Arends, M. J., Smith, S. K., Print, C. G. and Charnock-Jones, D. S. (2011). Activation of mutated K-ras in donor endometrial epithelium and stroma promotes lesion growth in an intact immunocompetent murine model of endometriosis. *Journal of Pathology* 224, 261-269.

Cottreau, C. M., Ness, R. B., Modugno, F., Allen, G. O. and Goodman, M. T. (2003). Endometriosis and its treatment with danazol or lupron in relation to ovarian cancer. *Clinical Cancer Research* 9, 5142-5144.

Defrere, S., Van Langendonckt, A., Vaesen, S., Jouret, M., Ramos, R. G., Gonzalez, D. and Donnez, J. (2006). Iron overload enhances epithelial cell proliferation in endometriotic lesions induced in a murine model. *Human Reproduction* 21, 2810-2816.

DeLair, D., Oliva, E., Koebel, M., Macias, A., Gilks, C. B. and Soslow, R. A. (2011). Morphologic Spectrum of Immunohistochemically Characterized Clear Cell Carcinoma of the Ovary: A Study of 155 Cases. *American Journal of Surgical Pathology* 35, 36-44.

Dinulescu, D. M., Ince, T. A., Quade, B. J., Shafer, S. A., Crowley, D. and Jacks, T. (2005). Role of K-ras and Pten in the development of mouse models of endometriosis and endometrioid ovarian cancer. *Nature Medicine* 11, 63-70.

Erzen, M., Rakar, S., Klancar, B. and Syrjanen, K. (2001). Endometriosis-associated ovarian carcinoma (EAOC): An entity distinct from other ovarian carcinomas as suggested by a nested case-control study. *Gynecologic Oncology* 83, 100-108.

Fukunaga, M., Nomura, K., Ishikawa, E. and Ushigome, S. (1997). Ovarian atypical endometriosis: Its close association with malignant epithelial tumours. *Histopathology* 30, 249-255.

Hapangama, D. K., Turner, M. A., Drury, J. A., Quenby, S., Hart, A., Maddick, M., Martin-Ruiz, C. and von Zglinicki, T. (2009). Sustained replication in endometrium of women with endometriosis occurs without evoking a DNA damage response. *Human Reproduction* 24, 687-696.

Hapangama, D. K., Turner, M. A., Drury, J. A., Quenby, S., Saretzki, G., Martin-Ruiz, C. and Von Zglinicki, T. (2008). Endometriosis is associated with aberrant endometrial expression of telomerase and increased telomere length. *Human Reproduction* 23, 1511-1519.

Heaps, J. M., Nieberg, R. K. and Berek, J. S. (1990). Malignant Neoplasms Arising in Endometriosis. *Obstetrics and Gynecology* 75, 1023-1028.

Horiuchi, A., Itoh, K., Shimizu, M., Nakai, I., Yamazaki, T., Kimura, K., Suzuki, A., Shiozawa, I., Ueda, N. and Konishi, I. (2003). Toward understanding the natural history of ovarian carcinoma development: a clinicopathological approach. *Gynecologic Oncology* 88, 309-317.

Hu, Q., Akatsuka, S., Yamashita, Y., Ohara, H., Nagai, H., Okazaki, Y., Takahashi, T. and Toyokuni, S. (2010). Homozygous deletion of CDKN2A/2B is a hallmark of iron-induced high-grade rat mesothelioma. *Laboratory Investigation* 90, 360-373.

Irving, J. A., Clement, P. B. (2011). Diseases of the Peritoneum. *Blaustein's Pathology of the Female Genital Tract. Sixth Edition.*

Itamochi, H., Kigawa, J. and Terakawa, N. (2008). Mechanisms of chemoresistance and poor prognosis in ovarian clear cell carcinoma. *Cancer Science* 99, 653-658.

Jacques, S. M. and Lawrence, W. D. (1990). Endometrial Adenocarcinoma with Variable-Level Myometrial Involvement Limited to Adenomyosis - a Clinicopathological Study of 23 Cases. *Gynecologic Oncology* 37, 401-407.

Jiang, X. X., Hitchcock, A., Bryan, E. J., Watson, R. H., Englefield, P., Thomas, E. J. and Campbell, I. G. (1996). Microsatellite analysis of endometriosis reveals loss of heterozygosity at candidate ovarian tumor suppressor gene loci. *Cancer Research* 56, 3534-3539.

Jiang, X. X., Morland, S. J., Hitchcock, A., Thomas, E. J. and Campbell, I. G. (1998). Allelotyping of endometriosis with adjacent ovarian carcinoma reveals evidence of a common lineage. *Cancer Research* 58, 1707-1712.

Jimbo, H., Hitomi, Y., Yoshikawa, H., Yano, T., Momoeda, M., Sakamoto, A., Tsutsumi, O., Taketani, Y. and Esumi, H. (1997). Evidence for monoclonal expansion of epithelial cells in ovarian endometrial cysts. *American Journal of Pathology* 150, 1173-1178.

Jones, S., Wang, T.-L., Shih, I.-M., Mao, T.-L., Nakayama, K., Roden, R., Glas, R., Slamon, D., Diaz, L. A., Jr., Vogelstein, B., Kinzler, K. W., Velculescu, V. E. and Papadopoulos, N. (2010). Frequent Mutations of Chromatin Remodeling Gene ARID1A in Ovarian Clear Cell Carcinoma. *Science* 330, 228-231.

Kalloger, S. E., Koebel, M., Leung, S., Mehl, E., Gao, D., Marcon, K. M., Chow, C., Clarke, B. A., Huntsman, D. G. and Gilks, C. B. (2011). Calculator for ovarian carcinoma subtype prediction. *Modern Pathology* 24, 512-521.

Kobayashi, H., Sumimoto, K., Moniwa, N., Imai, M., Takakura, K., Kuromaki, T., Morioka, E., Arisawa, K. and Terao, T. (2007). Risk of developing ovarian cancer among women with ovarian endometrioma: a cohort study in Shizuoka, Japan. *International Journal of Gynecological Cancer* 17, 37-43.

Kobayashi, H., Yamada, Y., Kanayama, S., Furukawa, N., Noguchi, T., Haruta, S., Yoshida, S., Sakata, M., Sado, T. and Oi, H. (2009). The Role of Hepatocyte Nuclear Factor-1 beta in the Pathogenesis of Clear Cell Carcinoma of the Ovary. *International Journal of Gynecological Cancer* 19, 471-479.

Koebel, M., Kalloger, S. E., Boyd, N., McKinney, S., Mehl, E., Palmer, C., Leung, S., Bowen, N. J., Ionescu, D. N., Rajput, A., Prentice, L. M., Miller, D., Santos, J., Swenerton, K., Gilks, C. B. and Huntsman, D. (2008). Ovarian Carcinoma Subtypes Are Different Diseases: Implications for Biomarker Studies. *PLoS Medicine* 5, 1749-1760.

Koerner, M., Burckhardt, E. and Mazzucchelli, L. (2006). Higher frequency of chromosomal aberrations in ovarian endometriosis compared to extragonadal endometriosis: a possible link to endometrioid adenocarcinoma. *Modern Pathology* 19, 1615-1623.

Kucera, E., Hejda, V., Dankovcik, R., Valha, P., Dudas, M. and Feyereisl, J. (2011). Malignant changes in adenomyosis in patients with endometrioid adenocarcinoma. *European Journal of Gynaecological Oncology* 32, 182-184.

Kumar, S., Munkarah, A., Arabi, H., Bandyopadhyay, S., Semaan, A., Hayek, K., Garg, G., Morris, R. and Ali-Fehmi, R. (2011). Prognostic analysis of ovarian cancer associated with endometriosis. *American Journal of Obstetrics and Gynecology* 204, 7.

Kuo, K. T., Mao, T. L., Jones, S., Veras, E., Ayhan, A., Wang, T. L., Glas, R., Slamon, D., Velculescu, V. E., Kuman, R. J. and Shih, I. M. (2009). Frequent Activating Mutations of PIK3CA in Ovarian Clear Cell Carcinoma. *American Journal of Pathology* 174, 1597-1601.

Kurman, R. J. and Shih, I.-M. (2010). The Origin and Pathogenesis of Epithelial Ovarian Cancer: A Proposed Unifying Theory. *American Journal of Surgical Pathology* 34, 433-443.

Kurman, R. J. and Shih, I. M. (2011). Molecular pathogenesis and extraovarian origin of epithelial ovarian cancer-Shifting the paradigm. *Human Pathology* 42, 918-931.

Lagrenade, A. and Silverberg, S. G. (1988). Ovarian-Tumors Associated with Atypical Endometriosis. *Human Pathology* 19, 1080-1084.

Lee, K. R. and Nucci, M. R. (2003). Ovarian mucinous and mixed epithelial carcinomas of mullerian (endocervical-like) type: A clinicopathologic analysis of four cases of an uncommon variant associated with endometriosis. *International Journal of Gynecological Pathology* 22, 42-51.

Lee, Y.-Y., Kim, T.-J., Kim, M.-J., Kim, H.-J., Song, T., Kim, M. K., Choi, C. H., Lee, J.-W., Bae, D.-S. and Kim, B.-G. (2011). Prognosis of ovarian clear cell carcinoma compared to other histological subtypes: A meta-analysis. *Gynecologic Oncology* 122, 541-547.

Lousse, J.-C., Defrere, S., Van Langendonckt, A., Gras, J., Gonzalez-Ramos, R., Colette, S. and Donnez, J. (2009). Iron storage is significantly increased in peritoneal macrophages of endometriosis patients and correlates with iron overload in peritoneal fluid. *Fertility and Sterility* 91, 1668-1675.

Lousse, J.-C., Van Langendonckt, A., Gonzalez-Ramos, R., Defrere, S., Renkin, E. and Donnez, J. (2008). Increased activation of nuclear factor-kappa B (NF-kappa B) in isolated peritoneal macrophages of patients with, endometriosis. *Fertility and Sterility* 90, 217-220.

Martini, M., Ciccarone, M., Garganese, G., Maggiore, C., Evangelista, A., Rahimi, S., Zannoni, G., Vittori, G. and Larocca, L. M. (2002). Possible involvement of hMLH1, p16(INK4a) and PTEN in the malignant transformation of endometriosis. *International Journal of Cancer* 102, 398-406.

Mayr, D., Amann, G., Siefert, C., Diebold, J. and Anderegg, B. (2003). Does endometriosis really have premalignant potential? A clonal analysis of laser-microdissected tissue. *Faseb Journal* 17, 693-+.

McConechy, M. K., Anglesio, M. S., Kalloger, S. E., Yang, W., Senz, J., Chow, C., Heravi-Moussavi, A., Morin, G. B., Mes-Masson, A.-M., Carey, M. S., McAlpine, J. N., Kwon, J. S., Prentice, L. M., Boyd, N., Shah, S. P., Gilks, C. B. and Huntsman, D. G. (2011). Subtype-specific mutation of PPP2R1A in endometrial and ovarian carcinomas. *Journal of Pathology* 223, 567-573.

Melin, A., Lundholm, C., Malki, N., Swahn, M. L., Sparen, P. and Bergqvist, A. (2011). Endometriosis as a prognostic factor for cancer survival. *International Journal of Cancer* 129, 948-955.

Milner, B. J., Allan, L. A., Eccles, D. M., Kitchener, H. C., Leonard, R. C. F., Kelly, K. F., Parkin, D. E. and Haites, N. E. (1993). P53 Mutation Is a Common Genetic Event in Ovarian-Carcinoma. *Cancer Research* 53, 2128-2132.

Mizuuchi, H., Nasim, S., Kudo, R., Silverberg, S. G., Greenhouse, S. and Garrett, C. T. (1992). Clinical Implications of K-Ras Mutations in Malignant Epithelial Tumors of the Endometrium. *Cancer Research* 52, 2777-2781.

Modesitt, S. C., Tortoler-Luna, G., Robinson, J. B., Gershenson, D. M. and Wolf, J. K. (2002). Ovarian and extraovarian endometriosis-associated cancer. *Obstetrics and Gynecology* 100, 788-795.

Murphy, A. A., Santanam, N. and Parthasarathy, S. (1998). Endometriosis: A disease of oxidative stress? *Seminars in Reproductive Endocrinology* 16, 263-273.

Nagle, C. M., Olsen, C. M., Webb, P. M., Jordan, S. J., Whiteman, D. C. and Green, A. C. (2008). Endometrioid and clear cell ovarian cancers - A comparative analysis of risk factors. *European Journal of Cancer* 44, 2477-2484.

Ness, R. B. and Cottreau, C. (1999). Possible role of ovarian epithelial inflammation in ovarian cancer. *Journal of the National Cancer Institute* 91, 1459-1467.

Ness, R. B., Grisso, J. A., Cottreau, C., Klapper, J., Vergona, R., Wheeler, J. E., Morgan, M. and Schlesselman, J. J. (2000). Factors related to inflammation of the ovarian epithelium and risk of ovarian cancer. *Epidemiology* 11, 111-117.

Nezhat, F., Cohen, C., Rahaman, J., Gretz, H., Cole, P. and Kalir, T. (2002). Comparative immunohistochemical studies of bcl-2 and p53 proteins in benign and malignant ovarian endometriotic cysts. *Cancer* 94, 2935-2940.

Nezhat, F., Datta, M. S., Hanson, V., Pejovic, T., Nezhat, C. and Nezhat, C. (2008). The relationship of endometriosis and ovarian malignancy: a review. *Fertility and Sterility* 90, 1559-1570.

Ngo, C., Chereau, C., Nicco, C., Weill, B., Chapron, C. and Batteux, F. (2009). Reactive Oxygen Species Controls Endometriosis Progression. *American Journal of Pathology* 175, 225-234.

Nyiraneza, C., Marbaix, E., Smets, M., Galant, C., Sempoux, C. and Dahan, K. (2010). High risk for neoplastic transformation of endometriosis in a carrier of lynch syndrome. *Familial Cancer* 9, 383-387.

Ogawa, S., Kaku, T., Amada, S., Kobayashi, H., Hirakawa, T., Ariyoshi, K., Kamura, T. and Nakano, H. (2000). Ovarian endometriosis associated with ovarian carcinoma: A clinicopathological and immunohistochemical study. *Gynecologic Oncology* 77, 298-304.

Okuda, T., Otsuka, J., Sekizawa, A., Saito, H., Makino, R., Kushima, M., Farina, A., Kuwano, Y. and Okai, T. (2003). p53 mutations and overexpression affect prognosis of ovarian endometrioid cancer but not clear cell cancer. *Gynecologic Oncology* 88, 318-325.

Orezzoli, J. P., Russell, A. H., Oliva, E., Del Carmen, M. G., Eichhorn, J. and Fuller, A. F. (2008). Prognostic implication of endometriosis in clear cell carcinoma of the ovary. *Gynecologic Oncology* 110, 336-344.

Palacios, J. and Gamallo, C. (1998). Mutations in the beta-catenin gene (CTNNB1) in endometrioid ovarian carcinomas. *Cancer Research* 58, 1344-1347.

Postoloff, A. V. and Rodenberg, T. A. (1955). Malignant Transition in Ovarian Endometriosis. *American Journal of Obstetrics and Gynecology* 69, 83-86.

Prowse, A. H., Fakis, G., Manek, S., Churchman, M., Edwards, S., Rowan, A., Koninckx, P., Kennedy, S. and Tomlinson, I. P. M. (2005). Allelic loss studies do not provide evidence for the "endometriosis-as-tumor" theory. *Fertility and Sterility* 83, 1134-1143.

Ren F, W. D., Jiang Y, Ren F (2011). Epigenetic inactivation of hMLH1 in the malignant transformation of ovarian endometriosis. *Archives of Gynecology and Obstetrics.* [Epub ahead of print].

Sampson, J. A. (1925). Endometrial carcinoma of the ovary, arising in endometrial tissue in that organ. *Archives of Surgery* 10, 1-72.

Sato, N., Tsunoda, H., Nishida, M., Morishita, Y., Takimoto, Y., Kubo, T. and Noguchi, M. (2000). Loss of heterozygosity on 10q23.3 and mutation of the tumor suppressor gene PTEN in benign endometrial cyst of the ovary: Possible sequence progression from benign endometrial cyst to endometrioid carcinoma and clear cell carcinoma of the ovary. *Cancer Research* 60, 7052-7056.

Schmeler, K. M. and Lu, K. H. (2008). Gynecologic cancers associated with Lynch syndrome/HNPCC. *Clinical & Translational Oncology* 10, 313-317.

Scott, R. B. (1953). Malignant Changes in Endometriosis. *Obstetrics and Gynecology* 2, 283-289.

Slavin, R. E., Krum, R. and Van Dinh, T. (2000). Endometriosis-associated intestinal tumors: A clinical and pathological study of 6 cases with a review of the literature. *Human Pathology* 31, 456-463.

Staats, P. N., Clement, P. B. and Young, R. H. (2007). Primary endometrioid adenocarcinoma of the vagina - A clinicopathologic study of 18 cases. *American Journal of Surgical Pathology* 31, 1490-1501.

Tan, D. S. P., Iravani, M., McCluggage, W. G., Lambros, M. B. K., Milanezi, F., Mackay, A., Gourley, C., Geyer, F. C., Vatcheva, R., Millar, J., Thomas, K., Natrajan, R., Savage, K., Fenwick, K., Williams, A., Jameson, C., El-Bahrawy, M., Gore, M. E., Gabra, H., Kaye, S. B., Ashworth, A. and Reis-Filho, J. S. (2011). Genomic Analysis Reveals the Molecular Heterogeneity of Ovarian Clear Cell Carcinomas. *Clinical Cancer Research* 17, 1521-1534.

Tashiro, H., Blazes, M. S., Wu, R., Cho, K. R., Bose, S., Wang, S. I., Li, J., Parsons, R. and Ellenson, L. H. (1997). Mutations in PTEN are frequent in endometrial carcinoma but rare in other common gynecological malignancies. *Cancer Research* 57, 3935-3940.

Toyokuni, S. (2009). Role of iron in carcinogenesis: Cancer as a ferrotoxic disease. *Cancer Science* 100, 9-16.

Uno, S., Zembutsu, H., Hirasawa, A., Takahashi, A., Kubo, M., Akahane, T., Aoki, D., Kamatani, N., Hirata, K. and Nakamura, Y. (2010). A genome-wide association study identifies genetic variants in the CDKN2BAS locus associated with endometriosis in Japanese. *Nature Genetics* 42, 707-U788.

Van Langendonckt, A., Casanas-Roux, F., Dolmans, M.-M. and Donnez, J. (2002a). Potential involvement of hemoglobin and heme in the pathogenesis of peritoneal endometriosis. *Fertility and Sterility* 77, 561-570.

Van Langendonckt, A., Casanas-Roux, F. and Donnez, J. (2002b). Iron overload in the peritoneal cavity of women with pelvic endometriosis. *Fertility and Sterility* 78, 712-718.

Van Langendonckt, A., Casanas-Roux, F., Eggermont, J. and Donnez, J. (2004). Characterization of iron deposition in endometriotic lesions induced in the nude mouse model. *Human Reproduction* 19, 1265-1271.

Veras, E., Mao, T.-L., Ayhan, A., Ueda, S., Lai, H., Hayran, M., Shih, I.-M. and Kurman, R. J. (2009). Cystic and Adenofibromatous Clear Cell Carcinomas of the Ovary Distinctive Tumors That Differ in Their Pathogenesis and Behavior: A Clinicopothologic Analysis of 122 Cases. *American Journal of Surgical Pathology* 33, 844-853.

Vestergaard AL, T. K., Knudsen UB, Munk T, Rosbach H, Poulsen JB, Guldberg P, Martensen PM. (2011). Oncogenic events associated with endometrial and ovarian cancers are rare in endometriosis. *Molecular Human Reproduction* [Epub ahead of print].

Wiegand, K. C., Lee, A. F., Al-Agha, O. M., Chow, C., Kalloger, S. E., Scott, D. W., Steidl, C., Wiseman, S. M., Gascoyne, R. D., Gilks, B. and Huntsman, D. G. (2011). Loss of BAF250a (ARID1A) is frequent in high-grade endometrial carcinomas. *Journal of Pathology* 224, 328-333.

Wiegand, K. C., Shah, S. P., Al-Agha, O. M., Zhao, Y., Tse, K., Zeng, T., Senz, J., McConechy, M. K., Anglesio, M. S., Kalloger, S. E., Yang, W., Heravi-Moussavi, A., Giuliany, R., Chow, C., Fee, J., Zayed, A., Prentice, L., Melnyk, N., Turashvili, G., Delaney, A. D., Madore, J., Yip, S., McPherson, A. W., Ha, G., Bell, L., Fereday, S., Tam, A., Galletta, L., Tonin, P. N., Provencher, D., Miller, D., Jones, S. J. M., Moore, R. A., Morin, G. B., Oloumi, A., Boyd, N., Aparicio, S. A., Shih, I.-M., Mes-Masson, A.-M., Bowtell, D. D., Hirst, M., Gilks, B., Marra, M. A. and Huntsman, D. G. (2010). ARID1A Mutations in Endometriosis-Associated Ovarian Carcinomas. *New England Journal of Medicine* 363, 1532-1543.

Wu, R., Hendrix-Lucas, N., Kuick, R., Zhai, Y., Schwartz, D. R., Akyol, A., Hanash, S., Misek, D. E., Katabuchi, H., Williams, B. O., Fearon, E. R. and Cho, K. R. (2007). Mouse model of human ovarian endometrioid adenocarcinoma based on somatic defects in the Wnt/beta-catenin and PI3K/Pten signaling pathways. *Cancer Cell* 11, 321-333.

Yamaguchi, K., Mandai, M., Oura, T., Matsumura, N., Hamanishi, J., Baba, T., Matsui, S., Murphy, S. K. and Konishi, I. (2010). Identification of an ovarian clear cell carcinoma gene signature that reflects inherent disease biology and the carcinogenic processes. *Oncogene* 29, 1741-1752.

Yamaguchi, K., Mandai, M., Toyokuni, S., Hamanishi, J., Higuchi, T., Takakura, K. and Fujii, S. (2008). Contents of endometriotic cysts, especially the high concentration of free iron, are a possible cause of carcinogenesis in the cysts through the iron-induced persistent oxidative stress. *Clinical Cancer Research* 14, 32-40.

Yamamoto, S., Tsuda, H., Miyai, K., Takano, M., Tamai, S. and Matsubara, O. (2011). Gene amplification and protein overexpression of MET are common events in ovarian clear-cell adenocarcinoma: their roles in tumor progression and prognostication of the patient. *Modern Pathology* 24, 1146-1155.

Yamashita, Y., Yatabe, Y., Akatsuka, S., Kajiyama, H., Kikkawa, F. ,Takahashi, T., and Toyokuni, S. (2011) MET amplification is a molecular hallmark in endometriosis-associated ovarian clear cell carcinoma and correlates with worse prognosis. *European Journal of Cancer* 47, S529-S529

Yantiss, R. K., Clement, P. B. and Young, R. H. (2000). Neoplastic and pre-neoplastic changes in gastrointestinal endometriosis - A study of 17 cases. *American Journal of Surgical Pathology* 24, 513-524.

Yoshikawa, H., Jimbo, H., Okada, S., Matsumoto, K., Onda, T., Yasugi, T. and Taketani, Y. (2000). Prevalence of endometriosis in ovarian cancer. *Gynecologic and Obstetric Investigation* 50, 11-15.

Zighelboim, I., Schmidt, A. P., Gao, F., Thaker, P. H., Powell, M. A., Rader, J. S., Gibb, R. K., Mutch, D. G. and Goodfellow, P. J. (2009). ATR Mutation in Endometrioid Endometrial Cancer Is Associated With Poor Clinical Outcomes. *Journal of Clinical Oncology* 27, 3091-3096.

17

Alteration in Endometrial Remodeling: A Cause for Implantation Failure in Endometriosis?

Saikat K. Jana, Priyanka Banerjee, Shyam Thangaraju,
Baidyanath Chakravarty and Koel Chaudhury
*Indian Institute of Technology, Kharagpur,
India*

1. Introduction

1.1 Implantation failure in endometriosis

The process of implantation is an interactive cascade of events between the embryo and the endometrium. It is a dynamic process consisting of three distinct phases. They are (i) apposition of embryo (ii) attachment with the epithelial lining of the endometrium and (iii) invasion into the endometrial stroma gaining access to the maternal circulatory system. Embryo implantation failure may occur due to embryonic defect or unsupportive endometrium. Advances in Assisted Reproductive Technology (ART) have made it possible to obtain good quality embryos; however, successful implantation remains the bottleneck for a successful pregnancy. The endometrium remodels before attaining a state of receptivity. Endometrium remains receptive during a limited period, when it is favourable for blastocyst attachment and implantation. In women, there is clinical evidence of a brief period of optimal uterine receptivity which allows for blastocyst implantation. This period, called the implantation window, is related to changes in the endometrial epithelial morphology. Inappropriate morphological development leads to unreceptive endometrium that causes defective endometrial /embryonic cross talk. This is generally agreed to be one of the main reasons for implantation failure. Endometriosis, characterized by benign growth of endometrial tissue outside the uterus, affects approximately 20%-48% of women during their reproductive years. The occurrence of aberrant hormonal, immunological, genetic and pathophysiological events associated with endometriosis is attributed to the heterogeneous etiology of the disease. The symptoms of endometriosis do not depend on the severity or stage of the disease. Women with even mildest degree of endometriosis can have a 3 - 4 fold reduction in their annual birth rate compared to normal non-endometriotic women.

Presence of endometriosis alters the characteristic of the endometrium. It also affects the expression of various factors and markers of receptivity during implantation window. All these result in dysfunctional endometrium. This can be a cause of higher implantation failure rates and lower pregnancy rates in endometriotic women due to failure of embryo implantation. However, alterations in endometrial remodeling in endometriosis resulting in impairment of the endometrial receptivity is still poorly understood. An understanding of endometrial receptivity in women with endometriosis is, therefore, crucial in understanding the fundamental causes of implantation failure which in turn, may have significant implications on fertility potential of these women.

2. Matrix turnover and angiogenesis during implantation

2.1 Matrix turnover in endometrium and implantation

The unique characteristic of the endometrial tissue is that it undergoes cyclic degeneration and regeneration in each menstrual cycle. The endometrium consists of a layer of columnar epithelium bedded on a layer of connective tissue. The extracellular matrix (ECM), which forms a component of the connective tissue, provides the scaffolding for the anchorage of the cells within the tissue (McIntush and Smith 1998) and presents a locale for cellular migration, division and differentiation (Birkedal-Hansen et al., 1993). The extensive remodeling of the connective tissue of the endometrium requires both the degradation and reformation of the ECM which is accomplished by highly regulated turnover of the ECM (Hulboy et al., 1997). This destruction of the ECM occurs by the action of a class of proteolytic enzyme identified as matrix metalloproteinases (MMP). MMPs and the tissue inhibitors of metalloproteinases (TIMP) regulate a number of aspects of reproductive physiology like dynamic remodeling of the ovary and endometrium throughout each menstrual cycle, implantation, embryonic development and parturition. There exists equilibrium between the MMPs and TIMPs action for controlling this turnover of the ECM. Any circumstances that may bring about interruption of this delicate balance leads to a number of pathological complexities related to pregnancy and infertility like luteinized unruptured follicle syndrome, ovarian cysts, endometriosis, uterine fibroids, inappropriate implantation resulting in tubal pregnancy or spontaneous abortion, premature rupture of fetal membranes, or carcinoma of the ovary or uterus (Curry and Osteen 2003).

Several studies have reported the diverse pattern of MMPs expression in the endometrium throughout the menstrual cycle. Since breakdown of the endometrial lining occurs during menstruation, several MMPs are reported to be highly expressed during this phase. However, their expression gradually falls off during rest of the cycle. Nevertheless various MMPs are observed to express at various phases of the cycling endometrium. Expression of MMP-2 remains consistent throughout the whole cycle along with TIMP-1 and TIMP-2. Endometrial MMP-9 expression shows a cyclical change in its distribution between glandular and stromal cells. It expresses in the endometrium throughout the cycle, however, its expression increases during midsecretory phase particularly in the glandular cells (Hulboy et al., 1997). Although the association of MMP-2 and -9 and their endogenous inhibitors in pathogenesis of infertile condition like endometriosis is well established (Salata et al., 2008), knowledge regarding their involvement in endometrial remodelling during implantation window in endometriotic women is limited.

2.2 Angiogenesis

Endometrial remodeling involves proliferation of its functional layer upon estrogen enhancement (Groothuis et al., 2007) and differentiation by the influence of progesterone from the luteinized follicles (Okada et al., 1999). This is followed by the degeneration of this superficial layer and again reconstruction of the new one. These constant cyclic changes of the endometrium are associated with angiogenesis and neovascularisation (Perrot-Applanat et al., 2000). Vascular endothelial growth factor (VEGF) is a prime angiogenic stimulus for vascular permeability based on its capability to bring on vascular leakage (Ferrara and Davis-Smyth 1997, Ferrara et al., 2003). VEGF regulated angiogenesis and neovasculogenesis of the endometrial tissue is elemental for the growth and differentiation of the endometrium for implantation and placentation (Giudice 1996, Perrot-Applanat 2000). Due to its control over the human reproductive cycle, VEGF is present in the stromal and glandular epithelium of the human endometrium throughout all phases of the menstrual cycle (Torry and Torry 1997, Smith 1998, Shifren et al., 1996, Charnock-Jones 1993, Popovici 1999, Lockwood 2002). However there exists a strong debate regarding its expression and angiogenesis. VEGF expression increased in the late secretory phase and heightened during menses (Torry and Torry 1997, Charnock-Jones 1993, Popovici 1999, Lockwood 2002, Bausero 1998). There is a marked increase even in the vascular network of the endometrium during the secretory phase over the proliferative phase (Ota 1998). But Nayak and Brenner reported that during proliferative phase there is a noted increase in the VEGF expression in stroma which shifts to glandular epithelium during the secretory phase (Nayak and Brenner 2002). However, contradictory report exist indicating that a gradual decline in angiogenesis occurs at the end of the cycle which rapidly increases with the start of a new cycle and reaching a maximum height during the mid cycle (Au and Rogers 1993). Other investigators have suggested that VEGF expression remains inconsistent (Sugino et al., 2002) or there is no change in the vascularity throughout the endometrial cycle (Rogers and Au 1993).

2.3 Regulation of matrix remodeling

It is suggested that inappropriate regulation of sex steroids may lead to defect in implantation. The role of estradiol in embryo implantation is a subject of controversy and its association with pregnancy outcome in IVF cycle is an area of research for many years (Kyrou et al 2009). Several studies have shown that midluteal decline of serum estradiol do not affect the endometrial development, embryo implantation and IVF outcome (Friedler et al., 2005; Narvekar et al., 2010; Hung et al., 2000). This may be due to the fact that during follicular phase, estradiol induces growth of follicles, preparation of endometrium and production of specific proteins, growth factors and receptors of estrogen and progesterone. Additionally, adverse effect of high estradiol level on endometrial receptivity is still under debate (Kyrou et al., 2009). A number of investigators found no effect of high estradiol levels on the treatment outcome of IVF/ICSI cycle (Sharara and McClamrock 1999, Kosmas et al., 2004). Some studies have, however, suggested that elevated levels of estradiol may be responsible for impaired endometrial receptivity (Simon et al., 1995; Valbuena et al., 2001; Kyrou et al., 2009). After ovulation, progesterone is the main contributory sex hormone executing the transformation of the endometrium during the secretory phase.

It is evidenced that expression of cyclooxygenase-2 (COX-2), a molecule associated with angiogenesis and cell differentiation, promotes the release of MMP-2 (Xiong et al., 2005) and -9 (Itatsu et al., 2009), and angiogenic factor VEGF (Wang *et al.* (2010). COX-2, on the other hand, is regulated by female sexual hormone estradiol and progesterone (Li et al., 2007). Since the process of angiogenesis during endometrial remodelling shares similarities with the process of angiogenesis during metastasis in cancer, estradiol may also be involved in the up-regulation of the gene expression of COX-2 and MMPs during embryo implantation. Involvement of COX-2 gene in embryo implantation is a subject of interest among the researchers working on endometrial receptivity, and is suggested to play an important regulatory role in successful implantation. However, little is known about its role in endometrial receptivity in women with endometriosis.

2.4 Endometrial receptivity markers

Inadequate uterine receptivity and poor embryo formation are two major factors responsible for implantation failure (Simon et al., 1998; Ledee-Bataille et al., 2002). Nowadays, using

ART procedure, clinicians can improve embryo formation considerably; however, no therapies are available to make the endometrium more receptive. Expression of various implantation markers and proteins lead to remodeling of the endometrial matrix thereby transforming the endometrium towards a receptive milieu. Several molecular repertoires expressed during the implantation window are considered to be useful markers of implantation. Expression of various markers including pinopodes $\alpha_v\beta_3$ integrin, LIF, L-selectin ligand and Mucin-1 throughout the different stages of implantation are considered to be responsible for endometrial receptivity.

2.4.1 Pinopodes

Pinopodes, also known as uterodomes, are large cytoplasmic protrusions from the endometrial epithelial surface and are several micrometers wide. These are specialized cell structures that are involved in adhesion and penetration of the blastocyst into the stroma. These structures project into the uterine lumen and are above the microvilli level. Their expression is limited to a maximum period of 2 days during the menstrual cycle corresponding to the presumed window of implantation (Stavreus-Evers et al., 2001). Endometrial pinopodes development is associated with the mid-luteal phase increased expression of leukaemia inhibitory factor (LIF) and its receptor (Aghajanova et al., 2003), progesterone (Stavreus-Evers et al., 2001) and integrin $\alpha v\beta_3$ (Lessey et al., 1992). Advocated as a marker of uterine receptivity, their expression, has been investigated solely by means of scanning electron microscopy (SEM) (Develioglu et al., 2000).

2.4.2 Integrins

Integrins are surface ligands, usually glycoproteins, belonging to the class of cell adhesion molecules (CAM). An integrin molecule consists of two different, non-covalently linked α and β subunits that are paired to form various heterodimers with distinct function (Hynes, 2002). At least 20 types of integrin heterodimer have been defined, which form from 14α and 9β subunits (Lindhard 2002). Integrins are unusual cell surface receptors in that they bind with low affinity and are present in large numbers, allowing for ligand motility without loss of attachment. Endometrial epithelial cells constitutively express certain integrins, whereas others are cycle dependent (Lessey 1992). $\alpha_v\beta_3$, an example of the latter is present on the apical surface of both luminal endometrial cells and human embryos. 41 different aberrant expressions of this integrin are reported in women with endometriosis (Lessey et al., 1994).

2.4.3 LIF

LIF is a member of the IL-6 family and is secreted by the endometrial epithelium, CD16– CD56 natural killer cells and type 2 T-helper cells. Animal and human studies indicate that LIF plays an important role in implantation and for pregnancy to occur (Lass et al., 2001). LIF protein can be detected by immunohistochemistry in the luminal, glandular and stromal epithelium. There is very little LIF expression in proliferative endometrium, but levels increase during the secretory phase, reaching a maximum between days 19 and 25, which coincides with the implantation window (Charnock-Jones 1994).

2.4.4 Mucins

Mucins are high molecular weight (MW) glycoproteins, which contain at least 50% of carbohydrate O-linked to a threonine/serine rich peptide core (Gendler et al., 1990). Among the 14 cloned human mucins, only Mucin-1 (MUC1) and to a lesser extent MUC6 have been found in the human endometrium (Gipson et al., 1997). Cell-cell and cell-matrix adhesion are inhibited in direct correlation to the length of the MUC-1 ectodomain (Hilkens et al., 1992; Wesseling et al., 1996).

2.4.5 L-Selectin ligand

Selectins are glycoproteins which also belong to the CAM family. The expression of selectin oligosaccharide-based ligands, such as MECA-79 or HECA-452, is up-regulated during the window of implantation (Genbacev et al., 2003). MECA-79 is immunolocalized in the luminal and glandular endometrial epithelium throughout the menstrual cycle, although the staining considerably intensifies during the mid-secretory phase. The physiological importance of the interaction between L-selectin and its oligosaccharide ligands has been investigated in the human endometrium (Genbacev et al., 2003).

Though several studies investigating endometrial receptivity during implantation window are documented, the mechanism responsible for implantation failure in endometriosis is still poorly understood. Expression of various cell adhesion molecules and pinopodes in women with endometriosis is explored in the present study. Since, COX-2 is reported to be physiologically involved in the process of angiogenesis (Matsumoto et al., 2002), and in view of the fact that angiogenesis is essential for endometrial remodeling, we were motivated to assess the expression of various angiogenic factors including VEGFR, MMP-2,-9 and their tissue inhibitors in women with endometriosis during the implantation window. Additionally, expression of COX-2 was studied to assess their associated regulatory role in the process of endometrial remodeling during implantation window.

2.5 Material and method

2.5.1 Subject selection

30 women with endometriosis and 20 without the disease were included in the study. Presence/absence of endometriosis was confirmed by diagnostic laparoscopy. It was ensured that these women had not received any kind of medical or hormonal treatment during the past three months. Women with history of chocolate cyst removal, previous history of any surgery, with other possible causes of pain or pelvic pathology including pelvic tuberculosis were excluded.

2.5.2 Sample collection

Blood samples collected from patients were allowed to clot and the serum separated by centrifugation at 3,000 rpm for 5 min at 4°C. Serum samples were stored at -20°C until further use. Endometrial biopsy was performed on the 7th day after confirmation of ovulation. The collected tissue was washed in phosphate buffer saline (PBS) and divided into three parts: one part was used for stromal and epithelial cells isolation for flow cytometric analysis of different molecular repertoires of the endometrium, the other part was fixed for immunohistochemistry (IHC) and scanning electron microscopy of these receptivity markers. From the third part, RNA was isolated immediately.

2.5.3 Isolation of cells and flow cytometric analysis

Endometrial tissue was first digested in 2% collagenase-1 (Invitrogen, Grand Island, NY, USA) in DMEM (Himedia, Mumbai, India) for 1.5 to 2 hrs at 37°C and then centrifuged to isolate the stromal cells. Undigested glands were then treated with 0.25% trypsin-0.02% EDTA (Himedia, Mumbai, India) for 4–8min, washed with 10% FBS-DMEM. Single epithelial cells were isolated by centrifugation, as described previously. Isolated cells were washed, RBC lysed using RBC lysis solution and fixed in 2% paraformaldehyde (20 min at RT). Single cell suspension thus obtained was divided into five parts; four parts were stained with mouse anti-human $\alpha_v\beta_3$ integrin, LIF (R&D Systems, Minneapolis, MN, USA), Muc-1 (Abcam, Cambridge, UK) and rat anti-human MECA-79 monoclonal antibody (Santa Cruz 1 Biotechnology, Inc., Santa Cruz, California, USA) according to instructions provided by the manufacturer in the manual. The fifth part remained unstained. Excess antibodies were washed out and the cells again incubated with fluorescein conjugated secondary goat anti-mouse and anti-rat IgG (R&D Systems, Minneapolis, MN, USA). After washing excess antibodies, the stained cells were analyzed using flow cytometer (BD FACS Calibur™, BD Biosciences, San Jose, CA, USA).

2.5.4 Immunohistochemistry

3-5 μm thick sections obtained from formaldehyde fixed, paraffin-embedded tissue were dehydrated in graded ethanol. After antigen retrieval, slides were blocked using 3% BSA in PBS and incubated with mouse anti-human αvβ3 integrin (R&D Systems, Minneapolis, MN, USA), Muc-1 (Abcam, Cambridge, UK), LIF and rat anti-human MECA-79 monoclonal antibody (Santa Cruz biotechnology, INC., Santa Cruz, California, USA). Excess primary antibody was washed with PBS and the sections were again incubated with anti-mouse and anti-rat biotinylated secondary antibody (Santa Cruz biotechnology, INC., Santa Cruz, California, USA) according to the manufacturer's protocol, before incubation with avidin biotinylated horseradish peroxidase (Santa Cruz biotechnology, INC., Santa Cruz, California, USA). Labeled cells were visualized with Diaminobenzidine (DAB) and sections counterstained with hematoxylin. Next, the slides were dehydrated using series of alcohol gradient and mounted using distrene, tricresyl phosphate (DPX) and xylene. The slides were then examined under bright field microscope (Carl Zeiss, Jena, Germany).

2.5.5 Scanning electron microscopy

Formaldehyde-fixed tissues were washed in PBS and dehydrated in a series of alcohol gradient (50%, 70%, 90%, 95%, 100%), each for 10 mins, dipped in HMDS (1,1,1,3,3,3-hexamethyl disilazane; SRL, Bombay, India) and air dried. Dried tissues were then mounted and coated with gold and the luminal endometrial surface thoroughly examined under SEM (Jeol JSM-5800 Scanning Microscope, Tokyo, Japan). Pinopode formation was also evaluated semi-quantitatively depending on their stage of development on the surface of the endometrium, and scored as (i) well-developed (ii) poorly developed and (iii) absent and on their abundance and scored as (i) abundant (ii) moderate (iii) few.

2.5.6 Real-time PCR

Levels of COX-2, MMP-2, -9, TIMP-1 and -2 gene expression were analyzed by real time PCR (RT-PCR), which was performed with ABI Prism 7000 Sequence Detection System (Applied Biosystems Inc., Carlsbad, California, USA) using syber green master mix (Applied Biosystems Inc., Carlsbad, California, USA). RT-PCR primers were designed using sequence data. Total RNA was isolated from tissue by RNA isolation kit (Trizol Reagent, Invitrogen, Carlsbad, California, USA) and 10 µl of total RNA isolated was subjected to reverse transcription for cDNA synthesis with High-Capacity cDNA Reverse Transcription Kits (Applied Biosystems, Carlsbad, California, USA), according to the manufacturer's instructions. After synthesis, 5 µl of cDNA was used for the RT-PCR mixed with syber green. At the end of each reaction, Cycle threshold (Ct) was manually set at the level that reflected the best kinetic PCR parameters, and melting curves were acquired and analyzed. Relative quantification was used to measure gene expression by relating the PCR signal.

2.5.7 Western blotting

The endometrial tissue was homogenized in tissue lysis buffer. The tissue lysate was then centrifuged at 15,000 g for 15 min and the protein concentration of the homogenates was determined by the GeNei™ Protein Estimation Kits (Bangalore Genei, India). 30 µg of homogenate protein were separated by SDS-polyacrylamide gel electrophoresis (SDS- PAGE). The separated proteins were electroblotted onto a Hybond PVDF membrane (GE Healthcare) at 30 volt for 13 hrs. After blocking the non-specific binding sites with non-fat dry milk in TBST buffer for 1 hr at room temperature, the blots were incubated overnight at 4°C with rabbit polyclonal antibody against COX-2, mouse monoclonal antibody against MMP-2,-9, TIMP-1 and -2 (Santa Cruz Biotechnology Inc, Santa Cruz, CA, USA), rabbit polyclonal antibody against VEGF, VEGFR1+VEGFR2 (Abcam, Cambridge, UK). The blots were then washed three times with TBST buffer, incubated for 1 hr at room temperature with horseradish peroxidase-linked goat anti-rabbit immunoglobulin G (IgG) and goat anti-mouse immunoglobulin G (IgG) (Santa Cruz Biotechnology Inc, Santa Cruz, CA, USA). After further washing, the immunoreactive proteins were revealed using the DAB as substrate.

2.5.8 Statistical analysis

Data were compared using independent two sample't' test and chi-square test, as applicable. Ky Plot version 2.0 beta 13 software and Graphpad Prism Software were used for this purpose. Statistical significance was defined as $p \leq 0.05$.

3. Result

The clinical characteristics such as age, BMI, endometrial thickness, serum estrogen and progesterone levels of women participating in this study are summarized in Table I.

Parameters	Endometriosis	Control	P value
Age	29.5±0.61	29.32±0.83	P>0.05
BMI	28.18 ± 0.7	26.51 ± 0.6	P>0.05
Endometrial thickness (cm)	9.25 ± 0.25	8.25 ± 0.41	P>0.05
Serum estrogen level (pg/ml)	258.5 ± 13.83	193.6 ± 14.66	P≤0.05
Serum progesterone level (ng/ml)	12.39 ± 1.28	26.43 ± 2	P≤0.05

(Mean ± SEM)

Table 1.

Low levels of immunoreactivity of the endometrial receptivity markers including $\alpha_v\beta_3$ integrin, LIF, L-selectin ligands (MECA-79) and Muc-1 were observed in women with endometriosis in contrast to strong immunoreactivity of controls. In addition, mean expression of these molecular markers detected by flow cytometric analysis shows a significantly lower expression both by the stromal and epithelial cells in women with endometriosis as compared to controls.

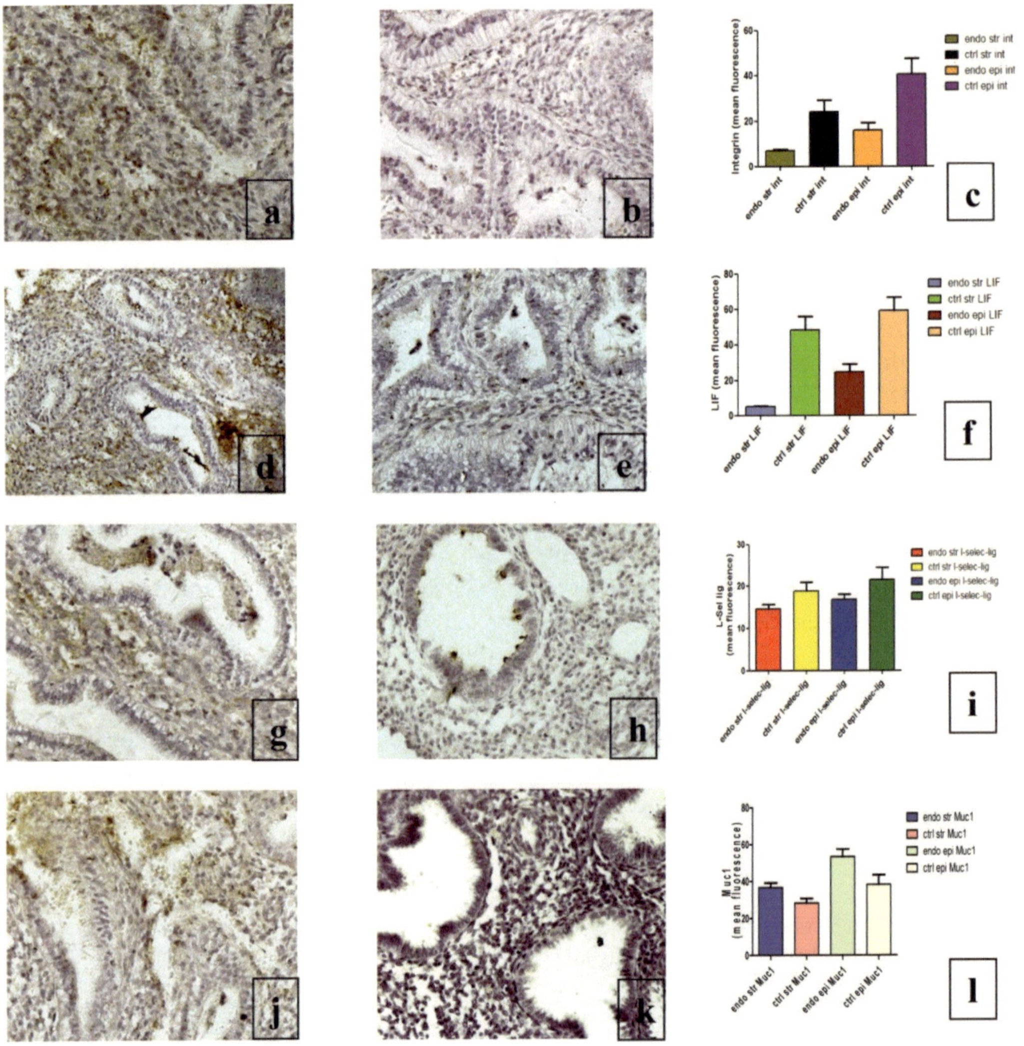

Fig. 1. Immunohistological images of different biochemical markers expression.
a. $\alpha_v\beta_3$ integrins in control **b.** $\alpha_v\beta_3$ integrins in women with endometriosis **c.** Graphical representation of $\alpha_v\beta_3$ integrin expression in the stromal and epithelial cells of endometrial tissues in endometriosis and control **d.** LIF in control **e.** LIF in women with endometriosis **f.** Graphical representation of LIF expression in the stromal and epithelial cells of endometrial tissues in endometriosis and control **g.** L-selectin ligand in control **h.** L-selectin ligand in women with endometriosis **i.** Graphical representation of L-selectin ligand expression in the stromal and epithelial cells of endometrial tissues in endometriosis and control **j.** Muc1 in control **k.** Muc1 in women with endometriosis **l.** Graphical representation of Muc1 expression in the stromal and epithelial cells of endometrial tissues in endometriosis and control.

Further, few poorly developed pinopodes were seen in women with endometriosis as compared to controls, which showed abundant well formed pinopodes (Figure 2, 3 and 4).

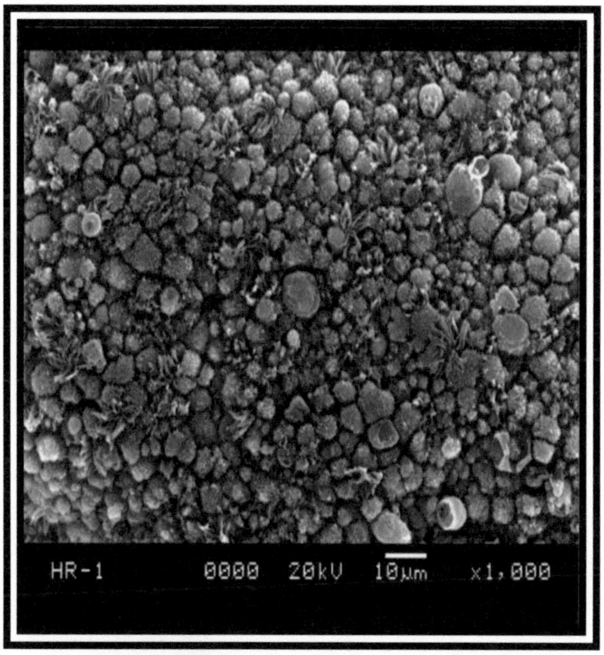

Fig. 2. Well developed pinopodes in control

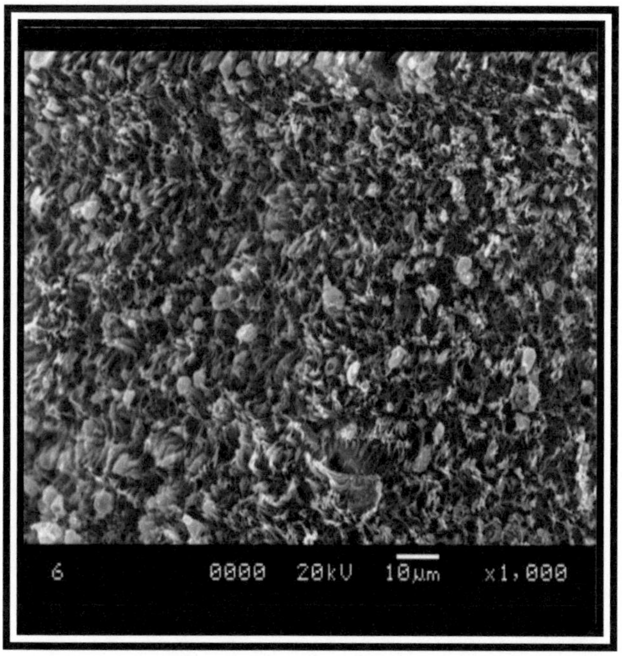

Fig. 3. Poorly developed pinopodes in endometriosis

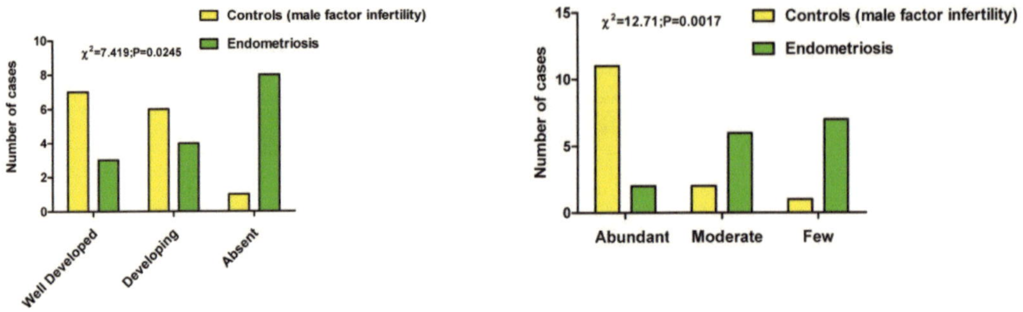

Fig. 4. Graphical representation of pinopode expression in the endometrial tissues in endometriosis and controls.

A significant increase in endometrial MMP-2, -9 and decrease in TIMP-1 and -2 expressions, were observed in women with endometriosis when compared to controls. Further, the endometrial expression of COX-2 was observed to be higher in women with endometriosis when compared with controls.

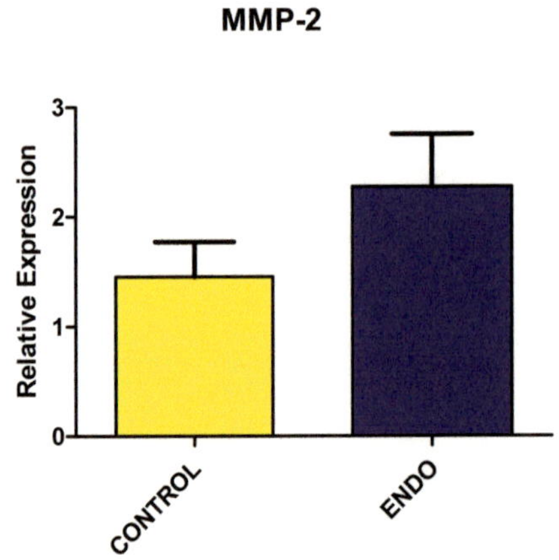

Fig. 5. Expression of MMP-2 gene in endometriosis and control

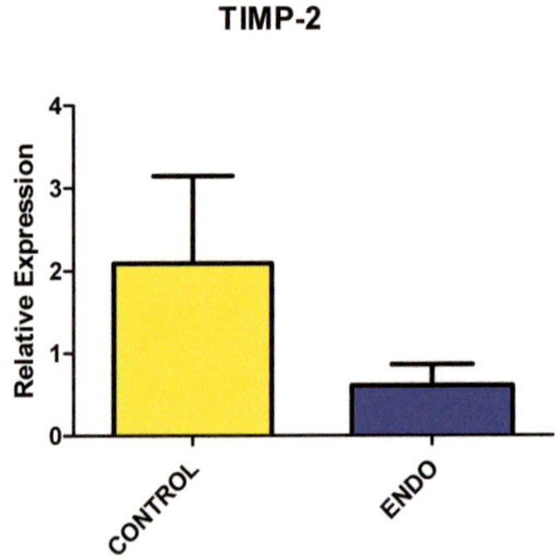

Fig. 6. Expression of TIMP-2 gene in endometriosis and control

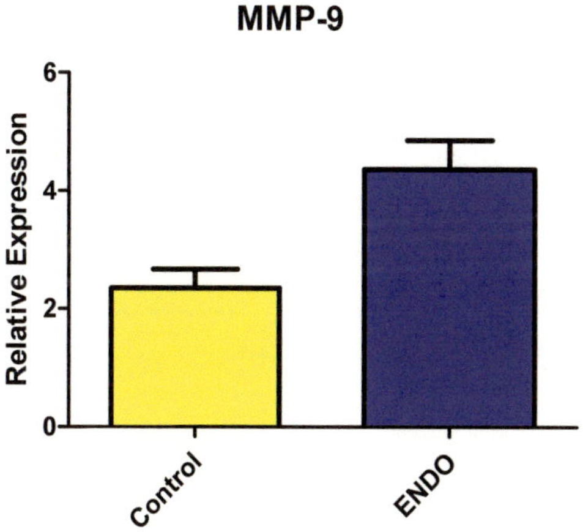

Fig. 7. Expression of MMP-9 gene in endometriosis and control

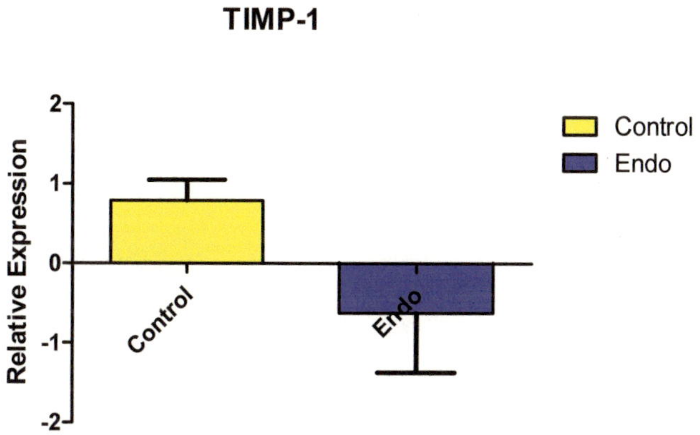

Fig. 8. Expression of TIMP-2 gene in endometriosis and control

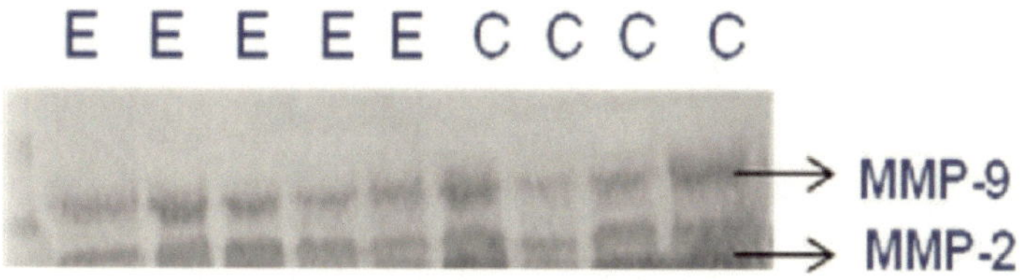

Fig. 9. Expression of MMP-2 and -9 in endometriosis and control

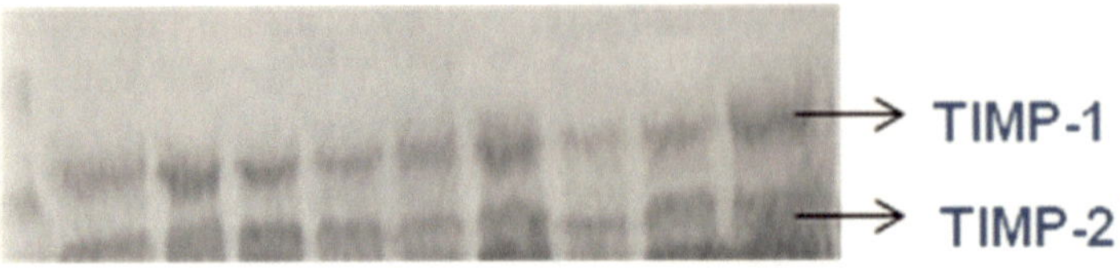

Fig. 10. Expression of TIMP-1 and -2 in endometriosis and control

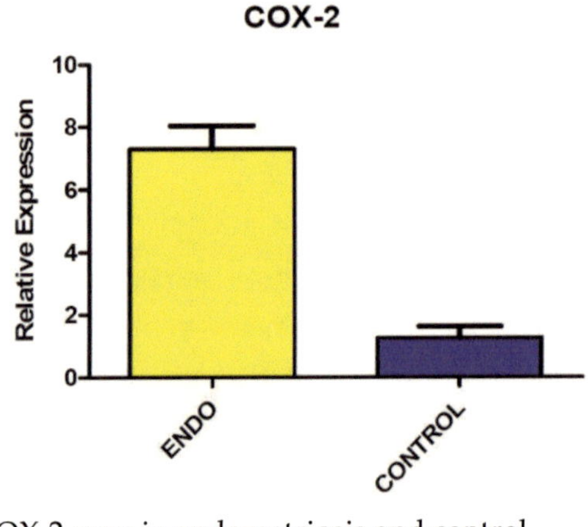

Fig. 11. Expression of COX-2 gene in endometriosis and control

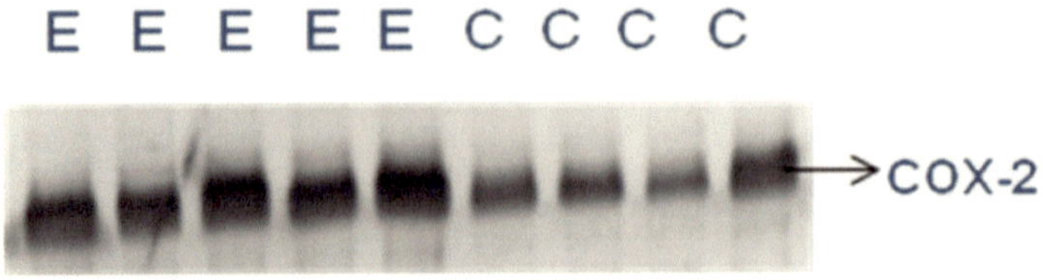

Fig. 12. Expression of COX-2 in endometriosis and control

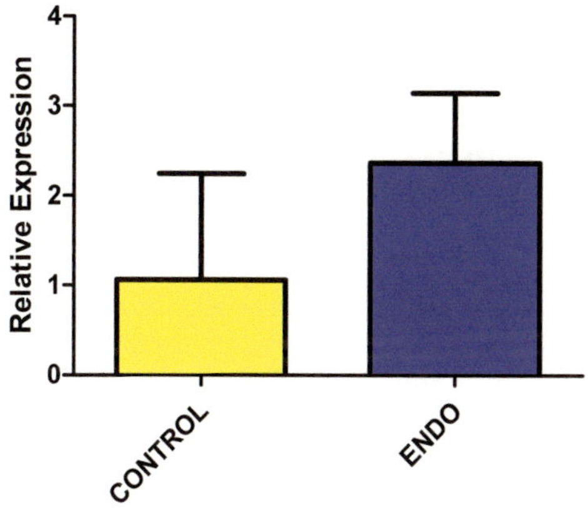

Fig. 13. Expression of VEGFR-1 gene in endometriosis and controls

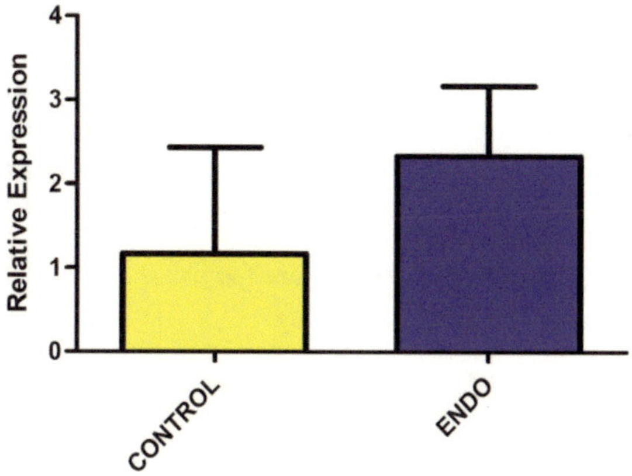

Fig. 14. Expression of VEGFR-2 gene in endometriosis and controls

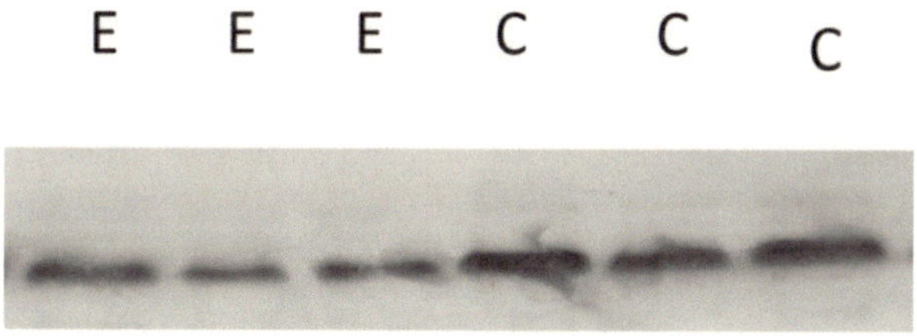

Fig. 15. Expression of endometrial VEGF in endometriotic women and control

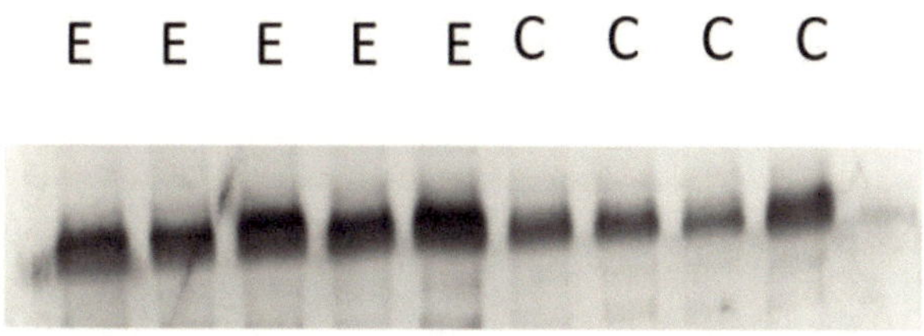

Fig. 16. Expression of endometrial VEGFR in endometriotic women and control

Endometrial expression of VEGF and its receptors VEGFR1 and VEGFR2 were observed to be lower and higher respectively in women with endometriosis when compared with controls.

4. Proposed molecular mechanism for implantation failure in endometriosis and future treatment strategies

In the present study, a hypothesis correlating various factors responsible for implantation failure in endometriosis is proposed (Figure 16). It is well established that endometriosis is an estrogen-dependent disorder. As mentioned earlier, estrogen regulates the expression of MMP-2 and MMP-9 in matrix turnover and VEGF mediated angiogenic activities in various physiological and pathological conditions. Based on our findings, we hypothesize that dysregulation of sex steroids induces over-expression of COX-2 in the endometrium of women with endometriosis. This, in turn, affects endometrial remodelling by up-regulating the expression of MMP-2 and -9, the major molecules responsible for matrix degradation and also increases the expression of VEGF and its receptors, considered to be key angiogenic molecules. This hypothesis is further evidenced by abnormal expression of implantation markers in these women suggesting poor endometrial receptivity and high rate of implantation failure. Molecules which can effectively control excessive endometrial matrix degradation by inhibiting over-expression of various factors responsible for matrix turnover and angiogenesis may be considered as a new therapeutic option for the treatment of endometriosis.

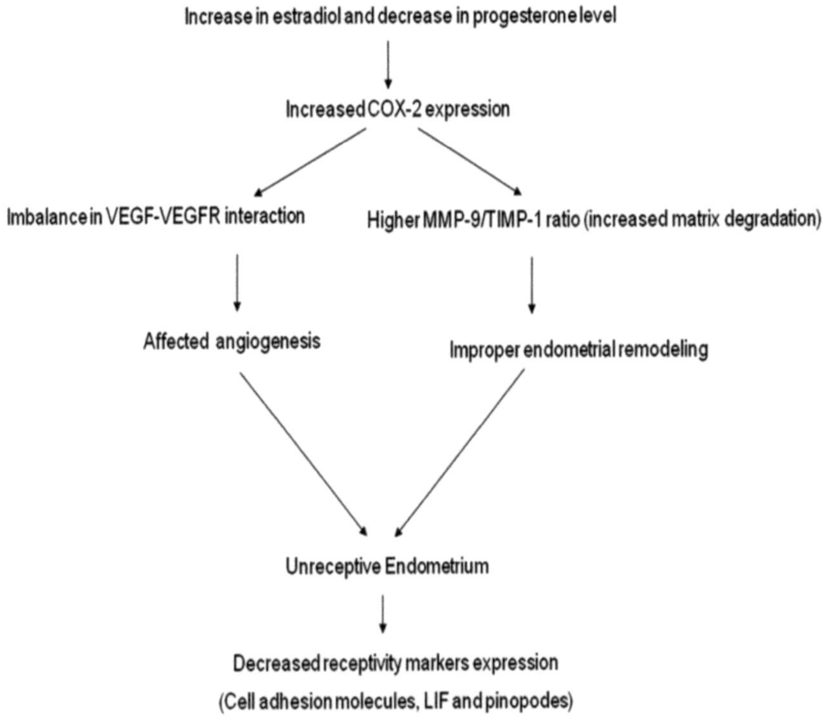

Fig. 16. Schematic representation of the molecular mechanism regulating the process of endometrial receptivity in endometriosis during implantation window

5. References

[1] Au, C.L. & Rogers, P.A. (1993). Immunohistochemical Staining of von Willebrand Factor in Human Endometrium During Normal Menstrual Cycle. *Human Reproduction*, Vol.8, No.1, (January 1993), pp. 17-23, ISSN 1460-2350

[2] Bausero, P.; Cavaille´, F.; Meduri, G.; Freitas, S. & Perrot-Applanat, M. (1998). Paracrine action of vascular endothelial growth factor in the human endometrium: Production and target sites, and hormonal regulation. *Angiogenesis*, Vol.2, No.2, (March 1998), pp. 167–182.

[3] Birkedal-Hansen, H.; Moore, W.G.I.; Bodden, M.K.; Windsor, L.J.; Birkedal-Hansen, B.; DeCarlo, A. *et al.* (1993). Matrix Metalloproteinases: A Review. *Critical Reviews in Oral Biology & Medicine*, Vol.4, No.2, (1993), pp. 197-250.

[4] Charnock-Jones, D.S.; Sharkey, A.M.; Fenwick, P.; & Smith, S.K. (1994). Leukaemia inhibitory factor mRNA concentration peaks in human endometrium at the time of implantation and the blastocyst contains mRNA for the receptor at this time. *Journal of Reproduction and Fertility*, Vol.101, No.2, (July 1994), pp. 421-426.

[5] Charnock-Jones, D.S.; Sharkey, A.M.; Rajput-Williams, J.; Burch, D.; Schofield, J.P.; Fountain, S.A. *et al.* (1993). Identification and localization of alternately spliced mRNAs for vascular endothelial growth factor in human uterus and estrogen regulation in endometrial carcinoma cell lines. *Biology of Reproduction*, Vol.48, No.5, (May 1993), pp. 1120-1128.

[6] Curry, T.E. Jr.; Osteen, K.G. (2003) The matrix metalloproteinase system: changes, regulation, and impact throughout the ovarian and uterine reproductive cycle. Endocrine Reviews, Vol.24, No.4, (Aug 2003), pp. 428-465.

[7] Ferrara, N.; Davis-Smyth, T. (1997) The biology of vascular endothelial growth factor. Endocrine Reviews, Vol.18, No.1, (Feb 1997), pp. 4-25.

[8] Ferrara, N.; Gerber, H.P.; & LeCouter, J. The biology of VEGF and its receptors. Nat Med 2003;9:669-76.

[9] Friedler S, Zimerman A, Schachter M, Raziel A, Strassburger D, Ron El R. The midluteal decline in serum estradiol levels is drastic but not deleterious for implantation after in vitro fertilization and embryo transfer in patients with normal or high responses. Fertility and Sterility 2005;83:54-60.

[10] Giudice L 1996 The endometrial cycle. In Reproductive Endocrinology, Surgery and Technology, pp 272–300. Eds EY Adashi, JA Rock & Z Rosenwaks. Philadelphia: Lippincolt-Raven Publishers.

[11] Perrot-Applanat M 2000 Hormonal regulation of vascular cell function: angiogenesis. In Encyclopedic Reference of Vascular Biology and Pathology pp 157–162. Ed A Bikfalvi. Heidelberg: Springer Verlag.

[12] Genbacev OD, Prakobphol A, Foulk RA, Krtolica AR, Ilic D, Singer MS. Trophoblast L-Selectin-Mediated Adhesion at the Maternal-Fetal Interface. Science 2003;299:405-8.

[13] Gendler SJ, Lancaster CA, Taylor-Papadimitriou J, Duhig T, Peat N, Burchell J. Molecular cloning and expression of human tumor-associated polymorphic epithelial mucin. J Biol Chem 1990;265:15286-93.

[14] Gipson IK, Ho SB, Spurr-Michaud SJ, Tisdale AS, Zhan Q, Torlakovic E. Mucin genes expressed by human female reproductive tract epithelia. Biol Reprod 1997;56:999-1011.

[15] Groothuis PG, Dassen HH, Romano A, Punyadeera C. Estrogen and the endometrium: lessons learned from gene expression profiling in rodents and human. Hum Reprod Update 2007;13:405-17.

[16] Hilkens J, Ligtenberg MJL, Vos HL, Litvinov SV. Cell membrane-associated mucins and their adhesion-modulating property. Trends in Biochemical Sciences 1992;17:359-63.

[17] Hulboy DL, Rudolph LA, Matrisian LM. Matrix metalloproteinases as mediators of reproductive function. Molecular Human Reproduction 1997;3:27-45.

[18] Hung Yu Ng E, Shu Biu Yeung W, Yee Lan Lau E, Wai Ki So W, Chung Ho P. A rapid decline in serum oestradiol concentrations around the mid-luteal phase had no adverse effect on outcome in 763 assisted reproduction cycles. Human Reproduction 2000;15:1903-8.

[19] Itatsu K, Sasaki M, Yamaguchi J, Ohira S, Ishikawa A, Ikeda H *et al.* Cyclooxygenase-2 Is Involved in the Up-Regulation of Matrix Metalloproteinase-9 in Cholangiocarcinoma Induced by Tumor Necrosis Factor-{alpha}. Am J Pathol 2009;174:829-41.

[20] Kosmas IP, Kolibianakis EM, Devroey P. Association of estradiol levels on the day of hCG administration and pregnancy achievement in IVF: a systematic review. Hum Reprod 2004;19:2446-53.

[21] Kottur A, Rao K, Srinivas M, Gupta N, Shetty N, Narvekar S. The degree of serum estradiol decline in early and midluteal phase had no adverse effect on IVF/ICSI outcome. J Hum Reprod Sci. 2010 Jan-Apr; 3(1): 25–30.

[22] Kyrou D, Popovic-Todorovic B, Fatemi HM, Bourgain C, Haentjens P, Van Landuyt. L .Does the estradiol level on the day of human chorionic gonadotrophin administration have an impact on pregnancy rates in patients treated with rec-FSH/GnRH antagonist? Human Reproduction 2009;24:2902-9.

[23] Lass A, Weiser W, Munafo A, Loumaye E. Leukemia inhibitory factor in human reproduction. Fertil Steril 2001;76:1091-6.

[24] Lessey BA, Castelbaum AJ, Sawin SW, Buck CA, Schinnar R, Bilker W . Aberrant integrin expression in the endometrium of women with endometriosis. J Clin Endocrinol Metab 1994;79:643-9.

[25] Li Y, Pu D, Li Y. The expression of cyclooxygenase-2 in cervical cancers and Hela cells was regulated by estrogen/progestogen. Journal of Huazhong University of Science and Technology -- Medical Sciences -- 2007;27:457-60.

[26] Lockwood CJ, Krikun G, Koo AB, Kadner S, Schatz F. Differential effects of thrombin and hypoxia on endometrial stromal and glandular epithelial cell vascular endothelial growth factor expression. J Clin Endocrinol Metab 2002;87:4280-6.

[27] McIntush EW, Smith MF. Matrix metalloproteinases and tissue inhibitors of metalloproteinases in ovarian function. Rev Reprod 1998;3:23-30.

[28] Nayak NR, Brenner RM. Vascular proliferation and vascular endothelial growth factor expression in the rhesus macaque endometrium. J Clin Endocrinol Metab 2002;87:1845-55.

[29] Okada H, Sanezumi M, Nakajima T, Okada S, Yasuda K, Kanzaki H. Rapid down-regulation of CD63 transcription by progesterone in human endometrial stromal cells. Mol Hum Reprod 1999;5:554-8.

[30] Ota H, Igarashi S, Tanaka T. Morphometric evaluation of stromal vascularization in the endometrium in adenomyosis. Hum Reprod 1998;13:715-9.

[31] Perrot-Applanat M, Ancelin M, Buteau-Lozano H, Meduri G, Bausero P. Ovarian steroids in endometrial angiogenesis. Steroids 2000;65:599-603.

[32] Popovici RM, Irwin JC, Giaccia AJ, Giudice LC. Hypoxia and cAMP Stimulate Vascular Endothelial Growth Factor (VEGF) in Human Endometrial Stromal Cells: Potential Relevance to Menstruation and Endometrial Regeneration. Journal of Clinical Endocrinology & Metabolism 1999;84:2245.

[33] Rogers PA, Au CL, Affandi B. Endometrial microvascular density during the normal menstrual cycle and following exposure to long-term levonorgestrel. Hum Reprod 1993;8:1396-404.

[34] Salata IM, Stojanovic N, Cajdler-Å□uba A, Lewandowski KC, LewiÅ„ski A. Gelatinase A (MM-2), gelatinase B (MMP-9) and their inhibitors (TIMP 1, TIMP-2) in serum of women with endometriosis: Significant correlation between MMP-2, MMP9 and their inhibitors without difference in levels of matrix metalloproteinases and tissue inhibitors of metalloproteinases in relation to the severity of endometriosis. Gynecological Endocrinology 2008;24:326-30.

[35] Sharara FI, McClamrock HD. Ratio of oestradiol concentration on the day of human chorionic gonadotrophin administration to mid-luteal oestradiol concentration is predictive of in-vitro fertilization outcome. Human Reproduction 1999;14:2777-82.

[36] Shifren JL, Tseng JF, Zaloudek CJ, Ryan IP, Meng YG, Ferrara N *et al.* Ovarian steroid regulation of vascular endothelial growth factor in the human endometrium: implications for angiogenesis during the menstrual cycle and in the pathogenesis of endometriosis. J Clin Endocrinol Metab 1996;81:3112-8.

[37] SimÃ³n C, Cano F, Valbuena D, RemohÃ- J, Pellicer A. Implantation: Clinical evidence for a detrimental effect on uterine receptivity of high serum oestradiol concentrations in high and normal responder patients. Human Reproduction 1995;10:2432-7.

[38] Smith SK. Angiogenesis, vascular endothelial growth factor and the endometrium. Hum Reprod Update 1998;4:509-19.

[39] Sugino N, Kashida S, Karube-Harada A, Takiguchi S, Kato H. Expression of vascular endothelial growth factor (VEGF) and its receptors in human endometrium throughout the menstrual cycle and in early pregnancy. Reproduction 2002;123:379-87.

[40] Torry DS, Torry RJ. Angiogenesis and the expression of vascular endothelial growth factor in endometrium and placenta. Am J Reprod Immunol 1997;37:21-9.

[41] Valbuena D, Martin J, de Pablo JL, Remohí J, Pellicer A, Simón C. Increasing levels of estradiol are deleterious to embryonic implantation because they directly affect the embryo. Fertility and Sterility 2001;76:962-8.

[42] Wang Y, Zhao AM, Lin QD. Role of cyclooxygenase-2 signalling pathway dysfunction in unexplained recurrent spontaneous abortion. *Chin Med J (Engl)* 2010;123:1543-1547.1

[43] Wesseling J, van der Valk SW, Hilkens J. A mechanism for inhibition of E-cadherin-mediated cell-cell adhesion by the membrane-associated mucin episialin/MUC1. Mol Biol Cell 1996;7:565-77.

[44] Xiong B, Sun TJ, Hu WD, Cheng FL, Mao M, Zhou YF. Expression of cyclooxygenase-2 in colorectal cancer and its clinical significance. World J Gastroenterol 2005;11:1105-8.

18

Pathomechanism of Infertility in Endometriosis

Hendi Hendarto
Dept. of Obstetric & Gynecology Faculty of Medicine, University of Airlangga / Dr. Soetomo Hospital, Surabaya, Indonesia

1. Introduction

Endometriosis is defined as the presence of endometrial-like tissue outside the uterus, which induces a chronic, inflammatory reaction (Kennedy *et al.*, 2005). Infertility is one of clinical manifestation of endometriosis showed by the difference of fecundity. At our tertiary hosital pelvic endometriosis is frequently found in infertile women: 23,8 % (1987), 37,2 % (1993) and 50 % (2002) cases of diagnostic laparoscopy (Samsulhadi, 2002).

An association between endometriosis and infertility has repeatedly been reported in the literature, but an absolute cause-effect relationship has not yet been confirmed. The controversy regarding whether endometriosis is a cause of infertility or an incidental finding is ongoing (ASRM, 2006; Gupta *et al.*, 2008). Many theories of endometriosis which may impair fertility have been suggested during the years, and new hypotheses and approaches to the problem have arisen with the application of assisted reproduction techniques (Garrido *et al.*, 2002). Data on the impact of endometriosis on the results of in-vitro fertilization and embryo transfer (IVF-ET) treatment are not consistent. Several theories have been proposed to identify the pathomechanism of infertility in endometriosis. None of these theories can completely explain these association. Based on many reports the possible mechanisms that could cause infertility in endometriosis are pelvic adhesion and endometrioma and also excess production of inflammatory factors in micro environment that both play a role in alteration fertility function. Severe endometriosis is associated with pelvic adhesions leading to a possible mechanic or anatomic disturbance of fertility, in the other hand a mild stage may have a direct and indirect negative effect on folliculogenesis, oocyte development, sperm function, embryogenesis, and endometrium receptivity (Barnhart *et al.*, 2002). Our aim in the present review is to describe an update on several approaches of the pathomechanism of infertility in endometriosis, based on its impact on a number of pathologic conditions, such as: pelvic adhesion and endometrioma, abnormal folliculogenesis and impaired oocyte function, altered sperm function, reduced embryo quality, and impaired endometrium receptivity.

2. Pelvic adhesion and endometrioma

The mechanisms by which endometriosis impairs fertility have not been completely determined but are likely varied. Ovarian involvement and adhesion that block tubal motility and pick-up of the egg could be a main causative of mechanical interference on fertility especially in severe endometriosis due to a possible mechanic or anatomic disturbance such as extensive pelvic adhesions. Pelvic endometriosis, the most common form of the disease, could be associated with increased secretion of pro-inflammatory cytokines, impaired cell-mediated immunity and neo-angiogenesis. Barnhart *et al.* (2002) found that compared with women with mild endometriosis, women with severe endometriosis have a statistically significantly lower pregnancy rate and implantation rate, have fewer oocytes obtained at ovarian retrieval, and have a lower peak estradiol concentration (Barnhart *et al.,* 2002).

Adhesion formation involves three important components: 1) acute inflammatory response, 2) fribinolysis, and 3) metalloproteinases and their tissue inhibitors. Celluler mediators within the peritoneal fluid can potentially modulate inflammatory responses over a large surface area due to the liquid nature of the peritoneal fluid. There are three important pro-inflammatory cytokines involved in adhesion formation: interleukine (IL)-1, IL-6 and Tumor Necrosis Factor (TNF)-α (Cheong *et al.,* 2002). Endometriosis is associated with signs of pelvic peritoneal inflammation including increased volume of peritoneal fluid, increased concentration of peritoneal fluid macrophages, and increased peritoneal fluid concentrations of IL-6, IL-8, TNF-α and other cytokines and growth factors. Indeed, these cytokines have been reported to increase the endometrial–peritoneal adhesion *in vitro* (D'Hooghe and Debrock, 2002). Pelvic adhesion secondary to endometriosis is the most accepted reason for infertility, presumably via dysfunction of the fallopian tube or ovary. Inflammatory cytokines, IL-6, IL- 8 and TNF-α produced by endometrial cells probably contribute to the adhesion process. IL-8 has been shown to stimulate the adhesion of endometrial cells to fibronectin. TNF-α has also been reported to promote endometrial stromal cell proliferation *in vitro* and endometrial stromal cell adhesion to extracellular matrix components (Garcia-Velasco and Arici, 1999). These pelvic adhesion inhibits ovum capture after ovulation.

Cysts of endometriosis (endometriomas) may become adherent to the uterus, bowel or pelvic side wall. Any of these anatomic distortions can result in infertility. The presence of an ovarian endometrioma greater than 1 cm in diameter is classified as stage III (moderate) or more in the revised American Society for Reproductive Medicine (ASRM) classification of endometriosis, but unfortunately, the staging system does not correlate well with a woman's chance of conception following therapy (ASRM, 2006). The impact of an ovarian endometrioma on infertility remains controversial, despite the number of studies that have been performed. Suzuki *et al* (2005) found that endometriosis, even after diagnostic laparoscopy with treatment when necessary, clearly affects the number of oocytes as well as the number of transferred embryos but not embryo quality and the related parameters of pregnancy, as indicated by the fertilization rate, embryo quality, implantation rate, pregnancy rate, and live birth rate, irrespective of the presence of an ovarian endometrioma (Suzuki *et al,* 2005). Nakahara (1998) found that the proportion of apoptotic bodies in the membrana granulosa cells and the cumulus cells from patients with endometrioma is significantly higher than that in patients without endometrioma. Based on these studies endometrioma prove the existence of a more advance stage of endometriosis than the non existence of endometrioma. The existence of endometrioma is considered one of the indicators of endometriosis in the ovary due to the increase of the apoptosis in the follicle and gave, in turn, the follicle an atretic status. Consequently, patients with endometriosis with endometrioma had smaller numbers of follicles developed, oocytes harvested, and mature oocytes (Nakahara *et al*, 1998).

In women with endometriosis, pelvic adhesions contain estrogen and progesterone receptors, and produce basic fibroblastic growth factor and vascular endothelial growth factor, implying a regulation of pelvic adhesion formation by steroid hormone. Zang (2010) found that both the percentage and the density of protein gene product (PGP) 9.5-positive nerve fibres in ovarian endometriotic lesions were significantly higher in women with ovarian endometriosis who had pelvic adhesions than in those women with ovarian endometriosis and no pelvic adhesions (Zang et al., 2010). It is suggested that ovarian endometriotic lesions may be innervated through mediating effects of peritoneal inflammatory cytokines and growth factors including IL-1, IL-6 and TNF-a, in women with pelvic adhesions, thus leading to an increase of nerve fibres in ovarian endometriotic lesions in women with ovarian endometriosis (Zang *et al.*, 2010).

3. Abnormal folliculogenesis and impaired oocyte function

Infertility associated with the advanced stages of endometriosis may be explained by pelvic adhesion and endometrioma as described above. The mechanism of infertility associated with endometriosis without adhesion and endometrioma, such as minimal or mild endometriosis as well as the negative impact of all stages of the disease on infertility is poorly understood. Many possibilities have been suggested, ranging from abnormal folliculogenesis to impaired endometrium receptivity (Arici *et al.*, 1999). Peritoneal fluid, a biologic fluid present in the abdominal cavity, has been a focus of research on endometriosis because of the extent of information it potentially carries about the disease. The proximity of peritoneal fluid to endometriotic lesions shows the milieu in which the immune mediators associated with the local inflammation of endometriosis can be studied. It has been suggested that such alterations in cytokines and growth factors interfere with folliculogenesis, ovulation and fertilization (Arici *et al.*, 1999).

The local microenvironment of peritoneal fluid surrounding the endometriotic implant is immunologically dynamic and links the reproductive and immune systems. Peritoneal fluid contains a variety of free floating cells, including macrophages, mesothelial cells, lymphocytes, eosinophils and mast cells (Oral *et al.*, 1996). The peritoneal fluid of women with endometriosis have confirmed an increased number, concentration and activation of macrophages which may induce proliferation of cells that are involved in inflammation through secretion of factors such as IL- 1, IL-6, and TNF-α (Oral *et al.*, 1996a). Other studies similary found that levels of cytokines, such as, IL-6, IL-8 and TNF-α increased in the peritoneal fluid of women with endometriosis (Arici *et al.*, 1996), meanwhile endometriotic implants also secreted various cytokines including IL-1, IL-6, IL-8, TNF-α in the peritoneal cavity in patients with endometriosis (Oral *et al.*, 1996b). Cytokines, which are produced by many cell types in peritoneal fluid, play a diverse role as toxic effect in constructing the peritoneal environment that induces the development and progression of endometriosis and endometriosis-associated infertility (Harada *et al.*, 2001).

Peritoneal fluid bathed the ovaries, hypothetically the inflammatory components in peritoneal fluid in women with endometriosis might diffuse into the ovarian follicles, or by paracrine mechanisms (Carlberg *et al.*, 2000) impair the granulosa cell function, oocyte maturation and folliculogenesis. Folliculogenesis is growth and development process of ovarian follicle consist of oocyte, granulosa and theca cells might result in mature and fertilizable oocyte (Rajkovic, 2006). The alteration of oocyte, granulosa, theca cells development and molecular follicular communication may impact on folliculogenesis. Carlberg (2000) found that granulosa cells of women with endometriosis have an up-regulated production of IL-1β, IL-6, IL-8, TNF-α which might be related to the reduced fertilization rate previously observed in endometriosis women (Carlberg *et al.*, 2000). Beside that women with endometriosis were reported having higher granulosa cell apoptosis rate and a lower percentage of G2/M phase granulosa cells compared with other group of infertile women. This result strongly suggest that the cytokines produced in endometriosis women may be responsible for the disturbance of the cell cycle in the granulosa cells as in other cells and in turn have pathogenic effects on folliculogenesis (Toya *et al.* 2000) . Nakahara (1998) found that higher incidence of apoptotic bodies correlates with a lower quality of oocytes in individual follicles. This study showed that the incidence of apoptotic bodies in membrana granulosa ovaries of patients with endometriosis undergoing the IVF-ET procedure was increased as the stage of the revised AFS classification advanced. It means that the quality of oocytes from patients with endometriosis decreases in proportion to advancing stages of the revised AFS classification and determine the degree of disturbance for folliculogenesis in the ovaries of the patients with endometriosis (Nakahara, 1998).

Our previous study postulated that apoptosis of granulosa cells caused disturbance in oocyte growth and maturation and associated with decreased growth differentiation factor-9 (GDF-9) production (Hendarto *et al.*, 2010). Oocyte-derived GDF-9 is obligatory for normal folliculogenesis and female fertility (Erickson and Shimasaki, 2001). Elvin (1999) reported that mouse GDF-9 can bind to receptors on granulosa cells, and plays multifunctional roles in oocyte-granulosa cell communication and regulation of follicular differentiation and function (Elvin *et al.*, 1999). In our study we found that the presence of GDF-9 in follicular fluid of preovulatory follicle was confirmed by western blotting analysis in a band of 53 kDa, and compared with the level in women with no endometriosis, GDF-9 level in the follicular fluid of women with severe endometriosis was lower. This might impair folliculogenesis, leading to reduced oocyte quality (Hendarto *et al.*, 2010). Our other study also comfirmed that oocyte-granulosa cell communication has already been altered showed by increasing the concentration of granulosa cell-derived kit-ligand in follicular fluid of infertile women with endometriosis (in publication process).

The cytoskeleton of metaphase II oocytes were influenced by rich pro-inflammatory factor present in peritoneal fluid of patients with endometriosis. By exposure of cryopreserved mouse oocytes to the peritoneal fluid from women with endometriosis, Mansour (2010) reported that in the endometriosis group, the cytoskeleton had a higher frequency of abnormal meiotic spindle and chromosomal misalignment, indicating severe damage compared with the control groups. The meiotic spindle plays a critical role in maintaining chromosomal organization and formation of the second polar body. Disorganization of the meiotic spindle can result in chromosomal dispersion, failure of normal fertilization, and abnormal development. Alterations of the spindle may be one of the many causes related to infertility and/or recurrent pregnancy loss in patients with endometriosis (Mansour *et al.*, 2010). Reactive oxygen species (ROS) have been detected in peritoeal fluid of endometriosis patients but are not significantly elevated compared with the control and idiopathic infertility groups (Bedaiwy *et al.*, 2002). Reactive oxygen species have detrimental effects on oocytes, they are able to diffuse and pass through cell membrane and alter most types of cellular molecule such as lipids, proteins and nucleic acids. The consequences are mitochondrial alterations, embryo cell block, ATP depletion and apoptosis (Guerin, 2001).

Based on several studies above it is proposed that pro-inflammatory factors and ROS in follicular fluid women with endometriosis may diffuse and impact autocrine-paracrine communication of ovarian follicles causing cell-cycle alteration and an increased apoptosis in granulosa cells. Beside that, the presence of pro-inflammatory factors and ROS could influence the oocyte such as abnormal meiotic spindle, chromosomal misalignment and decreased GDF-9 production. Both may impair oocyte-granulosa cell communicatin and cause abnormal folliculogenesis and, in turn, result in reduced oocyte quality. Futher studies are needed. (see figure 1)

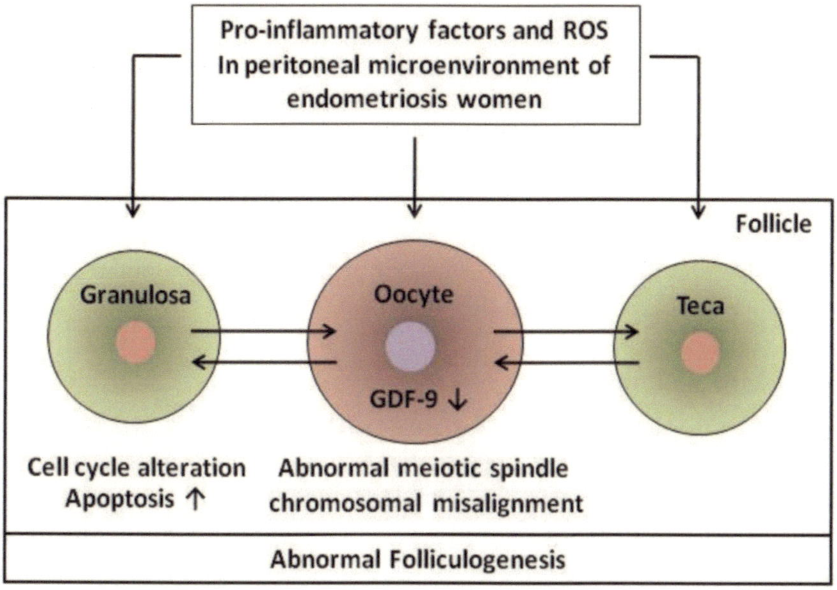

Fig. 1. Abnormal folliculogenesis in endometriosis (Hendarto, 2011)

4. Altered sperm function

Spermatozoa have to stay for a certain period of time in the female genital tract that normally favors capacitation, the ability to reach and fertilize the oocyte. The endometriosis-associated immuno-inflammatory changes in peritoneal fluid may have some adverse effects on spermatozoa (Carli *et al.*, 2007). Eisermann (1989) reported that levels of TNF-α of up to 800 U/ml in peritoneal fluid from infertile women with endometriosis higher than fertile women without endometriosis. In this concentration,

TNF-α caused a significant reduction in both progressive and total sperm motility when compared with controls group. Suggests that this may be a mechanism for the infertility observed in women with minimal endometriosis (Eisermann *et al.*, 1989). In the other study stated that the toxic effects of TNF-α could be the result of its ability to stimulate apoptosis in sperm cells through initiation of a caspase cascade. Exposing spermatozoa to pathological concentrations of TNF-α can result in significant loss of sperm function and genomic integrity. Infliximab, an TNF-α inhibitor, could potentially be used to help treat female infertility caused by endometriosis in those with elevated levels of TNF-α in their peritoneal fluid (Said *et al.*, 2005).

Another theory describing pathological effect of endometriosis on sperm function is the role of reactive oxygen species. Oxidative stress has been shown to exert toxic effects on sperm, damaging the sperm cell membrane, inducing DNA damage, and mediating sperm apoptosis (Agarwal *et al.*, 2006). Mansour (2009) found that progressive sperm DNA damage was significantly higher in samples incubated with peritoneal fluid from patients with endometriosis than those from healthy women. Spermatozoa are particularly susceptible to ROS-induced damage because their plasma membranes contain large quantities of polyunsaturated fatty acids and their cytoplasm contains low concentrations of the scavenging enzymes (Saleh *et al.*, 2002)

Reeve (2005) reported that significantly more spermatozoa bound per unit area to the ampullary epithelium of the uterine tubes taken from women with endometriosis, could potentially hinder fertilization by reducing the number of free spermatozoa in the tubal lumen that are available to take part in fertilization. Numerous studies have shown that spermatozoa that bind to the endosalpinx retain their viability, motility and fertilizing capacity longer than spermatozoa incubated alone or with other cell types. The aberrant expression of integrin in the endometrium of women with endometriosis would be speculated to increased sperm binding (Reeve *et al.*, 2005).

5. Reduced embryo quality

Use of IVF-ET as a therapeutic tool in endometriosis women with infertility could result in information about this disease and reproductive process aspects, such as folliculogenesis, fertilization, embryo development and implantation. The outcome of patients with endometriosis undergoing IVF-ET showed not only the influence of endometriosis on IVF result but also the possible pathomechanisms of infertility in endometriosis (Garrido et al., 2000). The impact of endometriosis in embryo development and quality is still on debate. Various embryo scoring system have been described to assess the developmental potential of embryos, but the most commonly used systems are the blastomeres cleavage rate, the shape and size of the blastomeres and the amount of anucleated fragment (Martynow et al., 2007)

Pellicer (1995) found a significantly reduced number of blastomeres in embryos from endometriosis patients compared with controls, and endometriosis patients had a poor IVF-ET outcome in terms of a reduced pregnancy rate per cycle, reduced pregnancy rate per transfer and reduced implantation rate per embryo replaced (Pellicer et al., 1995). Simon (1994) showed that patients who received embryos derived from endometriosis ovaries showed a significantly reduced ability to implant compared with the remaining groups (Simon et al., 1994). These result above suggest that infertility in endometriosis patients may be related to alterations within the oocyte which, in turn, result in reduced embryos quality (Pellicer et al., 1995).

Endometriosis induces an inflammatory state by activation of macrophages, releasing ROS and cytokines (Gupta *et al.*, 2008). Macrophages, cytokines and other products present in the peritoneal fluid from patients with endometriosis could be responsible for a change in the peritoneal environment that generates embryotoxic activity. Torres (2002) found embryotoxicity was increased in women with endometriosis, but there was little correlation with severity of the disease. These study also found a significant increase in embryotoxicity in the presence of high cytokine concentrations, especially with IL-6 (Torres et al., 2002). Other study by Pellicer found progesterone concentrations in follicular fluid increased with the severity of endometriosis that may be related to the release of the cytokines. The result of the study also showed that IL-6 concentration was significantly increased in follicular fluid of patients with endometriosis, whereas VEGF accumulation in follicular fluid was significantly decreased in women with endometriosis compared with controls. The increased IL-6 means that the immune system may be activated as a marker of altered follicular function that result in reduced oocyte and embryo quality. The decreased VEGF concentration needs further investigation, but in IVF, elevated VEGF concentrations have been shown to be related to good follicular vascularization and health. The study by Pellicer concluded profound differences in the follicular environment of the oocytes of women with endometriosis, compared with those of healthy patients. It may be suspected as a marker of altered follicular function that result in reduced oocyte and embryo quality.

6. Impaired endometrium receptivity

There are controversial information regarding implantation alteration in endometriosis-associated infertility. Various studies described three causative factors: an oocyte/embryo impairment, endometrial defect and altered endometrial-embryonic cross-talk (Garrido *et al.*, 2002). Implantation depends on an interaction of the trophoblast with the uterine epithelium, whereas a receptive endometrium is characterized by abundant secretory activity such as the presence of several integrins including the αvβ3 integrin. Lessey (1994) reported that the majority of women with abnormal αvβ3 integrin expression had endometriosis stage I or II and stated that αvβ3 integrin expression could be a useful marker of mild endometriosis (Lessey *et al.*, 1994). Inconsistent result pointed by Surrey (2010) that a high prevalence of aberrant endometrial αvβ3 vitronectin expression was noted in a group of infertile endometriosis patients who are IVF candidates but there were no significant differences in ongoing pregnancy or implantation rates in those patients who failed to express integrin αvβ3 vitronectin who were treated with a 3-month course of a GnRH agonist before an IVF cycle in comparison to untreated controls. Endometrial αvβ3 integrin expression did not predict which patients would benefit from prolonged administration of a GnRH agonist before initiation of controlled ovarian hyperstimulation for IVF (Surrey *et al.*, 2010)

The detection of pinopodes as a possible marker of receptivity in humans has been extensively studied. Pinopodes are specialized cell surface formations presumably involved in the adhesion of blastocysts to the luminal epithelium. Scanning electron microscopy in sequential endometrial biopsies showed that pinopodes formed briefly (1–2 days) and that their numbers correlate with implantation (Nikas *et al.*, 1999). Garcia-Velasco (2001) found pinopode expression in women with endometriosis did not differ from that of patients without endometriosis undergoing artificial cycles. Similarly, the clinical outcome in these women was comparable to that of the general population included in the oocyte donation program and this study stated that pinopode expression is not altered, suggesting that endometrial receptivity in women with this disease remains unaltered (Garcia-Velasco *et al.*, 2001).

Endometrial aspects and molecular studies on the receptivity status of endometrium resulted in conflicting data. Several studies suggest that an altered follicular microenvironment could be responsible for a defective folliculogenesis, and subsequently reduced oocyte/embryo quality, and in turn, result in altered embryo implantation but the debate still ongoing (Garrido *et al.*, 2002).

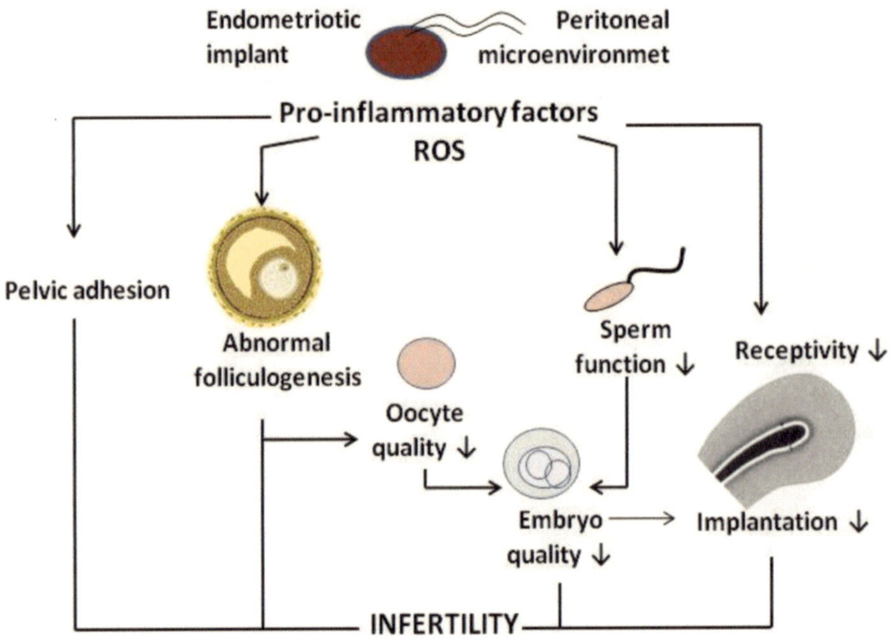

Fig. 2. Pathomechanism of infertility in endometriosis (Hendarto, 2011)

7. Summary

We have reviewed various studies with regard to the understanding of pathomechanism of infertility in endometriosis, based on its impacts on number of pathologic conditions, such as: pelvic adhesion and endometrioma, abnormal folliculogenesis and impaired oocyte function, altered sperm function, reduced embryo quality, and impaired endometrium receptivity. The controversy regarding whether endometriosis is a cause of infertility or an incidental finding is ongoing.

Based on several studies reviewed above showed that peritoneal microenvironment of women with endometriosis which contain pro-inflammatory factor and ROS is the main causative factor of the pathomechanism of infertility in endometriosis. They have a key role through autocrine-paracrine communication alteration in the mechanism of pelvic adhesion, abnormal folliculogenesis, reduced oocyte/embryo quality, reduced sperm fuction and implantaion impairment (see figure 2). We hope that the increase of our understanding on the above pathomechanism can increase our attention to the improvement of the complex management of infertility in endometriosis.

8. Acknowledgments

The author would like to thank Prof Lila Dewata and Prof Samsulhadi for their assistance in the preparation of the manuscript.

9. References

Agarwal, A., Gupta, S., & Sikkab, S. (2006). The role of free radicals and anti oxidants in reproduction. *Curr. Opin. Obstet. Gynecol.*, Vol. 18, pp. 325–332, ISSN 1040-872x.

Agarwal, A., Sharma, R.K., Nallella, K.P., & Thomas, A.J. Jr., Alvarez, J.G., Sikka, S.C. (2006). Reactive oxygen species as an independent marker of male factor infertility. *Fertil. Steril.*, Vol. 86, pp. 878–85, ISSN 1556-5653.

American Society for Reproductive Medicine (ASRM). (2006). Endometriosis and infertility. The Practice Committee of The American Society for Reproductive Medicine. *Fertil. Steril.*, Vol. 86, pp. 156-60, ISSN 1556-5653.

Arici, A., Tazuke, S.I., Attar, E., Kliman, H.J., Olive, D.L. (1996). Interleukin-8 concentration in peritoneal fluid of patients with endometriosis and modulation of interleukin-8 expression in human mesothelial cells. *Mol. Hum. Reprod.*, Vol. 2, pp. 40 –5, ISSN 1460-2407.

Barnhart, K.M., Dunsmoor, R., Su, M.S., & Coutifaris, C. (2002). Effect of endometriosis on in vitro fertilization. *Fertil. Steril.*, Vol. 77, pp. 1148-1155, ISSN 1556-5653.

Bedaiwy, M.A., Falcone, T., Sharma, R.K., Goldberg, J.M., Attaran, M., Nelson, D.R., et al. (2002). Prediction of endometriosis with serum and peritoneal fluid markers: a prospective controlled trial. Hum. Reprod., Vol. 17, pp. 426–31, ISSN 1460-2350.

Carlberg, M., Nejaty, J., Froysa, B., Guan, Y., Soder, O., & Bergqvist, A. (2000). Elevated expression of TNFα in cultured granulosa cells from women with endometriosis. *Hum. Reprod.*, Vol. 15, pp. 1250-5, ISSN 1460-2350.

Carli, C., Leclerc, P., Metz, C.N., & Akoum, A. (2007). Direct effect of macrophage migration inhibitory factor on sperm function: possible involvement in endometriosis-associated infertility. *Fertil. Steril.*, Vol. 88, pp. 1240–7, ISSN 1556-5653.

Cheong, Y.C., Shelton, J.B., Laird, S.M., Richmond, RM., Kudesia, G., Li, T.C., Ledger, W.L. (2002). IL-1, IL-6 and TNF-α concentrations in peritoneal fluid of women with pelvic adhesions. *Hum. Reprod.*, Vol. 17, pp. 69-75, ISSN 1460-2350.

D'hooghe, T.M., Debrock, S. (2002). Endometriosis, retrograde menstruation and peritoneal inflammation in women and in baboons. *Hum. Reprod. Update.*, Vol. 8, pp. 84-88, ISSN 1460-2369.

Eisermann, J., Register, K.B., Strickler, R.C., & Collins, J.L. (1989).The Effect of Tumor Necrosis Factor on Human Sperm Motility In Vifro. *J. of Andrology.*, Vol. 10, pp. 270-4, ISSN 1939-4640.

Elvin, J.A,. Clark, A.T., Wang, P., Wolfman, N.M., & Matzuk, M. (1999). Paracrine action of growth differentiation factor-9 in mammalian ovary. *Mol. Endocrinol.*, Vol. 13, pp. 1035–48, ISSN 1944-9917.

Erickson, G.F., & Shimasaki, S. (2001). The physiology of folliculogenesis: the role of novel growth factors. *Fertil. Steril.*, Vol. 76, pp. 943–9, ISSN 1556-5653.

Garcia-Velasco, J.A., Arici, A. (1999). Interleukin-8 stimulates the adhesion of endometrial stromal cells to fibronectin. *Fertil. Steril.*, Vol. 72, pp. 336-341, ISSN 1556-5653.

Garcia-Velasco, J.A., Nikas, G., Remohı´, J., Pellicer, J.A., & Simon, C. (2001). Endometrial receptivity in terms of pinopode expression is not impaired in women with endometriosis in artificially prepared cycles. *Fertil. Steril.*, Vol. 75, pp. 1231–3, ISSN 1556-5653.

Garrido, N., Navarro, J., Remohi, J., Simon, C., & Pellicer, A. (2000). Hormonal follicular environment and embryo quality in women with endometriosis. *Hum. Reprod. Updat.e*, Vol. 6, No. 1, pp. 67-74, ISSN 1460-2369.

Garrido, N., Navarro, J., Garcia-Velasco, J., Remohi, J., Pellicer, A., & Simon, C. (2002). The endometrium versus embryonic quality in endometriosis-related infertility. *Hum. Reprod. Update.*, Vol. 8, pp. 95-103, ISSN 1460-2369.

Guerin, P., El Mouatassim, S., & Menezo, Y. (2001). Oxidative stress and protection against reactive oxygen species in the pre-implantation embryo and its surroundings. *Hum. Reprod. Update.*, Vol. 7, pp. 175–89, ISSN 1460-2369

Gupta, S., Goldberg, J.M., Aziz, N., Goldberg,E., Krajcir,N., & Agarwal, A. (2008). Pathogenic mechanisms in endometriosis-associated infertility. *Fertil. Steril.*, Vol. 90, pp. 247–57, ISSN 1556-5653.

Harada, T., Iwabe, T., & Terakawa, N. (2001). Role of cytokines in endometriosis. *Fertil.Steril.*, Vol. 76, pp. 1–10, ISSN 1556-5653.

Hendarto, H., Prabowo, P., Moeloek, F.A., & Soetjipto. (2010). Growth differentiation factor 9 concentration in the follicular fluid of infertile women with endometriosis. *Fertil. Steril.*, Vol. 94, pp. 758–60, ISSN 1556-5653.

Kennedy, S., Bergqvist, A., Chapron, C., D'Hooghe, T., Dunselman, G., Greb, R., Hummelshoj, L., Prentice, A., Saridogan, E. (2005). ESHRE guideline for the diagnosis and treatment of endometriosis. *Hum. Reprod.*, Vol. 21, pp. 2698–2704, ISSN 1460-2350.

Lessey, B.A., Castelbaum, A.J., Sawin, S.W., Buck, C.A., Schinnar, R., Bilker, W., & Strom, B.L. (1994) Aberrant integrin expression in the endometrium of women with endometriosis. *J. Clin. Endocrinol. Metab.*, Vol. 79, pp. 643–649, ISSN 0021-972x

Mansour, G., Aziz, N., Sharma, R., Falcone, T., Goldberg, J., & Agarwal,A. (2009). The impact of peritoneal fluid from healthy women and from women with endometriosis on sperm DNA and its relationship to the sperm deformity index. *Fertil. Steril.*, Vol. 92, pp. 61–7, ISSN 1556-5653.

Mansour, G., Sharma, R.K., Agarwal, A., & Falcone, T. (2010). Endometriosis-induced alterations in mouse metaphase II oocyte microtubules and chromosomal alignment: a possible cause of infertility. *Fertil. Steril.*, Vol. 94, pp. 1894–9, ISSN 1556-5653.

Martynow, M.D., Jedrzejczak, P., Pawelczyk, L. (2007). Pronuclear scoring as a predictor of embryo quality in *in vitro* fertilization program. *Fol. Histo. et Cytobiol.*, Vol. 45, pp. 87-91, ISSN 0239-8508.

Nakahara, K., Saito, H., Saito, T., Ito, M., Ohta, N., Takahashi, T. et al. (1997). Ovarian fecundity in patients with endometriosis can be estimated by the incidence of apoptotic bodies. *Fertil. Steril.*, Vol. 69, pp. 931–5, ISSN 1556-5653.

Nikas, G. (1999). Pinopodes as markers of endometrial receptivity in clinical practice. *Hum. Reprod.*, Vol. 14, pp. 99 -106, ISSN 1460-2350.

Omwandho, C.O.A., Konrad, L., Halis, G.I., Oehmke, F., & Tinneberg, H.R. (2010). Role of TGF-bs in normal human endometrium and endometriosis. *Hum. Reprod.*, Vol. 25, pp. 101–109, ISSN 1460-2350.

Oral, E., Olive, D.L., & Arici, A. (1996a). The peritoneal environment in endometriosis. *Hum. Reprod. Update.*, Vol. 2, No. 5, pp. 385-398 , ISSN 1460-2369.

Oral, E., Seli, E., Bahtiyar, M., Olive, D., & Arici, A. (1996b). Growth regulated alpha expression in the peritoneal environment with endometriosis. *Obstet. Gyneco.l*, Vol. 88, pp.1050-6, ISSN 0020-7292.

Pellicer, A., Oliveira, N., Ruiz, A., Remohí, J., & Simón, C. (1995). Exploring the mechanism(s) of endometriosis-related infertility: an analysis of embryo development and implantation in assisted reproduction. *Hum. Reprod*, Vol. 10, pp. 91-97, ISSN 1460-2350.

Rajkovic, A., Pangas, S.A., & Matzuk, M.M. (2006). Follicular Development: Mouse, sheep and human models. In: *Knobil and Neill's Physiology of Reproduction*, Neill JD, pp 383-424. 3rd ed. Elsevier, ISBN: 978-0-12-515400-0, Los Angeles.

Reeve, L., Lashen, H., & Pacey, A.A. (2005). Endometriosis affects sperm–endosalpingeal interactions. *Hum. Reprod.*, Vol. 20, 448–451, ISSN 1460-2350

Said, T.M., Agarwal, A., Falcone, T., Sharma, R.K., Mohamed, A.. Bedaiwy, M.A., & Liang, L. (2005). Infliximab may reverse the toxic effects induced by tumor necrosis factor alpha in human spermatozoa: an in vitro model. *Fertil. Steril.*, Vol. 83, 1665–73, ISSN 1556-5653.

Saleh, R.A., Agarwal, A. (2002). Oxidative stress and male infertility: from research bench to clinical practice. *J. Androl.*, Vol. 23, pp. 737–752, ISSN 0196-3635.

Samsulhadi. (2002). Endometriosis: Dari biomolekuler sampai masalah klinis (Endometriosis : from biomoleculer to clinical application). *Majalah Obstetri dan Ginekologi*, Vol.10, pp. 43-50.

Simón, C., Gutiérrez, A., Vidal, A., Santos M.J dr los., Tarín J.J, Remohí, J., Pellicer, A. (1994). Outcome of patients with endometriosis in assisted reproduction: results from in-vitro fertilization and oocyte donation. *Hum. Reprod.*, Vol. 9 , pp. 725-729, ISSN 1460-2350.

Surrey, E.S., Lietz, A.K., Gustofson, R.L., Minjarez, D.A., & Schoolcraft, W.B. (2010). Does endometrial integrin expression in endometriosis patients predict enhanced in vitro fertilization cycle outcomes after prolonged GnRH agonist therapy? *Fertil. Steril.*, Vol. 93, pp. 646–51, ISSN 1556-5653.

Suzuki, T., Izumi, S., Matsubayashi, H., Awaji, H., Yoshikata, K., Makino, T. (2005). Impact of ovarian endometrioma on oocytes and pregnancy outcome in in vitro fertilization. *Fertil. Steril.,* Vol. 83, pp. 908-13, ISSN 1556-5653.

Torres, M.J.G., Acien, P., Campos, A., Velasco, I. (2002). Embryotoxicity of follicular fluid in women with endometriosis. Its relation with cytokines and lymphocytes populations. Hum. Reprod., Vol. 17, pp. 777-781, ISSN 1460-2350.

Toya, M., Saito, H., Ohta, N., Saito, T., Kaneko, T., & Hiroi, M. (2000). Moderate and severe endometriosis is associated with alterations in the cell cycle of granulosa cells in patients undergoing in vitro fertilization and embryo transfer. *Fertil. Steril.,* Vol. 73, pp. 344 -50, ISSN 1556-5653.

Zhang, X., Yao, H., Huang, X., Lu, B., Hong Xu, H., & Zhou, C. (2010). Nerve fibres in ovarian endometriotic lesions in women with ovarian endometriosis. *Hum. Reprod.,* Vol. 25, pp. 392–397, ISSN 1460-2350.

19

Analysis of Differential Genes of Uyghur Women with Endometriosis in Xinjiang

Aixingzi Aili, Ding Yan, Hu Wenjing, Yang Xinhua and Hanikezi Tuerxun
Xinjiang Medical University, China

1. Introduction

Endometriosis (EM) is a common and important health problem, it is estimated to be present in 10%-15% of women in the reproductive age group and 25%-35% of infertile women. In the First Affiliated Hospital of Xinjiang Medical University in China, 447 cases primaily diagnosed with surgically confirmed endometriosis between January 2000 to September 2005, among them 349 cases of endometriosis were Han Chinese (78.1%) and 69 cases Uyghur women with endometriosis (15.3%).

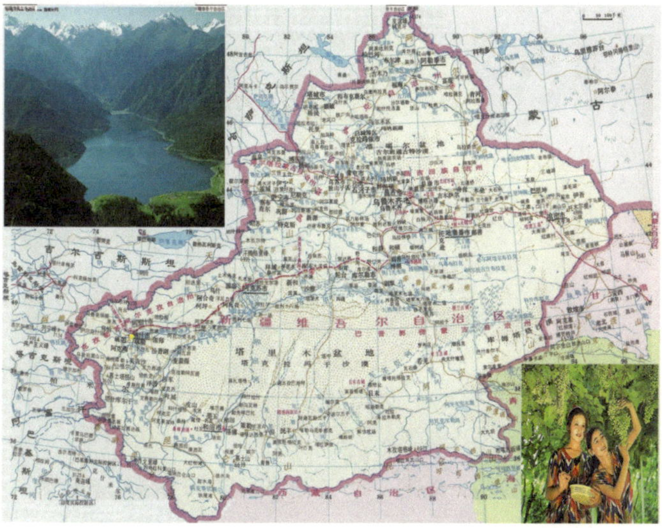

Fig. 1.

Xinjiang is the biggest province of China inhabited by ethnic minorities in which Uyghur people are accounted for more than 40% of the total population. In recent years, the number of the Uyghur women with endometriosis have been increased in Xinjiang, however still clearly less than Han chinese with endometriosis. The data from pathology deparment of the First Affiliated Hospital of Xinjiang Medical University between 1992 and 1996 showed that there were only three Uyghur women with endometriosis (5.76%) among 52 cases. Between 2000 and 2001, only 4 Uyghur women with endometriosis (3.1%) among 128 patients. Between 2003 and 2010, there were 73 Uyghur women (13.45%) with endometriosis in 565 cases. In Kashi, the Uyghur is occupied more than 80% of population. In the last 8 years, there were only 16 Uyghur women with endometriosis among 600 cases of endometriosis in People's Hospital of Kashi. It was demonstrated that the number of Uyghur women with endometriosis dramaticaly lower than Han chinese.

We performed At1asTMcDNA Expression Arrays (Clontech # 7854-1) cDNA microarray (containing 22,000. DNA)to compare the differential expression genes between ectopic endometrium of Uyghur and Han chinese women with endometriosis. Our study aimed to explore the molecular pathogenesis of endometriosis ethnic differences, so as to determine the cause of endometriosis of Uyghur women in Xinjiang.

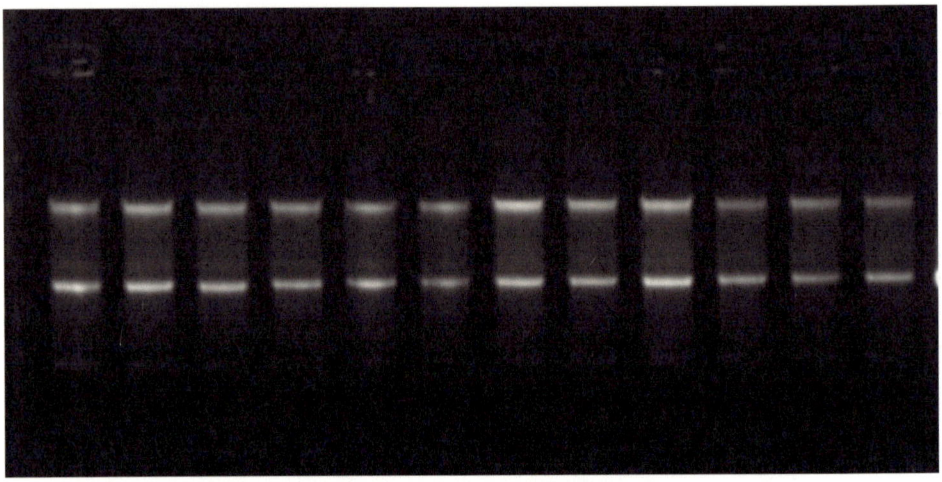

Fig. 2. Total RNA results.

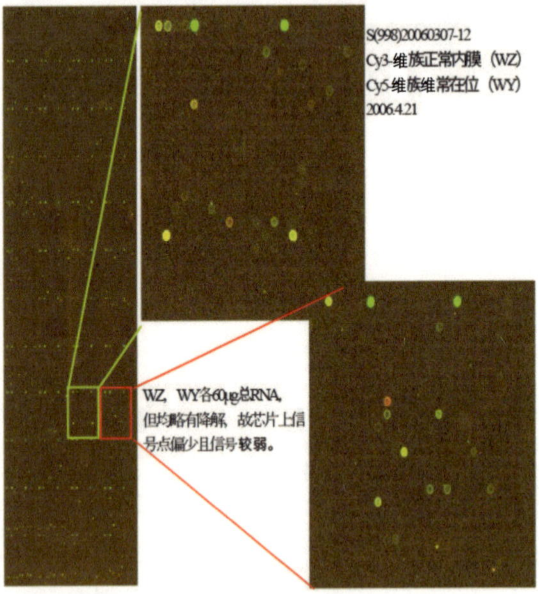

Fig. 3. Uyghur with and without endometriosis ectopic endometriosis hybrid.

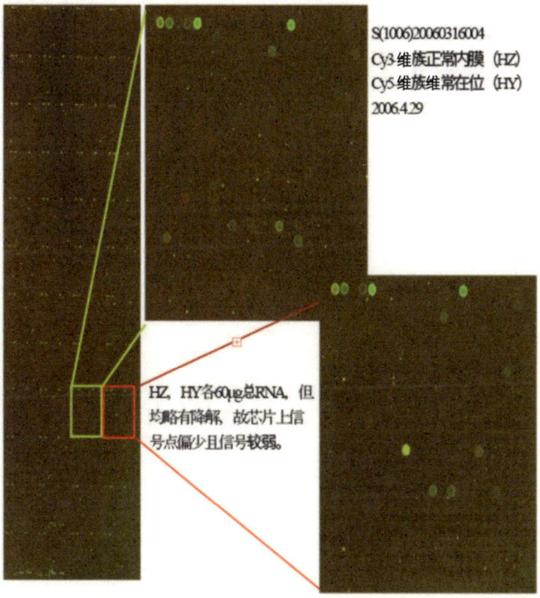

Fig. 4. Han with and without endometriosis ectopic endometriosis hybrid.

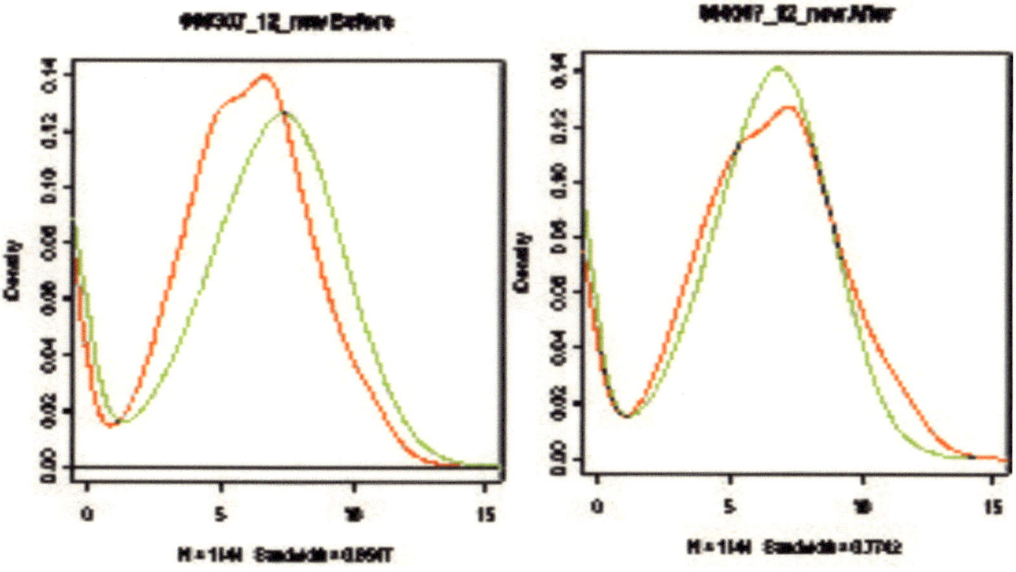

Fig. 5. Uyghur with and without endometriosis ectopic endometriosis hybrid before and after correction signal strength distribution.

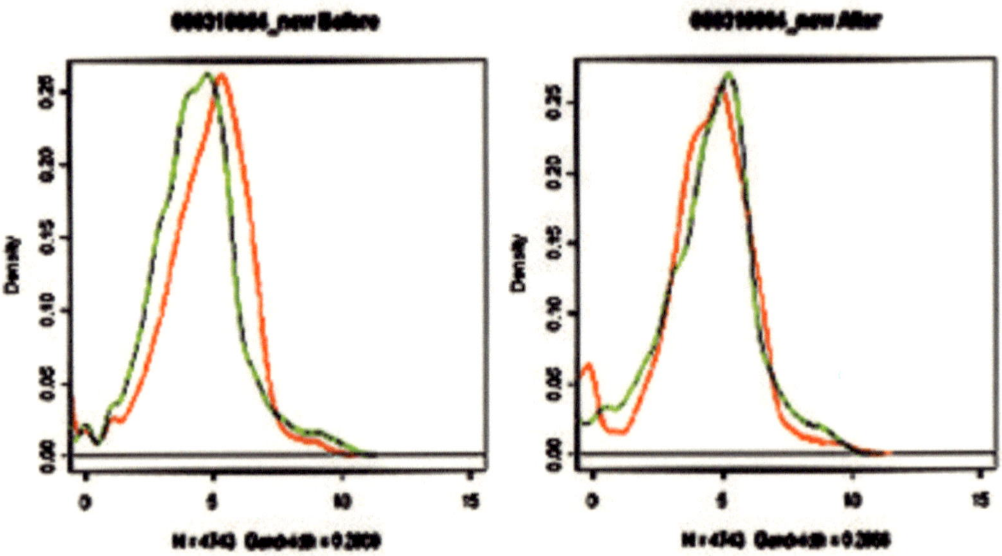

Fig. 6. Han with and without endometriosis ectopic endometriosis hybrid before and after correction signal strength distribution.

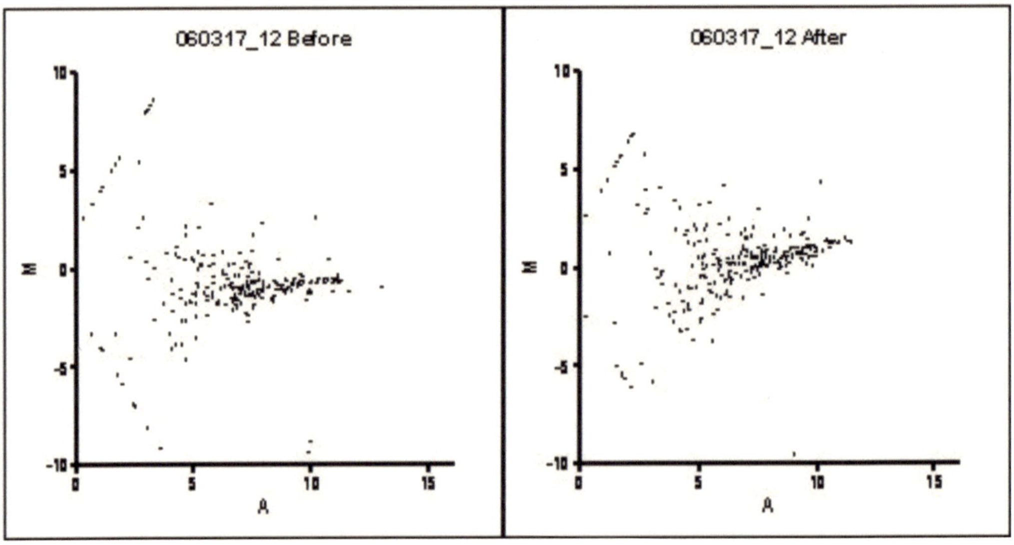

Fig. 7. Uyghur with and without endometriosis ectopic endometriosis hybrid before and after correction signal scatter.

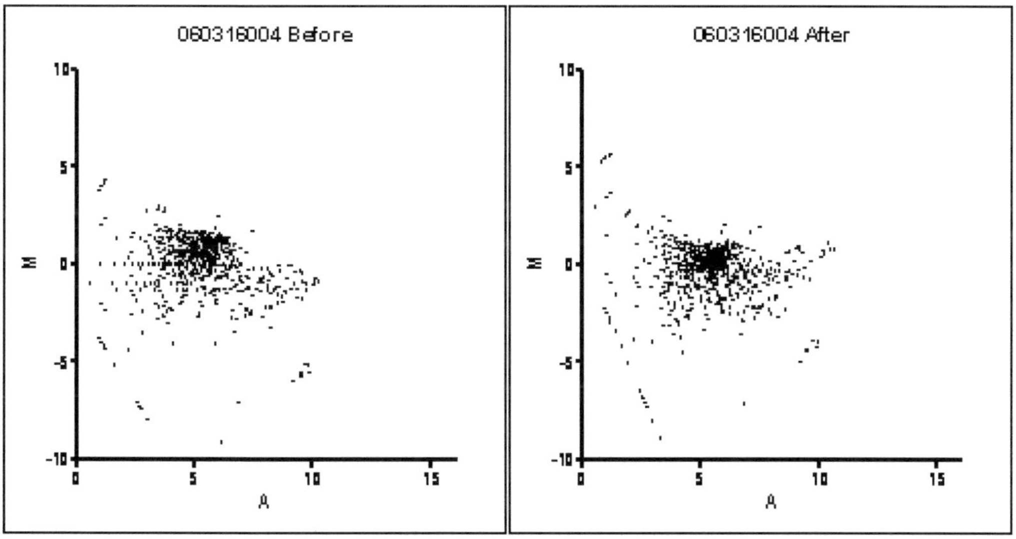

Fig. 8. Han with and without endometriosis ectopic endometriosis hybrid before and after correction signal scatter.

ID	Name	Cy5/Cy	Description
4340	FOS	3.649786	V-fos FBJ murine osteosarcoma viral oncogene homolog
7224	DCN	2.250099	Decorin
10599	VIM	1.629836	Vimentin
1900	GNG5	1.211619	Guanine nucleotide binding protein (G protein), gamma 5
1527	XCL1	1.169442	Small inducible cytokine subfamily C, mendometriosisber 1 (lymphotactin)
13167	IGFBP7	1.114798	Insulin-like growth factor binding protein 7
1651	RPS23	1.093641	Ribosomal protein S23
22665	TIMP3	-1.15294	Tissue inhibitor of metalloproteinase 3
13265	COL3A1	-1.55893	Collagen, type III, alpha 1 (Ehlers-Danlos syndrome type IV, autosomal dominant)
21389	RPL29	-1.63396	Ribosomal protein L29
8626	GAPD	-2.01536	Glyceraldehyde-3-phosphate dehydrogenase
22689	GAPD	-2.30404	Glyceraldehyde-3-phosphate dehydrogenase
22785	GAPD	-2.71698	Glyceraldehyde-3-phosphate dehydrogenase

Table 1. Uyghur with and without endometriosis ectopic endometriosis differential genes.

ID	Name	Rate of Cy5/Cy3	Description
18428	FTL	4.340706	ESTs, Weakly similar to FRHUL ferritin light chain [H.sapiens]
8586	APOE	3.768085	Apolipoprotein E
7998	CD74	3.623251	CD74 antigen (invariant polypeptide of major histocompatibility complex, class II antigen-associated
21034	CTSD	2.992721	Cathepsin D (lysosomal aspartyl protease)
20900	IGL@	2.941947	H.sapiens mRNA for IgG lambda light chain V-J-C region (clone Tgl9)
18699	BIN3	3.235432	Bridging integrator 3
10633	CTSB	2.736133	Cathepsin B
16743	IGKV1-9	2.482954	Immunoglobulin kappa variable 1-9
10901	IGHG3	2.24961	Immunoglobulin heavy constant gamma 3 (G3m marker)
17716	ZFHXI B	2.221742	Zinc finger homeobox 1 b
15732	ACTA2	1.939791	Actin, alpha 2, smooth muscle, aorta
6876	HLA-G	1.795164	HLA-G histocompatibility antigen, class I, G
9464	HLA-A	1.617767	Major histocompatibility complex, class I, A
12611	ITM2C	1.60875	Integral mendometriosisbrane protein 3
9202	DLGAP4	1.56221	KIAA0964 protein
6875	WNT7A	1.55996	Wingless-type MMTV integration site family, mendometriosisber 7A
6494	FTH1	1.55145	Ferritin, heavy polypeptide 1
6952	TMSB10	1.539032	Thymosin, beta 10
22794	ACTB	1.51553	Actin, beta
22769	ACTB	1.495315	Actin, beta
10474	FLJ14950	1.489821	Hypothetical protein FLJ14950
13167	IGFBP7	1.486395	Insulin-like growth factor binding protein 7
18071	HUMMHC W1A	1.460991	Cw1 antigen
22698	ACTB	1.45868	Actin, beta
12651	SPARC	1.441213	Secreted protein, acidic, cysteine-rich (osteonectin)
22696	RPL5	1.421712	Ribosomal protein L5
13180	LOC51237	1.416254	Hypothetical protein
14701	HSU79274	1.391079	Protein predicted by clone 23733
22793	ACTB	1.374773	Actin, beta
5712	GPX3	1.370492	Glutathione peroxidase 3(plasma)
22985	ACTB	1.342603	Actin, beta
22674	ACTB	1.333726	Actin, beta
22697	ACTB	1.33342	Actin, beta
21176	KPT13	1.327325	Keratin 13
22889	ACTB	1.325337	Actin, beta
22700	CYC1	1.325323	Cytochrome c-1
23193	LOC389643	1.323453	LOC389643

Table 2. Han with and without endometriosis ectopic endometriosis differential genes.

ID	Name	Rate of Cy5/Cy3	Description
9988	ACTB	1.293784	Actin, beta
20299	IL1 RN	1.283803	Interleukin 1 receptor antagonist
16687	TP73	1.277275	Tumor protein p73
22986	ACTB	1.267406	Actin, beta
22770	ACTB	1.258614	Actin, beta
10599	VIM	1.251847	Vimentin
22865	ACTB	1.233357	Actin, beta
22345	LOC440552	1.232367	similar to OK/SW-CL.16
8173	MARK2	1.227909	ELKL motif kinase
22962	ACTB	1.219306	Actin, beta
21216	SLPI	1.215856	Secretory leukocyte protease inhibitor
22690	ANKT	1.213863	Nucleolar protein
23200	LOC389622	1.212664	LOC389622
22961	ACTB	1.212137	Actin, beta
22673	ACTB	1.210056	Actin, beta
22890	ACTB	1.208872	Actin, beta
19718	SULT1C2	1.207869	Sulfotransferase family, cytosolic, 1C, mendometriosisber 2
12903	HSPA5BP1	1.179906	Hypothetical protein FLJ20539
22785	PDGFRA	1.159421	Platelet-derives growth factor receptor
1900	GNG5	1.125384	Guanine nucleotide binding protein (G protein), gamma 5
20231	SERF2	1.112907	Small EDRK-rich factor 2
15491	ZNF14	1.104864	Zinc finger protein 14 (KOX 6)
9735	KIAA0635	1.100348	Hypothetical protein FLJ13621
16540	CDW92	1.092801	CDw92 antigen
22762	COPEB	1.08944	Core promoterelendometriosisent binding protein
22866	ACTB	1.083347	Actin, beta
8626	GPX3	1.078504	Glutathione peroxidase 3(plasma)
1401	ELAVL3	1.077059	ELAV (endometriosisbryonic lethal, abnormal vision, Drosophila)-like 3 (Hu antigen C)
19581	GNG5	1.057676	Guanine nucleotide binding protein (G protein), gamma 5
7186	ID3	1.057184	Inhibitor of DNA binding 3, dominant negative helix-loop-helix protein
17362	FKBP14	1.036957	Hypothetical protein FLJ20731
9824	MTBP	1.030879	Mdm2, transformed 3T3 cell double minute 2, p53 binding protein (mouse) binding protein, 104kD
8364	ARHGDIA	1.029915	Rho GDP dissociation inhibitor (GDI) alpha
21961	RPS23	1.025033	Ribosomal protein S23
1580	NELF	1.017617	DKFZP586J1624 protein
22665	GAPD	-1.003765	Glyceraldehyde-3-phosphate dehydrogenase
22761	GAPD	-1.001544	Glyceraldehyde-3-phosphate dehydrogenase
17133	GAPD	-4.29046	Glyceraldehyde-3-phosphate dehydrogenase

Table 2. Han with and without endometriosis ectopic endometriosis differential genes. (Continuation)

ID	Name	Rate of Cy5/Cy3	Description
7979	PAEP	-5.57639	Progestagen-associated endometrial protein (placental protein 14, pregnancy-associated endometrial a
1813	TIMP3	-2.748361	Tissue inhibitor of metalloproteinase 3 (erythroid potentiating activity, collagenase inhibitor)

Table 2. Han with and without endometriosis ectopic endometriosis differential genes. (Continuation)

2. The incidence of endometriosis of Uyghur ethnic group in Xinjiang

The incidence of endometriosis has no precise information. Researchs have found that Asian women with endometriosis have a higher prevalence, and its disease risk :OR:8.6(95%CI 11.4—20.7). There was an exploratory study suggested that there might be an associated risk of endometriosis for those women who have worked as a flight attendant, service station attendant, or health worker, particularly a nurse. But they have not been reported the correlation between nationality, religion and other factors with endometriosis.

Clinical and epidemiological survey found that endometriosis has a genetic predisposition and significant family aggregation, and it loss of heterozygosity of 40% -70%. Dingyan(researcher in Xinjiang) found that no evidence was found to suggest an association between GSTM1-null genotype and endometriosis in the Hans chinese and Uyghurs. An association was found between GSTT1 -null genotype and endometriosis in the Hans chinese, but not in the Uyghurs. The two ethnic groups have different genetic predisposing factors to the development of endometriosis. There were significant difference in the frequencies of these two points among the Han chinese, European and Uyghur in Xinjiang. In Uyghur the distribution of CYP 1 A 1 /MspI genotypes were different from Han chinese and European.

3. The spectrum of microarray applications on endometriosis

A large number of microarray gene-specific cDNA are fixed on a glass or silica using the hybridization principles to detect the mRNA of the different sources. This study shows the different organization, different cells and tissues in different developmental stages that have differentially expressed genes. Development of molecular mechanisms provide theoretical basis for gene diagnosis and treatment of cutting-edge biotechnology. The theory proposed by Sampson in 1927 suggests that endometrial tissue is released into the peritoneal cavity via retrograde menstruation. The shed tissue then implants and grows ectopically. This theory is supported by the fact that up to 76% -90% of women experience retrograde menstruation ; and yet, endometriosis only affects 10% -15% of women. Reference to foreign literature, different individuals sample of patient with endometriosis geometric mixed, different individuals sample of patient without endometriosis geometric mixed, to eliminate non-specific genetic differences between individuals, and search for specific associated genes with endometriosis. By the gene microarray expression profiling 22,000 points compare ectopic endometrium and normal ectopic endometrial of the Uyghur and Han chinese with endometriosis, 11 differential genes expressed in ectopic endometrium were screened out between Uyhgur women with or without endometriosis respectively, FOS, DCN, VIN, GNGS, XCL 1, IGFBP7, PRS23, TIMP3, COL3A1, PRL29, GAPD; GAPD expression in the three loci, including FOS, DCN, VIN, GNGS, XCL1, IGFBP7, PRS23 were up-regulated, and TIMP3, COL3A1, PRL29, GAPD were down-regulated. The Han chinese group were significantly different genes, 58 of which TIMP3, PAEP, GADP were down-regulated, but GADP expressed in three loci shows different range. And from a different CD74, ACTA2, GPX3 and other 55 genes were upregulated, ACTB appear in 17 loci, GNGS appear in two loci. The same genes difference between the two groups is VIM, GNGS, PRS23, GAPD, TIMP3, including GAPD, TIMP3 are down-regulated. We get different genes according to their main function and are divided into the following categories: immune-related genes,proto-oncogenes and tumor suppressor genes,cell receptor,ion channels and transport protein; cytoskeleton and sports-related protein, apoptosis-related protein; DNA synthesis and repair, recombinant protein, DNA binding, transcription and transcription factors,cell signaling and transmission white and some unknown functional genes.

4. The possible role of clinically relevant different gene in endometriosis pathogenesis

The difference in the screened genes, tissue inhibitor of metalloproteinase 3 (TIMP-3) both in the Han chinese and Uyghur with endometriosis were down-regulated. The study of Zhou Honghui found that TIMP-3 down-regulation is remarkable in the secretory phase than proliferative phase. TIMP is a metalloproteinase (MMPs) inhibitors by the endometrial cells of MMPs which plays an important role in the invasion of the peritoneum and other connective tissue. Increased endometrial MMPs and TIMP down-regulation with the development of endometriosis is closely related. Because of TIMP up-regulation and MMPs down-reglation, ectopic endometrial of endometriosis is more invasive than normal force, and develop to the peritoneal endometriotic lesions.Angiogenesis is considered as a major process in the pathogenesis of endometriosis. Many factors are involved in this complex mechanism, and the vascular endothelial growth factor (VEGF) is an important mediator of angiogenesis; it is a potent endothelial cell mitogen, morphogen, and vascular permeability-inducing agent. VEGF binds to either of two tyrosine kinase receptors, the fm5-like tyrosine kinase (flt) and the kinase domain receptor (KDR or Flk-1). Peritoneal endometriotic lesions with high proliferative activity are also accompanied by high angiogenic activity, as reflected by higher expression of VEGF-A in stroma and glandular epithelium and VEGFR-2 in blood vessels. In our recent study, we showed that the vascular density and the expression of VEGF and its receptor VEGFR-2 (Flk-1) are significantly higher in deeply infiltrating endometriosis affecting the ovary, bladder and mainly the rectosigmoid, compared with the ectopic endometrium.

Controlled clinical analyses of angiogenesis in human endometriotic lesions are limited, because it is not possible to monitor the lesions without repeated laparoscopies. Thus, research into the fundamental mechanisms by which menstrual endometrium adheres, invades and establishes a functional vasculature to persist in an ectopic site, as well as the development of new therapeutical approaches, is best performed in experimental animal models. In contrast to humans and non-human primates, estrous animals do not shed their endometrial tissue and therefore do not develop endometriosis spontaneously. However, endometriosis can be induced by transplanting endometrial tissue to ectopic sites, and the establishment of an experimental model of endometriosis may be a good way to study the endometriosis angiogenesis process, and allow evaluation of the balance of the many factors involved.

This study by glyceraldehyde 3-phosphate dehydrogenase (GAPD) gene in Han chinese and Uyghurs with endometriosis group are down-regulated, GAPD genes are housekeeping gene family, Gene bank No. NM-002046, is a basic enzyme in the human body.It is a key enzyme of a series of biochemical reactions of the glycolysis, which generate ATP for the source of human cells energy, a variety of cells are present in the body, involved in glucose metabolism in glycolysis, in 12p13.

In Han and Uyghur groups the same set of common up-regulated genes are GNGS, VIM and PRS23. Abundance or localization changes in endometrial tissue were validated by immunohistochemistry and Western blotting. In addition, multiple charge and size isoforms were observed for VIM in endometriosis patients that was below the level of detection in healthy women.

Our experiment confirmed endometriosis may be related to multiple factors similar as diabetes, asthma, cancer-related disease, genetics and aberrant regulation in the endometrium and endometriotic. Lower different genes expression on Uyghur women with endometriosis compared to Han Chinese women with endometriosis may be the essential factor for relatively lower incidence of endometriosis on Uyghur women. Most genes we found on the endometrium of both Uyghur and Han Chinese women with endometriosis were the cytoskeleton, adhesion, invaded and immune related gene,patially explained the mechanism of malignant biological behaviors.

5. References

[1] O Down MJ, Philipp EE. The history of obstetrics and gynecology. New York: The Parthenon Publishing group, 2000,523.

[2] Jinghe Lang. The new progress on endometriosis research, Chinese journal of obstetrics and gynecology. 2005, 40:3-4.

[3] Stephen K, Simon B, Daniel EW. Genetics and infertility II affected sib-pair analysis in endometriosis. Hum Reprod Update, 2001,7(4): 411-418

[4] Eskenazi B, Warner ML. Epidemiology of endometriosis. Obstet Gynecol Clin North Am, 1997,24(2):235-258.

[5] Zondervan KT. The genetic basis of endometriosis. Curr Opin Obstet Gynecol, 2001,13(3):309-314.

[6] Qiaozhi Lin, Baozheng Wu .Endometriosis. Qiaozhi Lin's gynecology oncology. Beijin, People's Publishing House, the third edition, 2000,697-713.

[7] Eskenazi B, Warner ML. Epidemiology of endometriosis. Obstet Gynecol Clin North Am, 1997,24(2):235-258.

[8] Yan Ding, Zhifang Chen, Jianyong ChenThe Study on the differential genes expression on women with endometriosis in Xinjiang. Chinese journal of obstetrics and gynecology., 2004,39(2):101-104。

[9] Hawkins T, Venkatesh B, Rokhsar D, et al. Whole-genome shotgun assembly and analysis of the genome of Fugu rubripes. Science, 2002, 297:1301-1310.

[10] Jinghe Lang. The basic and clinical research of endometriosis. Beijin; Beijing union medical university press , 2003:35-50.

[11] Yali Li, Huilan Zhang. Endometriosis [J]. Chin J Pract Gynecol Obstet, 2002,18:131-172.

[12] Jane M, Borthwick D, Stephen C, et al. Determination of the trans- cript profile of human endometrium[J]. Molecular Human Reproduc- tion, 2003,9:19-33.

[13] Honghui Zhou, Yali Li, Jie Li, Screening differential genes expression associated with endometriosis with expression gene chip. Progress in Obstetrics and Gynecology, 2004, 13(6):406-409.

[14] Majid MA, Smith VA, Rasty DL, et al. Adenovirus mediated gene dilivery of tissue inhibitor of metalloproteinases-3 induces death in retinal pigment epithilial cells[J]. Br J Ophthalamol, 2002,86:97-101.

[15] Gao Y, Zhou S, Jiang W, et al. Effects of ganopoly on the immune functions in advanced-stage cancer patients. Immunol Invest, 2003,32 (3):201-215.

[16] Hsu MJ, Lee SS, Lee ST, et al. Signaling mechanisms of enhanced neutrophil phagocytosis and chemotaxis by the polysaccharide purified from Ganoderma lucidum. Br J Pharmacol, 2003,139(2):289- 298.

[17] Liu B, Aronson N, N Jr. Structure of human G protein gene GNG5[J]. Biochem Biophys Res Commun, 1998,251:88.

[18] Gough NR, Adler ENDOMETRIOSIS, Ray LB. Focus issue:targeting signaling pathways for drug discovery[J]. Sci STKE, 2004,(225):EG5.

[19] Perrenu J, Lilienlxaum A, Vasseur M, et al. Nucleotide Sequence of the vimentin gene [J]. 1988,62(1):7.

[20] Ferram S, Cartnizzare A, Battin R, et al. Human vimentin is readed on the short arm of chromosome 10[J]. Am J Hum Gene, 1987,4(14): 616.

[21] Nikcolic B, Nully E B, Mir H et al. Basic acid residue cluster within nuclear targeting sequence is assential for cytoplasma plectin- bimentin network junctions[J]J Cell Biol, 1996,134(6):1455.

[22] Hermann H, Aebi H. Intermediate filaments and their associates: multi-talented structural elements specifying cytoarchitecture and cytodynamics[J]. Curr Opin Cell Biol, 2000,12:79-90.

[23] Quax W, Meera khan P, Quax-jeuken Y. The structure of the vimentin gen[J]. Cell, 1983,35(1)215.

[24] Mingtong Xu,Lin Lv, Zhinu Zhong, People leptin gene cloning and sequence determined [J]. Sen University of Medical Sciences. 2000,21(2):104。

[25] Zoppi N, Oardella R, De Paepe A, et a1. Human fibroblasts with mutations in COL5A1 and COL3A1 genes do not organize collagens and fibronectin in the extracellular matrix, down—regulate alpha2betal integrin, and recruit alphavbeta3 instead of alphasbetal integrin[J]. J Biol Chem, 2004,279(18):18157-18168。

[26] Thomas EJ, Campbell G. Molecular genetic defects in endometriosis. Gynecol Obstet Invest, 2000,50(supl 1)44-50.
[27] Sendometriosisino C, Sendometriosisino A, Pietra G, et al. Role of major histocompatibility complex class I expression and natural killer-like T cells in the genetic control of endometriosis. Fertil Steril, 1995,64:909-916.
[28] Xin Wang, Chunyu Liu, Endometriosis [J]. People leptin gene cloning and sequence determined , 2002,37(6):346- 348.

20

Primary Afferent Nociceptors and Visceral Pain

Victor Chaban
Charles R. Drew University of Medicine and Science and University of California, Los Angeles, USA

1. Introduction

Patients with chronic pelvic pain frequently have pain from several pelvic organs. The most common diagnoses include endometriosis, interstitial cystitis, irritable bowel disease, pelvic floor tension myalgia, vulvar vestibulitis, and vulvodynia. Frequently, pain does not correlate with pathologic findings at the time of laparoscopy in the case of endometriosis, while vulvodynia, irritable bowel syndrome and pelvic floor tension myalgia and neuropathy may have no clearly demonstrable pathologic tissue changes. Most diagnoses associated with chronic pelvic pain have a high rate of recurrence and all are considered to be chronic conditions with a relapsing course. Endometriosis is a complex, poorly understood chronic illness of women in their reproductive age and pain is the major concern of women with this disease. Despite a successful reduction of pain using during the novel treatments pain returns in up to 75% of treated women. Pain is strongly associated with this disease and the lack of awareness to its pathology is further illustrated by the fact that the average time duration between the onset of pain and the diagnosis of endometriosis is 3 to 11 years despite the fact that 25-30% of women with chronic pelvic pain suffer from this disease. In women with endometriosis (mainly of reproductive age) alterations in the limbic and sympathetic nervous system and hypothalamic-pituitary-adrenal axis mediate a cycle of hypervigilance for pain sensations from pelvic organs, which can lead to descending induction of pathologic changes in pelvic organs. Chronic pelvic pain patients frequently have multiple diagnoses. Vicero-somatic and viscero-viseral hyperalgesia and allodynia result in the spread of a perception of pain from an initial site to adjacent areas. Chronic pelvic pain patients may initially have only one pain source in the pelvis, such as the uterus in dysmenorrhea or endometriosis implants, but a multitude of mechanisms involving the peripheral and central nervous system can lead to the development of painful sensations from other adjacent organs. Often the etiology of visceral pain is not clear, as there are many symptoms of the reproductive system, gastrointestinal and urinary tracts, musculoskeletal, neurological and psychological systems that often co-occur in the same patient. The variation of pain symptoms and pain perception and behavioral responses to pain in these patients is poorly understood. The treating clinician is often tempted to take a unidimensional approach and focus on one organ system and ignore the psychological and behavioral manifestations of the chronic pain.

The incidence of persistent, episodic, or chronic visceral pain are more prevalent in females thus defining the site(s) and mechanisms through which female steroid hormones modulate visceral nociception is an important step in understanding the gender differences in pain perception and in designing appropriate therapies for females. One such mechanism may be the convergence of nociceptive stimuli and estrogen input on the primary afferent neurons which innervate viscera. Based on our results, it is likely that estrogen receptors (ERs) expressed in primary afferent neurons modulate nociceptive signaling. Our recent data suggest that estrogen acting on primary afferent nociceptors modulates the response to pro- and anti-nociceptive signals associated with the clinical presentation of functional disorders such as endometriosis.

1.2 The nociception of endometriosis

Endometrial tissues outside the uterus can cause severe pain and this pain can be diminished with therapies that suppress estrogen production (Berkley *et al.* 2005). The mechanism of endometriosis-induced nociceptive signaling is poorly understood and in some cases pain can be exacerbated by co-morbidity with other chronic pelvic pain syndromes such as irritable bowel syndrome, painful bladder syndrome, vulvodynia and fibromyalgia. It has also been shown that ectopic implants develop sensory nerve supply both in women and in animal models of endometriosis. Sensory input arriving from the visceral organ to the spinal cord divergences at the level of primary sensory neurons which further transmit considerable information from periphery to the central nervous system. Visceral pain may be manifestation from a single organ such as uterus or may arise from algogenic conditions affecting more than one organ (Malykhina 2007). This type of pain is important not only because it is difficult to diagnose its clinical conditions but also for its therapeutic implications. It is quite possible to modulate pain from one viscus to another. Recent study by Giamberardino and others showed that the treatment of the endometriotic lesions results in the improvement of spontaneous and referred urinary symptoms (Giamberardino *et al.* 2010).

Cross-sensitization in the pelvis implies the transmission of noxious stimuli from one organ to another through an adjacent normal structure resulting in functional (rarely organic) changes. Pelvic organ cross-sensitization is considered as one of the factors contributing to chronic pelvic pain (Pezzone *et al.* 2005). Chronic pelvic pain (CPP) syndrome affects up to 25% of reproductive age women and results in dysmenorrhea, menstrual irregularities, back pain and reduced fecundity. One of the most common causes of CPP is endometriosis. Chronic pain adversely affects mood, social and professional life and general well being. Thus, assessing the impact of the pain on various domains of a patient's existence has become an important focus in the clinical management. Most women with complaints of pelvic pain will undergo laparoscopy to both diagnose and treat these diseases, but laparoscopy is often is unsuccessful due to lack of intraperitoneal pathology or altered pain processing. Pain out of proportion to identifiable pathology is the most immediate and dramatic consequence of disorders associated with CPP and is responsible for a highly negative impact on quality of life and substantial workforce loss. Results of a national survey determined that 15% of women in the United States have experienced CPP and only 10% of these consulted a gynecologist and 75% did not consult a health care provider of any type. Due to the alarming situation and unmet need, the USA and other countries have launched a call for more focused research on improving the diagnosis and treatment of CPP syndrome.

There is often no clear relationship between the severity of the chronic pelvic pain and pathology in the pelvic viscera, including reproductive tract (ovaries and uterus). It is still poorly understood how endometriosis is associated with pain symptoms in different organs and how this nociceptive signaling is ameliorated by a hypoestrogenic state. One of the possible explanation can be that endometrial implants' sensory nerve supply and its potentially estradiol-modulated influence on the nociception.

Several researchers have investigated the presence of nerve fibers in endometriotic lesions in both human and animal study. Using different types of specific immunohistochemical neuronal markers such as substance P (SP) and calcitonin gene related peptide (CGRP) sensory nerve fibers markers) in human peritoneal endometriotic lesions from women with visually and biopsy proven endometriosis, investigators have demonstrated multiple, small unmyelinated nerve fibers are present in peritoneal endometriotic lesions, and these peritoneal endometriotic lesions contain both Aδ and C nerve fibers. Accumulating evidence has shown these nerve fibers may play a critical role in pain production in patients with endometriosis, and a close histological relationship has been identified between these nerve fibers and endometriosis associated pain. Tulandi *et al.* (2001) reported that the distance between endometriotic glands and nerve fibers in endometriotic lesions from women with pain was closer than in women with no pain. The density of nerve fibers in peritoneal endometriotic lesions was much greater than in normal peritoneum in women with no endometriosis. The nerve fiber density in endometriotic lesions can be markedly reduced by hormonal drugs such as gonadotropin releasing hormone (GnRH) analogues and combined oral contraceptives, which have been used efficaciously to treat endometriosis-associated pain, indicating that modulation of these nerve fibers might alter pelvic nociception. The fact that peritoneal endometriotic lesions are innervated by sensory Aδ, sensory C nerve fibers raises the intriguing questions, what kind of role do these nerve fibers play in the mechanisms by which endometriotic lesions produce pain and hyperalgesia, and how do they modulate pain perception in these condition?

The demonstration of Aδ and C sensory fiber innervations to peritoneal endometriotic lesions, suggesting these innervations contributes to both visceral hyperalgesia and pelvic pain that occur in patients with endometriosis brings up the interesting questions, how do these sensory fibers transmit and modulate visceral nociception in endometriosis? Immunohistochemical staining of these nerve fibers in endometriosis showed co-localization of SP, CGRP, implicating SP and CGRP might be involved in modulation of visceral nociception. Endometriosis is an inflammatory disease, which is known to contain pro-inflammatory cytokines, prostaglandins, and other neuroactive agents that could readily activate the CGRP- and SP-positive C-fiber nociceptive afferents found in the endometriotic lesions.

When these sensory nerve fibers are stimulated by inflammatory substances, neurotransmitters such as SP, CGRP can be secreted from sensory nerve endings. SP and CGRP can contribute to the inflammatory response by causing vasodilation, plasma extravasation and cellular infiltration by interacting with endothelial cells, arterioles, mast cells, neutrophils and immune cells. SP can also act on mast cells in the vicinity of sensory nerve endings to evoke de-granulation and the release of TNF-α, histamine, prostaglandin D2 (PGD2) and leukotriene, providing a positive feedback. CGRP has a wide range of biological activities, including sensory transmission, regulation of glandular secretion, and inhibiting SP degradation by a specific endopeptidase to enhance SP release, thereby amplifying the effects.

Dorsal root ganglion (DRG) neurons can be activated or modulated by the activation of chemosensitive receptors on peripheral terminals and ATP has been implicated in sensory transduction of noxious stimuli by activating purinergic P2X receptors (Dunn *et al.* 2001). Once released into the intercellular areas, the action of ATP is mediated by primarily P2X3 receptors which are expressed on primary afferent fibers and cell bodies within DRG (Burnstock 2001). The capsaicin-sensitive primary afferent neurons of small- and medium-diameter neurons mediate nociceptive-like behaviors suggesting that TRPV1 expressing neurons are nociceptors. Activation of purinergic (P2X3) and transient potential receptors family vcanilloid-1 (TRPV1) receptors results in the depolarization and opening of voltage-gated Ca^{2+}channels (VGCC) (Koshimizu *et al.* 2000). A sensation of pain is produced by depolarization of the peripheral nerve terminals.

1.3 Estrogen receptors and nociceptive signaling in primary afferent neurons

Defining the site(s) and mechanisms through which sex estrogen modulates visceral nociception is an important step in understanding the mechanisms in pain perception associated with endometriosis and in designing appropriate therapies. One such mechanism may be the convergence of nociceptive stimuli and estrogen input on the primary afferent neurons which innervate viscera (i.e. uterus). Estrogen may modulate female sensitivity to clinical and experimentally induced pain. Based on our preliminary results, it is likely that estrogen receptors (ERs) expressed in primary afferent neurons modulate chemical signaling associated with nociception. Nociception is a balance of pro- and anti-nociceptive inputs that is subject to regulation depending on the normal state of the organism. Sensitization of primary afferent neurons to stimulation may play a role in the enhanced perception of visceral sensation and pain. Chest pain from coronary heart disease, endometriosis, acute and recurrent/chronic pelvic pain in women or abdominal are all visceral pain sensations that may result in part from sensitization (Berkley *et al.* 2001; Mayer *et al.* 2001). Mechanisms of peripheral sensitization may involve increased transduction that is secondary to repeated stimulation or an increase in the excitability of the afferent nerves by molecules that decrease the excitation threshold (Zimmermann 2001)

The cell bodies of primary visceral spinal afferent neurons are located in DRG. Direct activation of chemosensitive receptors and ion channels on their peripheral terminals and modulation of neuronal excitability activates extrinsic primary afferent nerves. Nociceptors belong predominantly to small and medium size DRG neurons whose peripheral processes detect potentially damaging physical and chemical stimuli. The terminals of primary visceral afferent neurons are described as having no organs end or morphological specialization, but respond to different chemical stimuli. Visceral nociceptive C-fibers activated by ATP released by noxious stimuli from cells in target organs, have been implicated as mediators of noxious stimulus intensities (Burnstock 2000). Alteration in signal transduction of primary afferent neurons can result in enhanced perception of the visceral sensation that is common in patients with different disorders resulting in elevated pain perception. Acute and recurrent/chronic pelvic pain in women and abdominal pain from IBS are illustrative examples of visceral pain that undergo sensitization (Giamberardino *et al.* 2010).

Peripheral sensitization can develop in response to sustain stimulation, inflammation, and nerve injury. Visceral pain is different from cutaneous pain based on clinical, neurophysiological and pharmacological characteristics (Chang and Heitkemper 2002). The pathophysiology of visceral hyperalgesia is less well-known than its cutaneous counterpart, and our understanding of visceral hyperalgesia is colored by comparison to cutaneous hyperalgesia, which is believed to arise as a consequence of the sensitization of peripheral nociceptors due to long-lasting changes in the excitability of spinal neurons. Endometriosis is currently defined as a chronic functional syndrome characterized by recurring symptoms of abdominal discomfort or pain. In the context of visceral pain, the TRPV1 receptor is a sensory neuron-specific cation channel which plays an important role in transporting thermal and inflammatory pain signals. Evidence for TRPV1's role is that mice lacking TRP1 receptor gene have deficits in thermal- or inflammatory-induced hyperalgesia (Davis *et al.* 2000). Activation of both TRPV1 and P2X receptors induce mobilization of $[Ca^{2+}]_i$ in cultured DRG neurons (Gschossmann *et al.* 2000).

Sex hormones and 17β-estradiol (E2) in particular may directly influence the functions of primary afferent neurons since both ERs are present on small-diameter DRG neurons (Papka and Storey-Workley 2002). Despite the broad spectrum of E2 effects in the nervous system, the mechanisms of hormonal pain modulation remain unclear. There are two subforms: estrogen receptor-α (ERα) and estrogen receptor-β (ERβ) which were traditionally thought of as ligand-activated transcription factors. However, recent work has demonstrated multiplicity of E_2 actions (membrane, cytoplasmic and nuclear) (Nadal *et al.* 2001). ER distributed through CNS and PNS including regions that mediate nociception. For example, ERs are expressed in dorsal horn neurons of the spinal cord and DRG neurons. DRG neurons express both ERα and ERβ *in vivo* (Papka and Storey-Workley 2002) and *in vitro* (Chaban 2010). These findings suggest that E2 may modulate sensory input at the primary afferent level. E2 can alter gene transcription, resulting in pro-nociceptive (reducing β-endorphin expression) or anti-nociceptive (increasing enkephalin expression) changes of endogenous opioid peptides , opioid receptors (Micevych and Sinchak 2001) and, by increasing levels of CCK, an anti-nociceptive and anti-opioid molecule (Micevych *et al.* 2002).

E2 can modulate cellular activity by altering ion channel opening and second messenger signaling by stimulating G-proteins (Chaban *et al.* 2003) , the signal transduction pathways traditionally associated with membrane receptor activation. Many of these effects have been ascribed to membrane-associated receptors. The results from other laboratories (Lee *et al.* 2002) and our data (Chaban *et al.* 2003) indicate that E2 is acting to modulate L-type VGCC. The cloned TRPV1 receptor is a nonselective cation channel with a high permeability for Ca^{2+}. TRPV1's are distributed in peripheral sensory nerve endings and are involved in the transduction of different stimuli in sensory neurons. TRPV1 functions as molecular integrator of painful chemical and physical stimuli (noxious heat (>43° C) and low pH). Various inflammatory mediators such as prostaglandin E_2 (PGE_2) and bradykinin potentiate TRPV1. The potentiation of TRPV1 activity can be quantified by measuring the differences of capsaicin-induced Ca^{2+} concentration changes before and after receptor activation (Petruska *et al.* 2000). Significantly, a subset of DRG neurons respond to both capsaicin and ATP indicating that there may be cross-activation of these receptors that may underlie the sensitization of visceral nociceptors. Capsaicin-induced TPRV1 receptor-mediated changes in $[Ca^{2+}]_i$ may represent a level of DRG activation to noxious cutaneous stimulation while ATP-induced changes in $[Ca^{2+}]_i$ may reflect the level of DRG neuron sensitization to noxious visceral stimuli since ATP is released by noxious stimuli and tissue damage near the primary afferent nerve terminals (Burnstock 2001).

Most of the published reports about sex and hormone-related differences in pain have addressed the modulatory effect of E2 on central nervous system mechanisms of nociception (Aloisi *et al.* 2000). Recent studies demonstrate that E2 has a significant role in modulating viscerosensitivity, indicating that E2-induced alterations in sensory processing may underlie sex-based differences in functional pain syndromes (Al-Chaer and Traub 2002). However, reports of E2 modulation of visceral and somatic nociceptive sensitivity are inconsistent. For example, elevated E2 levels have been reported to increase the threshold to cutaneous stimuli but decrease the percentage of escape responses to ureteral calculosis (Bradshaw and Berkley 2002). Additionally, nociceptive sensitivity increases when E2 levels are elevated (Holdcroft 2000; Bereiter 2001). Indeed in most clinical studies, women report more severe pain levels, more frequent pain and longer duration of pain than men. To help resolve these inconsistencies we propose to study E2 actions on the primary afferents.

Primary DRG neurons culture has been a useful model system for investigating sensory physiology and putative nociceptive signaling (Chaban *et al.* 2003). ATP-induced intracellular calcium concentration ($[Ca^{2+}]_i$) transients in cultured DRG neurons have been used to model the response of nociceptors to painful stimuli. In our laboratory we showed that E2, acting at the level of the plasma membrane, attenuates both ATP -induced $[Ca^{2+}]_i$ and capsaicin- induced $[Ca^{2+}]_i$ influx and that the expression of both P2X3 and TRPV1 depend on the expression of both ERs. Within the context of our hypothesis visceral nociception and nociceptor sensitization appear to be regulated by P2X3 and TRPV1. Estrogen attenuates DRG neurons response to ATP and capsaicin suggesting that visceral afferent nociceptors can be modulated by sex steroids at a new site at the level of primary afferent neurons. Our data suggest that E2 by itself appears to be anti-nociceptive but interferes with anti-nociceptive actions of other pain-modulating drugs (such as opioids). Thus, E2 acting on primary afferent nociceptors modulates the response to pro- and anti-nociceptive signals. Within the context of our cross-sensitization hypothesis, inflammation sensitizes non-inflamed viscera that are innervated by the same DRG and/or cross-sensitization occurs as a result of intra-DRG release of sensitizing mediators such as ATP or substance P in the DRG (Matsuka *et al.* 2001; Chaban 2008; Chaban 2010).

Lumbosacral DRG neurons (levels L6-S1) from wild type mice (WT) express estrogen receptors (ERα and ERβ), purinergic P2X3, vanilloid TRPV1, SP and methabotropic glutamate ($mGluR_{2/3}$) receptors. In our recent studies we also tested the difference in how somatic and visceral afferents are modulated by E2. Both short-term and long-term exposure to E2 significantly decreased the ATP and capsaicin-induced increase in $[Ca^{2+}]_i$.

2. Materials and methods

2.1 Animals

We have used 6~8 week female C57BL/6J, B6.129P2-Esr1^{tm1Ksk}/J, and B6.129P2-Esr2^{tm1Unc}/J mice were obtained the Jackson Laboratory (Bar Harbor, ME, USA). Upon arrival, mice were group housed in microisolator caging and maintained on a 12-h light/dark cycle in a temperature-controlled environment with access to food and water ad libitum. To test whether estrogen receptor α (ERα) or estrogen receptor β (ERβ) are involved in estradiol (E_2)-induced modification of $[Ca^{2+}]_i$ Wile type, estrogen receptor alpha knock-out (ERαKO) and estrogen receptor beta knock-out (ERβKO) mice will be used. The wild type, ERαKO and ERβKO mice will be obtained from the supplier and allowed to recover for two weeks. These studies were carried out in accordance with the guidelines of the Institutional Animal

Care and Use committee at the University of California and the NIH Guide for the Care and Use of Laboratory Animals.

2.2 Animal breeding

Experiments were performed on age-matched (8–10 wk old) heterozygous mutant mice lacking the gene male (ERα−/−) and female (ERα−/−) for ERα (ERα−/−), and the deficiency ERβ (ERβ−/−) mice were bred into heterozygous mutant female mice (ERβ−/−) and homozygous male mutant mice (ERβ−/−) (Jackson Laboratory, Bar Harbor, ME, USA). Mice were housed in climate-controlled rooms, and standard rodent chow and water were available *ad libitum* and were housed in accordance with the NIH Guide for the Care and Use of Laboratory Animals

2.3 Primary culture of DRG neurons

The isolation procedure and primary culture of mouse lumbosacral DRG has been published in detail (Chaban, Mayer et al. 2003). DRG tissues were obtained from c57/black 6J (The Jackson Laboratory; 30 g), ERαKO and ERβKO (Taconic; 20 g) transgenic types. Briefly, lumbosacral adult DRGs (level L1-S1) from Wt, ERαKO and ERβKO mice will be collected under sterile technique and placed in ice-cold medium Dulbecco's Modified Eagle's Medium (DMEM; Sigma Chemical Co., St. Louis, MO). Adhering fat and connective tissue will be removed and each DRG will be minced with scissors and place immediately in a medium consisting of 5 ml of DMEM containing 0.5 mg/ml of trypsin (Sigma, type III), 1 mg/ml of collagenase (Sigma, type IA) and 0.1 mg/ml of DNAase (Sigma, type III) and kept at 37°C for 30 minutes with agitation. After dissociation of the cell ganglia, soybean trypsin inhibitor (Sigma, type III) will be used to terminate cell dissociation. Cell suspension will be centrifuged for one minute at 1000 rpm and the cell pellet will be resuspended in DMEM supplemented with 5% fetal bovine serum, 2 mM glutamine-penicillin-streptomycin mixture, 1 μg/ml DNAase and 5 ng/ml NGF (Sigma). Cells will be plated on Matrigel® (Invitrogen)-coated 15-mm coverslips (Collaborative Research Co., Bedford, PA) and kept at 37° C in 5% CO_2 incubator for 24 hrs, given fresh media and maintained in primary culture until used for experimental procedures.

2.4 Western blot analysis

The expressions of TRPV1 and of P2X3 receptors in L1~S1 DRGs were studied by using Western blot analyses. Tissues from wild type (C57BL/6J), ERαKO, and ERβKO mice were quick frozen in tubes on dry ice during collection. L1~S1 DRG were combined, homogenized by mechanical disruption in ice-cold RIPA buffer plus protease inhibitors and incubated on ice for 30 minutes. Homogenates were then spun at 5000 g for 15 minutes and supernatants collected. Total protein was determined on the supernatants using the BCA microtiter method (Pierce, Rockford, Ill., USA). Samples containing equal amounts of protein (40μg) were electrophoresed under denaturing conditions using Novex Mini-cell system (San Diego, Calif., USA) and reagents (NuPage 4–12% Bis-Tris gel and MOPS running buffer). After electrophoretic transfer onto nitrocellulose membrane using the same system, the membrane was blocked with 5% non-fat dry milk (NFDM) in 25 mM TRIS buffered saline, pH 7.2, plus Tween 20 (TBST) for 1 hour at room temperature, followed by incubation with polyclonal rabbit antibody against TRPV1-N terminus (1:1000, Neuromics) and P2X3 receptor (1:1000, Neuromics) for overnight at 4°C. The membrane was then washed in TBST plus NFDM, and incubated with secondary antibody, HRP conjugated and rabbit IgG (Santa Cruz Biotechnology) at 1:5,000 in the same buffer for 2 hours at room temperature. Following a final wash in TBST without NFDM, the membrane was incubated with ECL+ (Amersham, Arlington Heights, Ill., USA) substrate for HRP. Membranes were probed with primary antibody and corresponding secondary antibodies, signals were scanned and quantified by Image J version 1.28U and NIH Image 1.60 scan software. Following enhanced chemiluminescence (ECL) detection of proteins, the membranes were stripped and rehybridized with β-actin antibody as a loading control. At least three independent cell preparations were used.

2.5 Immunohistochemistry (IHC)

DRG tissues were obtained from C57/black 6J (The Jackson Laboratory; 30 g), ERαKO and ERβKO (Taconic; 20 g) transgenic types. Following decapitation, DRG from bilateral spinal levels L1-S2 were removed and fixed in 4% paraformaldehyde for overnight at 4°C, according to procedures approved by National Institutes of Health policy on Humane Care and Use of Laboratory Animals. DRGs were rinsed in Delbecco's Phosphate Buffered Saline (DPBS) before cryoprotection in sucrose (20%, 4°C) for two days, after which excess liquid was removed. DRG were quick snap frozen in 2-methylbutane, and store them at -70°C. Each DRG was mounted in Tissue-Tek® OCT embedding medium (Sakura Finetek), and sectioned at -20°C in a MICROM H505E cryostat. Sections were cut at 20μm and store 4°C until required. Sections of DRGs were collected in PBS. Endogenous tissue peroxidase activity was quenched by soaking the sections for 10 min in 3% hydrogen peroxide solution in 0.01 M PBS. The specimens were washed and then treated for 60 min in blocking solution, 0.01 M PBS containing 0.5% Triton X-100 and 1% normal donkey serum (NDS) at room temperature. They were processed for wild type (n=4), ERαKO (n=4), or ERβKO (n=4) immunohistochemistry by the free floating method using polyclonal rabbit TRPV1 antibody (1:50000, Neuromics) or P2X3 receptor antibody (1:15000, Neuromics) for overnight at 4°C, washed in 0.01 M phosphate-buffered saline (PBS) and 0.01M Tris Buffered Saline (TBS), followed by incubation in solutions of donkey anti-rabbit fluorophore-conjugated secondary antibodies (1:200, Invitrogen) in 0.01M Tris Buffered Saline (TBS) for 3 hours at room temperature. Cells showing no apparent or only faint membrane/intracellular labeling were considered to be negative for TRPV1 or P2X3. TRPV1-positive cells included those with strong plasma membrane labeling that formed a discernible clustered pattern, and those with strong intracellular labeling that formed a punctuate pattern. Some neurons showed both strong plasma membrane and intracellular labeling. P2X3-positive neurons showed diffuse membrane/intracellular labeling. Mounted sections were air dried and coverslipped with Aqua Poly Mount (Polisciences, Warrington, PA). Images from at least three sections in each level were taken using Leica DMLB M130X microscope. The total numbers of DRG neurons expressing TRPV1 and P2X3 were counted. TRPV1- or P2X3-positive neurons were categorized according to their labeling patterns and were expressed as a percentage of the total number of TRPV1- or P2X3-positive cells. Immunohistochemical signal percent was measured by computerized image analysis (Image Pro-Plus, Media Cybernetics, Silver Spring, MD, USA).

2.6 $[Ca^{2+}]_i$ fluorescence imaging

Ca^{2+} fluorescence imaging was carried out as previously described (Gschossmann *et al.* 2000, Chaban *et al.* 2001). DRG neurons were loaded with fluorescent dye Fura-2 AM (Invitrogen) for 45 min at 37°C in HBSS supplemented with 20 mM HEPES, pH 7.4. The coverslips will be mounted on a fast-perfusion chamber P-4 (World Precision Instrument) and placed on a stage of Olympus IX51 inverted microscope. Observations were made at room temperature (20-23°C) with 20X UApo/340 objective. A fast superfusion system will be used to perfuse the cells with HBSS and rapidly apply E2 and other chemicals. Fluorescence intensity at 505 nm with excitation at 334 nm and 380 nm was captured as digital images (sampling rates of 0.1-2 s). Regions of interest were identified within the soma or neuritis from which quantitative measurements will be made by re-analysis of stored image sequences using Slidebook® Digital Microscopy software. $[Ca^{2+}]_i$ was determined by ratiometric method of Fura-2 fluorescence from calibration of series of buffered Ca^{2+} standards. We applied E2 acutely for five minutes onto the experimental chamber or the culture medium for 48 hours to study the prolonged effect of E2. Repeated applications of drugs were achieved by superfusion in a rapid mixing chamber into individual neurons for specific intervals (100-500 ms). Cells were perfused with experimental media (2 ml/min) using a Rainin® peristaltic pump.

2.7 Retrograde labeling

DRG neurons innervating viscera were identified by retrograde labeling. Briefly, mice were anesthetized with isoflurane. For colonic afferents, the descending colon was exposed and Fluorogold (5% solution in PBS; Molecular Probes, Eugene, OR) was injected into the intestinal muscle wall (10 μl injections of into five to six different sites) using a Hamilton syringe (Hamilton Co., Reno, NV) with a 26-gauge needle. In another experiments we used uterus-specific DRG neurons in which tetramethylrhodamine (TMR) dye was injected in the uterus. Injection sites were carefully swabbed, the colon and uterus were extensively rinsed with 0.9% sodium chloride solution and sealed with New Skin to prevent dye leakage. The abdomen was sutured and the animals monitored for signs of pain or discomfort during the survival period. All animals were allowed to survive one week to allow for maximal transport of retrograde markers and housed in groups of two under 12/12 hours light cycle with food and water available *ad libitum.*

2.8 Statistical analysis

The amplitude of $[Ca^{2+}]_i$ response represents the difference between baseline concentration and the transient peak response to drug stimulation. Significant differences in response to chemical stimulation will be obtained by comparing $[Ca^{2+}]_i$ increases during the first stimulation with the second. A cell will be judged responsive if E2 inhibits the second $[Ca^{2+}]_i$ transient by >30% of the first. This criterion was empirically derived in preliminary experiments. All of the data are expressed as the mean ± SEM. Statistical analysis was performed using Statistical Package for the Social Sciences 12.0 (SPSS, Chicago, IL, USA). To assess the significance among different groups, data were analyzed with one-way ANOVA followed by Schéffe post hoc test. A $P < 0.05$ was considered statistically significant.

3. Results

3.1 Role of P2X3 receptors in estrogen-induced nociceptive signaling in sensory neurons

P2X3 and TRPV1 receptors expression were examined by western blot analysis of lysates from wild type, ERαKO, and ERβKO DRG tissues using a P2X3 specific primary antiserum (Fig.1 (a)). An intense band representing a ~64 kDa protein ($P2X_3$) and a ~130 kDa (TRPV1) was seen in DRG lysates from wild type animals. There was a dramatic decrease in intensity of this band using lysates made from the both knock out DRG tissues when compared with wild type control animals (>4 fold decrease of control Fig.1). When the density in the control group was standardized to 1.0, the average densities were 0.172 ± 0.08 of ERαKO and 0.262 ± 0.10 of ERβKO in $P2X_3$ receptors, and 0.59 ± 0.06 of ERαKO and 0.391 ± 0.04 of ERβKO in TRPV1 receptors, suggesting that both $P2X_3$ and TRPV1 protein decreased in DRG, $P<0.05$, n=10.

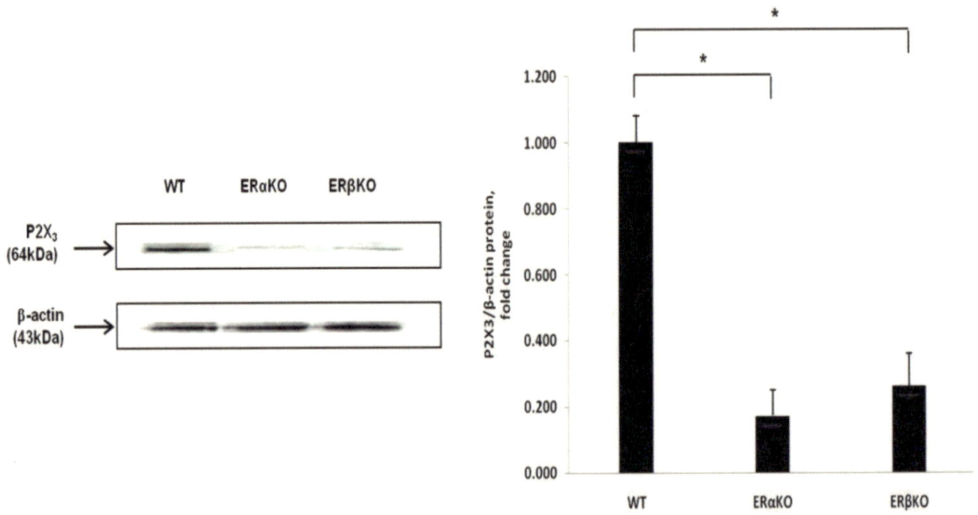

Fig. 1. Western blot analysis of DRG lysates shows reduced expression of P2X3 and TRPV1 in both knock-out mice.

Our study show that nociceptive capsaicin-sensitive TRPV1 receptors and ATP-sensitive $P2X_3$ receptors express in DRG neurons. DRGs section were immunostained with primary antibodies against $P2X_3$ and TRPV1. Neuronal profiles from each four mouse with ERαKO, ERβKO as well as wild type mice were quantified for each fluorescent probe. Both $P2X_3$ and TRPV1 receptors present in DRGs (Fig. 2).

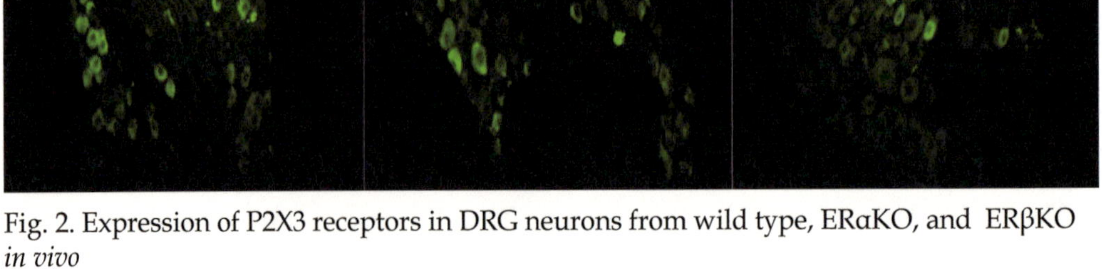

Fig. 2. Expression of P2X3 receptors in DRG neurons from wild type, ERαKO, and ERβKO *in vivo*

In our next experiments we evaluated P2X3 receptors modulation by ATP and E2 in sensory neurons. DRG neurons were loaded with fluorescent dye Fura-2 AM for one hour at 37°C in HBSS supplemented with 20 mM HEPES, pH 7.4. The coverslips were placed on a stage of Olympus IX51 inverted microscope. A fast superfusion system was used to perfuse the cells with HBSS and rapidly apply E_2 and other chemicals. Fluorescence intensity was captured as digital images (sampling rates of 0.1- 2s). Regions of interest were identified within the soma from which quantitative measurements were made by re-analysis of stored image sequences using Slidebook® Digital Microscopy software. $[Ca^{2+}]_i$ was determined by ratiometric method.

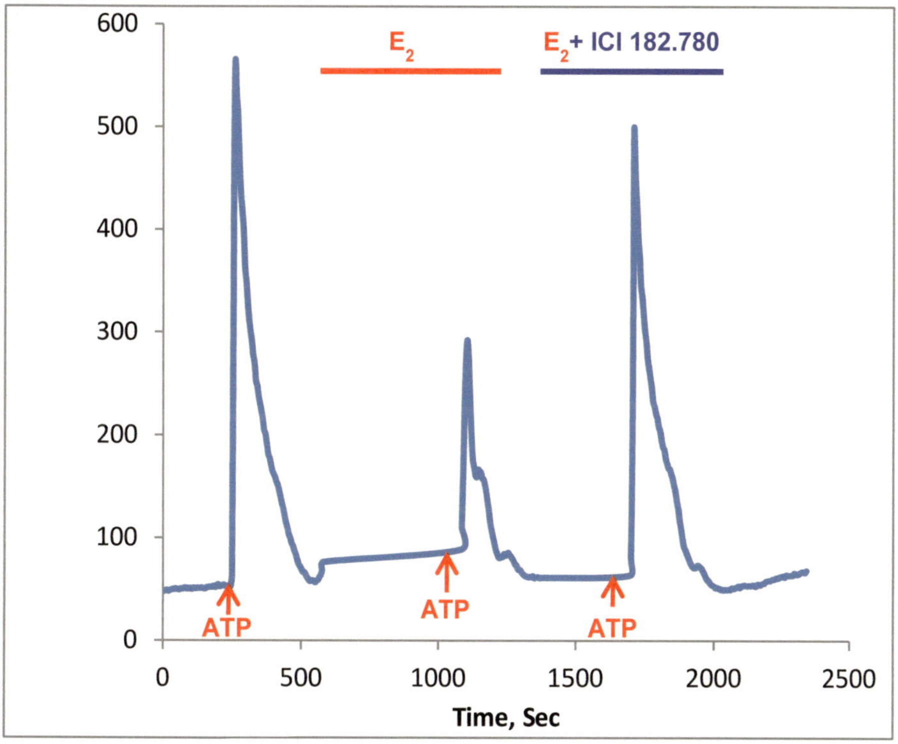

Fig. 3. 17 β-Estradiol (E2) significantly reduced ATP-induced $[Ca^{2+}]_i$ signaling *in vitro*. This effect was blocked by ER antagonist ICI 182 780

3.2 Role of TRPV1 receptors in estrogen-induced nociceptive signaling in sensory neurons

We found that nociceptive (small diameter) DRG neurons also express capsaicin-sensitive vanilloid (TRPV1) receptors. TRPV1positive neurons were categorized according to their labeling patterns and were expressed as a percentage of the total number of TRPV1 -positive cells. Immunohistochemical signal from ERαKO, ERβKO and WT mice was measured by computerized image analysis (Fig. 4)

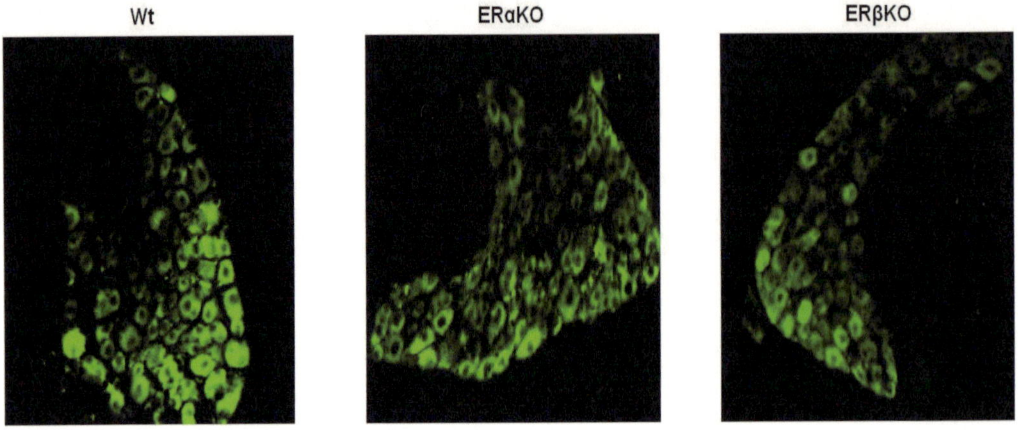

Fig. 4. Expression of TRPV1 receptors in dorsal root ganglion neurons from Wt, ERαKO, and ERβKO *in vivo*.

Capsaicin-induced TPRV1 receptor-mediated changes in $[Ca^{2+}]_i$ may represent a level of DRG activation to noxious cutaneous stimulation while ATP-induced changes in $[Ca^{2+}]_i$ may reflect the level of DRG neuron sensitization to noxious visceral stimuli since ATP is released by noxious stimuli and tissue damage near the primary afferent nerve terminals . In the view of this fact, TRPV1 receptor expression and activity might be considered as markers for a specific subtype of sensory neurons, and their activation by exogenous stimuli (e.g. capsaicin) could be a useful tool to exam the possible modulatory effects of pain-related substances.

3.3 Primary afferent sensory neurons receive input from different visceral organs

An important test of our hypothesis will be to establish that E2 modulates visceral afferents. A corollary of that hypothesis was that cutaneous pain may be differently modulated compared with visceral pain. We have proposed that E2 preferentially acts on visceral afferents to modulate the nociception. In a series of experiments using retrograde tract

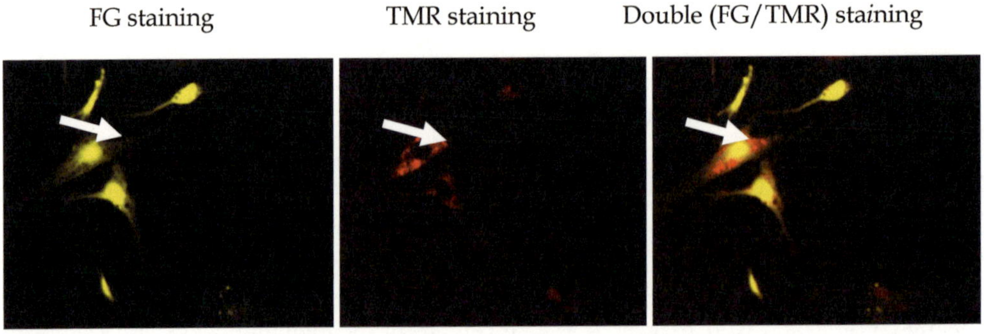

Fig. 5. Identification of colon-specific (with FG), uterus-specific (with TMR) and DRG receiving input from both organs *in vitro*

tracing we identified cutaneous and visceral afferent neurons *in vivo and in vitro*. We also found a subset of DRG neurons which innervate both visceral organs: uterus and colon.

4. Conclusion

Endometriosis is one of the most common benign gynecological diseases, characterized by the presence of endometrial tissue outside the uterine cavity, most commonly implanted over visceral and peritoneal surfaces within the female pelvis. Clinical studies have shown that it may occur in up to 10-15% of women of reproductive age. Symptoms of endometriosis are usually associated with pelvic pain, including recurrent painful periods, painful intercourse, and painful defecation during menstruation, chronic lower abdominal pain and hypersensitivity. Unfortunately, understanding of the mechanisms of endometriosis-associated pain and its management in women is currently insufficient. Studies have shown possible mechanisms of chronic pelvic pain associated with endometriosis could be due to persistent nociceptive input from endometrial tissues that lead to peripheral and central sensitisation resulting in increased responsiveness of dorsal root ganglion and dorsal horn neurons. Indeed, recent studies in human and animals have shown that peritoneal endometrial lesions are richly innervated by Aδ and C sensory nerve fibers, which positively stained by substance P or calcitonin gene-related peptide.

Several lines of evidence indicated that there is a close relationship between nerve fiber density and endometriosis-associated pain. There is a significant increase in nerve fiber density in women with endometriosis who reported pelvic pain, suggesting these nerve fibers may play an important role in the mechanisms of pain generation. Accumulating literatures described that SP presents in the myometrium and is involved in the inflammatory and pain responses, suggesting a possible role of SP nerve fibers in the generation of pain related to endometriosis. SP, which is synthesized and contained in 20-30% of DRG neurons, is involved in the transmission of nociceptive information to the central nerve system. SP is contained primarily in, and co-released from, small-diameter primary afferent fibers on noxious stimulation. Activation of nociceptive C and Aδ primary afferent fibers by electrical, chemical, or mechanical stimulation has been reported to release SP. Visceral nociceptive C-fibers can be activated by SP, representing an endogenous system regulating inflammatory, immune responses, and visceral hypersensitivity. SP afferent fibers play an important role in the pathogenesis of visceral hyperalgesia, suggesting critical role of SP in regulation of pelvic nociception associated with endometriosis. ATP is a peripheral mediator of pain which contributes to the activation of sensory afferents by activating ATP receptors following inflammation or nerve injury. It may correlate with SP release and play an important role in modulating nociception in primary sensory neurons. Local injections of ATP and ATP analogs to the rat hindpaw elicit spontaneous pain behaviors, hyperalgesia and allodynia which can be augmented by inflammation, indicating ATP might be involved in visceral hyperalgesia associated with endometriosis. Although these findings reveal the greater abundance of primary sensory nerve fibers clearly present within the peritoneal endometrial lesions in patients diagnosed with endometriosis, and these nerve fibers may play an important role in pain generation associated with endometriosis, pain mechanisms associated with endometriosis are still not well known, and the role of these primary sensory nerve fibers has not been specifically determined.

Our data support the idea that E2 modulates nociceptive responses in pelvic pain syndromes such as endometriosis, however, whether E_2 is pro- or anti-nociceptive remains unresolved. Within the context of our hypothesis visceral nociception and nociceptor sensitization appear to be regulated by P2X3 and TRPV1. E2 modulates DRG neurons response to ATP and capsaicin suggesting that visceral afferent nociceptors are modulated by E2 in the DRG. The DRG is an important site of visceral afferent convergence and cross-sensitization. We have demonstrated that 17-β estradiol (E2), the most common form of estrogen act on functional properties of P2X3 and TRPV1 receptors in DRG neurons *in vitro*. DRG neurons from Wt and knock-out mice responded to P2X3 and TRPV1 activation. We also studied the long-term (chronic) exposure to E2 on sensory neurons that mimics the temporal pattern of circulating E2 levels in cycling female rodents which is equivalent to an E2 primal action on animal reproductive behavior. The localization of ER in DRG neurons and the attenuation of ATP/capsaicin- induce $[Ca^{2+}]_i$ strongly suggest that E2 modulates visceral pain processing peripherally. Moreover, E2 appears to have different actions on nociceptive signaling depending on the input. Adult DRG neurons in short-term culture retain the expression of receptors (P2X and TRPV1) which mediate the response to putative nociceptive signals. They continue to respond to ER agonists mimicking *in vivo* activation. An important advantage is that these neurons can be studied apart from endogenous signals. Our data clearly showed the new role of nociceptors in pathophysiological aspects of chronic pelvic pain and potential way of designing future therapies.

5. References

Al-Chaer, E. D. and R. J. Traub (2002). "Biological basis of visceral pain: recent developments." Pain 96(3): 221-225.

Aloisi, A. M., I. Ceccarelli, et al. (2000). "Gonadectomy and persistent pain differently affect hippocampal c-Fos expression in male and female rats." Neurosci Lett 281(1): 29-32.

Bereiter, D. A. (2001). "Sex differences in brainstem neural activation after injury to the TMJ region." Cells Tissues Organs 169(3): 226-237.

Berkley, K. J., A. Cason, et al. (2001). "Vaginal hyperalgesia in a rat model of endometriosis." Neurosci Lett 306(3): 185-188.

Berkley, K. J., A. J. Rapkin, et al. (2005). "The pains of endometriosis." Science 308(5728): 1587-1589.

Bradshaw, H. B. and K. J. Berkley (2002). "Estrogen replacement reverses ovariectomy-induced vaginal hyperalgesia in the rat." Maturitas 41(2): 157-165.

Burnstock, G. (2000). "P2X receptors in sensory neurones." Br J Anaesth 84(4): 476-488.

Burnstock, G. (2001). "Purine-mediated signalling in pain and visceral perception." Trends Pharmacol Sci 22(4): 182-188.

Chaban, V. V. (2008). "Visceral sensory neurons that innervate both uterus and colon express nociceptive TRPv1 and P2X3 receptors in rats." Ethn Dis 18(2 Suppl 2): S2-20-24.
Chaban, V. V. (2010). "Peripheral sensitization of sensory neurons." Ethn Dis 20(1 Suppl 1): S1-3-6.
Chaban, V. V., E. A. Mayer, et al. (2003). "Estradiol inhibits ATP-induced intracellular calcium concentration increase in dorsal root ganglia neurons." Neuroscience 118(4): 941-948.
Chang, L. and M. M. Heitkemper (2002). "Gender differences in irritable bowel syndrome." Gastroenterology 123(5): 1686-1701.
Davis, J. B., J. Gray, et al. (2000). "Vanilloid receptor-1 is essential for inflammatory thermal hyperalgesia." Nature 405(6783): 183-187.
Dunn, P. M., Y. Zhong, et al. (2001). "P2X receptors in peripheral neurons." Prog Neurobiol 65(2): 107-134.
Giamberardino, M. A., R. Costantini, et al. (2010). "Viscero-visceral hyperalgesia: characterization in different clinical models." Pain 151(2): 307-322.
Gschossmann, J. M., V. V. Chaban, et al. (2000). "Mechanical activation of dorsal root ganglion cells in vitro: comparison with capsaicin and modulation by kappa-opioids." Brain Res 856(1-2): 101-110.
Holdcroft, A. (2000). "Hormones and the gut." Br J Anaesth 85(1): 58-68.
Koshimizu, T. A., F. Van Goor, et al. (2000). "Characterization of calcium signaling by purinergic receptor-channels expressed in excitable cells." Mol Pharmacol 58(5): 936-945.
Lee, D. Y., Y. G. Chai, et al. (2002). "17Beta-estradiol inhibits high-voltage-activated calcium channel currents in rat sensory neurons via a non-genomic mechanism." Life Sci 70(17): 2047-2059.
Malykhina, A. P. (2007). "Neural mechanisms of pelvic organ cross-sensitization." Neuroscience 149(3): 660-672.
Matsuka, Y., J. K. Neubert, et al. (2001). "Concurrent release of ATP and substance P within guinea pig trigeminal ganglia in vivo." Brain Res 915(2): 248-255.
Mayer, E. A., B. D. Naliboff, et al. (2001). "Basic pathophysiologic mechanisms in irritable bowel syndrome." Dig Dis 19(3): 212-218.
Micevych, P. E., V. V. Chaban, et al. (2002). "Oestrogen modulates cholecystokinin: opioid interactions in the nervous system." Pharmacology & toxicology 91: 387-397.
Micevych, P. E. and K. Sinchak (2001). "Estrogen and endogenous opioids regulate CCK in reproductive circuits." Peptides 22: 1235-1244.
Nadal, A., M. Diaz, et al. (2001). "The estrogen trinity: membrane, cytosolic, and nuclear effects." News Physiol Sci 16: 251-255.
Papka, R. E. and M. Storey-Workley (2002). "Estrogen receptor-alpha and -beta coexist in a subpopulation of sensory neurons of female rat dorsal root ganglia." Neurosci Lett 319(2): 71-74.
Petruska, J. C., J. Napaporn, et al. (2000). "Subclassified acutely dissociated cells of rat DRG: histochemistry and patterns of capsaicin-, proton-, and ATP-activated currents." J Neurophysiol 84(5): 2365-2379.

Pezzone, M. A., R. Liang, et al. (2005). "A model of neural cross-talk and irritation in the pelvis: implications for the overlap of chronic pelvic pain disorders." Gastroenterology 128(7): 1953-1964.

Zimmermann, M. (2001). "Pathobiology of neuropathic pain." Eur J Pharmacol 429(1-3): 23-37.

21

Embryo Quality and Pregnancy Outcome in Infertile Patients with Endometriosis

Veljko Vlaisavljević, Marko Došen and Borut Kovačič
Department of Reproductive Medicine and Gynecologic Endocrinology, Clinics for Gynecology and Perinatology, University Clinical Center Maribor, Slovenia

1. Introduction

Investigation of one complex pathological condition is definitively a challenging task, but trying to find the connection(s) between two is even more difficult. This is very true in the case of infertility and endometriosis. Both conditions have numerous symptoms, very diverse clinical pictures and multifactorial etiologies. The first step toward understanding the connection between the two is to prove the correlation between them. The next task is to try to understand the mechanisms by which they affect each other, which involves examination and comparison of numerous variables specific for each condition. The results are still the subject of many controversies.

1.1 Endometriosis and infertility

At present, there is little debate that endometriosis and infertility are actually associated. For example, early retrospective studies (Hasson, 1976; Drake & Grunet, 1980; Strathy et al., 1982) and one more recent prospective study (Mahmood & Templeton, 1991) performed in women who underwent laparoscopy (for various reasons) showed that endometriotic lesions were significantly more frequent in women who were treated for infertility than in those who requested laparoscopy for tubal sterilization. Prevalence of endometriosis in infertile women ranged from 21 - 48% which was in clear contrast to the prevalence of 1.3 - 5% in fertile women (Hasson, 1976; Drake & Grunet, 1980; Strathy et al., 1982). Another line of evidence of the existence of a link between endometriosis and infertility came from studies in women who underwent donor insemination because of severe male infertility. In these studies, women with endometriosis had significantly fewer conceptions per procedure than women without this condition (Hammond et al., 1986; Yeh & Seibel, 1987). In studies where peritoneal endometriosis was induced in rabbits (Schenken & Asch, 1980), primates (Schenken et al., 1984) and rodents (Vernon & Wilson 1985; Barragan et al., 1992) it was clearly demonstrated that endometriosis was strongly associated with infertility regardless of localization and/or extension of the lesions.

While it is relatively easy to document the link between the two conditions, defining precise pathophysiologic mechanisms and proving a causal relationship between endometriosis and infertility is much more difficult.

In severe cases of endometriosis, the seriously distorted anatomy of pelvic organs is the obvious cause of impaired fertility. In the absence of pelvic adhesions and scarring, when only mild to moderate endometriotic lesions are present, finding the cause and the consequence is anything but an easy task. Many confounding factors make these studies both controversial and difficult to interpret. One of the main problems is the choice of the appropriate control group. The common practice has been to choose women with tubal factor infertility or those with unexplained infertility as controls. The problem with this choice is our inability to identify women with inherently reduced potential for conception (fertilization and implantation) and to exclude them from the control group. Also, the common practice is to make observations on the patients with endometriosis who are treated by one of the techniques of assisted reproductive technologies (ART). This practice is problematic because the use of ART creates a non-physiologic environment and many subtle but important *in vivo* effects of endometriosis on the process of conception may be hidden in *in vitro* conditions.

Hypotheses on mechanisms by which mild to moderate endometriosis could impair fertility potential are numerous and will be mentioned here only briefly. One group of investigators tested hypotheses that endocrine abnormalities in women with mild and moderate endometriosis might be the cause of reduced fertility. As was already conveniently summarized in the literature (Garrido et al., 2000; Hunter et al., 2004), proposed mechanisms were hypersecretion of prolactin in patients with endometriosis (Muse et al., 1982), impaired folliculogenesis (Tummon et al., 1988), altered ovulation (Dmowski et al., 1986) and luteal phase defects (Grant, 1966). The other line of investigation was directed towards immune dysfunctions as potential causes of infertility in patients with endometriosis. Proposed mechanisms were chronic inflammatory reaction and altered immune responses induced by endometriosis (Harada et al., 2001), including increased production of cytokines and other soluble immunomodulators in the peritoneal fluid. These altered immune responses could further affect motility and velocity of the sperm, lead to sperm phagocytosis (Soldati et al., 1989), accelerate ovum transport (Croxato et al., 1978), impair the process of fertilization (Mahadevan et al., 1983), display direct embryo toxicity (Damewood et al., 1990) or adversely affect the process of implantation (Yovich et al., 1985; Matson & Yovich, 1986). Unfortunately, results of these studies were usually contradicting and no definitive conclusion could be made so far. It is likely that there is more than one answer to this complex problem.

2. Endometriosis and embryo quality

Among investigators who reported poorer results of IVF-ET outcome in patients with endometriosis, there is a general agreement on few final consequences in contrast to numerous possible pathophysiologic mechanisms leading to it.

These include:

1. Impairment of the quality of oocytes (resulting in lower fertilization rates) and/or
2. Decrease in the implantation capacity of embryos (Pellicer et al., 2001).

An indirect marker of oocyte quality and a possible predictor of embryo's implantation capacity is the quality of the developing embryo. As such, this parameter could be used for assessment of the effects of endometriosis on fertility.

2.1 Measures of embryo quality

Quality of the embryo may be described using many direct and indirect measures. For example, parameters which could be used for indirect assessment of embryo quality are number of embryos on Day 2, total number of blastocysts, number of frozen blastocysts, but also the implantation rate and early pregnancy loss rate. The only direct measure of embryo quality is embryo quality score based on morphological characteristics of a developing embryo. However, this parameter is quite difficult to use in practice. One reason for this difficulty is the absence of uniformity of scoring systems used by different laboratories. Another is a consequence of two facts: (1) quality score is a categorical variable and (2) it is (still) a common practice to transfer more than one embryo (blastocyst) at a time. In other words, if two or more embryos of different qualities have been transferred, it is not possible to calculate "the mean embryo quality score" or to determine exactly which one of transferred embryos has eventually implanted.

Researchers who would come across this issue tried to overcome it in various ways. The simplest was to exclude from the study those patients in whom embryos with different quality scores were transferred (La Sala et al., 2005). The main drawback of this approach was a significant reduction of observed cycles, i.e. of the sample size. Also, this tactic prevented incorporation of some other important variables (namely the number of transferred embryos) in the final analysis. On the other hand, some of the authors (Lambers et al, 2007) used a cumulative embryo score, previously introduced by Steer (Steer et al., 1992). Cumulative embryo score was defined as an additive parameter (i.e. following the transfer of two embryos with scores of 1 and 3, the total score of embryos transferred was 4). Other investigators (Winter et al., 2002) assessed embryo quality with relation to the number of embryos transferred and the possibility of elective transfer. According to this system, embryos were scored 1 in the case of an elective transfer of one or two embryos (highest score); elective transfer of 3 embryos yielded a score of 2; if two or three embryos had been transferred non-electively, the score was 3, and if only a single embryo was transferred non-electively, it was scored 4 (worst score).

In our research, we adopted yet another approach. If multiple embryos of different quality were transferred, we assumed that (1) implanting embryo was the best quality embryo (the so-called leading embryo) and (2) the leading embryo determined embryo quality score of the entire group of transferred embryos. The first assumption was well documented in the literature (Hourvitz et al., 2006) and the second one was additionally tested in our sample.

2.2 Relevant studies encompassing the measures of embryo quality

Despite the fact that important hypothesis blames defective early embryo development for poorer IVF-ET outcome in patients with endometriosis, relatively few studies have analyzed the association between quality of transferred embryo(s) and endometriosis. We will briefly present several important studies on the subject.

A group of Spanish investigators conducted three separate retrospective analyses of the success of their IVF-ET and oocyte donation program in patients and donors with and without endometriosis (Pellicer at al., 1995). In the segment of the study on early embryonic development, which was performed on 36 women with endometriosis and on 34 with tubal infertility used as a control group, they explored the embryos grown in vitro for 72 hours before embryo transfer. Embryo quality assessment system included the number of blastomeres and the degree of fragmentation after 48 and 72 hours in culture. If embryos presented only one or two blastomeres 72 hours after oocyte retrieval, it was considered that an embryo arrest had occurred. After 72 hours in culture, there was a significant decrease in the number of blastomeres in endometriosis compared to tubal infertility patients (5.4 ± 0.1 versus 6.1 ± 0.3 blastomeres, respectively, $p<0.04$) and a significant increase in the percentage of arrested embryos (57.4 ± 2.3 in patients with endometriosis versus 45.2 ± 5.8 in control group, $p<0.05$). In order to control for the influence of semen parameter on embryo quality, researchers further subdivided groups of patients taking into account the quality of semen. If abnormal semen was used for in vitro fertilization, higher degree of embryonic arrest was observed in comparison to the group with normal semen parameters (55.6 ± 6.4 vs. 20.3 ± 7.9 ($p<0.01$), respectively, in the group with tubal infertility; 61.8 ± 2.6 vs. 47.5 ± 2.8 ($p<0.003$), respectively, in the group with endometriosis). Also, if the semen used had normal characteristics, significantly more arrested embryos were noted in patients with endometriosis compared to patients with tubal infertility ($p<0.001$). Further insight into the problem was attained when the same researchers analyzed pregnancy outcome of oocyte donation with regards to the origin of donated oocytes. This segment of the research incorporated a total of 178 embryo transfers in 141 women. If oocytes were donated by donors without endometriosis, implantation and ongoing pregnancy rates were comparable in both recipients with and those without endometriosis. If oocytes were collected from donors with endometriosis, significantly lower implantation rates were reported in recipients ($p<0.05$). The authors of this study concluded that infertility in patients with endometriosis may be related to oocyte alterations which result in embryos of lower quality and reduced implantation ability, although the impact of hostile (anti-implantatory) environment on embryos of normal developmental potential cannot be ruled out.

Another study which reported negative impact of endometriosis on embryo quality was the prospective case control study in which researchers included 37 patients with "true" endometriomas and 56 patients without any complex ovarian cysts as controls (Yanushpolsky et al., 1998). All endometriomas were larger than 1 cm in diameter and would be classified as stage III endometriosis according to The ASRM-revised classification of endometriosis (The American Fertility Society, 1985). Only patients with complex "chocolate" cysts in which CA 125 levels in cyst fluid were >100.000 U/ml ("true" endometriomas) were included in the study. Embryo quality was expressed as the number of embryos reaching at least four-cell stage on the second day after oocyte retrieval. Quality of the embryos in the group of patients with endometriomas was significantly reduced compared to controls ($p=0.09$). Also, in patients with endometriomas, significantly fewer oocytes were retrieved ($p=0.06$) and early pregnancy loss rate (biochemical pregnancies and early clinical spontaneous miscarriages combined) was significantly higher ($p=0.04$). Interestingly, fertilization rate and implantation rate were not significantly different between the studied groups.

A group of Norwegian investigators also confirmed detrimental effect of endometriosis on embryo quality (Tanbo, 1995). They analyzed 215 women (385 cycles) whose main indication for IVF-ET was unexplained infertility (ovulatory women, with patent tubes and normal uterine cavity, normal laparoscopy and normal sperm characteristics), 143 women (285 cycles) with endometriosis as the only indication and 180 women (353 cycles) with tubal infertility (control group). Cleavage rate and failure of cleavage were used as criteria of embryo quality. Significantly lower cleavage rates were observed in both unexplained infertility and endometriosis groups compared with the tubal infertility group. Total failure of cleavage was 19.2% in unexplained infertility, 14.3% in endometriosis and 3.6% in tubal infertility group ($p<0.0001$). Since there were no differences in sperm characteristics between the groups, the authors speculated that lower cleavage rates could be a consequence of inferior oocyte quality in unexplained infertility and endometriosis group.

In an interesting study of authors from U.S.A. a total of 235 preimplantation embryos were retrospectively analyzed (Brizek et al., 1995). These embryos were obtained from 56 IVF-ET cycles performed in 30 women. Sixteen patients had endometriosis as the main indication for the procedure and the remaining 14 were controls without endometriosis who were chosen randomly from other diagnosis categories. The incidence of specific phenotypes ranging from normal 2PN zygote to different types of abnormal embryos was then recorded on days 1 and 2 following fertilization. An increased incidence of aberrant development of embryos derived from women with endometriosis was demonstrated. There were three abnormal phenotypes on day 1 and two abnormal phenotypes on day 2 which were significantly more prevalent in patients with endometriosis. However, there was no statistical difference in the number of normal embryos in patients with endometriosis compared to controls on day 1 or day 2. Despite the fact that the effect of endometriosis was observed in the developmental dynamics of the fertilized ovum, no gross endometriosis-specific morphological changes in oocytes recovered from endometriosis group could be seen.

In contrast to previously cited observations, several other studies failed to show negative influence of endometriosis on the parameters of embryo quality. A group of authors from the U.S.A. conducted a retrospective analysis of 284 IVF-ET cycles from patients with a sole diagnosis of endometriosis, or tubal factor, or unexplained infertility (Arici et al., 1996). All of the patients had laparoscopy prior to the IVF procedure. The criteria for the diagnosis of unexplained infertility were confirmed ovulatory cycles, normal tubal patency on hysterosalpingography, normal sperm analyses. The severity of endometriosis was graded as defined by the Revised American Fertility Society classification (The American Fertility Society, 1985) and patients were further divided into two subgroups as minimal to mild (stages I and II) and moderate to severe (stages III and IV). Quality of embryos was assessed on the day of the transfer in line with the system used by the authors' center according to their morphology as observed under the inverted microscope (morphological grades I to V). In the final analysis, the researchers used "the average embryo quality score" for the given subgroup of patients, which was probably calculated as the arithmetical average of all embryo quality scores expressed as grades I to V. No statistically significant difference in "average embryo score" among subgroups were noted (1.8 ± 0.5 in the minimal to mild endometriosis group vs. 2.0 ± 0.6 in the moderate to severe endometriosis group vs. 1.9 ± 0.5 in the tubal infertility group vs. 1.8 ± 0.6 in the unexplained infertility group; $p>0.05$). Surprisingly, when the data were analyzed according to the stage of endometriosis, in the group with moderate to severe endometriosis (stages III and IV) a significantly higher fertilization rate was observed compared to the group with minimal to mild endometriosis (stages I and II) (78.4% vs. 66.8%, respectively; $p=0.001$). However, implantation rates were low and not significantly different between these subgroups (5.5% in the group with moderate to severe endometriosis vs. 2.8% in the group with minimal to mild endometriosis, $p=0.46$).

Another study which failed to show negative impact of endometriosis on embryo quality was conducted by Swedish researchers (Bergendal et al., 1998). The analysis included a total of 65 IVF-ET cycles in 48 patients with endometriosis as the only apparent cause of infertility and 98 cycles in 98 patients in whom tubal factor was the only apparent cause of infertility (controls). The embryos were graded according to criteria set by the authors' center (morphology and cleavage stage) with embryo quality scores raging from 1 to 3, with 3 being the best score. The average score of the whole subgroup (defined as arithmetical average of all scores) was used in the final analysis. Despite the fact that fertilization rate was significantly higher in patients with tubal infertility compared to patients with endometriosis (78.3 ± 18.3% vs. 60.1 ± 31.7%, respectively; $p=0.00001$), no difference was noted in cleavage rates (87.9 ± 19.1% in the tubal factor group vs. 85.2 ± 22.1% in the endometriosis group; $p=0.43$) or morphological score of embryo for ET (2.5 ±0.39 in the tubal infertility group vs. 2.4 ± 0.4 in the endometriosis group; $p=0.45$).

In yet another study which reported results on the impact of endometriosis on embryo quality (Dmowski et al., 1995), a retrospective analysis of 237 consecutive IVF-ET cycles in patients with and without endometriosis was conducted. In the group without endometriosis, indications for IVF-ET were tubal disease, pelvic adhesions, male factor, unexplained infertility, ovarian dysfunction ant other factors. In this study, the number of oocytes cleaved was taken as the indirect measure of embryo quality. The authors reported there was no difference between groups in the number of fertilized and cleaved oocytes, but no exact numerical values for these variables were included in the published report. The lack of properly defined control group (endometriosis vs. all other indications) and the absence of further details on development of transferred embryos warrant caution for interpretation, at least in the segment of the study pertaining to embryo quality.

2.3 Our study

We conducted a retrospective clinical study which encompassed 346 stimulated IVF or ICSI cycles with the transfer of one or two blastocysts performed at the Department of Reproductive Medicine and Gynecological Endocrinology at the University Medical Centre of Maribor, Slovenia.

The primary objective of our study was to examine possible differences in direct and indirect indicators of embryo quality between women with endometriosis as the only indication for the treatment and an adequate control group of women with tubal factor only. Possible differences in various other outcomes of IVF-ET cycles between these two groups were also analyzed. The secondary goal was to examine the influence of embryo quality on various outcomes of IVF-ET cycles against all other important variables as controls in the group of women with endometriosis.

2.3.1 Materils and methods

Data used in this analysis were received from the centre's database on couples treated for infertility from 2003 to 2010. If there any data for any variable was missing from the database, the patient's documentation (paper records) was checked. If it was still impossible to find the missing data, the patient was excluded from further analysis. Patients included were under 43 years of age and prior to entering an IVF/ICSI treatment, underwent all tests prescribed by the protocol for clinical examination of infertile couples.

The observed cycles were divided into two groups: 173 cycles were performed in patients with endometriosis as the only indication for treatment and 173 cycles in women with tubal factor infertility (control group). The patients from tubal factor group were individually matched with women with endometriosis by age group (<30, 30-34, 35-39, >39 years), number of retrieved oocytes (<5, 5 or more) and number of transferred embryos (1, 2 or 3).

Patients were most frequently stimulated according to the protocol involving gonadotrophin-releasing hormone agonists (GnRH-a) (almost exclusively using the long protocol). In the few remaining patients, the protocol with gonadotrophin-releasing hormone antagonists (GnRH-ant) was applied. GnRH agonists used were triptorelin (Diphereline®, Ipsen Pharma Biotech, France), gosereline (Zoladex®, Zeneca Pharmaceuticals, England) or busereline (Suprefact®, Sanofi Aventis, France). Cetrorelix (3 mg) (Cetrotide®, Merck Serono, Switzerland) was used as a GnRH antagonist. Follicle growth was predominantly stimulated by recombinant FSH (Gonal F®, Merck Serono, Switzerland), while human menopausal gonadotrophin (HMG) (Menopur ®, Ferring Pharmaceuticals, Switzerland) was used occasionally. On the day when at least two follicles reached an average diameter of 18 mm, final maturation of the oocyte was stimulated by the urinary human HCG (Profasi®, Merck Serono, Switzerland, using a dose of 10,000 IU) or human recombinant HCG (Ovitrelle®, Merck Serono, Switzerland, 250 mg dose). A detailed description of the laboratory procedures can be found elsewhere (Kovacic et al., 2009). Approximately 36 hours (36 ± 1) following the administration of HCG, oocytes were recovered by ultrasound-guided trans-vaginal follicle aspiration. Fertilization was performed through IVF or ICSI. Medicult® media (MediCult, Denmark) were used for oocyte culturing. Pursuant to the protocol of our centre, only one or maximally two blastocysts were transferred on the fifth, exceptionally on the fourth day following follicle aspiration. Labotec® catheter (Labotec, Germany) was used for blastocyst transfer. In line with the legislation in force at the time of the study, the couple was allowed to decide on the number of embryos to be transferred. Embryos were transferred only after both partners signed the official consent form for the transfer of embryos. A day after the follicle aspiration, all patients started receiving didrogesterone (30 mg/day) (Dabroston®, Belupo, Croatia) or micronized progesterone (600 mg/day) (Utrogestan®, Laboratories Besins International, France) for luteal support.

Quality of transferred blastocysts was evaluated by a blastocyst classification system based on morphological criteria, developed by our centre (Kovacic et al., 2004). This classification is a modification of the earlier, well established blastocyst evaluation system (Gardner & Schoolcraft, 1999). The classification used in our laboratory takes into consideration four parameters: blastocoel expansion, inner cellular mass (ICM) form, morphology and cohesion of the trophoectoderm (TE) as well as the degree of embryo fragmentation. There are 8 grades of quality of blastocysts (B1 to B8) in this system, with B1 being the best quality score and B8 the worst. The data on blastocyst quality expressed in this way had to be transformed before entering the statistical model. The transformation was performed in two steps. First, the blastocysts from B1 category were designated as optimal quality blastocysts, while those in categories B2–B8 were classified as being of suboptimal (non-optimal) quality. In the second step, in cases where blastocysts of different quality were transferred, the subgroup with blastocysts of different quality was merged with the subgroup in which all transferred blastocysts were of optimal quality. In this way, for the final statistical analyses we had a subgroup with blastocysts of suboptimal quality only and a subgroup with at least one blastocyst of optimal quality. All other possibilities for regrouping were also tested, but it was concluded that the chosen transformation of data showed the best fit with this model. This conclusion was expected, because it was in line with the assumption that in those cases in which multiple embryos of different quality were transferred and only one of implanted, the higher quality embryo (so-called leading embryo) had the highest probability of implantation.

In our analysis we made a distinction between premenstrual pregnancy loss (loss of conceptus prior to the first measurement of βhCG level 14 days after ovulation or embryo transfer), biochemical pregnancy (loss of conceptus after the first measurement of βhCG level but before the ultrasound (US) confirmation of implantation) and early clinical miscarriage (pregnancy loss after US confirmation of viable pregnancy but before the beginning of the second trimester) (Došen et al., 2011). Biochemical pregnancies and early clinical miscarriages are commonly identified together as early pregnancy losses (EPL).

Basic demographic and clinical characteristics are presented as mean ± standard deviation (SD) or median with 1st and 3rd quartile and analyzed by independent-samples t-test if normally distributed or by Mann-Whitney test if skewed. Categorical data are expressed as proportions and analyzed by chi-squared test. The results are presented as odds ratios and their 95% confidence intervals (CI). P value of under 0.05 was considered to be statistically significant. Statistical analysis was performed using STATISTICA® software, version 8.0 (StatSoft Inc., OK, USA).

2.3.2 Results

2.3.2.1 Differences in embryo quality indicators and other parameters between the groups

Average age of the patients was 32 years (in the group of women with endometriosis 32.6 ± 3.5, the youngest patient was 25 and the oldest 42 years old; in the group with tubal infertility 32.5 ± 3.9, the youngest patient was 22 and the oldest 43 years old).

Analysis of differences in quality score of transferred blastocysts between patients with endometriosis and tubal factor infertility showed marginal statistical significance, if all the scores (B1-B8) were analyzed together (chi-square=14.03, p=0.051). Further analysis was undertaken to identify the subgroups of the same blastocyst quality score in which possible significant difference was present. The results are presented in Table 1.

Blastocyst quality score	Endometriosis group (N=173)	Tubal factor group (N=173)	P value
B1	195 (24.8)	201 (25.2)	0.873
B2	54 (6.9)	70 (8.8)	0.161
B3	106 (13.5)	114 (14.3)	0.653
B4	85 (10.8)	71 (8.9)	0.198
B5	47 (6.0)	46 (5.8)	0.851
B6	105 (13.4)	140 (17.5)	0.022
B7	41 (5.2)	25 (3.1)	0.038
B8	153 (19.5)	132 (16.5)	0.127
Total	786 (100.0)	799 (100.0)	

Table 1. Comparison of embryo quality scores between the studied groups

Since a significant difference was present only in the subgroups of transferred blastocysts of very low quality (scores B6 and B7), this finding doesn't provide any further insight into the problem.

Analysis of indirect embryo quality indicators showed no statistically significant differences between the groups. The results are presented in Table 2.

Variable[a]	Endometriosis group (N=173)	Tubal factor group (N=173)	P value
No. of embryos on Day 2	7.5 ± 0.30	7.5 ± 0.29	0.890
No. of blastocysts	3.7 ± 0.21	4.0 ± 0.20	0.317
No. of frozen blastocysts	2.0 ± 0.18	2.4 ± 0.20	0.210

[a] Data are expressed as mean ± standard error.

Table 2. Comparison of indirect indicators of embryo quality between the studied groups.

Analysis of outcomes of IVF-ET cycles also failed to show any statistically significant differences between the groups. Results are presented in Table 3.

The outcome	Endometriosis group (N=173)	Tubal factor group (N=173)	P value
Implantation rate (%)	40.6 (112/276)	47.1 (130/276)	0.123
Clinical pregnancy rate (%)	49.7 (86/173)	54.3 (94/173)	0.389
Clinical miscarriage rate (%)	4.6 (8/173)	6.4 (11/173)	0.479
Early pregnancy loss* rate (%)	8.7 (15/173)	11.6 (20/173)	0.373
Live birth rate (%)	40.0 (64/173)	45.1 (74/173)	0.351

*Biochemical pregnancies and clinical miscarriages combined

Table 3. Comparison of IVF-ET cycles outcomes between the studied groups

In the additional analysis of some of the other important parameters, no significant differences were noted between the groups.

Variable	Endometriosis group (N=173)	Tubal factor group (N=173)	P value
No. of oocytes retrieved (N)	11.2 ± 0.41	11.1 ± 0.39	0.773
No. of fertilized oocytes (N)	7.6 ± 0.31	7.5 ± 0.29	0.859
Fertilization rate (%)	69.4 ± 1.39	69.0 ± 1.38	0.847
Male factor present (%)	96 (55.5)	84 (48.6)	0.197

Table 4. Comparison of variables of IVF-ET cycles between the studied groups

2.3.2.2 Blastocyst quality and other possible predictors of various outcomes

The other objective of our investigation was to define the influence of blastocyst quality on various outcomes of IVF-ET cycles against all other important variables as controls in the group of women with endometriosis.

In our analysis, we incorporated 11 parameters as possible predictors of four main outcomes of stimulated IVF-ET cycles. The encompassed parameters were:

- patient's age,
- fertilization method (IVF or ICSI),
- type of gonadotrophin used for stimulation (human menopausal gonadotrophin (HMG) or recombinant follicle stimulation hormone (FSH)),
- number of retrieved oocytes,
- number of fertilized oocytes,
- fertilization rate,
- number of embryos on Day 2,
- number of blastocysts (embryos on Day 5),
- number of transferred blastocysts,
- number of frozen blastocysts and
- embryo quality score of transferred blastocysts.

Several examined predictors were transformed in categorical variables, as will be explained below. The six observed outcomes were:

- positive βhCG 14 days after ET,
- clinical pregnancy rate,
- live births rate,
- biochemical pregnancy rate,
- early clinical miscarriage rate, and
- early pregnancy loss rate (EPL - biochemical pregnancies and early clinical miscarriages taken together).

The relationship between continuous predictors and the number of implanted blastocysts was analyzed using Spearman correlation, while the effect of categorical predictors on the number of implanted blastocysts was tested by Mann-Whitney test or Kruskal-Wallis one-way analysis of variance. For all other outcome variables, the effect of possible predictors was analyzed using univariate logistic regression model. Before the incorporation of possible predictors in the multiple regression model, correlations among variables were tested to detect possible multicolinearity and to choose appropriate variables for the final analysis. The impact of possible predictors on the number of live born infants was evaluated using analysis of variance or chi-squared test, as appropriate. For post-hoc comparison of continuous variables, Bonferroni correction of alpha was used, while Keppel modification of Bonferroni correction was used for categorical variables.

Because of the low number of events per variables (EPV) for early clinical miscarriages, biochemical pregnancies and EPLs included in the logistic regression (Vittinghoff & McCulloch, 2007), a multiple model for analyzing the relative contribution of each predictor was constructed only for these three outcomes: **positive** βhCG 14 days following embryo transfer, clinical pregnancy rate and live births rate.

After testing all parameters for multicolinearity, a problem was detected in these pairs of variables: the number of retrieved oocytes/the number of fertilized oocytes, the number of retrieved oocytes/the number of embryos on Day 2, the number of fertilized oocytes/the number of embryos on Day 2 and the number of blastocysts/the number of frozen blastocysts. Accordingly, these pairs of variables were not included in the multiple regression model.

2.3.2.2.1 *Positive βhCG*

A univariate logistic regression model suggested a statistically significant correlation between the positive βhCG 14 days after ET and these indirect indicators of embryo quality: the number of embryos on Day 2 (OR=1.091; 95% CI 1.004 - 1.185, P<0.039), the number of blastocysts (OR=1.303; 95% CI 1.138 - 1.491, P<0.001), the number of frozen blastocysts (OR=1.436; 95% CI 1.208 - 1.708, P<0.001) and the embryo quality score of transferred blastocyst (in the form of two subgroups: the one with blastocysts of suboptimal quality only and the other with at least one blastocyst of optimal quality) (OR=5.339; 95% CI 2.782 - 10.246, P<0.001). A statistically significant correlation in univariate model was also noted for the age of the woman (OR=0.857; 95% CI 0.781 - 0.940, P=0.001), the number of retrieved oocytes (OR=1.069; 95% CI 1.006 - 1.135, P=0.030) and the number of fertilized oocytes (OR=1.088; 95% CI 1.003 - 1.180, P=0.041).

After controlling for the all other independent possible predictors in the multiple logistic regression model, the predictors of positive βhCG 14 days after ET in patients with endometriosis identified as statistically significant were the embryo quality score of transferred blastocyst (OR=4.278; 95% CI 1.976 - 9.265, P<0.001) and the age of the woman (OR=0.848; 95% CI 0.757 - 0.950, P=0.005).

2.3.2.2.2 *Clinical pregnancy rate*

Application of a logistic regression in univariate model showed that there was a statistically significant correlation between the clinical pregnancy rate and these indirect measures of embryo quality: the number of blastocysts (OR=1.278; 95% CI 1.122 - 1.457, P<0.001), the number of frozen blastocysts (OR=1.376; 95% CI 1.170 - 1.618, P<0.001) and the embryo quality score of transferred blastocyst (in the form of two subgroups: the one with blastocysts of suboptimal quality only and the other with at least one blastocyst of optimal quality) (OR=4.708; 95% CI 2.466 - 8.986, P<0.001). A statistically significant correlation in univariate model was also noted for the age of the woman (OR=0.875; 95% CI 0.781 - 0.941, P=0.001) and the number of retrieved oocytes (OR=1.069; 95% CI 1.007 - 1.134, P=0.027).

After controlling for all other independent possible predictors in the multiple logistic regression model, the predictors of the clinical pregnancy rate in patients with endometriosis identified as statistically significant were the embryo quality score (OR=3.485; 95% CI 1.608 - 7.553, P=0.002) and the age of the woman (OR=0.861; 95% CI 0.770 - 0.963, P=0.009).

2.3.2.2.3 *Live births*

A univariate logistic regression model indicated that there was a statistically significant correlation between the live births rate and these indirect measures of embryo quality: the number of blastocysts (OR=1.313; 95% CI 1.139 - 1.513, P<0.001), the number of frozen blastocysts (OR=1.402; 95% CI 1.183 - 1.661, P<0.001) and the embryo quality score of transferred blastocyst (in the form of two subgroups: the one with blastocysts of suboptimal quality only and the other with at least one blastocyst of optimal quality) (OR=3.316; 95% CI 1.693 - 6.496, P<0.001). A statistically significant correlation in univariate model was also noted for the age of the woman (OR=0.861; 95% CI 0.780 - 0.950, P=0.03).

After controlling for all other independent possible predictors in the multiple logistic regression model, the predictors of the live births rate in patients with endometriosis identified as statistically significant were the age of the woman (OR=0.851; 95% CI 0.756 - 0.958, P=0.07) and the number of frozen blastocysts (OR=1.319; 95% CI 1.034 - 1.683, P=0.026).

3. Conclusion

It is generally accepted that endometriosis and infertility are associated. However, the mechanisms connecting these complex conditions are still elusive. Results of different studies on virtually every aspect of this subject are controversial. Despite controversy, there is general agreement on relatively few final consequences of these pathophysiologic processes - endometriosis impairs the quality of oocytes with resulting lower fertilization rates and/or decreases implantation capacity of embryos (Pellicer et al., 2001).

One of indirect markers of oocyte quality and a possible predictor of embryo's implantation capacity is the quality of the developing embryo. As such, this parameter could be valuable for the assessment of influence of endometriosis on fertility of affected individuals. There are several indicators of embryo quality. Some of them are indirect measures of quality (the number of embryos on Day 2, the number of blastocysts, the number of frozen blastocysts, but also the implantation rate), while the only direct measure is the embryo quality score based on morphological characteristics of a developing embryo.

Our study showed no statistically significant difference of quality score of transferred blastocysts, indirect measures of embryo quality, common outcomes of IVF-ET cycles (implantation rate, clinical pregnancy rate, clinical miscarriage rate, early pregnancy loss rate and live births rate) or other analyzed parameters (male factor present, number of oocytes retrieved, number of fertilized oocytes, fertilization rate method of fertilization) between the group of infertile patients with endometriosis and the group with tubal factor infertility only.

In the further analysis of our data, we also showed that in infertile patients suffering only from endometriosis, embryo quality was a statistically significant positive predictor of positive βhCG measurement (if embryo quality was expressed in the form of embryo quality score, OR=4.278; 95% CI 1.976 - 9.265, P<0.001), clinical pregnancy rate (if embryo quality was expressed in the form of embryo quality score, OR=3.485; 95% CI 1.608 - 7.553, P=0.002) and live births rate (if embryo quality was expressed in the form of number of frozen blastocysts, OR=1.319; 95% CI 1.034 - 1.683, P=0.026). As expected, the patient's age was a statistically significant negative predictor of the success of IVF-ET cycles (positive βhCG measurement, clinical pregnancy rate and live births rate) in the observed group of patients.

Endometriosis is still an insufficiently explained condition. Numerous controversies still surrounding this complex disease indicate an obvious need for further clinical studies, meta-analyses and explanation of its pathophysiologic mechanisms. Should a consensus be reached on a precise methodology, future studies would definitely be more informative and results easier to use in clinical practice.

4. References

Arici, A.; Oral, E.; Bukulmez O.; Duleba, A.; Olive, DL. &, Jones, EE. (1996). The effect of endometriosis on implantation: results from the Yale University in vitro fertilization and embryo transfer program. *Fertil Steril*, 65: 603-7.

Barragán, JC.; Brotons, J.; Ruiz, JA. & Acien, P. (1992). Experimentally induced endometriosis in rats: effect on fertility and the effects of pregnancy and lactation on the ectopic endometrial tissue. *Fertil Steril*, 58: 1215–19.

Bergendal, A.; Naffah, S.; Nagy, C.; Bergqvist, A.; Sjöblom, P. & Hillensjö, T. (1998). Outcome of IVF in patients with endometriosis in comparison with tubal factor infertility. J Assist Reprod Genet, 15: 530-4.

Brizek, CL.; Schlaff, S.; Pellegrini, VA.; Frank, JB. & Worrilow, KC. (1995). Increased incidence of aberrant morphological phenotypes in human embryogenesis - an association with endometriosis. *J Assist Reprod Genet*, 12: 106-12.

Croxato, HB.; Ortiz, ME.; Guiloff, E.; Ibarra, A.; Salvatierra, AM.; Croxatto, HD. & Spilman, CH. (1978). Effect of 15 (S)-15-methyl prostaglandin F2a on human oviductal motility and ovum transport. *Fertil Steril*, 30: 408-14.

Damewood, MD.; Hesla, JS; Schlaff, WD.; Hubbard, M.; Gearhart, JD. & Rock, JA. (1990). Effect of serum from patients with minimal to mild endometriosis on mouse embryo development in vitro. *Fertil Steril*, 54: 917-20.

Dmowski, WP.; Radwanska, E.; Binor, Z. & Rana, N. (1986). Mild endometriosis and ovulatory dysfunction: effect of danazol treatment on success of ovulation induction. *Fertil Steril*, 46: 784-9.

Dmowski, WP.; Rana, N.; Michalowska, J.; Friberg, J.; Papierniak, C. & el-Roeiy. A. (1995). The effect of endometriosis, its stage and activity, and of auto antibodies on in vitro fertilization and embryo transfer success rates. *Fertil Steril*, 63: 555-62.

Dosen, M.; Vlaisavljevic, V. & Kovacic, B. (2011). Early miscarriage after single and double blastocyst transfer - An analysis of 1020 blastocyst transfers. Zdravniski Vestnik, 80: I-72-87.

Drake, TS. & Grunert, GM. (1980). The unsuspected pelvic factor in the infertility investigation. *Fertil Steril*, 34: 27–31.

Gardner, DK. & Schoolcraft, WB. (1999). In vitro culture of human blastocysts. In: *Toward Reproductive Certainty: Fertility and Genetics Beyond,* Jansen, R. & Mortimer, D., pp. 378-88, Partenon Publishing UK, Carnforth

Garrido, N.; Navarro, J.; Remohi, J.; Simon, C. & Pellicer, A. (2000). Follicular hormonal environment and embryo quality in women with endometriosis. *Hum Reprod Update*, 6; 67-74.

Grant, A. (1966). Additional sterility factors in endometriosis. *Fertil Steril*, 17: 514-9.

Hammond, MG.; Jordan, S. & Sloan, CS. (1986). Factors affecting pregnancy rates in donor insemination program using frozen semen. *Am J Obstet Gynecol*, 155: 480–5.

Harada, T.; Iwabe, T. & Terakawa, N. (2001). Role of cytokines in endometriosis. *Fertil Steril*, 76: 1-10.

Hasson, HM. (1976). Incidence of endometriosis in diagnostic laparoscopy. *J Reprod Med*, 16: 135–8.

Hourvitz, A.; Lerner-Geva, L.; Elizur, SE.; Baum, M.; Levron, J. & David B. (2006). Role of embryo quality in predicting early pregnancy loss following assisted reproductive technology. *RBM Online*, 13(4): 504–9.

Hunter, MI.; Huang, A. & DeCherney, AH. (2004). Endometriosis and ART. In: *Textbook of Assisted Reproductive Techniques. Laboratory and Clinical Perspectives,* Gardner, DK.; Weissman, A.; Howles, CM. & Shoham Z., pp. 761-9, Taylor & Francis UK, London.

Kovacic, B.; Vlaisavljevic, V.; Reljic, M. & Cizek-Sajko M. (2004). Developmental capacity of different morphological types of day human morulae and blastocysts. *RBM Online*, 8: 687–94.

Kovacic, B.; Cizek Sajko, M. & Vlaisavljevic, V. (2010). A prospective, randomized trial on the effect of atmospheric versus reduced oxygen concentration on the outcome of intracytoplasmic sperm injection cycles. *Fertil Steril*, 94(2): 511-9.

Lambers, MJ.; Mager, E.; Goutbeek, J.; McDonnell, J.; Homburg, R. & Schats R. (2007). Factors determining early pregnancy loss in singleton and multiple implantations. *Hum Reprod*, 22: 275–9.

La Sala, GB.; Nicoli, A.; Villani, MT.; Gallinelli, A.; Nucera, G. & Blickstein, I. (2005). Spontaneous embryonic loss rates in twin and singleton pregnancies after transfer of top- versus intermediate-quality embryos. *Fertil Steril*, 84: 1602–5.

Mahadevan, MM.; Trounson, AO. & Leeton, JF. (1983). The relationship of tubal blockage, infertility of unknown cause, suspected male infertility and endometriosis to success of in vitro fertilization and embryo transfer. *Fertil Steril*, 40: 755-62.

Mahmood, TA. & Templeton, AA. (1991). Folliculogenesis and ovulation in infertile women with mild endometriosis. *Hum Reprod*, 6: 227–231.

Matson, PL. & Yovich, JL. (1986). The treatment of infertility associated with endometriosis by in vitro fertilization. *Fertil Steril*, 46: 432-4.

Muse, K.; Wilson, EA. & Jawar, MJ. (1982). Prolactin hyperstimulation in response to thyrotropin-releasing hormone in patients with endometriosis. *Fertil Steril*, 38: 419-22.

Pellicer, A.; Oliveira, N.; Ruiz, A.; Remohí, J. & Simón, C. (1995). Exploring the mechanism(s) of endometriosis-related infertility: an analysis of embryo development and implantation in assisted reproduction. *Hum Reprod*, 10(Suppl 2): 91-7.

Pellicer, A.; Navarro, J.; Bosch, E.; Garrido, N.; Garcia-Velasco, JA.; Remohí, J. & Simón C. (2001). Endometrial quality in infertile women with endometriosis. *Ann N Y Acad Sci*, 943: 122-30.

Schenken, RS. &, Asch, RH. (1980). Surgical induction of endometriosis in the rabbit: effects on fertility and concentrations of peritoneal fluid prostaglandins. *Fertil Steril*, 34: 581-7.

Schenken, RS.; Asch, RH.; Williams, RF & Hodgen GD. (1984). Etiology of infertility in monkeys with endometriosis: luteinized unruptured follicle, luteal phase defects, pelvic adhesions and spontaneous abortions. *Fertil Steril*, 41: 122–30.

Steer, CV.; Mills, CL.; Tan, SL.; Campbell, S. & Edwards, RG. (1992). The cumulative embryo score: a predictive embryo scoring technique to select the optimal number of embryos to transfer in an in-vitro fertilization and embryo transfer programme. *Hum Reprod*, 7: 117–9.

Strathy, JH.; Molgaard, CA; Coulam, CB. & Melton, LJ. (1982). Endometriosis and infertility: A laparoscopic study of endometriosis among fertile and infertile women. *Fertil Steril*, 38: 667–72.

Soldati, G.; Piffaretti-Yanez, A.; Campana, A.; Marchini, M.; Luerti, M. & Balerna, M. (1989). Effect of peritoneal fluid on sperm motility and velocity distribution using objective measurements. *Fertil Steril*, 52: 113-9.

Tanbo, T.; Omland, A.; Dale, PO. & Abyholm, T. In vitro fertilization/embryo transfer in unexplained infertility and minimal peritoneal endometriosis. (1995). *Acta Obstet Gynecol Scand*, 74: 539-43.

The American Fertility Society. Revised American Fertility Society classification of endometriosis. (1985). *Fertil Steril*, 43: 351-2.

Tummon, IS.; Maclin, VM.; Radwanska, E.; Binor, Z. & Dmowski, WP. (1988). Occult ovulatory dysfunction in women with minimal endometriosis or unexplained infertility. *Fertil Steril*, 50: 716-20.

Vernon, MW. & Wilson, EA. (1985). Studies on the surgical induction of endometriosis in the rat. *Fertil Steril*, 44: 684–94.

Vittinghoff, E. & McCulloch, CE. (2007). Relaxing the rule of ten events per variable in logistic and Cox regression. *Am J Epidemiol*, 165(6): 710-8.

Winter, E.; Wang, J.; Davies, MJ. & Norman, R. (2002). Early pregnancy loss following assisted reproductive technology treatment. *Hum Reprod*, 17: 3220–3.

Yanushpolsky, EH.; Best, CL.; Jackson, KV.; Clarke, RN.; Barbieri, RL. & Hornstein, MD. (1998). Effects of endometriomas on oocyte quality, embryo quality and pregnancy rates in in vitro fertilization cycles: a prospective, case-controlled study. *J Assist Reprod Genet*, 15: 193-7.

Yeh, J. & Seibel, MM. (1987). Artificial insemination with donor sperm: A review of 108 patients. Obstet Gynecol, 70: 313–6.

Yovich, JL.; Yovich, JM.; Tuvik, AI.; Matson, PL. & Willcox DL. (1985). In-vitro fertilization for endometriosis. *Lancet*, 2(8454): 552.

22

Endometriosis and Infertility: The Role of Oxidative Stress

Ionara Barcelos[1] and Paula Navarro[2]
[1]*University of West Parana,*
Da Vinci - Reproductive Medicine,
[2]*University of Sao Paulo,*
University of Sao Paulo - Ribeirao Preto,
Brazil

1. Introduction

Several reports have supported the concept of reduced fecundity in women with endometriosis (Garrido et al., 2002; 2000). Contradictory data have been reported for in vitro fertilization (IVF) outcomes in patients with endometriosis (Garrido et al., 2002; Garcia-Velasco & Arici, 1999; Kumbak et al., 2008; Fernando et al., 2008). Some studies suggest lower fertilization, implantation, and pregnancy rates in women with endometriosis (Barnhardt et al., 2002; Al-Fadhli et al., 2006), possibly owing to impaired oocyte quality with consequent poor embryo quality, or to endometrial defects or defective interactions between the endometrium and the embryo (Kumbak et al., 2008, Brizek et al., 1995; Pellicer et al., 1995).

Oocyte quality depends on proper cytoplasmic and nuclear maturation (Kim et al., 1998), with the latter requiring the presence of normal cell spindles that guide chromosome segregation during meiosis (Wang & Keefe, 2002; Mandelbaum et al., 2004; De Santis et al., 2005; Volarcik et al., 1998; Van Blerkom & Davis, 2001). The cell spindle of the oocyte is extremely sensitive to several factors, including oxidative stress (Liu et al., 2003; Navarro et al., 2004; 2006), which might be involved in the etiopathogenesis of infertility related to endometriosis (Campos Petean et al, 2008; Mansour et al, 2009; Jozwik et al., 1999; Carbone et al., 2003).

The oxidative balance of the reproductive female tract depends on some types of free radicals and on different antioxidant mechanisms that neutralize them. There are two major groups of free radicals: reactive oxygen species and reactive nitrogen species.

2. Reactive Oxygen Species (ROS)

The ROS have physiological and pathological functions in the female reproductive tract. Fertility problems related to ROS have etiopathogenic factors in common (Agarwal et al., 2005). These reactive species are generated through enzymatic and non-enzymatic organic reactions. Biological reactions, through electron transference or through oxigenase, that use oxygen (O_2) as substrate, generate large amounts of ROS. As the mithocondrial respiratory chain is the major O_2 cell intake system, the majority of ROS are produced by this system under physiological conditions (Fujii et al., 2005). The **superoxide radical (O_2^-)** is formed when electrons leak from the electron transport chain ($O_2 + e^- \rightarrow O_2^-$) (Agarwal et al., 2005). The dismutation of superoxide results in the formation of **hydrogen peroxide (H_2O_2)** ($2\ O_2^- + 2\ H^+ \rightarrow H_2O_2 + O_2$) (Agarwal et al., 2005). The same can also be generated by reduction of O_2^- ($O_2^- + e^- + 2\ H^+ \rightarrow H_2O_2$) (Babior, 1997). The **hidroxyl (OH^-) ion** is formed by the acquisition of 1 electron by **H_2O_2** ($H_2O_2 + e- + H^+ \rightarrow OH + H_2O$) (Babior, 1997). The hydroxyl ion is highly reactive and can modify purines and pyrimidines and cause strand breaks resulting in DNA damage (Agarwal et al., 2005).

3. Antioxidants

Under normal conditions, all organisms have enzymatic and non-enzymatic mechanisms capable of neutralizing pro-oxidants species and/or repair damages caused by reactive species, converting them to H_2O, to prevent overproduction. Many antioxidants of low molecular weight such as vitamins and polyphenols are usually found in nutrients, although enzymatic neutralization of reactive species is the most effective mechanism (Agarwal et al., 2005; Fujii et al., 2005).

4. Non-enzymatic antioxidants

Also known as synthetic antioxidants or dietary supplements, this group influences in an exogenous way the antioxidant defense system of the organism. The most common are: vitamins C and E, selenium, zinc, taurine, hypotaurine, glutathione, β-carotene, and carotene.

Vitamin E may block the initiation of lipid peroxidation as well as its propagation phase (Bornoden, 1994).

Glutathione is the major non-protein sulfhydryl component of mammalian cells and has an important role in cellular protection from oxidative stress (Meister, 1983). Glutathione synthesis increases throughout oocyte development and maturation until the periovulatory follicle stage (Perreault et al., 1988). After fertilization, glutathione participates in the sperm decondensation process, while the oocyte activation process occurs, and the sperm head turns into the male pronucleus (Calvin et al., 1986; Perreault et al., 1984, 1988; Yoshida, 1992, 1993). A study performed with bovine oocytes has shown the important role of COCs during the in vitro maturation process. Through gap junctions, cumulus oophorus cells (COCs) might mediate glutathione synthesis by the oocytes, a crucial enzyme for the cytoplasmic and nuclear maturation process. This intimate relation between COCs and oocytes apparently occurs due to the presence of gap junctions (De Matos et al., 1997).

5. Enzymatic antioxidants

The enzymatic defenses responsible for ROS neutralization are mainly represented by superoxide dismutase (SOD), catalase, glutathione peroxidase (GPx), depending or not on selenium and glutathione reductase (GR) (Fujii et al., 2005):

- **Superoxide dismutase (SOD):**

The superoxide anion is produced by a one-electron reduction of an oxygen molecule and initiates a radical chain reaction. It is believed that SOD, which dismutates the superoxide anion to hydrogen peroxide ($2\ O_2^- + 2\ H+ \rightarrow H_2O_2 + O_2$), plays a central role in antioxidant reactions. Three isozymes are produced by mammals (Fujii et al., 2005):

- SOD1 encodes Cu,Zn-SOD, which is largely cytosolic;
- SOD2 encodes Mn-SOD, a mitochondrial isoform;
- SOD3, which encodes the extracellular form (EC-SOD), structurally similar to CuZn-SOD.

One of the striking phenotypes of SOD1-deficient mice is female infertility, suggesting a potential role of this enzyme in female fertility. SOD2 is inducible under various oxidative stress and inflammatory conditions. EC-SOD is present at high levels in the epididymis, seminiferous tubules of the testis, as well as the lungs (Fujii et al., 2005).

The presence of SOD was evidenced in human follicular fluid (FF) and the identification of high concentrations of SOD in FF was associated with oocytes that were not fertilized (Sabatini et al., 1999). Data of a recently published study showed that SOD activity decreased with age in women, but increased in women with endometriosis and ovulatory dysfunction (Matos et al., 2009). When the cause of infertility was male factor, the success of ART was associated with increased SOD activity. Variations in SOD activity emphasize the importance of oxidative stress in the oocyte maturation process, and are suggested to be a potential biomarker of ART success (Matos et al., 2009).

A recent study has established a threshold level in FF which ROS may be considered toxic for viable embryo formation and pregnancy outcome. ROS, lipid peroxidation and total antioxidant capacity were estimated. The upper cut-off ROS level beyond which viable embryo formation is not favorable was found to be approximately 107 cps/400 microl FF. This level, determined in women with tubal factor infertility, was further validated in women with endometriosis and PCOS and correlated with fertilization and pregnancy rate and embryo quality (Jana et al., 2010).

- **Peroxidases:**

Catalase exclusively detoxifies hydrogen peroxide and has no requirement for an electron donor **($2\ H_2O_2 \rightarrow 2\ H_2O + O_2$)**. It plays a role in organs such as the liver, but its specific function in the genital tract is largely unknown (Fujii et al., 2005).

Glutathione is a tripeptidyl molecule and is present in either the reduced (GSH) or the oxidized state (GSSG). It plays pleiotropic roles, which include the maintenance of cells in a reduced state and the formation of conjugates with some harmful endogenous and xenobiotic compounds. In addition, GSH serves as an electron donor for GPx that reduces peroxide **($2GSH + H_2O_2 \rightarrow GSSG + 2\ H_2O$)**. At least four selenium-containing GPx isozymes are produced in mammals (Fujii et al., 2005):

The cytosolic form, GPX1, is widely distributed in tissues and has been the most extensively investigated form. However, GPX1-knockout mice show no abnormality in phenotype including reproductive capability (Ho et al., 1997);

- GPX2 encodes a gastrointestinal form, and no specific function for it is known in reproduction
- GPX3 is present in plasma and in epididymal fluid
- GPX4 encodes an isoform that specifically detoxifies phospholipid hydroperoxide and is thus referred to as PhGPx, and is expressed at high levels in the testis. A defect in GPX4 has been suspected to be a cause of male infertility triggered by selenium deficiency, although direct evidence for its requirement is missing (Hansen & Deguchi, 1996).

In a reaction promoted by peroxidase, GSH is oxidized to GSSG. Regeneration of GSH is, therefore, crucial for the ability of cells to fight exposure to oxidant metabolites. GSH levels are maintained by de novo synthesis that is catalyzed by two enzymes, γ- glutamylcysteine synthetase (γ-GCS) and glutathione synthetase (GS). The reduction of GSSG is catalyzed by **glutathione reductase** (GR) using NADPH as an electron donor **(2 GSSG + NADPH + H^+ → 2GSH + $NADP^+$)**. GR is also inhibited by compounds produced in response to nitrosative stress, such as nitrosoglutathione. In the female reproductive system, GSH is assumed to play a role by reducing oxidative stress either by direct interaction with ROS, by the **glutathione redox system**, or by donating an electron to GPx (Fujii et al., 2005).

High levels of SeGPx were found in follicles that held oocytes with the potential to be fertilized and lower levels were related to fertilization failure (Paszkowski et al., 1995).

6. Endometriosis and oxidative stress

Some authors have suggested that endometriosis might be associated with oxidative stress (Agarwal et al., 2003; Szczepanska et al., 2003; Gupta et al., 2006). In pelvic endometriosis there might be an activation of macrophages in the peritoneal environment leading to increased production of reactive oxygen and nitrogen species, cytokines, prostaglandins, growth factors and, therefore, oxidative stress generating lipid peroxidation and its degradation products and other products formed by its interactions with low density lipoproteins and other proteins. Peroxidized lipids, when decomposed, generate products such as malondialdehyde (MDA) and could be recognized as foreign bodies, leading to an antigenic response with consequent production of antibodies (Halliwell, 1994; Murphy et al., 1998). This process would induce oxidative damage to red blood cells and to endometrial and peritoneal cells which would stimulate recruitment and activation of a larger number of mononuclear phagocytes, maintaining oxidative damage to the pelvic environment (Van Langendonckt et al., 2002). Oxidative stress compromises mesothelial cells and might induce adhesion sites for endometrial cells, contributing to development and progression of the endometriosis focus (Alpay et al., 2006).

In a recent study by our group, blood samples were collected during the early follicular phase of the menstrual cycle for the analysis of serum MDA, GSH and total hydroxyperoxide levels by spectrophotometry and of vitamin E by high performance liquid chromatography. A positive association between infertility related to endometriosis, advanced disease stage and increased serum hydroxyperoxide levels was demonstrated, suggesting an increased production of reactive species in women with endometriosis. These data, taken together with the reduction of serum vitamin E and GSH levels, suggest the occurrence of systemic oxidative stress in women with infertility associated with endometriosis (Andrade et al., 2010).

The activation of polymorphonuclear leucocytes and macrophages observed in endometriosis patients might be induced by several factors, including damaged red blood cells, apoptotic endometrial cells, cellular debris and some other inflammatory cells. In endometriosis these actions of peritoneal macrophages appear to be stimulated *in vitro* by the immune response or by agents such as α and γ-interferon, increasing inducible nitric oxide synthase (NOS) expression, producing more nitric oxide and nitrite and nitrate compounds (Agarwal et al., 2005). However, we obtained no conclusive data concerning nitric oxide, peroxidized lipids and ROS levels in the peritoneal fluid of patients with and without endometriosis (Agarwal et al., 2003; Amaral et al., 2005).

In women with endometriosis and adenomyosis, we also observe a greater expression of Mn-SOD and CuZn-SOD in the endometrium throughout the menstrual cycle, as well as aberrant expression of GPx and xanthine peroxidase (XO), in topic and ectopic endometrium. SOD activity seems to be significantly higher in the ectopic endometrium of endometriomas than in the topic endometrium (Alpay et al., 2006). However, this increase in the expression of antioxidant enzymes in the topic and ectopic endometrium of endometriosis patients could be a primary event or secondary to an increase of ROS, which needs to be evaluated. If, on the one hand, we have no conclusive data concerning the pattern of expression of the most important oxidant and antioxidant enzymes in topic and ectopic endometrium, on the other hand, we have not found, so far, any studies that have evaluated the expression of these enzymes in granulosa cells of patients with endometriosis, whose anomalies could contribute to the impairment of folliculogenesis and of the acquisition of oocyte competence to permit fertilization and support embryo development.

The above data suggest a trend to a greater production of free radicals in endometriosis patients associated with a potential alteration of antioxidant capacity. This may contribute to oxidative stress which could be related to the pathogenesis and progression of endometriosis.

Another very interesting aspect of endometriosis is its enigmatic association with infertility, observed in 25 to 30% of women with this affection. Until now, little is known about the mechanisms involved in the pathogenesis of infertility, especially in minimal and mild endometriosis, where there is no significant alteration of pelvic anatomy.

New approaches to the treatment of infertility related to this disorder have included the increasingly more common application of ART. The introduction of *in vitro* fertilization (IVF) for the treatment of infertility secondary to endometriosis has become an important tool for the study of the potential effects of endometriosis on specific stages of the reproductive process, including folliculogenesis, fertilization, embryo development and implantation. Contradictory data have been reported for IVF outcomes in patients with endometriosis (García-Velasco & Arici, 1999; Garrido et al., 2000). This discrepancy seems to be multifactorial since IVF outcomes might be affected by different variables, such as ovulation induction protocol, patient selection criteria, laboratory procedures, and embryo transfer technique, among other factors.

As previously said, contradictory data have been reported for IVF outcomes in patients with endometriosis (Garrido et al., 2002; Garcia-Velasco & Arici, 1999; Kumbak et al., 2008; Fernando et al., 2008). Some studies suggest lower fertilization, implantation, and pregnancy rates in women with endometriosis (Barnhart et al., 2002; Al-Fadhli et al., 2006), possibly owing to impaired oocyte quality with consequent poor embryo quality, or to endometrial defects or defective interactions between the endometrium and the embryo (Kumbak et al., 2008, Brizek et al., 1995; Pellicer et al., 1995). Conflicting findings of some alterations in topic endometrium of endometriosis patients could explain, at least partially, the disturbance of the interaction between embryo and endometrium, generating anomalies in the implantation process (García-Velasco & Arici, 1999; Garrido et al., 2000). However, similar implantation rates in oocyte donation cycles have been recorded for women with endometriosis and control subjects, suggesting the crucial role of oocyte quality in impaired implantation processes (Pellicer et al., 1995; 2001; Díaz et al., 2000; Garrido et al., 2000; Katsoff et al., 2006). According to some authors, impaired oocyte quality would be responsible for compromising (Brizek et al., 1995) or completely blocking embryo development (Pellicer et al., 1995) in women with endometriosis, reinforcing the role of poor oocyte quality in the outcome of ART procedures in this group of patients.

Studies that intended to evaluate indirectly oocyte quality in patients with endometriosis analyzed multiple paracrine factors present in FF, such as interleukins, vascular endothelial growth factor (VEGF), and tumor necrosis factor (TNF), as well as granulosa cells apoptosis, leucocyte number and activity, among other indirect predictors of oocyte quality (Garrido et al., 2000, 2002). However, few studies have evaluated oocyte quality in patients with endometriosis by more objective morphological criteria.

Oocyte quality depends on factors related to the acquisition of nuclear and cytoplasmic competence. Although involving different processes, nuclear and cytoplasmic maturation are connected events that occur simultaneously in determined situations, although cytoplasmic molecular programming starts in the oocyte growth phase (Ferreira et al., 2009).

Nuclear competence depends on the anatomic and functional integrity of the meiotic spindle, a temporary and dynamic structure responsible for chromosomal segregation during meiosis (Wang & Keefe, 2002; Navarro et al., 2005). Meiotic anomalies might contribute to cell development failure by different paths, such as the inability of the oocyte to complete the maturation process in order to be fertilized, or the occurrence of variable errors of the meiotic maturation process that do not stop fertilization but might compromise embryo development pre or post implantation, as well as the future viability of the fetus (Armstrong, 2001; Chaube et al., 2005; Mansour et al., 2009). On the other hand, there is evidence that oxidative stress might promote meiotic anomalies and pre-implantation embryo development (Liu et al., 2003; Navarro et al., 2004, 2006; Agarwal et al., 2006; Mansour et al., 2009). Oxidative stress also seems to induce genomic and mitochondrial DNA damage (Aitken et al., 2001), which leads directly to reduced fertility (Guerin et al., 2001). Recently it was demonstrated that the peritoneal fluid of endometriosis patients promotes anomalies in oocyte cytoskeleton and increases embryo apoptosis, preventable by antioxidant supplementation (L-carnitine) in the culture medium, as shown in a study using mice as the experimental model (Mansour et al., 2009), suggesting that oxidative stress might be involved in the etiopathogenesis of poor oocyte quality in patients with this disease. In some recent studies, sperm incubated with peritoneal fluid of endometriosis patients showed increased DNA fragmentation and the extent of fragmentation increased according to endometriosis stage and infertility duration. Similarly, oocytes incubated with peritoneal fluid of endometriosis patients presented increased DNA damage and the extent of damage was proportional to the period of exposure. As expected, embryos incubated with peritoneal fluid also showed DNA fragmentation as indicated by an increase of apoptosis. The increase of DNA damage in spermatozoa, oocytes and embryos seems to be responsible for the numerous abortions and for fertilization and implantation failure among endometriosis patients (Mansour et al., 2009).

Our group was the first to assess the meiotic spindle and chromosome distribution of in vitro-matured (IVM) oocytes obtained from stimulated cycles of endometriosis patients and to compare them with a control group consisting of couples with male or tubal factors of infertility. We showed that, although IVM rates were similar for the two groups evaluated, a higher proportion of telophase I oocytes tended to occur in the endometriosis group. The number of oocytes was too low to detect statistically significant differences. However, this finding suggests a potential delay or impairment of meiosis I during IVM in the context of endometriosis. The mechanisms underlying this finding remain unclear. Recent studies demonstrated significant DNA damage and increased anomalies in the microtubules and chromosomes of oocytes incubated with PF from endometriosis patients (Mansour et al, 2009; Carbone et al., 2003), which were prevented by supplementation of the culture medium with the antioxidant L-carnitine, suggesting that impaired oocyte quality in endometriosis may be mediated by oxidative stress (Carbone et al., 2003). Although the data were obtained from frozen/thawed MII mouse oocytes and may not necessarily be extrapolated to human oocytes, they support our hypothesis that oxidative stress might be involved in the delay or impairment of meiosis I in oocytes of women with endometriosis (Barcelos et al., 2009), a possibility that requires more in-depth evaluation in future studies.

Unpublished data from our group suggest that this finding is also confirmed in in vivo matured oocytes of patients with moderate and severe endometriosis. However, we did not find well designed studies evaluating different pro and antioxidants markers in this group of patients, co-relating them with ART outcome as indirect predictors of oocyte quality.

If we have very little evidence correlating endometriosis and meiotic oocyte anomalies, data about the potential association between endometriosis and oocyte cytoplasmic maturation markers are even rarer. The gene expression of the antioxidant enzymatic system is one of the markers of oocyte cytoplasmic maturation, playing an important role by minimizing the hazardous effects of oxidative stress (Cetica et al., 2001). It has already been demonstrated that catalase, SOD and GPx are found in oocytes and COCs. GSH is one of the oocyte cytoplasmic maturation markers that have been intensely investigated. Some studies show that an adequate expansion of COCs, which is considered to be an oocyte maturation marker, is partially dependent on the intracellular concentration of GSH (Furnus et al., 1998). Intracellular GSH levels increase as the oocyte develops from germinal vesicle to metaphase II (Ali et al., 2003). After fertilization, the total amount of intracellular GSH correlates with spermatic chromatin decondensation, with consequent oocyte activation and also with the transformation of the sperm head to male pronucleus (De Matos & Furnus, 2000). However, no studies have evaluated the expression of this enzyme or of the entire GSH redox system in COCs of patients with infertility related to endometriosis. Matos et al. (2009) suggested a positive correlation between the SOD activity of COCs of infertile women submitted o ovarian stimulation for ART due to male factor and ART outcomes. In this same study an increase in SOD activity was observed in in vitro culture of COCs from infertile women with endometriosis. However, the authors analyzed the COCs of only six patients.

Some authors have associated minimal endometriosis with impaired steroidogenesis in granulosa cells, represented not only by a reduced baseline activity of aromatase, but also by a lower production of progesterone in non-stimulated and stimulated cycles (Harlow et al., 1996; Gomes et al., 2008). A functional failure of oocytes due to abnormal follicular function could be a result of this disease (Wardle et al., 1985). The antioxidants not only have an anti-apoptotic effect on preovulatory in vitro cultured follicles (Tsai-Turton & Luderer, 2006), but are also involved in the regulation of steroidogenic enzyme function dependent on cytochrome P450 (Verit et al., 2007). Some studies have suggested that ascorbic acid (Murray et al., 2001), as well as SOD (Lapolt & Hong, 1995) may have inhibitory effects on aromatase, an enzyme responsible for the conversion of androgens to estrogens, which could induce storage of androgens in the follicular fluid, leading to follicular atresia (Verit et al., 2007). As mentioned earlier, some recent data have demonstrated an increase of SOD activity in COCs (in vitro culture) of infertile women with endometriosis (Matos et al., 2009). Since no studies on endometriosis patients have evaluated antioxidant enzyme expression in luteinized granulosa cells and their correlation with steroidogenic enzymes dependent on cytochrome P450 expression, involved in ovarian steroidogenesis, our group has performed studies evaluating these possible associations.

7. Endometriosis, steroidogenesis and folliculogenesis

Some studies have shown an increase of luteinized unruptured follicle syndrome (LUF) and of the incidence of lutheal phase defects in women with endometriosis (Cheesman et al., 1983; Holtz et al., 1985; Saracoglu et al., 1985; Kaya & Oral, 1999). Other recent studies have shown a polymorphism of the progesterone gene and resistance to the action of progesterone in endometriosis tissues (Bulun et al., 2006; Van Kaam et al., 2007), supporting the hypothesis of impaired progesterone production and/or action in endometriosis (Bulun et al., 2006; Harlow et al., 1996). Some data show impaired steroidogenesis of granulosa cells associated with minimal endometriosis, represented not only by a reduction of basal aromatase activity, but also by a lower production of progesterone in stimulated as well as non-stimulated cycles (Harlow et al, 1996). Therefore, ovulatory dysfunction induced by impairment of ovarian steroid secretion as well as inadequate lutheal function might be important for the pathogenesis of infertility associated with endometriosis. A function defect in the oocyte due to abnormal follicle function might be the result of this ovulatory dysfunction (Wardle et al., 1985). Supporting this hypothesis, clinical studies involving IVF and some programs of oocyte donation have pointed out the importance of impaired oocyte quality in the pathogenesis of infertility associated with endometriosis (Pellicer et al., 1998; Garrido et al., 2002).

3β-Hydroxysteroide dehydrogenase/delta 5-delta 4-isomerase (3β-HSD) is an important enzyme associated with the biosynthesis of progesterone. Bar Ami (1994) evaluated the fertilization capacity related to the competence of granulosa cells and COCs to secrete progesterone. COCs from fertilized oocytes presented a 1.9 times higher progesterone level ($p<0.001$) on days 0-3 and a 1.6 times higher level ($p<0.02$) on days 3-5 of culture when compared to the levels in COCs of non-fertilized oocytes. Nevertheless, in COCs of fertilized oocytes, the activity of 3β-hydroxysteroid dehydrogenase was significantly higher after oocyte aspiration and also 3 to 5 days later compared to non-fertilized oocytes. These results suggest that, in stimulated cycles, in follicles that hold mature COCs there is a synchrony and correlation between competence to perform progesterone secretion by COCs as well as by granulosa cells and the potential of these oocytes to be fertilized. Such correlation suggests and supports the intimate relation of enzymatic activity of 3β-hydroxysteroid dehydrogenase and progesterone production with oocyte fertilization capacity, which may suggest the important role of this enzyme as coadjuvant in the acquisition of oocyte competence. The reduction of the gene expression and/or activity of this enzyme could lead to a lower production of progesterone and impairment of the lutheal phase.

Aromatase is present in granulosa cells and actually plays a fundamental role in follicle maturation and in the establishment of oocyte quality (Erickson et al., 1989; Foldesi et al., 1998; Speroff & Fritz, 2005). But, if on the one hand we find evidence of increased aromatase expression in ectopic endometrium, on the other, there are poor and inconclusive data concerning the expression of this enzyme by luteinized granulosa cells, suggesting a lower activity of this enzyme, but with no confirmation of an associated lower gene expression.

It is known that oocyte quality results from a complex and synchronized process that lasts several months, from primordial follicle to pre-ovulatory follicle. This process starts in a gonadotropin-independent way and later becomes gonadotropin dependent. In this last phase, oocyte, granulosa cells and FSH interact synergically. Granulosa cell multiplication and the specific way they respond first to FSH and later to LH in order to produce intra-follicle steroids are crucial events in this process (Speroff & Fritz, 2005). We know that there are gap junctions between granulosa cells, which is evidence that there are molecular interactions between them and possibly with the oocyte itself, through signaling molecules such as growth and differentiation factor-9 (GDF-9) and bone morphogenetic protein-15 (BMP 15) (Albertini & Barrett, 2003; Combelles et al., 2004; Thomas & Vanderhyden, 2006; Hutt & Albertini, 2007). However, little information is available about the communication between granulosa cells and the oocyte.

Granulosa cells differentiate into mural and cumulus cells during folliculogenesis, a fact that has stimulated the study of their potential as mesenchymal stem cells. To date there are no studies comparing the gene expression of mural granulosa cells and COCs and, possibly, since they are cells with distinct function and differentiation, there might be genes with different patterns of expression. When they reach the pre-antral follicle stage, granulosa cells can synthetize all three types of steroids (androgens, progestagens and estrogens) (Speroff & Fritz, 2005). However, the proportions and timing of their production are crucial. It is known that FSH and also LH have hormonal receptors on granulosa cells and there is a synergism between these receptors and intra-follicle hormonal production to permit the development of a follicle that holds a mature oocyte (Costa et al., 2004; Speroff & Fritz, 2005; Silva et al., 2008). Androgens, for instance, are necessary at low concentrations at the very beginning of follicle development, as a substrate for estradiol production. According to the two cells theory, theca cells convert C21 components (cholesterol) to androgen, which is a substrate for the aromatase of granulosa cells that converts androgens (C19) to estrogens (C18). The transformation of an androgenic environment to an estrogenic one is crucial in order to produce an oocyte capable of ovulation (Speroff & Fritz, 2005). In granulosa cells, aromatase plays an essential role in folliculogenesis and in estradiol production and its expression increases with follicle development (Tetsuka &Hillier, 1997; Guet et al., 1999) under the influence of FSH (Speroff & Fritz, 2005). Therefore, aromatase is a crucial enzyme in granulosa cells which is responsible for the formation of an estrogenic follicle microenvironment, essential for development and maturation (Speroff & Fritz, 2005). Nevertheless, it is important to state that aromatase is the final point of the entire ovarian steroidogenic cascade and the only enzyme capable of converting androgens to estrogens. Therefore, if its activity is impaired, that specific follicle will have difficulty in acquiring a normal pre-ovulatory state.

Intra-follicle hormonal relations are essential for the success of the entire ovulatory process both in natural cycles and in cycles stimulated for ART. Regarding maturation, Costa et al. (2004) analyzed cycles stimulated with exogenous gonadotropins without using a GnRH analogue and found that the follicles that held mature oocytes presented an increase in the progesterone/testosterone (P/T) ratio), in the progesterone/estradiol (P/E2) ratio and in the estradiol/testosterone (E/T) ratio in follicular fluid when compared to immature oocytes, suggesting a decrease in C21 to C19 conversion, but not in aromatase activity. Silva et al. (2008) analyzed these same ratios in follicles of women submitted to stimulated cycles using a GnRH analogue and observed that the action of the analogue remained intact and its most important effect was a decrease in intra-follicle androgen, with higher rates of fertilization and maturation.

In vitro studies using granulosa cell culture of women with endometriosis submitted to ovarian hyperstimulated cycles showed that these cells present impaired aromatase activity. Harlow et al. (1996) investigated aromatase activity in patients with minimal and mild endometriosis using granulosa cell culture in which estrogen production was evaluated after adding testosterone to the culture medium. They found a decrease in aromatase activity in patients with endometriosis compared to control. Researchers from the same group (Cahill et al., 2003) using the same technique found a lower sensitivity to LH in granulosa cells of patients with endometriosis.

Abreu et al. (2006) found a reduction of estradiol production in *in vitro* luteinized mural granulosa cells of women with endometriosis, after 24 hours of cell culture. Under baseline conditions or when the culture medium was supplemented with a lower concentration of testosterone ($2x10^{-6}$M), estradiol production was lower in the endometriosis group. However, when the concentration of testosterone (an aromatase precursor) added to the culture medium was increased ($2x10^{-5}$M), there was no difference between the endometriosis and control groups concerning estradiol production. In another study performed by Abreu et al. (2009) no difference in aromatase gene expression (CYP19A1) was observed in luteinized mural cells of women with endometriosis and controls submitted to

ART. However, data obtained by the analysis of gene expression of mural granulosa cells of patients with endometriosis cannot be necessarily extrapolated to cumulus oophorus cells (COCs).

We found evidence that COCs might contribute to oocyte cytoplasmic maturation (Tanghe et al., 2002) through a net of gap junctions between COCs and between these and the oocyte (Furger et al., 1996). Nevertheless, the presence of COCs is important for fertilization to occur (Tanghe et al., 2002) because it attracts selected spermatozoa and promotes their capacitation and penetration. On the other hand, it should be emphasized that COCs protect the oocyte against apoptosis induced by oxidative stress (Tatemoto et al., 2000), which occurs when there is a large number of ROS compared to the anti-oxidants available. Some studies have suggested that analysis of gene expression of COCs might be used as an indirect predictor of oocyte quality and of the outcome of ART procedures, which could lead to distinct clinical applications (Hamamah et al., 2006; Assou et al., 2006, 2008; Hamel et al., 2008; Tesfaye et al., 2009; Haouzi & Hamamah, 2009).

In the female reproductive system, ROS and anti-oxidants play physiological roles during folliculogenesis, oocyte maturation, lutheal regression and fertilization (Agarwal et al., 2006). For example, an increase in ROS production in granulosa cells (Jancar et al., 2007) and on oxidative damage to DNA marker (8-hydroxy-20-deoxyguanosine) levels in granulosa cells and COCs (Seino et al., 2002) was associated with lower fertilization, poor embryo quality and reduction of implantation rates. Nevertheless, oxidative stress also seems to be associated with the etiopathogenesis of reproduction, as is the case in endometriosis (Guerin et al., 2001; Van Langendonckt et al., 2002; Agarwal et al., 2003; Barcelos et al., 2008), idiopathic infertility and polycystic ovary syndrome (Gonzalez et al., 2006).

Considering this substantial involvement of ROS and oxidative stress in fertilization and reproduction modulation, it is accepted that anti-oxidant enzymes on COCs modulate oocyte maturation and might be related to specific conditions that limit the success of ART. Some studies have shown that superoxide dismutase (La Polt & Hong, 1995) might have inhibitory effects on aromatase, suggesting a potential correlation between gene expression of one of the major anti-oxidant enzymatic system and aromatase expression.

8. References

Abreu LG, Romão GS, Dos Reis RM, Ferriani RA, De Sá MF, De Moura MD. Reduced aromatase activity in granulosa cells of women with endometriosis undergoing assisted reproduction techniques. Gynecol Endocrinol. 2006 Aug;22(8):432-6.

Agarwal A, Gupta S, Sharma R. Role of oxidative stress in female reproduction. Reprod Biol Endocrinol. 2005; 3:28.

Agarwal A, Said TM, Bedaiwy MA, et al. Oxidative stress in an assisted reproductive techniques setting. Fertil Steril. 2006; 86(3):503-12.

Agarwal A, Saleh RA, Bedaiwy MA. Role of reactive oxygen species in the pathophysiology of human reproduction. Fertil Steril. 2003, 79(4):829-843.

Aitken RJ, Krausz C. Oxidative stress, DNA damage and the Y chromosome. Reproduction 2001;122:497–506.

Albertini DF, Barrett SL. Oocyte-somatic cell communication. Reproduction. 2003 61:49-54. 2003.

Al-Fadhli R, Kelly SM, Tulandi T, Tanr SL. Effects of different stages of endometriosis on the outcome of in vitro fertilization. J Obstet Gynaecol Can 2006;28:888-91.

Ali AA, Bilodeau JF, Sirard MA. Antioxidant requirements for bovine oocytes varies during in vitro maturation, fertilization and development. Theriogenology. 2003 Feb;59(3-4):939-49.

Alpay Z, Saed GM, Diamond MP. Female infertility and free radicals: potential role in adhesions and endometriosis. J Soc Gynecol Investig. 2006; 13(6):390-8.

Amaral VF, Bydlowski SP, Peranovich TC, Navarro PA, Subbiah MT, Ferriani RA. Lipid peroxidation in the peritoneal fluid of infertile women with peritoneal endometriosis. Eur J Obstet Gynecol Reprod Biol. 2005 Mar 1;119(1):72-5.

Andrade AZ, Rodrigues JK, Dib LA, Romão GS, Ferriani RA, Jordão Junior AA, Navarro PA. Serum markers of oxidative stress in infertile women with endometriosis. Rev Bras Ginecol Obstet. 2010 Jun;32(6):279-85.

Armstrong DT. Effects of maternal age on oocyte developmental competence. Theriogenology. 2001; 55(6):1303-22.

Assou S, Anahory T, Pantesco V, Carrourl T, Pellestor F, Klein B, Reyftmann L, Dechaud H, De Vos J, Hamamah S. The human cumulus-oocyte complex gene-expression profile Hum Reprod. 2006 July ; 21(7): 1705–1719.

Assou S, Haouzi D, Mahmoud K, Aouacheria A, Guillemin Y, Pantesco V, Rème T, Dechaud H, De Vos J, Hamamah S. A non-invasive test for assessing embryo potential by gene expression profiles of human cumulus cells: a proof of concept study. Mol Hum Reprod. 2008 ;14(12):711-9.

Babior BM. Superoxide: a two-edged sword. Bras J Biol Res. 1997; 30(2): 141-55.

Bar-Ami S. Increasing progesterone secretion and 3 beta-hydroxysteroid dehydrogenase activity of human cumulus cells and granulosa-lutein cells concurrent with successful fertilization of the corresponding oocyte. J Steroid Biochem Mol Biol. 1994 Dec;51(5-6):299-305.

Barcelos ID, Vieira RC, Ferreira EM, Araújo MC, Martins W de P, Ferriani RA, Navarro PA. Meiotic abnormalities of oocytes from patients with endometriosis submitted to ovarian stimulation. Rev Bras Ginecol Obstet. 2008 Aug;30(8):413-9.

Barcelos ID, Vieira RC, Ferreira EM, Martins WP, Ferriani RA, Navarro PA. Comparative analysis of the spindle and chromosome configurations of in vitro-matured oocytes from patients with endometriosis and from control subjects: a pilot study. Fertil Steril. 2009 Nov;92(5):1749-52. Epub 2009 Jun 12.

Barnhart K, Dungsmoor-Su R, Coutifaris C. Effect of endometriosis on in vitro fertilization. Fertil Steril. 2002; 77(6): 148-55.

Bornoden W. Antioxidant nutrients and protection from free radicals. In: Kotsonis FN, Mackey M, Hjelle JJ (eds). Nutritional Toxicolgy. New York, Raven Press 1994; 19-48.

Brizek CL, Schlaff S, Pellegrini VA, Frank JB, Worrilow KC. Increased incidence of aberrant morphological phenotypes in human embryogenesis--an association with endometriosis. J Assist Reprod Genet 1995;12:106-12.

Bulun SE, Ping Yin YHC, Imir G, et al. Progesterone resistance in endometriosis: link to failure to metabolize estradiol. Mol Cell Endocrinol 2006;248:94–103.

Cahill DJ, Harlow CR, Wardle PG. Pre-ovulatory granulosa cells of infertile women with endometriosis are less sensitive to luteinizing hormone. Am J Reprod Immunol. 2003 Feb;49(2):66-9.

Calvin HI, Grosshans K, Blake EJ. Estimation and manipulation of glutathione levels in prepuberal mouse ovaries and ova: relevance to sperm nucleus transformation in the fertilized egg. Gamete Res 1986.

Campos Petean C, Ferriani RA, Dos Reis RM, Dias de Moura M, Jordao AA, Jr., Navarro PA. Lipid peroxidation and vitamin E in serum and follicular fluid of infertile women with peritoneal endometriosis submitted to controlled ovarian hyperstimulation: a pilot study. Fertil Steril 2008.

Carbone MC, Tatone C, Delle Monache S, Marci R, Caserta D, Colonna R et al. Antioxidant enzymatic defences in human follicular fluid: characterization and age-dependent changes. Mol Hum Reprod 2003;9:639-43.

Cetica PD, Pintos LN, Dalvit GC, Beconi MT. Antioxidant enzyme activity and oxidative stress in bovine oocyte in vitro maturation. IUBMB Life. 2001 Jan;51(1):57-64.

Chaube SK, Prasad PV, Thakur SC, et al. Hydrogen peroxide modulates meiotic cell cycle and induces morphological features characteristic of apoptosis in rat oocytes cultured in vitro. Apoptosis. 2005; 10(4):863–874.

Cheesman KL, Cheesman SD, Chatterton Jr RT, Cohen MR. Alterations in progesterone metabolism and luteal function in infertile women with endometriosis. Fertil Steril 1983;40(5):590–5.

Combelles CM, Carabatsos MJ, Kumar TR, Matzuk MM, Albertini DF. Hormonal control of somatic cell oocyte interactions during ovarian follicle development. Mol Reprod Dev. 2004 Nov;69(3):347-55.

Costa LO, Mendes MC, Ferriani RA, Moura MD, Reis RM, Silva de Sá MF. Estradiol and testosterone concentrations in follicular fluid as criteria to discriminate between mature and immature oocytes. Braz J Med Biol Res. 2004 Nov;37(11):1747-55. Epub 2004 Oct 26.

de Matos DG, Furnus CC, Moses DF. Glutathione synthesis during in vitro maturation of bovine oocytes: role of cumulus cells. Biol Reprod. 1997 Dec;57(6):1420-5.

de Matos DG, Furnus CC. The importance of having high glutathione (GSH) level after bovine in vitro maturation on embryo development effect of beta-mercaptoethanol, cysteine and cystine. Theriogenology. 2000 Feb;53(3):761-71.

De Santis L, Cino I, Rabellotti E, Calzi F, Persico P, Borini A et al. Polar body morphology and spindle imaging as predictors of oocyte quality. Reprod Biomed Online 2005;11:36-42.

Díaz I, Navarro J, Blasco L, et al. Impact of stage III-IV endometriosis on recipients of sibling oocytes: matched case-control study. Fertil Steril. 2000;74(1):31-4.

Erickson GF, Garzo VG, Magoffin DA. Insulin-like growth factor-I regulates aromatase activity in human granulosa and granulosa luteal cells. J Clin Endocrinol Metab. 1989 Oct;69(4):716-24.

Fernando S, Breheny S, Jaques AM, Halliday JL, Baker G, Healy D. Preterm birth, ovarian endometriomata, and assisted reproduction technologies. Fertil Steril 2008.

Ferreira EM, Vireque AA, Adona PR, Meirelles FV, Ferriani RA, Navarro PA. Cytoplasmic maturation of bovine oocytes: structural and biochemical modifications and acquisition of developmental competence. Theriogenology. 2009 Mar 15;71(5):836-48. Epub 2009 Jan 3. Review.

Földesi I, Breckwoldt M, Neulen J. Oestradiol production by luteinized human granulosa cells: evidence of the stimulatory action of recombinant human follicle stimulating hormone. Hum Reprod. 1998 Jun;13(6):1455-60.

Fujii J, Iuchi Y, Okada F. Fundamental roles of reactive oxygen species and protective mechanisms in the female reproductive system. Reprod Biol Endocrinol. 2005; 3:43.

Furger C, Cronier L, Poirot C, Pouchelet M. Human granulosa cells in culture exhibit functional cyclic AMP-regulated gap junctions. Mol Hum Reprod. 1996 Aug;2(8):541-8.

Furnus CC, de Matos DG, Moses DF. Cumulus expansion during in vitro maturation of bovine oocytes: relationship with intracellular glutathione level and its role on subsequent embryo development. Mol Reprod Dev. 1998 Sep;51(1):76-83

García-Velasco J, Arici A. Is endometrium or the oocyte/embryo affected in endometriosis? Hum Reprod. 1999; 14 (Suppl. 2):77-89.

Garrido N, Navarro J, Garcia-Velasco J, Remohi J, Pellice A, Simon C. The endometrium versus embryonic quality in endometriosis-related infertility. Hum Reprod Update 2002;8:95-103.

Garrido N, Navarro J, Remohi J, Simon C, Pellicer A. Follicular hormonal environment and embryo quality in women with endometriosis. Hum Reprod Update 2000;6:67-74.

Gomes FM, Navarro PA, de Abreu LG, Ferriani RA, dos Reis RM, de Moura MD. Effect of peritoneal fluid from patients with minimal/mild endometriosis on progesterone release by human granulosa-lutein cells obtained from infertile patients without endometriosis: a pilot study. Eur J Obstet Gynecol Reprod Biol. 2008;138(1):60-5.

González F, Rote NS, Minium J, Kirwan JP. Reactive oxygen species-induced oxidative stress in the development of insulin resistance and hyperandrogenism in polycystic ovary syndrome. J Clin Endocrinol Metab. 2006 Jan;91(1):336-40. Epub 2005 Oct 25.

Guérin P, El Mouatassim S, Ménézo Y. Oxidative stress and protection against reactive oxygen species in the pre-implantation embryo and its surroundings. Hum Reprod Update. 2001; 7(2):175-89.

Guet P, Royère D, Paris A, Lansac J, Driancourt MA. Aromatase activity of human granulosa cells in vitro: effects of gonadotrophins and follicular fluid. Hum Reprod. 1999 May;14(5):1182-9.

Gupta S, Agarwal A, Kraicir N, et al. Role of oxidative stress in endometriosis. Reprod Biomed Online. 2006; 13(1):126-34.

Halliwell B. Free radicals, antioxidants and human disease: curiosity, cause or consequence? Lancet. 1994; 344(8924):721-4.

Hamamah S, Matha V, Berthenet C, Anahory T, Loup V, Dechaud H, Hedon B, Fernandez A, Lamb N. Comparative protein expression profiling in human cumulus cells in relation to oocyte fertilization and ovarian stimulation protocol. Reprod Biomed Online. 2006;13(6):807-14.

Hamel M, Dufort I, Robert C, Gravel C, Leveille MC, Leader A, Sirard MA. Identification of differentially expressed markers in human follicular cells associated with competent oocytes. Hum Reprod. 2008;23(5):1118-27.

Hansen JC, Deguchi Y: Selenium and fertility in animals and man – a review. Acta Vet Scand 1996, 37:19-30.

Haouzi D, Hamamah S. Pertinence of Apoptosis Markers for the Improvement of In Vitro Fertilization (IVF). Curr Med Chem. 2009;16(15):1905-16.

Harlow CR, Cahill DJ, Maile LA, et al. Reduced preovulatory granulosa cell steroidogenesis in women with endometriosis. J Clin Endocrinol Metab 1996;81:426–9.

Ho YS, Magnenat JL, Bronson RT, Cao J, Gargano M, Sugawara M, Funk CD: Mice deficient in cellular glutathione peroxidase develop normally and show no increased sensitivity to hyperoxia. J Biol Chem 1997, 272:16644-16651.

Holtz G, Williamson HO, Mathur RS, Landgrebe SC, Moore EE. Luteinized unruptured follicle syndrome in mild endometriosis assessment with biochemical parameters. J Reprod Med 1985;30(9):643–5.

Hu Y, Betzendahl I, Cortvrindt R, Smitz J, Eichenlaub-Ritter U. Effects of low O2 and ageing on spindles and chromosomes in mouse oocytes from pre-antral follicle culture. Hum Reprod 2001;16:737-48.

Hutt KJ, Albertini DF. An oocentric view of folliculogenesis and embryogenesis. Reprod Biomed Online. 2007 Jun;14(6):758-64.

Jana SK, K NB, Chattopadhyay R, Chakravarty B, Chaudhury K. Upper control limit of reactive oxygen species in follicular fluid beyond which viable embryo formation is not favorable. Reprod Toxicol. 2010 Jul;29(4):447-51.

Jancar N, Kopitar AN, Ihan A, Virant Klun I, Bokal EV. Effect of apoptosis and reactive oxygen species production in human granulosa cells on oocyte fertilization and blastocyst development. J Assist Reprod Genet. 2007 Feb-Mar;24(2-3):91-7.

Jozwik M, Wolczynski S, Szamatowicz M. Oxidative stress markers in preovulatory follicular fluid in humans. Mol Hum Reprod 1999;5:409-13.

Katsoff B, Check JH, Davies E, Wilson C. Evaluation of the effect of endometriosis on oocyte quality and endometrial environment by comparison of donor and recipient outcomes following embryo transfer in a shared oocyte program. Clin Exp Obstet Gynecol. 2006; 33(4):201-2.

Kaya H, Oral B. Effect of ovarian involvement on the frequency of luteinized unruptured follicle in endometriosis. Gynecol Obstet Invest 1999;48(2):123–6.

Kim NH, Chung HM, Cha KY, Chung KS. Microtubule and microfilament organization in maturing human oocytes. Hum Reprod 1998;13:2217-22.

Kumbak B, Kahraman S, Karlikaya G, Lacin S, Guney A. In vitro fertilization in normoresponder patients with endometriomas: comparison with basal simple ovarian cysts. Gynecol Obstet Invest 2008;65:212-6.

LaPolt PS, Hong LS. Inhibitory effects of superoxide dismutase and cyclic guanosine 30,50-monophosphate on estrogen production in cultured rat granulosa cells. Endocrinology 1995;136:5533–9.

Liu L, Trimarchi JR, Navarro P, Blasco MA, Keefe DL. Oxidative stress contributes to arsenic-induced telomere attrition, chromosome instability, and apoptosis. J Biol Chem 2003;278:31998-2004.

Mandelbaum J, Anastasiou O, Levy R, Guerin JF, de Larouziere V, Antoine JM. Effects of cryopreservation on the meiotic spindle of human oocytes. Eur J Obstet Gynecol Reprod Biol 2004;113 Suppl 1:S17-23.

Mansour G, Abdelrazik H, Sharma RK, Radwan E, Falcone T, Agarwal A. L-carnitine supplementation reduces oocyte cytoskeleton damage and embryo apoptosis induced by incubation in peritoneal fluid from patients with endometriosis. Fertil Steril. 91(5 Suppl):2079-86, 2009

Matos L, Stevenson D, Gomes F, Silva-Carvalho JL, Almeida H. Superoxide dismutase expression in human cumulus oophorus cells Molecular Human Reproduction, Vol.15, No.7 pp. 411–419, 2009

Meister A. Selective modification of glutathione metabolism. Science 1983; 220:472-477.

Murphy AA, Santanam N, Parthasarathy S. Endometriosis: A disease of oxidative stress? Semin Reprod Endocrinol. 1998; 16(4):263-73.

Murray AA, Molinek MD, Baker SJ, Kojima FN, Smith MF, Hillier SG, et al. Role of ascorbic acid in promoting follicle integrity and survival in intact mouse ovarian follicles in vitro. Reproduction 2001;121:89–96.

Navarro PA, Liu L, Ferriani RA, Keefe DL. Arsenite induces aberrations in meiosis that can be prevented by coadministration of N-acetylcysteine in mice. Fertil Steril 2006;85 Suppl 1:1187-94.

Navarro PA, Liu L, Keefe DL. In vivo effects of arsenite on meiosis, preimplantation development, and apoptosis in the mouse. Biol Reprod. 2004; 70(4):980-5.

Navarro PA, Liu L, Trimarchi JR, et al. Noninvasive imaging of spindle dynamics during mammalian oocyte activation. Fertil Steril. 2005; 83(Suppl 1):1197-205.

Paszkowski T, Traub AI, Robinson SY, McMaster D: Selenium dependent glutathione peroxidase activity in human follicular fluid. Clin Chim Acta 1995, 236:173-180).

Pellicer A, Navarro J, Bosch E, Garrido N, Garcia-Velasco JA, Remohí J, Simón C. Endometrial quality in infertile women with endometriosis. Ann N Y Acad Sci. 2001 Sep;943:122-30. Review.

Pellicer A, Oliveira N, Ruiz A, Remohi J, Simon C. Exploring the mechanism(s) of endometriosis-related infertility: an analysis of embryo development and implantation in assisted reproduction. Hum Reprod 1995;10 Suppl 2:91-7.

Pellicer A, Valbuena D, Bauset C, et al. The follicular environment in stimulated cycles of women with endometriosis: esteroid levels and embryo quality. Fertil Steril 1998;69:1135–41.

Perreault SD, Barbee RR, Slott VI. Importance of glutathione in the acquisition and maintenance of sperm nuclear decondensing activity in maturing hamster oocytes. . Dev Biol. 1988 Jan;125(1):181-6.

Perreault SD, Wolff RA, Zirkin BR. The role of disulfide bond reduction during mammalian sperm nuclear decondensation in vivo. Dev Biol. 1984 Jan;101(1):160-7.

Revised American Society for Reproductive Medicine classification of endometriosis: 1996. Fertil Steril. 1997 May;67(5):817-21. [No authors listed]

Sabatini L, Wilson C, Lower A, Al-Shawaf T, Grudzinskas JG Superoxide dismutase activity in human follicular fluid after controlled ovarian hyperstimulation in women undergoing in vitro fertilization. Fertil Steril 1999, 72:1027-1034.].

Saracoglu OF, Aksel S, Yeoman RR,Wiebe RH. Endometrial estradiol and progesterone receptors in patients with luteal phase defects and endometriosis. Fertil Steril 1985;43(6):851–5.

Seino T, Saito H, Kaneko T, Takahashi T, Kawachiya S, Kurachi H. Eight-hydroxy-2'-deoxyguanosine in granulosa cells is correlated with the quality of oocytes and embryos in an in vitro fertilization-embryo transfer program. Fertil Steril. 2002 Jun;77(6):1184-90.

Silva AL, Abreu LG, Rosa-e-Silva AC, Ferriani RA, Silva-de-Sá MF. Leuprolide acetate reduces both in vivo and in vitro ovarian steroidogenesis in infertile women undergoing assisted reproduction. Steroids. 2008 Dec 22;73(14):1475-84. Epub 2008 Aug 26.

Speroff L, Fritz MA. Regulation of the Menstrual Cycle. In: Speroff L & Fritz MA. Clinical Gynecologic Endocrinology and Infertility. 7 ed. Baltimore: Lippincott Williams & Wilkins p. 187-231: 2005.

Szczepanska M, Kozlik J, Skrzypczak J, et al. Oxidative stress may be a piece in the endometriosis puzzle. Fertil Steril. 2003; 79(6):1288-93.

Tanghe S, Van Soom A, Nauwynck H, Coryn M, de Kruif A. Minireview: Functions of the cumulus oophorus during oocyte maturation, ovulation, and fertilization. Mol Reprod Dev. 2002 Mar;61(3):414-24.

Tatemoto H, Sakurai N, Muto N. Protection of porcine oocytes against apoptotic cell death caused by oxidative stress during In vitro maturation: role of cumulus cells. Biol Reprod. 2000 Sep;63(3):805-10.

Tesfaye D, Ghanem N, Carter F, Fair T, Sirard MA, Hoelker M, Schellander K, Lonergan P Gene expression profile of cumulus cells derived from cumulus-oocyte complexes matured either in vivo or in vitro. Reprod Fertil Dev. 2009;21(3):451-61.

Tetsuka M, Hillier SG. Differential regulation of aromatase and androgen receptor in granulosa cells. J Steroid Biochem Mol Biol. 1997 Apr;61(3-6):233-9.

Thomas FH, Vanderhyden BC. Oocyte-granulosa cell interactions during mouse follicular development: regulation of kit ligand expression and its role in oocyte growth. Reprod Biol Endocrinol. 2006 Apr 12;4:19.

Tsai-Turton M, Luderer U. Opposing effects of glutathione depletion and follicle-stimulating hormone on reactive oxygen species and apoptosis in cultured preovulatory rat follicles. Endocrinology 2006;147:1224–36.

Van Blerkom J, Davis P. Differential effects of repeated ovarian stimulation on cytoplasmic and spindle organization in metaphase II mouse oocytes matured in vivo and in vitro. Hum Reprod 2001;16:757-64.

Van Kaam KJ, Romano A, Schouten JP, Dunselman GA, Groothuis PG. Progesterone receptor polymorphism +331G/A is associated with a decreased risk of deep infiltrating endometriosis. Hum Reprod 2007;22(1):129–35.

Van Langendonckt A, Casanas-Roux F, Donnez J. Oxidative stress and peritoneal endometriosis. Fertil Steril. 2002; 77(5):861-70.

Verit FF, Erel O, Kocyigit A, Association of increased total antioxidant capacity and anovulation in nonobese infertile patients with clomiphene citrate–resistant polycystic

Volarcik K, Sheean L, Goldfarb J, Woods L, Abdul-Karim FW, Hunt P. The meiotic competence of in-vitro matured human oocytes is influenced by donor age: evidence that folliculogenesis is compromised in the reproductively aged ovary. Hum Reprod 1998;13:154-60.

Wang WH, Keefe DL. Prediction of chromosome misalignment among in vitro matured human oocytes by spindle imaging with the PolScope. Fertil Steril 2002;78:1077-81.

Wardle PG, Mitchell JD, McLaughlin EA, Ray BD, McDermott A, Hull MG. Endometriosis and ovulatory disorder: reduced fertilization in vitro compared with tubal and unexplained infertility. Lancet 1985; 2(8449):236-9.

Yoshida M, Ishigaki K, Pursel VG. Effect of maturation media on male pronucleus formation in pig oocytes matured in vitro. Mol Reprod Dev 1992; 31:68-71.

Yoshida M. Role of glutathione in the maturation and fertilization ofpig oocytes in vitro. Mol Reprod Dev 1993; 35:76-81.

Section 4

Diagnosis and Treatment

23

Current Insights and Future Advances in Endometriosis Diagnostics

Michele Cioffi and Maria Teresa Vietri
*Department of General Pathology,
Faculty of Medicine and Surgery of Second University of Naples, Naples,
Italy*

1. Introduction

Endometriosis is a benign gynaecological disease characterized by the presence of endometrial glands and stroma outside the uterine cavity. This condition is mainly found in women of reproductive age, from all ethnic and social groups and it is associated with pelvic pain and infertility. Endometriosis is typically present in the pelvis such as on the ovaries and pelvic peritoneum, but may also involve the bowel, ureter or bladder. It regresses after menopause or ovariectomy, suggesting it could depend on the production and metabolism of sex steroids: high concentrations of estrogens were found in the endometriotic lesions, which grow and regress in an oestrogen-dependent way. Nevertheless, the pathogenesis and the molecular mechanism that underlie the development of endometriosis have troubled the investigators through many years, remaining an enigma. The disease is widely accepted to result from the ectopic implantation of refluxed menstrual tissues. In addition, immunologic changes, environmental, hormonal and genetic factors contribute to the multifactorial etiology of endometriosis.

Many studies are therefore focusing on identifying markers for the diagnosis and follow-up of endometriosis. Although the "gold standard" for the diagnosis of endometriosis is the laparoscopy, many reports have suggested that various serum, peritoneal fluid and tissue markers might be associated with endometriosis. In fact, the identification of more sensitive and specific markers of endometriosis should facilitate the development of accurate and non-invasive techniques for diagnosis and prognosis (Table 1). Furthermore, the inheritable susceptibility to endometriosis justifies the growing interest in identifying genes and/or genetic polymorphisms that could lead to an increased risk of disease. Identifying these polymorphisms may open to their use as genetic biomarkers of endometriosis.

Over the last 20 years, several proteomics technologies have been used to research novel proteins with a potential etiological role in endometriosis, and to identify candidate serum markers for this condition. While some molecules identified by proteomics technologies may have a relevant role in the pathogenesis of endometriosis, the research of potential serum markers for this condition is still far from any clinical application.

The early diagnosis of endometriosis could prevent the possible progression of endometriosis, resulting in more pain, infertility and in a declining quality of life.

For a clinical purpose, the identification of highly sensitive and specific diagnostic test of endometriosis should facilitate the development of accurate and non-invasive test diagnosis and prognosis.

PERITONEAL FLUID AND/OR SERUM MARKERS	Glycoproteins Growth factors Cytokines Autoantibodies Hormones Proteolytic enzymes and their inhibitors Soluble adhesion molecules Environmental contaminant
ENDOMETRIAL MARKERS	Cell adhesion molecules (CAMs) Proteolytic enzymes
ENDOMETRIAL TISSUE BIOCHEMICAL MARKERS	Aromatase P450 Hormone receptors
GENETIC MARKERS	Survivin gene expression p53 mutations Polymorphisms

Table 1. Markers for endometriosis

2. Peritoneal fluid and/or serum markers

Many serum and peritoneal fluid markers can be used to discriminate between patients with or without endometriosis (Table 2). Using markers with a high degree of sensitivity and specificity for endometriosis it is possible the development of peritoneal fluid and /or serum based diagnostics tools, therapeutic strategies and prognosis markers.

GLYCOPROTEINS	CA125 CA19-9
GROWTH FACTORS	Hepatocyte growth factor (SF/HGF) Fibroblast growth factor (FGF) Epidermal growth factor (EGF) Transforming growth factor-alpha (TGF-α) Transforming growth factor-beta (TGF-β) Vascular endothelial growth factor (VEGF) Epidermal growth factor receptor (EGF-R) Insulin-like growth factor I (IGF-I)
CYTOKINES	TNF-α IL-1 IL-6 IL-8 Monocyte chemoattractant protein (MCP)-1 Interferon-γ

Table 2. Peritoneal fluid (PF) and/or serum markers for endometriosis

AUTOANTIBODIES	Antiendometrial antibodies Autoantibodies to oxidized lipoproteins Thyroid peroxidase antibodies IgG anti-laminin-1 antibodies Anti-phospholipid antibodies
HORMONES	Luteinizing hormone (LH) Progesterone Estradiol Thyroid stimulating hormone (TSH) Follicle stimulating hormone (FSH) Leptin
PROTEOLYTIC ENZYMES AND THEIR INHIBITORS	Matrix metalloproteinases (MMPs) Tissue inhibitors for MMPs (TIMPs)
SOLUBLE ADHESION MOLECULES	Intercellular adhesions molecule-1 (sICAM-1) Human leukocyte class I antigens (sHLA-I) E-cadherin
ENVIRONMENTAL CONTAMINAT	Dioxin-like chemicals

Table 2. Peritoneal fluid (PF) and/or serum markers for endometriosis. (Continuation)

2.1 Glycoproteins

Some serum glycoproteins, more commonly known for its use in the diagnosis or monitoring of cancers, might also serve as a marker for endometriosis, although levels are usually elevated only in advanced stages and are therefore not suitable for routine screening.

2.1.1 CA125

CA125 is a 200,000 Da glycoprotein expressed on the surface of the coelomic epithelium, including the epithelium of the endocervix, endometrium, fallopian tube, pelvic peritoneum and placental tissues. Serum CA125 levels increase in patients with malignant and benign gynaecologic diseases, including endometriosis.

Despite the most important clinical use of CA125 is the monitoring of patients with ovarian cancer, high levels can be found in women with endometriosis. Many studies have assessed the role of CA125 serum levels in women affected with endometriosis. The sensitivity and specificity of serum CA125 assay varies with the stage of disease. Usually, high CA125 serum levels can be found both in most patients with advanced endometriosis and in few patients with early-stage disease. Therefore, the routine use of serum CA125 cannot be used as a diagnostic tool for endometriosis. Serum CA125 may be more useful in evaluating recurrent disease or the outcome of a surgical treatment. CA125 levels may also be useful in patients with advanced endometriosis and several studies have suggested the use of this marker in the preoperative diagnosis of endometriosis.

The patients with endometriosis often undergo repeated laparoscopic examinations to assess the progress during and after therapy or to determine the recurrence of disease. Therefore, CA125 may be useful in the management of endometriosis and some authors suggest its assessment in women with suspected endometriosis, in association with laparoscopy and biopsy. In addition, in literature was reported that measurement of serum CA125 levels might be useful in identifying patients with infertility that may have severe endometriosis and could benefit from early surgical treatment.

CA125 levels were assessed in the PF of patients with and without endometriosis. Although levels of CA125 in the PF were almost 10 times higher than serum levels, no differences were found between women with and without endometriosis. In addition, CA125 levels are measured also in other body fluids, such as menstrual discharge and the uterine fluid, but are not useful in clinical practice.

2.1.2 CA19-9

CA19-9 is a high-molecular-weight glycoprotein that was initially thought to be an oncofetal antigen. Serum CA19-9 levels were elevated in patients with some malignant tumour, such as gastrointestinal adenocarcinoma, pancreatic carcinoma, or lung carcinoma; thus, the measurement of serum CA19-9 levels is useful in the diagnosis of these tumours. In gynaecology, the serum CA19-9 levels are elevated in patients with malignant and benign ovarian tumours. Furthermore, a case of an ovarian chocolate cyst with a markedly elevated serum CA19-9 level has been reported. In addition, it has been reported that serum CA19-9 levels in women with endometriosis are significantly reduced during therapy compared with the basal levels before treatment. Serum CA19-9 levels in patients with endometriosis are significantly higher than those in patients without endometriosis and that serum CA19-9 levels increase in accordance with the advancement of the clinical stage of endometriosis. CA19-9 was also detected in the endometrial glandular epithelium in ovarian chocolate cysts by immunohistochemistry. These results reveal that the measurement of the serum CA19-9 levels, as well as the serum CA125 level, may prove to be a valuable tool for predicting the severity of endometriosis as diagnosed by laparoscopy.

2.2 Growth factors

The endometrium in endometriosis behaves like tumorous tissue and the growth factors involved in tumour proliferation, angiogenesis and invasiveness have been investigated for their expression in endometriosis. Indeed, the degree of endometriosis is positively correlated with the concentration in peritoneal fluid and serum of *Hepatocyte Growth Factor/Scatter Factor (HGF/SF)*, a multifunctional polypeptide that has been implicated in embryo development, tissue repair, and cancer growth, produced mainly by mesenchymal cells with activity mediated through the c-met receptor found principally on epithelial and endothelial cells (Zong et al., 2003).

Inflammatory macrophages and the inflammatory mediators they release could be related to the ectopic implantation of endometriosis: *Fibroblast Growth Factor (FGF), Epidermal Growth Factor (EGF), Transforming Growth Factor-alpha (TGF-α), Transforming Growth Factor-beta (TGF-β) and Tumor Necrosis Factor-alpha (TNF- α)*. It is been shown that these growth factors stimulate in vitro proliferation of endometrial stromal cells, suggesting that they could improve the implantation of endometrial cells.

Elevated serum levels of *Epidermal Growth Factor Receptor (EGF-R)*, involved in angiogenesis, suggest an active role for EGF in the development of endometriosis (Matalliotakis et al., 2003a, 2003b).

Insulin-like Growth Factor I (IGF-I) serum levels in patients with early stage endometriosis, and in healthy control, were significantly lower than the levels in patients with late stage endometriosis, suggesting that IGF-I is an important mediator in the development and/or maintenance of endometriosis or progression to late stage disease (Gurgan et al., 1999).

Many studies report that angiogenesis is probably involved in the pathogenesis of endometriosis. *Vascular endothelial growth factor (VEGF)*, also known as vascular permeability factor, is one of the most potent and specific angiogenic factors. VEGF has emerged as an important regulator of normal angiogenesis and pathological neovascularisation.

VEGF levels in both peritoneal fluid and serum were higher in women with endometriosis compared with controls. The cellular source of VEGF in peritoneal fluid has not yet been precisely defined. Some evidence suggests that the endometriotic lesions themselves produce this factor and that the activated peritoneal macrophages are able to synthesize and secrete VEGF (Matalliotakis et al., 2003a, 2003b).

2.3 Immunological markers

The immune system plays an important role in the pathogenesis of endometriosis, which begins, therefore, to be treated as an autoimmune disease. T-helper, T-suppressor and natural killer (NK) cells concentrations are altered in serum and peritoneal fluid of patients with endometriosis (Lebovic et al., 2001; Nothnick, 2001). In addition, IgG and IgA anti-endometrial antibodies have been detected in the sera and vaginal and cervical secretions of endometriosis patients. The presence of anti-phospholipids and anti-histones antibodies has been documented by some authors and questioned by others. These observations would believe that markers of immune reactivity, particularly cytokines, might be used as a diagnostic aid for endometriosis.

2.3.1 Cytokines

Macrophages are a major source of many cytokines involved in immune response, haematopoiesis, inflammation and many other homeostatic processes. Upon stimulation by microorganisms, microbial products or endogenous factors including cytokines, macrophages can *de novo* synthesize and release a large variety of cytokines (i.e. IL-1, IL-1ra, IL-6, IL-8, IL-10, IL-12, TNF-α, IFN-α, IFN-γ, MCP-1, MCP-3, MIF, M-CSF, G-CSF, GM-CSF, MIP-1, MIP-2, LIF, OSM, TGF-β). Some cytokines can up-regulate the production of cytokines by macrophages (IL-3, GM-CSF, IFN-γ) while others can inhibit it (IL-4, IL-10, IL-13, TGF-β). In addition, these cytokines can modulate most of the macrophage functions and cell surface marker expression. Other cytokines (chemokines such as MCP-1, 2, 3, MIP-1,2 and RANTES) contribute to the recruitment of circulating monocytes within tissues.

T lymphocytes are important regulatory cells that secrete several cytokines and participate actively in this inflammatory response. According to the pattern of cytokines secreted, the immune response is classified as cytotoxic or type 1 (IFN-γ, IL-2, IL-12) and humoral or type 2 (IL-4, IL-5, IL-10 and IL-13) (Barcelò et al., 2006).

The role of cytokines and growth factors in the pathophysiology of endometriosis is evident. They are probably responsible for the proliferation of endometrial cells and implantation of endometrial cells or tissue. In addition, cytokines increase the tissue remodelling through their influence on matrix metalloproteinases. Probably the most important effect of cytokines on ectopic endometrial tissue is an increase in angiogenesis of ectopic endometrial tissue and neovascularisation of the affected region. Therefore, cytokines play an important role in the initiation, propagation and regulation of immune and inflammation responses. The activation of immune cells results in a burst and cascade of inflammatory cytokines.

ELISA kits are available to assess the cytokines in the serum and peritoneal fluid (PF) of endometriosis patients. PF is rich with variable cellular components including macrophages, mesothelial cells, lymphocytes, eosinophils and mastcells. Approximately 85% of PF leukocytes are macrophages. It has been hypothesized that peritoneal macrophage activation is a key step in disease initiation and progression. Activated macrophages in the peritoneal cavity of women with endometriosis are potent producers of cytokines (Bedaiwy et al., 2002). Thus, PF contains a rich mixture of cytokines. Cytokines, such as TNF-α, IL-1, IL-6, IL-8, monocyte chemoattractant protein (MCP)-1 and IFN-γ, are elevated in the PF of women with endometriosis, suggesting that they are involved in the progression of the disease. The level of IL-1 in PF is positively correlated with the progression of endometriosis, but the serum level of IL-1 seems to have no correlation with endometriosis.

The Tumor Necrosis Factors (TNF) superfamily of cytokines represents a multifunctional group proinflammatory cytokines, which activate signalling pathways for cell survival, apoptosis, inflammatory responses, and cellular differentiation. Induction of cellular responses to TNF occurs through two receptors, TNFR1 (TNF Receptor-1 or CD120a) and TNFR2 (TNF Receptor-2 or CD120b). TNFR1 is activated in most human tissues by the binding of TNFα. On the other hand, TNFR2 is primarily expressed in immune cells and is activated by both TNFα and TNFβ (Kawasaki et al., 2002).

The main TNF is TNF-α, which is produced by neutrophils, activated lymphocytes, macrophages, NK cells and several non-hematopoietic cells. The TNF-α is involved in the normal physiology of the endometrial proliferation in the human endometrium. TNF-α is expressed predominantly in epithelial cells, especially in the secretory phase. The stromal cells stain for TNF-α mostly in the proliferative phase of the menstrual cycle. These data suggest that hormones influence the role of this cytokine.

Some reports found that concentrations of TNF-α in both serum and PF were very high at the early stage of the disease and decreased with the severity of the endometriosis. Moreover, the assessment of TNF-α levels in the PF can be used as a basis for non-surgical diagnosis of endometriosis.

The role of IL-6 in the pathogenesis of endometriosis has been widely studied. IL-6 is a regulator of inflammation and immunity, which may represent a physiological link between the endocrine and immune systems. IL-6 also modulates the secretion of other cytokines, promotes T-cell activation, differentiation of B cells and inhibits the growth of several human cell lines (Nothnick, 2001).

The data about IL-6 levels in the PF of patients with endometriosis are controversial. In fact, no statistically significant differences are reported between controls and endometriosis patients. In contrast, serum levels of IL-6 were significantly higher in women with endometriosis than in controls and the highest levels were found in women with chocolate cysts (Wieser et al., 2003; Iwabe et al., 2003).

2.3.2 Autoantibodies

Endometriosis is supposed to be an autoimmune disorder and many autoantibodies have been proposed as a diagnostic test. A variety of autoantibodies have been detected in endometriosis patients (thyroid peroxidase antibody, IgG anti-laminin-1 antibodies, anti-phospholipid antibodies and the novel anti-PDIK1L antibodies). The most commonly reported types are antiendometrial antibodies, autoantibodies against the oxidative-stress-induced, antigens to malondialdehyde-modified low-density lipoprotein (LDL) and oxidized low-density lipoprotein (Ox-LDL).

Some investigators have hypothesized that antiendometrial antibodies may cause infertility in some women with endometriosis by preventing the fertilized embryo from implanting in the uterus. In addition, increasing evidence suggests that oxidative stress occurs in the PF of women with endometriosis and oxidatively modified lipoproteins were found in the PF.

2.4 Hormones

Serum and PF hormones levels vary in patients affected with endometriosis. Luteinizing hormone (LH) levels are significantly higher in both serum and PF in patients with endometriosis than in normal controls (Illera et al., 2001). However, levels of prolactin, thyroid stimulating hormone (TSH) and follicle stimulating hormone (FSH) in the serum were no different between the different groups.

Recently it was reported that serum concentrations of leptin are increased in patients with endometriosis. This increase may play an anti-apoptotic role in activated endometrial stromal cells into the peritoneal cavity, stimulating endometrial cell implantation and cause infertility (Tanaka et al., 2003). Furthermore another study measured the serum concentration of leptin using a radioimmunoassay method, showing a significant association between leptin concentrations and stage of endometriosis (Viganò et al., 2002).

2.5 Proteolytic enzymes and their inhibitors

The physiological changes in endometriosis involve multiple steps of matrix remodelling. Endometriosis associated to abnormal matrix remodelling is affected by several molecular factors including proteolytic enzymes and their inhibitors, which mediate tissue turnover, and ovarian steroids, which normally regulate reconstruction of endometrium in the menstrual cycle.

The extracellular matrix (ECM) constitutes a well-organized network structure that surrounds the cells. The tissue remodelling involving ECM turnover is regulated by the pooled action of proteolytic enzymes, matrix metalloproteinases (MMP) and tissue inhibitors for MMP (TIMP). The inappropriate expression of MMP and TIMP is associated with tumorigenesis and metastasis, as well as with endometriosis.

Several MMP have been implicated in the development of endometriosis (Sillem et al., 2001). The levels of MMP and TIMP in patients with endometriosis are different depending on the method of measurement and collection of samples of different tissues at different stages of endometriosis. The values of TIMP-1 is determined by radioimmunoassay measurement in serum of patients with PF in endometriosis are lower than in controls. In contrast, the concentration of TIMP-1 was restored after treatment with gonadotropin releasing hormone. Another study reported that there was no significant difference in levels of cathepsin D, a proteolytic enzyme thought to promote digestion of ECM proteins in endometriosis, in serum from women with and without endometriosis.

2.6 Soluble adhesion molecules

It is thought that the retrograde flow of the menstrual debris to the peritoneal cavity plays an important role in the origin of endometriosis but the mechanism of endometrial cells implantation remains unknown. Recently many studies have reported the importance of adhesion molecules in this process.

Several adhesion molecules (CAM) are expressed in the human endometrium: i.e. integrins, cadherins and immunoglobulin superfamilies. These adhesion molecules show cyclical changes during the menstrual cycle. The major cell surface receptors of the ECM are the *integrins* that contain large (α) and small (β) subunits.

β1-integrins are known to mediate the interaction between the cell-cell and cell-extracellular matrices and are represented by very late activation (VLA) antigen molecules. It is well known that endometriosis is frequently associated with immunological abnormalities. However, only a few studies have been conducted on the adhesion molecules, particularly on β 1-integrins, in endometriosis. It has reported that integrins are expressed in the endometrium in endometriosis. The ability of endometriotic tissues to express integrins may explain the high recurrence rates in patients with endometriosis, as these samples retain their adhesion potency after retrograde menstruation and are thus able to establish cell-cell and cell-matrix interactions with the surrounding peritoneum.

The soluble forms of the *intercellular-adhesion molecule-1 (sICAM-1)* are secreted from the endometrium and endometriotic implants. Moreover, endometrium from women with endometriosis secretes a higher amount of this molecule than tissue from women without the disease. Consequently, a strong correlation exists between levels of sICAM-1 and the number of endometriotic implants in the pelvis. Therefore, it has been hypothesized that sICAM-1 may be useful in the diagnosis of endometriosis (Leng et al., 2002). Many investigators have reported a significant increase in serum concentration of sICAM-1 in patients with endometriosis. The sICAM-1 concentrations were higher in patients with stage I–II endometriosis, suggesting that studies on these soluble adhesion molecules can help clarify the pathogenic mechanisms of endometriosis. Elevated ICAM-1 levels were found in patients with severe endometriosis, but its sensitivity is not high and the concomitant use of the CA125 marker increases the sensitivity and specificity of detection (Somigliana et al., 2002).

The **E-cadherin** mediates cell-cell interaction and cells adhere preferentially to cells that express the same cadherin. Cadherins are distributed widely among animals and play a potentially significant role in morphogenetic events during embryogenesis. Cadherin is also expressed in the cell-to-cell boundaries of the endometrium. It is reported that E-cadherin expression on the endometrium was higher in the secretory phase than in the proliferative phase, although there is one report that the expression was unchanged during the cycle. Furthermore, the level of E-cadherin in serum of endometriosis patients was significantly higher than that of control group.

The level of E-cadherin in the serum of both III stage and IV stage endometriosis patients was higher than that of I and II stage patients. However, the difference between them was not statistically significant. E-cadherin may play a role on the morbidity of endometriosis and the serum E-cadherin assay might be helpful as a serum marker for the diagnosis and management of endometriosis (Fu & Lang, 2002).

2.7 Environmental contaminant

Environmental toxins, such as dioxins and polychlorinated biphenyls are some of the factors that have been suggested to play a significant role in the development of endometriosis. In fact, detection of environmental contaminant residues in serum and ovarian follicular fluid confirms this hypothesis. Dioxin-like chemicals, such as 2,3,7,8-tetrachlorodibenzo-p-dioxin (TCDD) and polyhalogenated aromatic hydrocarbons (PHAHs), may exert effects on the pathophysiology of endometriosis through a number of pathways: (1) activation of pro-carcinogens; (2) altered synthesis and metabolism of estradiol; (3) altered production of pro-inflammatory growth factors or cytokines and (4) alterations in tissue remodelling processes.

Exposure to HAHs and TCDD seems to be associated with a dose-dependent increase in the incidence and severity of endometriosis. TCDD may target peripheral blood and peritoneal and endometrial leukocyte populations inducing chronic expression of TNF-α and other inflammatory mediators resulting in increased adhesion, vascularization and proliferation of endometriotic cells. It has been suggested that an elevated concentration of TNF-a might participate in TCDD-mediated toxicity and contribute to the pathogenesis of endometriosis.

Dioxins may affect the expression of TNF-α via the induction of an inflammatory cytokine network, since the region of DNA that recognize the ligand-activated AhR, the dioxin-response element of DRE, is present in the genes of potent inducers of TNF-α including IL-1b, IL-6 and IFN-γ (Rier & Foster, 2003).

3. Endometrial markers

The adhesion of endometrial cells to the extracellular matrix (ECM) would be expected to play a central role in the pathogenesis of endometriosis. Various cell adhesion molecules (CAMs) have been investigated for their expression in endometriotic endometrium. Each cell type expresses a distinct pattern of integrins and other CAMs, including the cadherins, selectins and members of the immunoglobulin family that determines cell shape, maintains cell position and polarity and affects hormonal responsiveness. In addition, apoptosis might be mediated through loss of appropriate signals from the ECM through alternations in the integrin expression. Based on cell adhesion and the genes involving in adhesion and invasion aspects, cell adhesion molecules (CaMs) and proteolytic enzymes were investigated for their mechanisms in association with the progression of endometriosis.

4. Endometrial tissue biochemical markers

4.1 Aromatase P450

Aromatase P450 is the key enzyme for biosynthesis of oestrogen, which is an essential hormone for the establishment and growth of endometriosis. There is no detectable aromatase enzyme activity in normal endometrium; therefore, oestrogen is not locally produced in endometrium. Endometriosis tissue, however, contains very high levels of aromatase enzyme, which leads to production of significant quantities of oestrogen (Dheenadayalu et al., 2002). Moreover, one of the best-known mediators of inflammation and pain, prostaglandin E2 (PGE2), was found to be the most potent known inducer of aromatase activity in endometriotic stromal cells. The clinical significance of local aromatase activity that is induced strikingly by PGE2 in endometriotic tissue was exemplified recently by the successful use of an aromatase inhibitor to treat an unusually aggressive case of recurrent postmenopausal endometriosis that was resistant to any other surgical or hormonal modalities of treatment. Therefore, the aberrant expression of aromatase P450 in endometriotic tissue, in contrast to eutopic endometrium, justifies the local biosynthesis of estrogen that promotes the growth of these lesions and possibly mediates the resistance to conventional hormonal treatments, which is observed in a number of women with endometriosis. The molecular mechanisms that are responsible for aberrant aromatase P450 expression may provide insights into the etiology of endometriosis and lead to identification of molecular targets for the development of novel treatment strategies. Although endometrial aromatase P450 expression does not correlate with the disease stage, a recent study demonstrated that detection of aromatase P450 transcripts in the endometrium of endometriosis patients might be a potential qualitative marker of endometriosis.

4.2 Hormone receptors

The expression of receptors for the ovarian steroid hormones oestrogen and progesterone was studied immunohisto-chemically using monoclonal antibodies. The quantification of these receptors in the endometrium could be potentially useful in screening for this disease.

The eutopic endometrium of patients with endometriosis is different from endometrium of fertile controls regarding apoptosis, cytokines and other characteristics. Although cyclic changes were also detected in ectopic endometrium, different patterns of receptor expression suggested a difference in hormonal regulation between the two sites.

The concentrations of steroid receptors in ectopic endometrium increased gradually as the cycle progressed. Compared with eutopic endometrium, oestrogen and progesterone receptor concentrations were significantly lower in the proliferative phase, similar in the early secretory phase and significantly higher in the late secretory phase. The different patterns of receptor expression suggested different hormonal regulations between eutopic and ectopic endometrium.

There are two isoforms for oestrogen (ER) and progesterone (PR) receptors-ER-α and ER-β, PRA and PR-B. These isoforms exist in the endometrium and their function and content are different from one another. The different concentrations and biological activity of steroid receptor isoforms might lead to various hormonal responsiveness of ectopic endometrium. High concentrations of ER and PR in the ectopic endometrium during the secretory phase could explain the high proliferative activity of endometriotic tissue in this phase. Conversely, a decrease in ER and PR expression in ectopic implants during the secretory phase might lead to diminished proliferation. The expression of oestrogen and progesterone receptors may be regarded as an index of differentiation of the endometriotic implant. Consequently, ER and PR receptors may be used as markers of the activity of all subtypes of endometriotic lesions.

5. Genetic markers

Several genetic abnormalities or mutations have been suggested that might be related to endometriosis. Many technological approaches can help identify possible genetic markers of endometriosis. A number of technologies have emerged to facilitate progress in this direction (Taylor et al., 2002). Gene based technologies includes subtractive cDNA hybridization and cDNA microarray techniques.

5.1 Survivin gene expression

In endometriotic lesions, although derived from normal endometrium, decreased expression of adhesion molecules and increased expression of proteolytic enzymes may contribute to establishment of endometrial glands and stroma at ectopic sites, likely as behaviour of cancer cells. Normal epithelial cells undergo apoptosis when they separate from their primary tissue. However, spontaneous apoptosis of ectopic endometrial tissue is impaired in women with endometriosis, and its decreased susceptibility to apoptosis might participate in the growth, survival, and invasion of endometriotic tissue. Although there have been some reports on the induction of apoptosis in endometriotic lesions, there is no consensus on the mechanism of escape from apoptosis in endometriosis, and little is known on the correlation between survival activity and invasive phenotype in endometriotic cells. Among the regulators of cell death, inhibitor of apoptosis (IAP) proteins has recently emerged as modulators of an evolutionarily conserved step in apoptosis, which may potentially involve the direct inhibition of terminal effector caspases 3 and 7.

Survivin is a novel inhibitor of apoptosis and is expressed during fetal development and in cancer tissues, but its expression has not been reported in normal adult tissues or benign diseases. Survivin gene and protein expression was detected in normal human endometrium and that survivin could play an important role in physiological homeostasis during the normal menstrual cycle (Konno et al., 2000). The survivin is also expressed in ectopic endometriotic tissue; however, there has been no report on the biological significance of survivin in endometriosis, an aggressive tumour-like benign disease.

5.2 p53 mutations

Genomic alterations may represent important events in the development of endometriosis. Tumour suppressor genes play a role in the regulation of cell growth and prevention of carcinogenesis. The altered tumour suppressor genes might be related with the development of endometriosis. p53, a representative tumour suppressor, is involved in cell proliferation and progression of various tumour types (Akahane et al., 2007).

High frequency of p53 locus deletion was observed in the endometriosis specimens (Bischoff et al., 2002). The p53 protein abnormalities and chromosomal aberrations may be involved in malignant transformation of ovarian endometriosis (Mhawech et al., 2002). In contrast, some investigators have demonstrated the undetectable expression of p53 in the endometriosis specimens.

Although the real role of p53 polymorphism has not been clarified, it deserves more attentions in the study of endometriosis and the development of gene therapy. However, the real roles of these p53 gene polymorphisms upon endometriosis remain to be clarified. Lager cohort recruitment is request for its further clarification. After the elucidation of these issues, some tumour suppressor gene polymorphisms might become useful markers to predict the future development of endometriosis as well as the development and intervention of genetic therapy.

5.3 Polymorphisms

Some genetic polymorphisms, involved in sex steroids biosynthesis and metabolism, may be reasonably associated with an increased risk of endometriosis. Specific genes with polymorphisms have been investigated for an association with endometriosis. Some association studies implicated GALT (a gene involved in galactose metabolism) and GSTM1 and NAT2 (genes encoding for the detoxification enzymes) as possible disease susceptibility genes. Recent finding have added to the evidence for the involvement of GSTM1 and NAT2, but have cast doubt on the role of GALT. The CDKN1A gene codon 31-arginine/serine polymorphism is not associated with endometriosis. Polymorphisms of the arylhydrocarbon receptor (AHR) gene and related genes were examined, and in at least one study, no association was found.

The endometriosis regresses after menopause or ovariectomy, suggesting it could depend on the production and metabolism of sex steroids (Kitawaki et al., 2002): high concentrations of estrogens were found in the endometriotic lesions, which grow and regress in an oestrogen-dependent way.

The inheritable susceptibility to endometriosis justifies the growing interest in identifying genes and/or genetic polymorphisms that could lead to an increased risk of disease. Identifying these polymorphisms may open to their use as genetic biomarkers of endometriosis (Vietri et al., 2007a, 2007b). Some genetic polymorphisms, involved in sex steroids biosynthesis and metabolism, may be reasonably associated with an increased risk of endometriosis, like progesterone receptor (PR), AR, oestrogen receptor (AR), 17beta-hydroxysteroid dehydrogenase type 1 (HSD17B1), cytochrome P450 subfamily 17 (CYP17) and cytochrome P450 subfamily 19 (CYP19) (Guo, 2006). No doubt this list is likely to increase over the years. The most widely used approach for the identification of endometriosis-predisposing genetic polymorphisms are the genetic association studies, by which genetic susceptibility polymorphisms are identified through the identification and assessment of the difference in allele/genotype frequencies between patients and control subjects.

The **CYP17 genotype** contains a single nucleotide T>C polymorphism situated 34bp upstream of the translation initiation site. C allele may have great promoter activity, increasing the transcription of P450c17 alpha enzyme. This effect amplifies the production of precursor androgens that are subsequently converted to estrogens. In fact, C allele is associated with high levels of estradiol in young women. CYP19 gene lies on chromosome 15 and encodes cytochrome P450, a major component of aromatase. Aromatase is a key enzyme in the conversion of androgens to estrogens, and mediates the rate-limiting step in the metabolism of C_{19} androgens to estrogens. Different polymorphisms of CYP19 are present in the gene and have been related to variations of aromatase activity (Gennari et al., 2004). A silent SNP, C1558T, corresponding to the 3′ untraslated region of the mRNA, has been correlated to the level of aromatase mRNA in breast tumour cells. Another polymorphism, GA at Val80, has been previously associated with breast cancer risk. Few studies have been published on the association between CYP17 T>C polymorphism with risk of endometriosis, showing controversial data. Some studies connected C1558T polymorphism with endometriosis risk (Huber et al., 2005), while no report relates Val80 SNP to endometriosis.

The **CYP19 genotype** may play a role in increased risk of endometriosis lying on an environmental and genetic background. The polymorphisms of CYP19 are significantly represented in Val80 and C1558T in patients affected with endometriosis. Despite endometriosis is a multifactorial disease, identifying Val80 and C1558T polymorphisms of CYP19 could help to comprehend the mechanisms of endometriosis. The assessment of these polymorphisms could help to anticipate the diagnosis or expect it in asymptomatic women to elaborate a follow up program. Other than that, a follow up by ultrasound and blood markers could be proposed in these patients, in order to define unclear symptoms such as dysmenorrhoea and chronic pelvic pain.

6. Future scope

Endometriosis is associated with genetic and immunological influences and exposure to environmental factors. It seems to result from a complex sequence of events in which multiple gene loci interact with each other and the environment to produce the disease phenotype, but thus far little is known about the candidate genes involved (Balow & Kennedy 2005). Because of this complexity, endometriosis is ideally suited as a target for genome wide scanning. Mutations and single-nucleotide polymorphisms (SNPs) have been identified in a number of genes that might confer susceptibility to endometriosis, but their precise role remains to be determined.

Proteome analysis is now widely accepted as a complementary technology to genetic profiling and together enables a better understanding of diseases and the development of new treatments. Proteomics allows the simultaneous observation of alterations in protein expression that may be either a precursor to or causative in disease development or a consequence of the disease. These techniques check and identify proteins that are expressed differently in patients with endometriosis versus normal controls. More recently, protein arrays using antibodies enable the screening of thousands of proteins against one sample. In future, such arrays could measure the expressions of multiple proteins to reveal changes in their regulation and expression in disease states. Furthermore, by using protein chip arrays, differential analysis of protein expression in women with and without differential protein profiling technology can be developed into a powerful tool for endometriosis research.

The study of protein function and protein-protein interaction can clarify the biology of the disease more so than the application of genomics. This is because gene expression and biological effects are linked via complex protein synthesis and gene interaction pathways.

Genomics includes hybridization techniques (e.g. differential colony hybridization), subtractive techniques (e.g. hybridization and representational difference analysis), gel-based techniques (e.g. RNA arbitrarily primed or differential display), and sequencing based techniques (e.g. expression sequence tags and serial analysis of gene expression). Furthermore, the use of DNA microarrays allows the search for new gene expression markers of endometriosis by identifying differentially expressed genes in endometriosis implants compared with endometrial tissue. The aim of the technique is to identify changes in gene expression characterizing the disease state so that we can understand the disease's progression and identify novel therapeutic targets.

Apart from the better understanding of the pathophysiology and the metabolic pathways that lead to potential biomarkers for endometriosis, there are still issues to be clarified and applications to be achieved. Once a protein or small number of proteins have been shown to be differentially expressed in endometriosis, the next step will be to use this information to try to develop a non-invasive diagnostic test for endometriosis. This diagnostic test should ideally have good sensitivity and specificity as well as satisfactory positive and negative predicative values for the detection of endometriosis, and also be cost effective and readily available.

Genetic markers that are prognostic for endometriosis can be genotyped early in life and could predict individual response to various risk factors and treatment. Genetic predisposition revealed by genetic analysis for susceptibility genes can provide an integrated assessment of the interaction between genotypes and environmental factors, resulting in synergistically increased prognostic value of diagnostic tests. Thus, pre-symptomatic and early symptomatic genetic testing is expected to be the cornerstone of the paradigmatic shift from late surgical interventions to earlier preventative therapies. Thus, there is an urgent need for novel genetic markers that are predictive of endometriosis and endometriosis progression, particularly in treatment decisions for individuals who are recognized as having endometriosis.

Such genetic markers may enable prognosis of endometriosis in much larger populations compared with the populations that can currently be evaluated by using existing risk factors and biomarkers.

The availability of a genetic test may allow, for example, early diagnosis and prognosis of endometriosis, as well as clinical intervention to mitigate progression of the disease. The use of these genetic markers will also allow selection of subjects for clinical trials involving novel treatment methods.

The discovery of genetic markers associated with endometriosis will further provide novel targets for therapeutic intervention or preventive treatments of endometriosis and enable the development of new therapeutic agents for treating endometriosis.

7. Conclusions

One of the main objectives of the gynaecologist is to diagnose endometriosis without the use of laparoscopy or laparotomy. Currently, laparoscopy offers the most specific and sensitive technique for evaluating and monitoring endometriosis. Even so, microscopic or occult endometriosis may be misdiagnosed because of the inability to visualize some lesions. Attempts for early diagnosis and treatments of endometriosis have been weighed down by lack of proper methods to study and manage the disease. Furthermore, the need for non-invasive diagnostic methods is evident because the laparoscopy is a surgical procedure with potentially dangerous risks.

At present, there are no reliable markers for the diagnosis and prognosis of endometriosis and identification of serum and endometrial markers is decisive for disease diagnosis and follow-up of patients.

The diagnostic laboratories are using new genomic and proteomic technologies to develop novel diagnostic and therapeutic approaches for endometriosis. These technologies will facilitate the generation of molecular expression profiles and then identifying potential gene and protein targets. This will lead to available markers with high sensitivity and specificity for screening of endometriosis, then to the development of serum diagnostic tools, therapeutic strategies and prognosis markers.

The combination of immunological discoveries and recent advances in DNA technologies may provide the long sought screening tool with the desirable diagnostic accuracy for this puzzling disorder.

The identification of specific genetic alterations and protein profiles associated with endometriosis offers a unique opportunity to develop assays for early diagnosis and/or treatment. By identifying proteins in biological samples, a minimally invasive tool should be feasible to assess the presence of disease and monitor response to treatment and/or disease progression.

The promise for gene-based diagnostic tests for endometriosis and rational development of genetically targeted and molecular therapeutic strategies is, in principle, excellent. The evolving genomic and proteomic technologies remain poised to revolutionize the diagnosis and treatment of endometriosis, but have not yet lead to a single new therapy or tested biomarker. Many problems remain to be resolved and, while some of these are technical in nature, the most intractable ones have mainly to do with the complex and multifactorial character of the disease itself.

8. References

Akahane, T., Sekizawa, A., Purwosunu, Y., Nagatsuka, M. & Okai, T. (2007). The role of p53 mutation in the carcinomas arising from endometriosis, *Int J Gynecol Pathol,* Vol. 26, No. 3, (July 2007), pp. 345-351, ISSN 0277-1691

Balow, D.H. & Kennedy, S. (2005). Endometriosis: new genetic approaches and therapy, *Ann Rev Med,* Vol. 56, pp. 345-356, ISSN 0066-4219

Barcelò, B., Pons, J., Fuster, A., Sauleda, J., Noguera, A., Ferrer, J.M. & Agustì, A.G. (2006). Intracellular cytokine profile of T lymphocytes in patients with chronic obstructive pulmonary disease, *Clin Exp Immunol,* Vol. 145, No. 3, (September 2006), pp. 474-479, ISSN 0009-9104

Bedaiwy, M.A., Falcone, T., Sharma, R.K., Goldberg, J.M., Attaran, M., Nelson, D.R. & Agarwal A. (2002). Prediction of endometriosis with serum and peritoneal fluid markers: a prospective controlled trial, *Hum Reprod,* Vol. 17, No. 2, (March 2002), pp. 426-431, ISSN 0268-1161

Bischoff, F.Z., Heard, M. & Simpson, J.L. (2002). Somatic DNA alterations in endometriosis: high frequency of chromosome 17 and p53 loss in late-stage endometriosis, *J Reprod Immunol,* Vol. 55, No. 1-2, (May-June 2002), pp. 49-64, ISSN 0165-0378

Dheenadayalu, K., Mak, I. Gordts, S., Campo, R., Higham, J., Puttemans, P.; White, J., Christian, M., Fusi, L. & Brosens J. (2002). Aromatase P450 messenger RNA expression in eutopic endometrium is not a specific marker for pelvic endometriosis, *Fertil Steril,* Vol. 78, No. 4 (October 2002), pp. 825–829, ISSN 0015-0282

Fu, C. & Lang, J. (2002). Serum soluble E-cadherin level in patients with endometriosis, *Chin Med Sci J,* Vol. 17, No. 2, (June 2002), pp. 121–123, ISSN 1001-9294

Gennari, L., Nuti, R., & Bilezikian, J.P. (2004). Aromatase activity and bone homeostasis in men, *J Clin Endocrinol Metab,* Vol. 89, No. 12, (December 2004), pp. 5898-5907, ISSN 0021-972X

Guo, S.W. (2006). Association of endometriosis risk and genetic polymorphisms involving sex steroid biosynthesis and their receptors: a meta-analysis, *Gynecol Obstet Invest,* Vol. 61, No. 2, pp. 90-105, ISSN 0378-7346

Gurgan, T., Bukulmez, O., Yarali, H., Tanir, M. & Akyildiz, S. (1999). Serum and peritoneal fluid levels of IGF I and II and insulin-like growth binding protein-3 in endometriosis, *J Reprod Med,* Vol. 44, No. 5, (May 1999), pp. 450–454, ISSN 0024-7758

Huber, A., Keck, C.C., Hefler, L.A., Schneeberger, C., Huber, J.C., Bentz, E.K. & Tempfer, C.B. (2005). Ten estrogen-related polymorphisms and endometriosis: a study of multiple gene-gene interactions, *Obst Gynecol,* Vol. 106, No. 5, (November 2005), pp. 1025-1031, ISSN 0029-7844

Illera, J.C., Silvan, G., Illera, M.J., Munro, C.J., Lessey, B.A. & Illera, M. (2001). Measurement of serum and peritoneal fluid LH concentrations as a diagnostic tool for human endometriosis, *Reproduction,* Vol. 121, No. 5, (May 2001), pp. 761–769, ISSN 1470-1626

Iwabe, T., Harada, T., Sakamoto, Y., Iba, Y., Horie, S., Mitsunari, M. & Terakawa, N. (2003). Gonadotropin-releasing hormone agonist treatment reduced serum interleukin-6 concentrations in patients with ovarian endometriomas, *Fertil Steril,* Vol. 80, No. 2, (August 2003), pp. 300-304, ISSN 0015-0282

Kawasaki, H., Onuki, R., Suyama, E. & Taira, K. (2002). Identification of genes that function in the TNFα-mediated apoptotic pathway using randomized hybrid ribozyme libraries, *Nat Biotechnol,* Vol. 20, No. 4, (April 2002), pp. 376-80, ISSN 1087-0156

Kitawaki, J., Kado, N., Ishihara, H., Koshiba, H., Kitaoka, Y. & Honjo, H. (2002). Endometriosis: the patophysiology as an estrogen-dependent disease, *J Steroid Biology,* Vol. 83, No. 1-5, (December 2002), pp. 149-155, ISSN 0960-0760

Konno, R., Yamakawa, H., Utsunomiya, H., Ito, K., Sato, S. & Yajima, A. (2000). Expression of survivin and Bcl-2 in the normal human endometrium, *Mol Hum Reprod,* Vol. 6, No. 6, (June 2000), pp. 529-534, ISSN 1360-9947

Lebovic, D.I., Mueller, M.D. & Taylor, R.N. (2001). Immunobiology of endometriosis *Fertil Steril,* Vol. 75, No. 1, (January 2001), pp. 1-10, ISSN 0015-0282

Leng, J., Lang, J., Zhao, D. & Liu, D. (2002). Serum levels of soluble intercellular molecule 1 (sICAM-1) in endometriosis, *Zhonghua Yi Xue Za Zhi,* Vol. 82, No. 3, (February 2002), pp. 189–190, ISSN 0376-2491

Matalliotakis, I.M., Goumenou, A.G., Koumantakis, G.E., Athanassakis, I., Dionyssopoulou, E., Neonaki, M.A. & Vassiliadis, S. (2003). Expression of serum human leukocyte antigen and growth factor levels in a Greek family with familial endometriosis, *J Soc Gynecol Investig,* Vol. 10, No. 2, (February 2002), pp. 118–121, ISSN 1071-5576

Matalliotakis, I.M., Goumenou, A.G., Koumantakis, G.E., Neonaki, M.A., Koumantakis, G.E., Dionyssopoulou, E., Athanassakis, I. & Vassiliadis, S. (2003). Serum concentrations of growth factors in women with and without endometriosis: the action of anti-endometriosis medicines, *Int Immunopharmacol,* Vol. 3, No. 1, (January 2003), pp. 81–89, ISSN 1567-5769

Mhawech, P., Kinkel, K., Vlastos, G. & Pelte, M.F. (2001). Ovarian carcinomas in endometriosis: an immunohistochemical and comparative genomic hybridization study, *Int J Gynecol Pathol,* Vol. 21, No. 4 (October 2001), pp. 401-406, ISSN 0277-1691

Nothnick, W.B. (2001). Treating endometriosis as an autoimmune disease, *Fertil Steril,* Vol. 76, No. 2, (August 2001), pp. 223–231, ISSN 0015-0282

Rier, S. & Foster, W.G. (2003). Environmental dioxins and endometriosis, *Sem Reprod Med,* Vol. 21, No. 2, (May 2003), pp. 145-154, ISSN 1526-8004

Sillem, M., Prifti, S., Koch, A., Neher, M., Jauckus, J. & Runnebaum, B. (2001). Regulation of matrix metalloproteinases and their inhibitors in uterine endometrial cells of patients with and without endometriosis, *Eur J Obstet Gynecol Reprod Biol,* Vol. 95, No. 2, (April 2001), pp. 167–174, ISSN 0301-2115

Somigliana, E., Viganò, P., Candiani, M., Felicetta, I., Di Blasio, A.M. & Vignali, M. (2003). Use of serum-soluble intercellular adhesion molecule-1 as a new marker of endometriosis, *Fertil Steril,* Vol. 77, No. 5, (May 2003), pp. 1028–1031, ISSN 0015-0282

Tanaka, T., Utsunomiya, T., Bai, T., Nakajima, S. & Umesaki, N. (2003). Leptin inhibits decidualization and enhances cell viability of normal human endometrial stromal cells, *Int J Mol Med,* Vol. 12, No. 1, (July 2003), pp. 95–98, ISSN 1107-3756

Taylor, R.N., Lundeen, S.G. & Giudice, L,C. (2002). Emerging role of genomics in endometriosis research, *Fertil Steril,* Vol. 78, No. 4, (October 2002), pp. 694-698, ISSN 0015-0282

Vietri, M.T., Molinari, A.M., Iannella, I., Cioffi, M., Bontempo, P., Ardovino, M., Scaffa, C., Colacurci, N. & Cobellis, L. (2007). Arg72Pro p53 polymorphism in Italian women: no association with endometriosis, *Fertil Steril,* Vol. 88, No. 5, (November 2007), pp. 1468-1469, ISSN 0015-0282

Vietri, M.T., Cioffi, M., Sessa, M., Simeone, S., Bontempo, P., Trabucco, E., Ardovino, M., Colacurci, N., Molinari, A.M. & Cobellis, L. (2009). CYP17 and CYP19 gene polymorphisms in women affected with endometriosis, *Fertil Steril,* Vol. 92, No. 5, (November 2009), pp. 1532-1535, ISSN 0015-0282

Viganò, P., Somigliana, E., Matrone, R., Dubini, A., Barron, C., Vignali, M. & di Blasio, A.M. (2002). Serum leptin concentrations in endometriosis, *J Clin Endocrinol Metabol,* Vol. 87, No. 3, (March 2002), pp. 1085–1087, ISSN 0021-972X

Wieser, F., Fabjani, G., Tempfer, C., Schneeberger, C., Sator, M., Huber, J. & Wenzi R. (2003). Analysis of an interleukin-6 gene promoter polymorphism in women with endometriosis by pyrosequencing, *J Soc Gynecol Investig,* Vol. 10, No. 1, (January 2003), pp. 32-36, ISSN 1071-5576

Zong, LL., Li, Y.L. & Ha, X.Q. (2003). Determination of HGF concentration in serum and peritoneal fluid in women with endometriosis, *Di Yi Jun Yi Da Xue Xue Bao,* Vol. 23, No. 8, pp. (August 2003), 757-760, ISSN 1000-2588

24

Imaging Tools for Endometriosis: Role of Ultrasound, MRI and Other Imaging Modalities in Diagnosis and Planning Intervention

Shalini Jain Bagaria[1], Darshana D. Rasalkar[2] and Bhawan K. Paunipagar[2]
[1]*Department of Obstetrics & Gynecology, UCMS & GTB Hospital, Dilshad Garden,*
[2]*Department of Imaging and Interventional Radiology, The Chinese University of Hong Kong, Prince of Wales Hospital, Hong Kong*

1. Introduction

Endometriosis is the presence of endometrial glands as well as stroma at the locations outside uterus. It affects up to 10% of women. Grossly there are three forms of the disease, namely a) superficial endometrial implants, b) ovarian endometriomas or endometriotic cysts, and c) deep infiltrating endometriosis. All the three forms depict varied manifestation of a single disease and require a careful pre operative work up to know the extent and distribution of the disease precisely as it is critical to frame the plan of management.

The superficial implants are typically 2-3 mm in size rooted in the serosal tissue of the peritoneum. They initially appear as red highly vascular lesions. Later, repeated haemorrhage and inflammation triggers fibrosis and haemosiderin deposition in them causing raised powder burn lesions. It is hard to find such lesions by USG or MRI. Traditional method of diagnostic endoscopy still remains the golden standard of reference to diagnose and stage this form of disease.

Endometriomas of the ovary or chocolate cysts of the ovary contain degraded blood products. The dark and gelatinous material in them is surrounded by fibrous wall of variable thickness. Endomeriotic cysts are often bilateral and multiple. Both the USG and MRI play key role in its evaluation.

The deep infiltrating endometriosis (DIE) is defined as the implant penetrating into the retroperitoneal space or the wall of the pelvic organs to the depth of at least 5mm. (Knoninckx et al). They usually appear as solid nodules. These types of lesions permeate deep into the surrounding fibromuscular tissues and induce smooth muscle proliferation and fibrous reaction effecting development of solid nodules. In case of visceral involvement, they can infiltrate into the muscle layer from the serosal layer. The resulting smooth muscle proliferation can lead to stricture formation and later obstruction.

2. Natural history of the disease

The natural history of the symptomatic disease is uncertain. The lesions may either continue to be same or may evolve further or may regress. Its malignant transformation is uncommon and its exact incidence is not known. This is diagnosed only if there is no evidence of metastasis from any primary sites and the surrounding tissue has presence of benign as well as the malignant endometrial tissue.

3. Locations

The disease most commonly affects the ovaries and the pelvic peritoneum. DIE classically affects the rectovaginal septum and the uterine ligaments (69.2%), the vagina (14.5%), the rectosigmoid bowel (9.9%), and the bladder and ureter (6.4%) in the order of frequency. Rarely lungs and CNS may be involved.

4. Diagnostic modalities for evaluation of endometriosis

The diagnosis of endometriosis is conventionally made by laparoscopy but over the time the imaging techniques have evolved to greatly facilitate the pre operative diagnosis. Further laparoscopy has limited role in visualizing atypical non pigmented extraperitoneal sites of involvement and the areas especially concealed by pelvic adhesions.

By and large ultrasound is the first preliminary investigation done to assess the pelvic disease in reproductive age group. Although it has limited role in detection of superficial implants, it is useful in the diagnosis and treatment of endometriomas. MRI provides a good alternative with high specificity and sensitivity for detecting deep infiltrating (DIE) endometriosis as well as endometriomas. The main drawback of MRI is again inability to detect small peritoneal infiltrates (< 3mm). Introduction of fat saturated T1 weighted image on MRI has consistently improved its accuracy in distinguishing between ovarian mass with lipids from endometriomas.

Computed tomography usually gives ill defined results, thus is not very helpful. Conventional investigations like barium enema or intravenous urography may prove useful in detection of visceral endometriosis. Their use however is limited in current practice due to excessive radiation dose.

Further sections of this chapter will first discuss the various imaging modalities in detail followed by the characteristic appearance of diverse typical and atypical forms of endometriosis.

4.1 Ultrasound

Ultrasound as discussed is usually the first investigation done in subject suspected of any pelvic disease. USG has the advantage of having good resolution, easy accessibility, less expensive, and is free of ionizing radiation. Three modes are available- transabdominal, transvaginal and endorectal scanning.

For transabdominal scanning 3-5 MHz convex probe is used. Full bladder is must for this technique in order to properly visualize the uterus and the ovaries. It is very useful in cases of suspected bladder involvement and abdominal wall endometriosis. Kidneys should be examined for hydronephrosis

Transvaginal scanning (TVS) is done with probe of high frequency 6-7.5MHz positioned in vagina. Full bladder is not a pre requisite for this mode of USG and procedure is well accepted by most of the patients. TVS has superior image quality and resolution as compared to TAS. Thus it has high sensitivity (92%) and specificity (99%) in detecting endometriomas. The typical ultrasound findings include a cystic mass with diffuse, low-level echoes (figure 1).

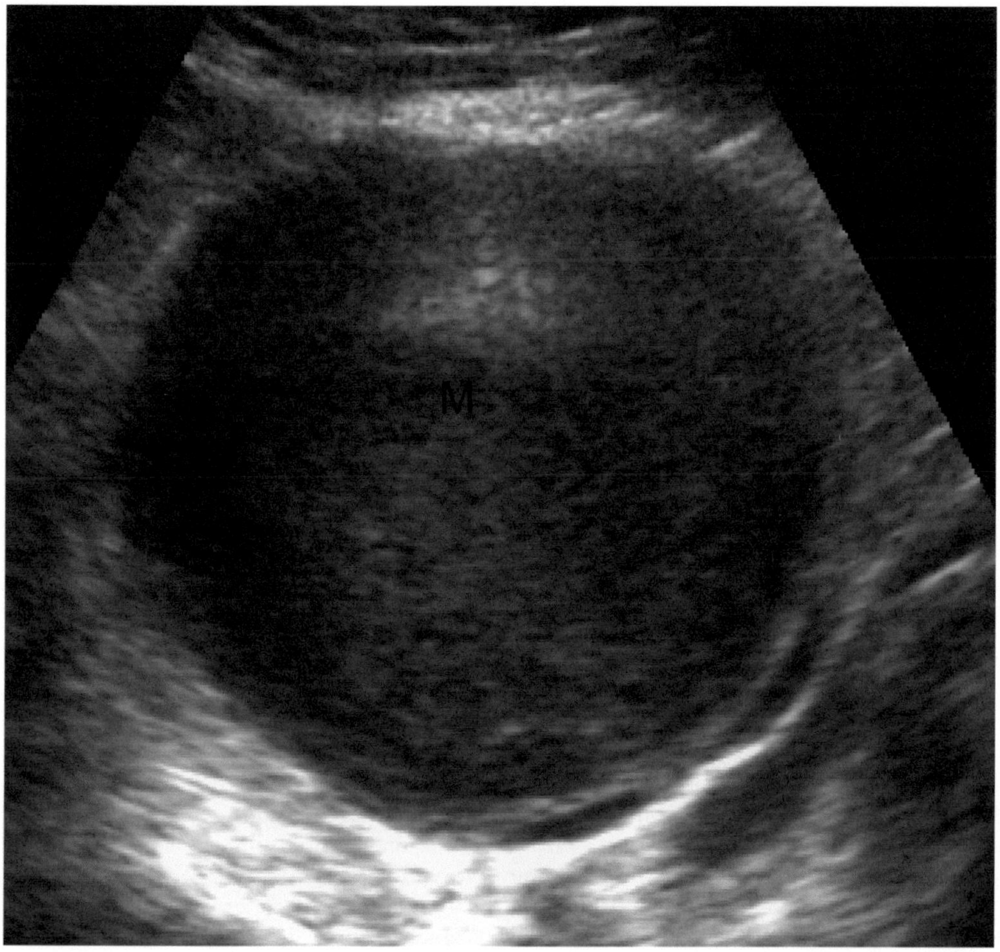

Fig. 1. Grey-scale Transvaginal ultrasound of an endometrioma(M). Note the characteristic diffuse, low-level echoes of the endometrioma giving a solid appearance

Depending on the age of the haemorrhage, the contents of the cyst, may vary in appearance. At times, an endometrioma may resemble a cystic-solid or entirely solid mass. Punctate echogenicities in the wall of endometriomas are less commonly seen but add specificity to the diagnosis. Endometriomas can be multilocular with internal thin or thick septations and thick irregular walls. Mild vascularity may be identified on color Doppler (figure 2). Color Doppler US shows no blood flow in the fine septations, whereas blood flow can often be detected in thick septations because of revascularization of chronic haematoma. Internal moving echos within endometrioma may reveal color signal.

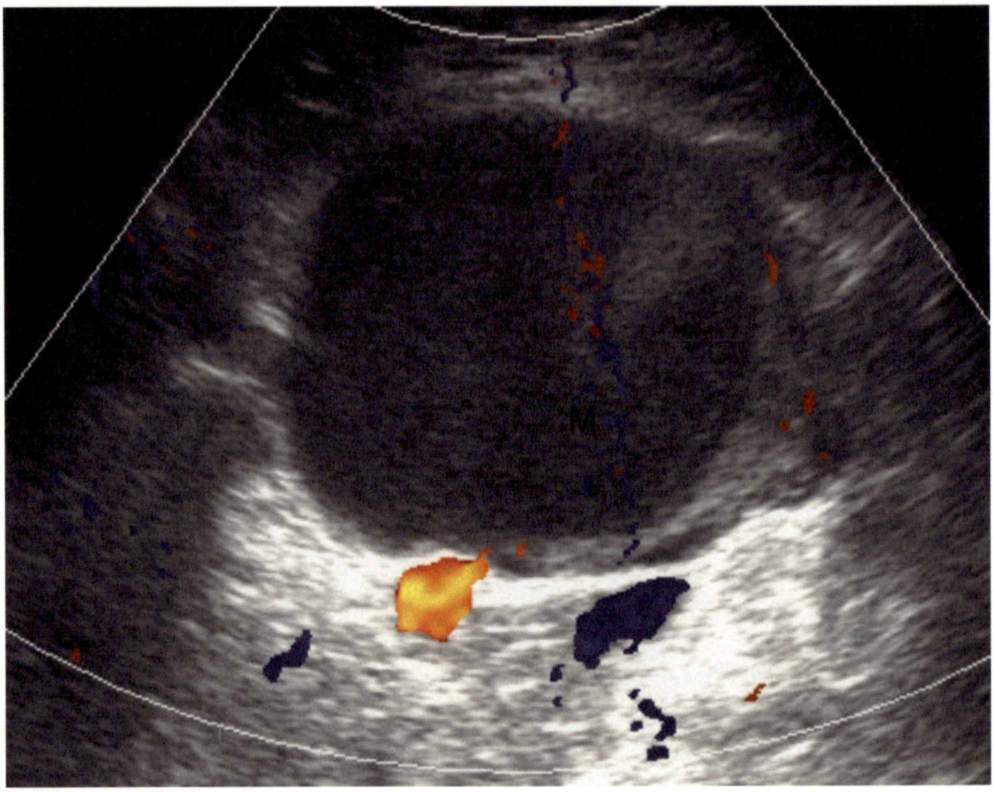

Fig. 2. Transvaginal ultrasound of an endometrioma color Doppler image showing mild peripheral vascularity. Internal color signals are likely related to moving internal echos.

Spectral Doppler reveal low-resistance waveforms which may not be helpful in differentiating endometriomas from other masses including malignancy.

Transrectal sonography uses biplane convex flexible rectal probe of 6.5MHz. The probe is flexible and can be advanced into the sigmoid colon to look for any signs of invasion by endometriosis. Patient preparation with rectal enema is required before endorectal sonography. The rectum and the surrounding area in the perimetry show five alternating hyper and hypoechoic layers respectively. The endometriotic deposits are visualized as triangular or round hypoechoic lesions on transrectal USG. It is superior to MRI with reported high sensitivity and specificity of 97% and 80%.

4.2 Magnetic resonance imaging

MRI is a non invasive intervention by which whole pelvis can be visualized in different planes. It can be very useful in patients in whom ultrasound findings are equivalent and in carefully selected high risk population. It is especially beneficial in identifying endometriomas, adhesions, superficial peritoneal implants and extraperitoneal lesions, particularly those in the rectovaginal space and uterosacral ligaments as well as in solid endometriotic nodules. In view of longer imaging times required for MRI, antiperistaltic medication to decrease the bowel movement can minimize motion related artifact and also enhances the visualization of the bowel involvement.

The signal intensity of MRI depends on the contents of the endometrial implants. The contents of these implants mainly include the proteins and degraded blood products, the ratio of which varies according to the stage of the haemorrhage and thus the variation in the signal intensity can be noted on MR images. The acute haemorrhage may give hypointense (dark) signal on the T1 and T2 weighted images. In contrast the lesions containing degraded blood products like methemoglobin, proteins and iron may be seen as hyperintense (bright) on T1 (figure 3) and hypointense (dark) on T2 weighted images(figure 4). Multiple high signal lesions, usually in the ovaries, on T1-weighted images, also are highly suggestive of endometriosis. The diagnostic MR imaging features of endometrioma include cystic mass with high signal intensity on T1-weighted images and loss of signal intensity on T2-weighted images. This phenomenon is referred to as "shading" as a result of high protein and iron concentration from recurrent hemorrhage in the endometrioma.

The advent of fat saturated T1 weighted technique has greatly enhanced the value of MRI in differentiating among endometriomas and lipid containing ovarian tumors like dermoid cysts. Use of contrast medium (Gadolinium) has not shown any advantage over plain MRI for the purpose but it may be useful when malignant lesion is suspected.

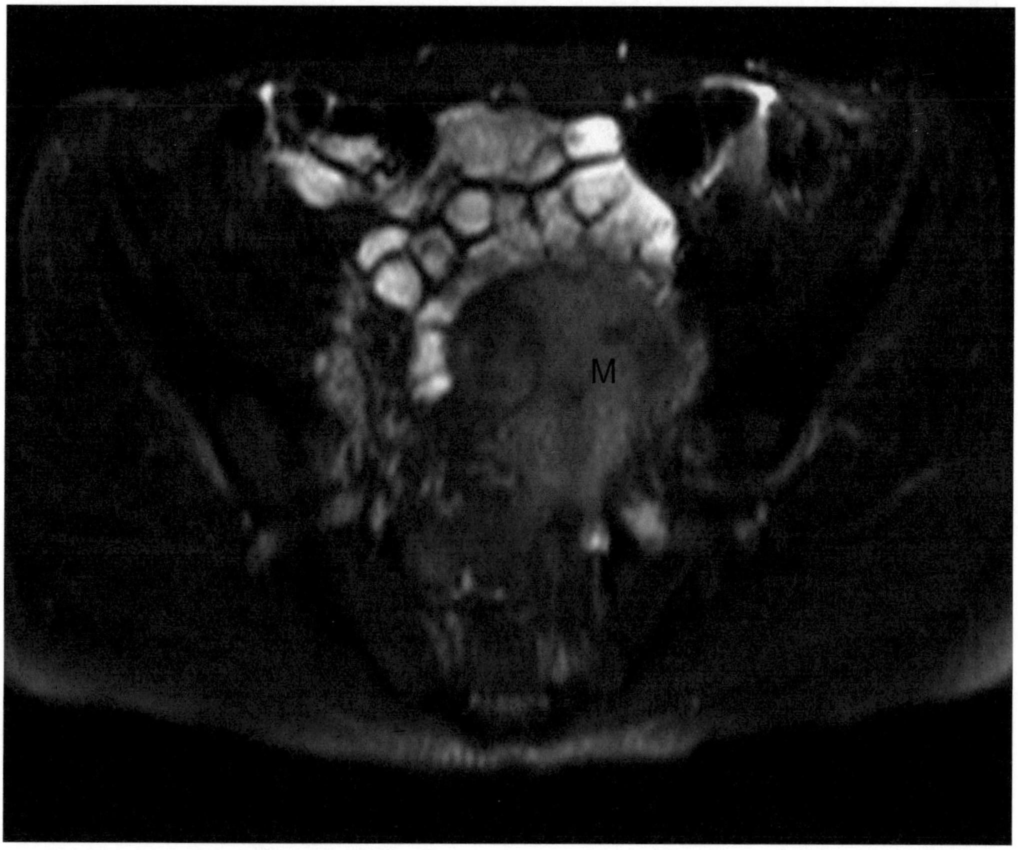

Fig. 3. Axial fat saturated T1Weighted image reveals T1 hyperintense lesions in the left ovary (M) suggestive a chocolate cyst/endrometrioma of the ovary.

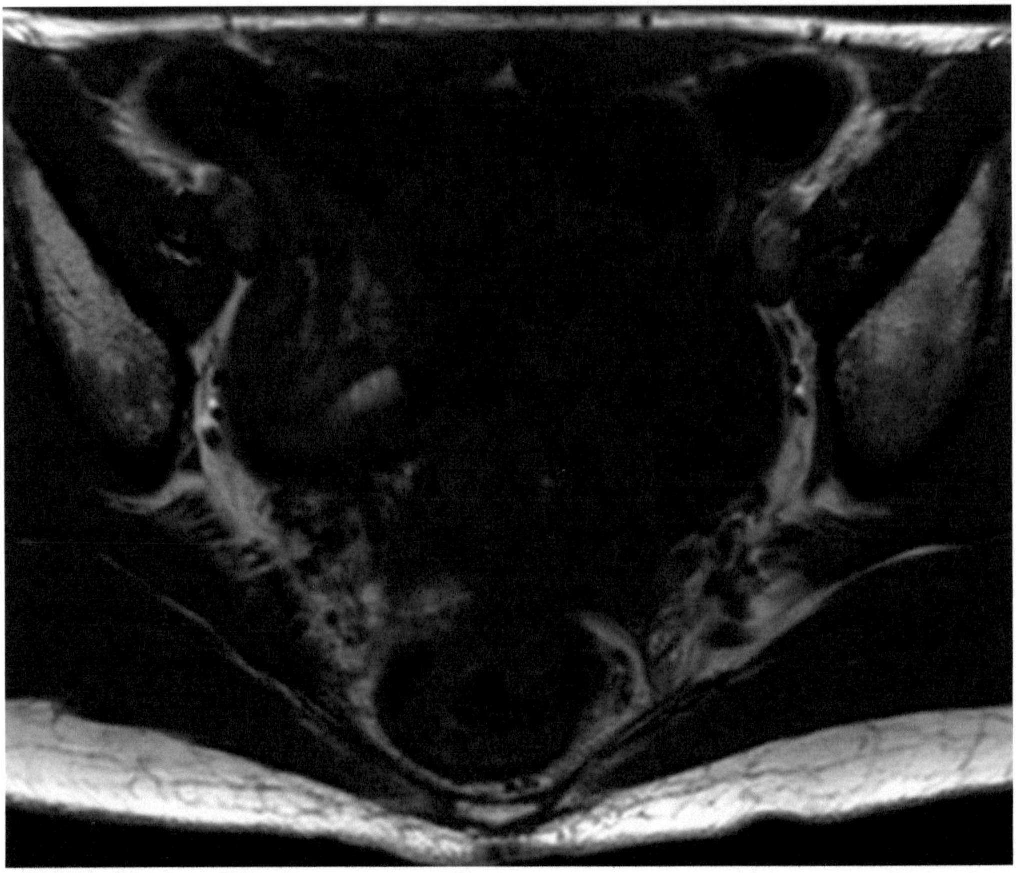

Fig. 4. Axial T2Weighted image showing the lesions are hypointense on T2W images.

The solid nodules of DIE appear as low intermediate signal on T1 weighted with punctuate areas of high signal and uniform low signals on T2 weighted images. The high signal zone is the consequence of foci of haemorrhage bounded by fibrous tissues. However it is difficult to identify superficial peritoneal implants on MRI.

Adhesions in the pelvis are one of the hallmarks of the disease. They appear as low signal areas of stranding. Adhesions are also suggested by the fixed retroverted uterus, angulated loops of bowel or displacement of the ovaries. Complications of endometriosis such as bowel implants and ureteral obstruction can often be detected on MRI.

It is now feasible to see the visceral deposits on MRI directly. Rather some studies claim MR imaging to be more specific than endorectal USG with sensitivity and specificity of 90-92% and 91 to 98% respectively (Gougoutas CA et al). MRI has valuable role in identification of nerve invasion (sciatic endometriosis) and abdominal wall lesions. The accuracy of MRI has been improved with the introduction of newer approach particularly endocavitary and phased array coils.

Role of MRI has been analyzed by various authors in the past. Stratton et al in a study reported 69% sensitivity and 75% specificity for detecting endometriosis confirmed on biopsy. MRI proposed diagnosis in nearly all patients with the severe form of the disease but by and large could recognize only small number of endometriotic areas as compared to surgery. Thus it is relatively less sensitive in determining the extent of the disease.

With this background in mind, the next section of the chapter will discuss in detail the features specific to different types of endometriosis on USG and MRI.

5. Different types of endometriosis

5.1 Superficial implants

Both USG and MRI has major limitation in diagnosing this type of endometriosis as already discussed. Endoscopy remains the standard practice to determine the extent of involvement by such lesions.

5.2 Endometriomas

Transvaginal sonography (TVS) is universally most frequently used imaging tool for evaluation of endometriomas. USG features of chocolate cysts are diverse. The classical appearance is that of a cystic structure with diffuse low level internal echoes and echogenic wall foci. The cyst may be unilocular or multilocular. It may contain thin or thick septa. Sometimes there may be wall nodularity. Wall nodularity if present requires further investigation to rule out malignancy. Imaging alone cannot exclude malignant neoplasm.

It is interesting to note that out of 20% of the endometriomas exhibiting wall nodularity, 35% had hyperechogenic wall foci (Patel et al). Effort should be made to distinguish between wall nodularity and the hyperechogenic foci within the wall. The latter when present in lesion with low level echoes and no features of malignancy is indicative of endometrioma.

Differential diagnoses of chocolate cyst include haemorrhagic cyst, dermoid cyst and cystic neoplasms. Dermoid cyst usually exhibit either echogenic shadow due to its fat content or acoustic shadowing due to calcium which aids in the diagnosis. To differentiate between haemorrhagic cyst and chocolate cyst can be a difficult task. The haemorrhagic cyst usually displays high level internal echoes within a thin walled cyst which may advance with time and emerge as a more complex cyst. Formation of fibrin may imitate thin septa but these lesions usually resolve on follow up.

The accuracy of USG can be further improved by color Doppler flow studies. Blood flow in the endometrioma is through the regularly spaced vessels running in the hilar region and the pericystic space.

MRimaging is another tool for identifying endometriomas. Due to the cyclical bleeding endometriomas contain blood products at different age. They are seen as bright or hyperintense lesions on T1 weighted image. On T2 they appear more hypointense or dark with foci of hyperintensity, imparting it the classical appearance of 'shading'. Shading is effect of degenerated blood products present at different stage within the same cyst. It can range from subtle layering to a complete signal void (black).

Since both the haemorrhagic cysts and the chocolate cyst contain blood products, it can be difficult to distinguish between them except for the fact that hemorrhagic cysts do not display shading, are mostly unilocular and resolve on interval imaging. In contrast dermoid cysts are easily diagnosed on MRI since they lose the signals and become dark on fat suppressed sequences.

After contrast administration, the periovarian peritoneal surface of the cyst can be enhanced which can help in identification of torsion ovary. Endometrioma in an enlarged but poorly enhancing ovary with peripherally located follicles is suggestive of torsion ovary on MRimaging.

5.3 Solid deep lesions

Solid deep lesions display low to intermediate signal intensity with punctuate areas of high signal intensity on T1 weighted images. Uniform low signal intensity is seen on T2 weighted images. The punctuate foci of high intensity are due to the zone of haemorrhage surrounded by abundant solid fibrous tissues. These may actually mimic metastatic lesions arising from intraperitoneal malignancies such as ovarian carcinomas. The two entities can be differentiated on T2 weighted images by the low signal intensity imparted by solid endometriomas often in combination with the presence of endometrial cyst.

Masses situated in the pouch of Douglas, posterior vaginal fornix and uterosacral ligaments may comprise of large fraction of glandular material with little fibrotic reaction, imparting hyperintense signals on T2 weighted images. Administration of contrast material will enhance such solid lesions, making it possible to distinguish it from necrosis or intramural hemorrhage.

Frequently the signal intensity may not be able to pick up the deep endometriosis of the uterosacral ligaments, especially if the punctuate foci of haemorrhage are missing in the lesion. In such case, the diagnosis is often made by correlating the thickening of the ligaments. Thickening more than 9mm in size or nodularity within the ligaments either bilateral or asymmetrical often give clue to the diagnosis.

5.4 Bladder endometriosis

Bladder endometriosis can be identified on MRI by deviation in signal intensity and gross anatomical anomalies in bladder wall thickness which can be localized or diffuse. Most of the times there are foci of high signal intensity in abnormally thickened bladder wall. Such findings may exist even if patients have normal cystoscopy result or without urinary symptoms. Bladder endometriosis infact infrequently infilterates the mucosa. Thus it is difficult to make out the lesions on cystoscopy. Advanced disease may present as ureteral obstruction and hydronephrosis.

5.5 Rectal endometriosis

Deep rectal involvement is less obvious on MRimaging due to the rectal contents which impart artifacts. Conventional MRI has infact sensitivity of only 33%. Results can be improved with the use of phased array coils, endovaginal coils and rectal contrast enema. MRI features that can be helpful in diagnosis include thickening of the rectal wall correlated with specific symptoms clinically, low signal intensity on T2 weighted images, and occasionally the presence of punctuate hyperintense foci of haemorrhage.

Endorectal sonography as dicussed earlier is superior to MR imaging for diagnosis of this entity. The deposits on bowel are seen as rounded hypoechoic areas.

5.6 Malignant transformation in endometriosis

Malignant transformation in endometrioma is a rare well-known complication of endometriosis, occurring in a younger age group with estimated incidence is less than 1% of women with ovarian endometriosis. The common histologic types are endometrioid adenocarcinoma and clear cell carcinoma arising from glandular elements and rare form is endometrial stromal sarcoma occurs arising from stromal elements. Loss of the T2 shading effect is more commonly detected in malignant than in benign endometriomas. The postulated reasoning for this is dilution of haemorrhagic fluid by tumor secretions, although is not specific to malignant endometrial cysts. Enhancing mural nodules within a cystic mass is another feature of malignant change in endometriosis. Typically mural nodules are enhancing, T1-weighted low and variable T2-weighted signal intensities. Dynamic subtraction images with a gradient- echo sequence often improve nodule enhancement. Again, enhancing mural nodules within endometriotic cysts, although seen more commonly in malignant endometriomas is not specific and has been reported in benign lesions.

5.7 Scar endometriosis

Solid endometriosis can also develop in a caesarian section scar. MRI is valuable in identifying these lesions. MRI characteristically shows high signal intensity on T1 and hypointensity on T2 weighted images. Fat saturated sequences are more helpful in the diagnosis specially in context of myometrium along the surgical scar.

6. Conclusion

The imaging techniques have revolutionized the pre operative diagnosis of endometriosis although the ultimate confirmation is by histopathology only. The major advantage of these tools is being non invasive method.

7. References

Gougoutas CA, Siegelman ES, Hunt J, et al. Pelvic endometriosis: various manifestations and MR imaging findings. AJR Am J Roentgenol2000; 175: 353-358.

Knonickx PR, Meulman C, Demeyere S, Lesaffre E, CornillieFJ. Suggestive evidence that pelvic endometriosis is a progressive disease, whereas deeply infiltrating endometriosis is associated with pelvic pain. Fertil Steril 1991; 55: 759-765.

Patel MD, Feldstein VA, Chen DC, Lipson SD et al. Endometriomas: diagnostic performance of US. Radiology 1999; 210: 739-745.

Stratton P, Winkel C, Premkumar A et al. Diagnostic accuracy of laparoscopy, magnetic resonance imaging, and histopathologic examination for the detection of endometriosis. Fertil Steril 2003; 79: 1078-1085

25

Pelvic Endometriosis: A MR Pictorial Review

Rosario Francesco Grasso, Riccardo Del Vescovo,
Roberto Luigi Cazzato and Bruno Beomonte Zobel
Department of Radiology, Campus Bio-Medico University of Rome, Italy

1. Introduction

Endometriosis is one of the most common benign gynaecological conditions. It is defined as the presence of ectopic endometrial glands and stroma outside the uterus. The ectopic endometrium responds to hormonal stimulation with a cyclic hemorrhage, resulting in a complex spectrum of symptoms.

Pain is the cardinal symptom of endometriosis, even though patients may experience several different types of pain, such as dysmenorrhea, deep dyspareunia, discomfort during defecation or while urinating, according to the anatomic location of this disorder. Endometriotic implants, pelvic adhesions and ovarian endometriomas are commonly associated with chronic pelvic pain. Haemorrhage into an endometrioma may result in acute pain. Infertility is another commonly associated complaint.

The exact prevalence of endometriosis is not well defined, as the diagnostic gold standard is represented by laparoscopy or laparotomy. It is estimated about 5-10%, including both symptomatic and asymptomatic women. Nulliparous women and women reporting short and heavy menstrual cycles are at increased risk [1]; these epidemiological findings support the metastatic implantation from retrograde menstruation hypothesis. Other theories include the metaplastic differentiation of serosal surfaces or müllerian remnant tissue, and the induction of undifferentiated mesenchyme to form endometriotic tissue due to released substances from the shed endometrium (induction theory) [2].

The most common locations of endometriosis are the ovaries and the pelvic peritoneum, followed in order of decreasing frequency by deep lesions of the pelvic subperitoneal space, the intestinal system and the urinary system. Deep pelvic endometriosis is a pathologically distinct entity: deep endometriotic lesions penetrate under the surface of peritoneum (infiltration > 5mm) and are tipically found in the uterosacral ligaments, rectum, rectovaginal septum, vagina or bladder, and induce a fibromuscolar hyperplasia that surrounds endometriosis foci [3].

The diagnosis of endometriosis still remains a challenge for clinicians, resulting from similarities in clinical symptoms to other benign or malignant gynaecological diseases.

Laparoscopy is the standard of reference in the diagnosis of endometriosis; histological analysis of biopsy specimens should confirm the diagnosis, even if it is not necessary.

On the other hand, laparoscopy is also required for staging the disease. The most widely used staging system is the 1985 Revised Classification of Endometriosis published by the

American Fertility Society [4]. The rAFS score takes into account the presence of ovarian and peritoneal implants (subdivided into superficial or deep), the severity of the adhesions and the presence or not of a complete posterior cul-de-sac obliteration (i.e. frozen pelvis). The rAFS staging system has shown poor correlation to the clinical severity of the disease, so requiring further refinement. Meanwhile a new staging system called ENZIAN score has been recently developed [5]; it is focused on the deep pelvic endometriosis that is the most severe form of the disease.

The clinical value of this staging system and its correlation to the reproductive prognosis of endometriosis patients should be assessed.

Therapeutic options are observation, medical treatment, surgery or a combination strategy.

The most widely used medical therapy of endometriosis includes oral contraceptives, androgenic agents, progestins, and gonadotropin releasing hormone (GnRH) analogs. The choice of a surgical option depends upon the severity of the disease. Surgery is the main therapeutic option in patients with deep pelvic endometriosis. Anterior cul-de-sac endometriosis involving the bladder can be treated with laparoscopic surgery. Preoperative staging of disease is necessary because in certain cases surgery should be performed by standard laparotomy (bladder endometriosis associated with bowel involvement). Treatment of posterior cul-de-sac endometriosis can be achieved with laparoscopy, but a vaginal or a laparotomic approach is needed when vaginal or severe bowel disease, respectively are present.

2. Pathologic features of endometriosis

The most common site of involvement is the ovary, but virtually all pelvic organs can be affected by the disease.

Ovarian endometriosis includes a superficial form, which appears as small punctuate foci measuring no more than 5 mm, and a 'deep' one; in the latter case the typical aspect is that of the "chocolate cyst" or "endometrioma". Chocolate cysts typically have thick, fibrotic walls, a dark-brown, viscous content and their diameter rarely exceed 15 cm.

Aspect of endometriotic peritoneal implants ranges from punctuate foci to small stellar patches; according to the age of the lesion and the amount of pigment, they could appear white, yellow, red, blue or brown (**Fig. 1**).

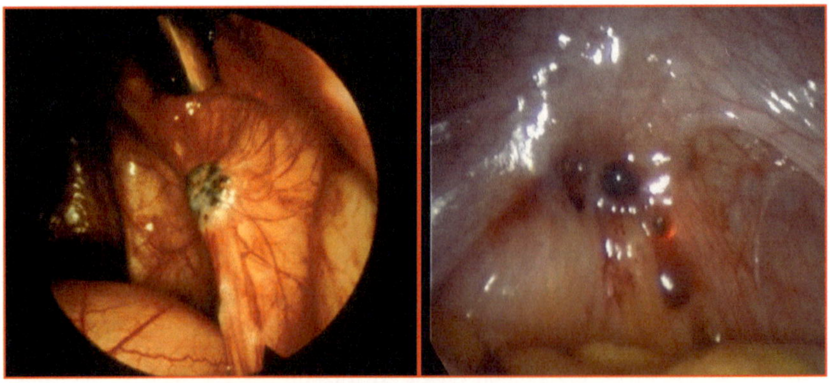

Fig. 1. Endometriotic nodules as they are seen in laparoscopy

When the peritoneal lesion invades the subserosal layers it progressively leads to extensive fibrosis, wall thickening of the pelvic organs, nodule formation and distortion of the normal pelvic anatomy due to a fibrous retraction; the most severe form is the so called "frozen pelvis", that consists of a huge amount of tissue involving the retro-uterine excavation and causing an extensive infiltration of the posterior pelvis (torus uteri, uterosacral ligaments, vaginal and rectal wall).

Microscopic appearance of endometriosis is composed of endometrial glands, stroma and occasionally histiocytes, due to an inflammatory response caused by cyclic hemorrhages within the implant. In rare cases endometriosis may lack glands (stromal endometriosis) [6].

3. Radiologic evaluation of endometriosis

Radiologists are often involved in the diagnosis and pre-operative assessment of the disease: an accurate pre-operative evaluation of the endometrial implants (location, size and depth of penetration) could help the surgeon to perform a radical surgical excision in cases in which severe fibrosis and adhesions hide deep lesions and impede laparoscopic evaluation.

Imaging methods that are used in the daily practice to diagnose endometriosis are ecotomografy, especially Transvaginal Ultrasound (TVUS) and Magnetic Resonance Imaging (MRI).

TVUS provides high resolution images of the pelvic organs, providing reliable information in patients with both acute and chronic pelvic pain [7].

The classic endometrioma on TVUS appears as an area of low and homogenous echoes.

TVUS has been reported to be the best method for discriminating between endometriotic and non-endometriotic cysts, with a sensitivity of 83% and a false positive rate of 7%. The addition of CA-125 evaluation does not improve the diagnostic accuracy of TVUS, thus indicating TVUS alone to be the least expensive instrument for identifying the presence of endometriomas [8,9].

The role of TVUS for the assessment of deep pelvic endometriosis has been recently reported, with conflicting results. TVUS is apparently more accurate than Rectal Endoscopic Ultrasound (RES) for predicting deep pelvic endometriosis in specific locations and should be the first line imaging method in this setting [10]. RES appears to be the best technique for evaluating the depth of bowel infiltration by endometriosis [11].

The role of MRI in the diagnosis of endometriosis has increased after 1987, when Nishimura *et al. [12]* demonstrated the value of this imaging method in the diagnosis of endometriomas. Then the use of MRI for the evaluation of deep endometriosis was proposed by Siegelman *et al. [13]*, who studied its role in analysing solid pelvic masses. More recently other investigators [14] showed the promising results of MRI for the specific evaluation of deep endometriosis.

Also dynamic MR imaging has been tested for this purpose, showing a good accuracy in the differential diagnosis of nodular endometriosis from other pathologic conditions of abdominal wall and pelvis [15].

4. MRI technique

In our experience, MRI studies are performed with a 1.5 T magnet (Magnetom Symphony; Siemens Erlangen, Germany) and a surface phased-array coil. Patient preparation requires intravenous injection of an antispasmodic drug prior to study in order to reduce artefacts from bowel motion.

On the basis of the characteristics of our system, the standard imaging protocol includes a coronal T2-weighted HASTE sequence (half-Fourier single shot turbo spin echo: TR 700 ; TE 89; section thickness 6.0 mm; field of view 350x450 mm; matrix 320; time of acquisition 21 s), transverse T1-weighted turbo spin echo sequences from the iliac crest to the pubic sinfisis (TR 771; TE 9.7; section thickness 4.0 mm; field of view 400 x 219 mm; matrix 512x512; time of acquisition 2:46), transverse, sagittal and coronal T2-weighted turbo spin echo sequences. These sequences allow an initial complete analysis of the pelvic region and a preliminary evaluation of endometriotic lesions, which appear as hyperintense lesions in T1-weighted sequences and mildly hypointense or hyperintense in T2 weighted sequences. The FLASH T1-weighted sequences with fat suppression in transverse, coronal and sagittal plane (Fast Low-Angle Shot 2D: TR 357; TE 4.76; FA 70°; section thikness 4.5 mm; field of view 300x300 mm; matrix 256x256; time of acquisition 1:31) (T1 flash 2d fat sat) are performed to evaluate adnexal masses because they allow a distinction between a fatty content lesion (for example a teratoma, which appear hypointense in fat-suppressed T1 weighted sequences) and endometriomal cyst (that exhibits a typical hyperintense signal in such sequences). Fat-suppressed MRI is also useful in enhancing the contrast between hemorrhagic implants and normal tissue.

Contrast-enhanced FLASH T1-weighted sequences (gadolinium Gd-DTPA 0.1 mmol/kg is administrated intravenously) are performed in selected cases, expecially when a mural nodule within a hyperintense endometrioma is observed. Finally, the contrast agent is administrated when the initial images carry the suspicion of ureteral infiltration. In such cases we perform FLASH 3D T1 weighted sequences in the coronal plane with MIP recostruction of 1 mm (MR Urography) (TR: 2.96; TE 1.21; section thickness 1.40 mm; field of view 350x490 mm; matrix 384; time of acquisition 20 sec).

5. Spectrum of MRI findings

The diagnosis of endometriosis by means of MRI is based on the combination of two aspects: presence abdominal areas with morphologic and signal intensity abnormalities. Endometriotic lesions appear hyperintense on T1-weighted images and mildly hypointense or hyperintense on T2-weighted images (**Fig. 2A, B**). Gradual variation of signal intensity on T2-weighted images has been described as the "shading" sign (**Fig. 2A**) and it is due to chronic bleeding with accumulation of high concentration of iron and protein in the endometrioma.

Fat saturation allows differentiation between hemorrhagic (endometriomas) and fatty (dermoid cyst) content of cystic lesions (**Fig. 3**). Moreover, it increases detection of small implants.

Use of contrast-enhanced imaging is required to identify solid enhancing nodules within endometriotic cysts when malignant transformation is suspected or to define the extent of inflammation associated with endometriosis.

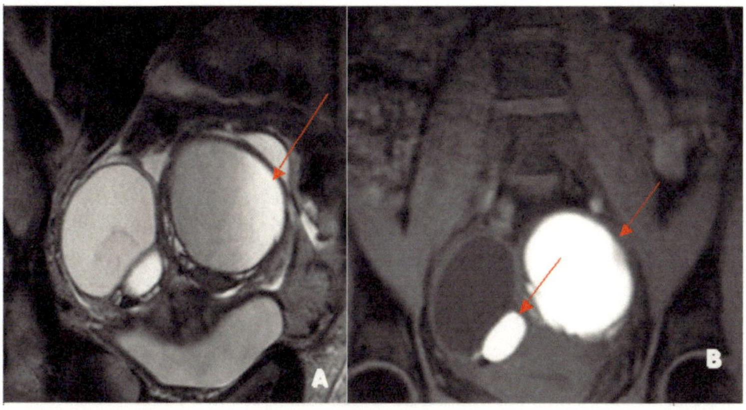

Fig. 2. Endometriotic lesions appear mildly hypointense or hyperintense on T2-weighted images (A) and hyperintense on T1-weighted images (arrows in B). Gradual variation of signal intensity on T2-weighted images has been described as "shading" sign and is due to chronic bleeding with accumulation of high concentration of iron and protein in endometriomas (arrows in A).

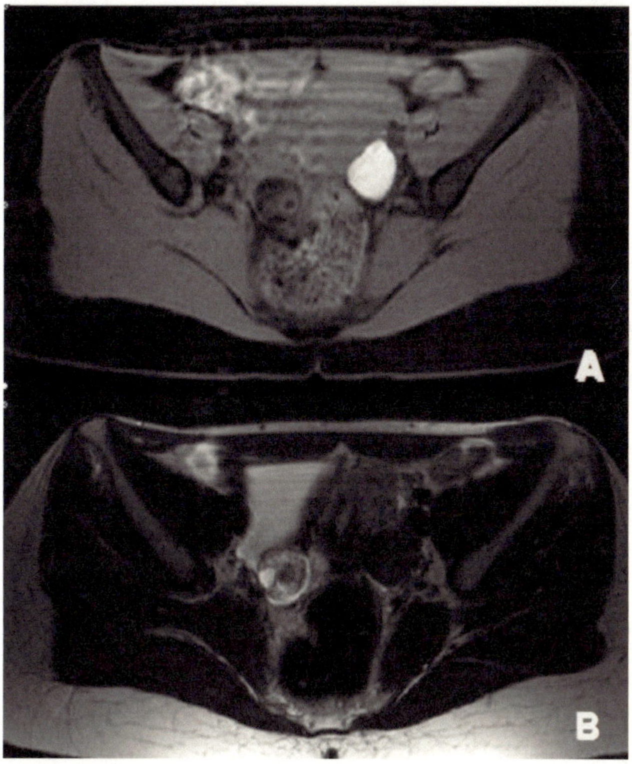

Fig. 3. T1-weighted-fat-suppressed image showing a hyperintense mass on the left ovary and a disomogenous hypointense mass on the right one (A). On T2-weighted sequence (B) the left mass appear hypointense. The left mass proved to be an endometrioma with recent hemorrhage; on the contrary, owing to its appeareance on fat-suppressed sequence, the right mass proved to be a dermoid syst.

5.1 Ovarian endometriosis

Adnexal localization is the most common clinical setting of endometriosis.

TVUS remains the first diagnostic method in the evaluation of the ovary, generally reserving MRI as a tool for resolving cases in which there is some doubt.

At MRI, a large endometrioma (>1 cm in diameter) appears as a homogeneously hyperintense mass on T1 weighted MR images and show a low signal intensity on T2 weighted MR images with areas of high signal intensity. The 'shading' sign is used to differentiate endometriomas from functional hemorrhagic cysts that do not show it, which usually disappears at subsequent MRI examinations.

Another diagnostic criteria for a definitive diagnosis of endometriomas is the presence of multiple T1 hyperintense cysts regardless of their T2 signal intensity [16].

Endometriomas are often bilateral (more than 50% of cases), multilocular or associated with interovarian adhesions; in the last case a typical MRI pattern called "kissing ovaries" could be noted (**Fig. 4**).

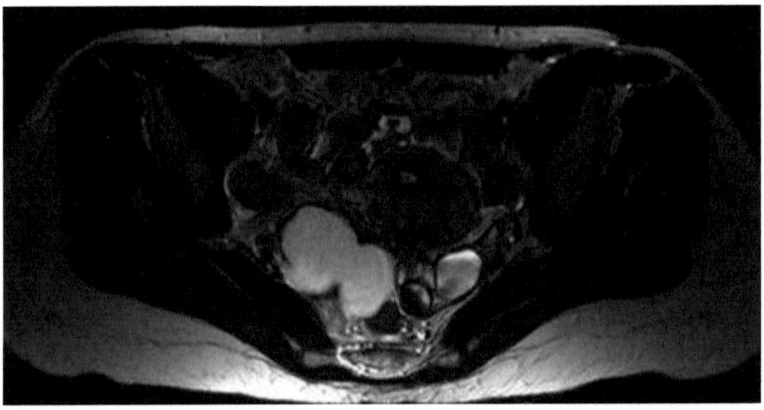

Fig. 4. T2-weighted image acquired on the transverse plane, showing hyperintense bilateral endometrioma masses on the ovaries that are closed up due to interovarian adhesions (Kissing ovaries).

Fat suppression is mandatory to differentiate endometriomas from cystic teratomas.

5.2 'Deep endometriosis'

Deep endometriotic lesions are classified according to the anatomic location in the anterior compartment (bladder) or in the posterior compartment (uterosacral ligament, vagina and bowel).

Multifocality is a major characteristic of deep endometriosis, thus requiring in some cases different surgical procedures (laparoscopy and/or laparotomy) to obtain a complete exeresis and a functional improvement.

5.3 Endometriosis of the bladder

Localization of disease in the bladder is estimated in < 1% of patients.

Uterus is usually anteflexed and the anterior cul-de-sac is obliterated due to extensive adhesions. The patient often complain pain, especially while urinating.

Two types of bladder endometriosis have been recognised. One develops exclusively after cesarean section and is considered to result from iatrogenic implantation of decidua. The other, a primary form, is found in women who have not previously undergone surgery on the uterus. Various hypotheses have been proposed to explain the pathogenesis in the latter case. Microscopically, the typical pattern is a focus of endometriosis scattered in the bladder wall. The main feature is the paucity of endometrial-type stroma [17].

MRI is reliable for the diagnosis of bladder endometriosis. Endocavitary coil MRI is reliable for establishing the depth of the lesions penetrating into the bladder wall [18].

On MRI images, bladder endometriosis can be diagnosed as a localized or diffuse bladder wall thickening, or as focal signal intensity abnormality. T2 and T1 weighted images can show a nodular hypointense mass usually located on the anterior upper or posterior bladder wall (**Fig. 5**).

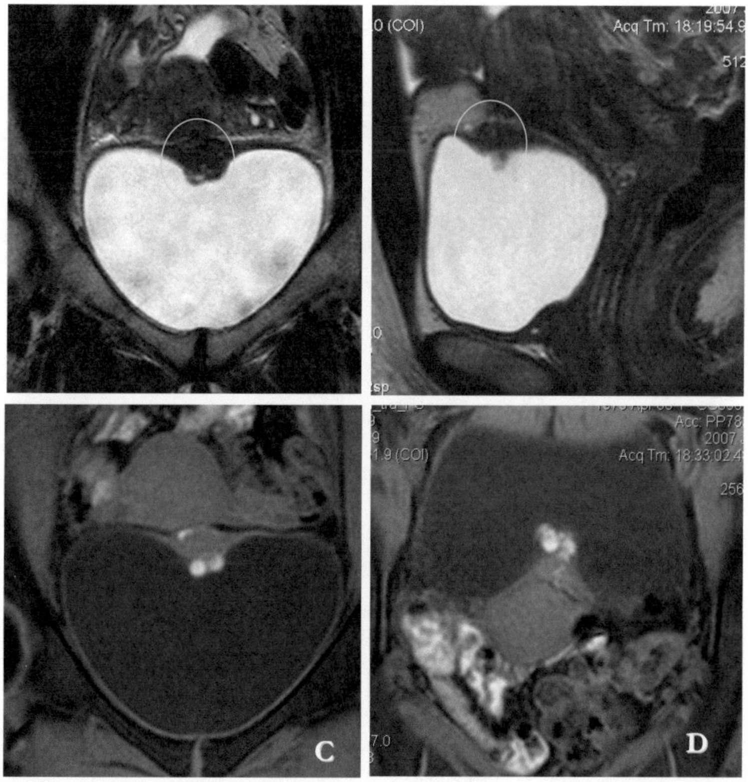

Fig. 5. Coronal (A) and sagittal (B) T2-weighted images showing localized bladder wall thickening in the anterior upper bladder wall (blue circles). On fat suppressed T1-weighted coronal (C) and axial (D) images some high signal intensity intra-lesion spots indicating recent haemorrage.

On fat suppressed T1-weighted FLASH 2d images, some high signal intensity intralesional spots are present in some cases.

5.4 Endometriosis of the uterosacral ligaments (USLs)

USLs are one of the most common targets of pelvic endometriosis, which is diagnosed more frequently in a clinical than in a surgical setting. USLs extend over a mean cranio-caudal distance of 21±8 mm. Three regions of origin have been found: cervix alone, vagina alone, cervix and vagina. Insertion points are the piriformis muscle, the sciatic foramen and the ischial spine [19].

This affliction often elicits pelvic pain, dyspareunia and painful bowel movement.

Women with endometriosis in this site present thick USLs due to endometriotic nodules and subsequently, fibrosis is responsible for cul-de-sac obliteration.

TVUS may provide quantitative information to manage patients with USLs endometriosis [20].

At MRI, involvement of USLs by endometriosis is diagnosed when the ligament appears thickened or shows irregular margins (**Fig. 6**) compared with the margins of the controlateral ligament. T2-weighted images identify all lesions as iso- or hypointense to myometrium, while T1-weighted images are less sensitive due to lesions isointensity to myometrium. The proximal portion of the ligament typically presents with asymmetric nodular thickening.

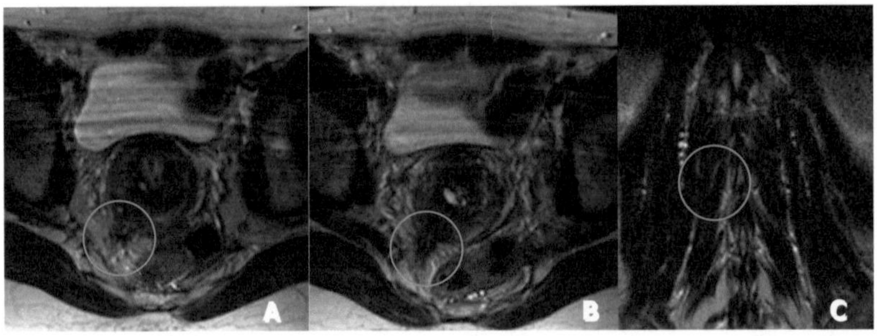

Fig. 6. Axial (A and B) and coronal (C) T2-weighted images showing irregular thickening of the right Utero-Sacral ligaments (blue circles). On the same image there is infiltration of the rectal serosa (blue circle).

Fat-suppressed T1-weighted images sometimes demonstrate hyperintense spots that correlate with hemorrhagic endometrial implants on the ligament (**Fig. 7**).

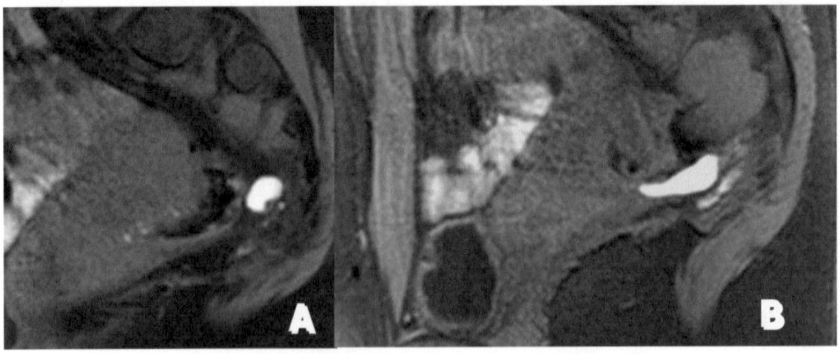

Fig. 7. Fat-suppressed T1-weighted images demonstrate hyperintense spots that correlate with hemorrhagic endometrial implants on the ligament (A, B).

In patients with USLs involvement adhesions could often develop thus, providing posterior displacement of the uterus and ovaries, angulation of bowel loops, elevation of the posterior vaginal fornix, and loculated fluid collections [21]. At MRI, adhesions are detected when low signal intensity is found within the ligaments.

5.5 Endometriosis of the vagina

Endometriosis of the vagina includes lesions infiltrating the anterior rectovaginal pouch, posterior vaginal fornix and retroperitoneal area between the anterior rectovaginal pouch and posterior vaginal fornix.

Patients tipycally refer dyspareunia.

MRI represents the ideal complement to physical examination and TVUS in order to predict lesion extension upward and posteriorly. Sometimes, the use of a water enema is used to predict the extension of the lesion toward the rectum.

In patients with vaginal endometriosis axial and sagittal T2-weighted Turbo Spin Echo images usually show hypointense nodules. Anterior attraction of the rectum toward the torus uteri and asymmetric thickening of the rectal wall are associated to rectal wall infiltration. Determining the depth of infiltration of the rectal wall allows the gynaecologist to discuss the surgical approach (nodulectomy vs bowel resection) with the colorectal surgeon. The use of the endorectal coil optimizes the finding of MRI [22].

T1-weighted images with fat suppression could demonstrate T1 isointensity of the nodule and some small hyperintense foci, suspected for micro-haemorragies (**Fig. 8 A**).

Most patients with vaginal involvement also demonstrate obliteration of the retrouterine excavation (**Fig. 8 B, C**); in such cases the extension of the pelvic focus may lead to ureteral infiltration and ureterohydronephrosis.

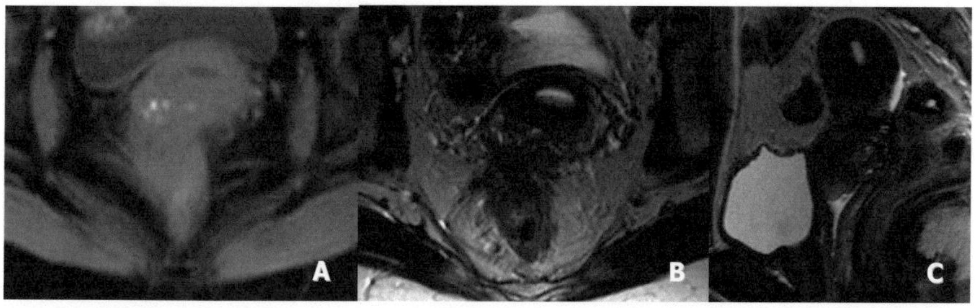

Fig. 8. T1-weighted image with fat suppression demonstrates isointensity of the nodule and some small hyperintense foci, suspected for micro-haemorragies (A). Axial (B) and sagittal (C) T2-weighted image show obliteration of retrouterine escavation by an hypointense nodule, with anterior attraction of the rectum toward the torus uteri and asymmetric thickening of the rectal wall.

5.6 Endometriosis of the bowel

Rectosigmoid endometriosis represents 70% of cases of intestinal endometriosis.

Clinical symptoms of patients with endometriosis of the recto-sigmoid colon are manifested as crampy pain, flatulence, painful tenesmus, constipation, diarrhoea and bowel obstruction.

Among patients with rectosigmoid endometriosis also dyspareunia is another common symptom. Endometriosis less frequently affects appendix, cecum and distal ileum.

The implants are usually serosal but they can erode through the subserosal layers and cause a fibromuscular hyperplasia of the muscularis propria. Due to the normal appearance of the mucosa in most patients with bowel endometriosis, diagnosis by colonoscopy is often false negative. The appearance of gastrointestinal implants on double-contrast barium enema images is characterized in most cases by a puckering or a crenulated appearance of the affected wall; when the lesion causes a circumferential narrowing of the rectosigmoid colon the differential diagnosis with a primary colon carcinoma is difficult.

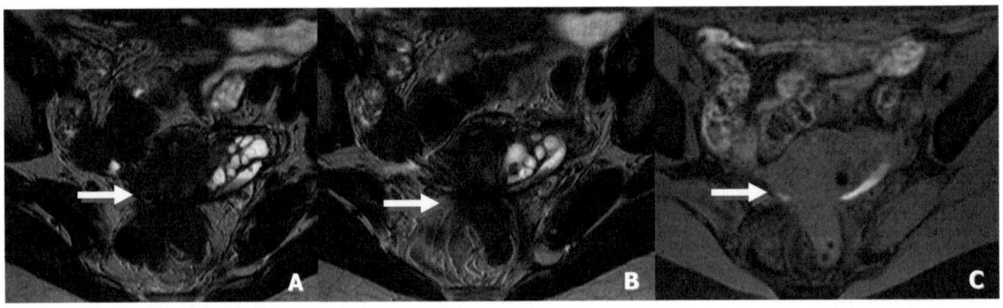

Fig. 9. Diagnostic criteria of bowel invasion at MRI are: colorectal wall thickening with traction of the rectum toward the torus uteri (A, B, C).

At MRI, bowel lesions show a signal intensity similar to fibromuscular tissue (hypointense), with occasional hyperintense foci of T1- and T2- weighted images. An asymmetric thickening of the lower surface of the sigmoid wall or a colorectal wall thickening with attraction of the rectum toward the torus uteri is a common sign (**Fig. 9**).

According to Roy C *et al* [23], the use of the contrast media helps in reaching the diagnosis of an invasion inside the muscular layer of the intestinal wall. In such cases a thin bright layer on T2-weighted images together with post-contrast enhancement on fat-suppressed T1-weighted images and obliteration of fatty tissue plane between the nodule and the intestinal wall, represents the diagnostic clue of muscular layers involvement. Combined pelvic-phased array and endovaginal coils improve the diagnostic power in the detection of intestinal wall invasion, when compared to phased array alone.

5.7 Malignant transformation

A limited number of endometriosis patients (<5%) will develop ovarian cancer.

Women with endometriosis-associated cancer are typically pre-menopausal, have high incidence of endometrioid and clear cell histologies, and have early stage disease [24].

The association between endometriosis and intra-peritoneal cancer still remains unclear. Probably, women with endometriosis are more susceptible to malignant transformation because of a deficit in their immune system that enables the endometriosis to flourish. Also estrogen may play a role, so endometriosis should be closely monitored in women in the reproductive age [25].

The typical morphologic appearance of an endometriosis-associated carcinoma is that of a unilateral large cystic mass containing hemorrhagic fluid and mural nodules. Signal intensity is low on T1-weighted images and variable on T2-weighted images. Contrast enhancement of a mural nodule at fat-suppressed T1-weighted sequences is the most important finding for a diagnosis of malignant shift. The "shading" sign within the cystic mass is rarely observed on T2-weighted images because of the diluition of the hemorrhagic fluid caused by tumor secretions. Accordingly, disappearance of the "shading" sign within the mass on T2-weighted images is a diagnostic clue to its malignancy [26].

6. Conclusions

MRI is progressively becoming a widely employed technique in the diagnosis and preoperative staging of endometriosis. It should be performed in selected patients according to the results of TVUS and the severity of symptoms. This imaging method has the advantage to cover the entire pelvis thus, helping the surgeon to achieve a complete resection and prevent post-surgical recurrence.

7. References

[1] Missmer SA & Cramer DW. The epidemiology of endometriosis. Obstetrics and Gynecology Clinics of North America 2003 ; 30 : 1-19

[2] Olive DL, Schwartz LB. Endometriosis. N Engl J Med 1993; 328:1759–1769

[3] Chapron C, Fauconnier A, Vieira M, Barakat H, Dousset B, Pansini V, Vacher-Lavenu MC, Dubuisson J.B.. Anatomical Distribution of deeply infiltrating endometriosis : surgical implications and proposition for a classification. Hum Reprod 2003; 18:157-161.

[4] Revised American fertility Society classification of endometriosis: 1985. Fertil Steril 1985; 43: 351-352.

[5] Tuttlies F. et al. ENZIAN-Score, eine Klassifikation der tief infiltrierenden Endometriose: Zentralbl Gynacol 2005; 127: 275-282.

[6] Clement PB. Diseases of the peritoneum. In: Kurman RJ, ed. Blaustein's pathology of the female genital tract. 4th ed New York, NY: Springer-Verlag, 1994; 660-680.

[7] Okaro E, Valentin L. The role of ultrasound in the management of women with acute and chronic pelvic pain. Best Practice and Research Clinical Obstetrics and Gynaecology 2004, Vol 18 No 1 1 pp 105-123.

[8] Mais V, Guerriero S, Ajossa S, Angiolucci M, Paoletti AM, Melis GB. The efficiency of transvaginal ultrasonography in the diagnosis of endometrioma. Fertil and Steril 1993, 60:776-780.

[9] Guerriero S, Mais V, Ajossa S, Paoletti AM, Angiolucci M, Melis GB. Transvaginal ultrasonography combined with CA-125 plasma levels in the diagnosis of endometrioma. Fertil and Steril 1996, 65:293-298.

[10] Bazot M., Malzy P., Cortez A., Roseau G., Amouyal P., Darai E. Accuracy of transvaginale sonosgraphy and rectal endoscopic sonography in the diagnosis of deep infiltrating endometriosis. Ultrasound Obstet Gynecol 2007; 30:994-1001.

[11] Chapron C, Vieira M., Chopin N, Balleyguier C, Barakat H, Dumontier I, Roseau G, Fauconnier A, Foulot H, Dousset B. Accuracy of rectal endoscopic ultrasonography and magnetic resonance imaging in the diagnosis of rectal involvement for patients presenting with deeply infiltrating endometriosis. Ultrasound Obstet Gynecol 2004; 24:175-179.

[12] Nishimura K, Togashi K, Itoh K, Fujisawa I, Noma S, Kawamura Y, Nakano Y, Itoh H, Torizuka K, Ozasa H. Endometrial cysts of the ovary: MR imaging. Radiology. 1987 Feb;162(2):315-8.

[13] Siegelman ES, Outwater E, Wang T, Mitchell DG. Solid pelvic masses caused by endometriosis: MR imaging features. AJR Am J Roentgenol. 1994 Aug;163(2):357-61.

[14] Bazot M, Darai E, Hourani R, Thomassin I, Cortez A, Uzan S, Buy JN. Deep pelvic endometriosis: MR imaging for diagnosis and prediction of extension of disease. Radiology. 2004 Aug;232(2):379-89

[15] Onbas O, Kantarci M, Alper F, Kumtepe Y, Durur I, Ingec M, Gursan N, Okur A. Nodular endoimetriosis: dynamic MR imaging. Abdominal Imaging 2007, 32: 451-456.

[16] Togashi K, Nishimura K, Kimura I et al . Endometrial cysts: diagnosis with MR imaging. Radiology 1991. 180: 73-78.

[17] Fedele L, Piazzola E, Raffaelli R, Bianchi S. Bladder endometriosis: deep infiltrating endometriosis or adenomyosis?. Fertil and Steril. 1998; 69: 972-974.

[18] Halleguier C, Chapron C, Dubuisson J B, Kinkel K, Fauconnier A, Vieira M et al.. Comparison of Magnetic Resonance Imaging and Transvaginal Ultrasonography in diagnosing bladder endometriosis. The journal of the American Association of Gynecologic Laparoscopy 2002; 9 (1) 15-23.

[19] Umek W H, Morgan D M, Ashton-Miller J A, DeLancey J O L. Quantitative analysis of uterosacral ligament origin and insertion points by magnetic resonance imaging. The American College of Obstetricians and Gynecologists. 2004; vol 103, no. 3, 447-451.

[20] Ohba T, Mizutani H, Maeda T, Matsuura K, Okamura H. Evaluation of endometriosis in uterosacral ligaments by transrectal ultrasonography. Human Reproduction 1996; vol 11 no.9 2014-17.

[21] Zawin M, McCarthy S, Scoutt L, Comite F. Endometriosis: appearance and detection at MR imaging. Radiology 1989; 171:693–696

[22] Kinkel K, Chapron C, Balleyguier C, Fritel X, Dubuisson JB, Moreau JF. Magnetic resonance imaging characteristics of deep endometriosis. Hum Reprod. 1999 Apr;14(4):1080-6.

[23] Roy C, Balzan C, Thoma V, Sauer B, wattiez A, Leroy J. Efficiency of MR imaging to orientate surgical treatment of posterior deep pelvic endometriosis. Abdom Imaging 2008; XX:1-9.

[24] S. C. Modessitt, G. Tortolero-Luna, J. B. Robinson. D.M. Gerhenson, J.K. Wolf Ovarian and Extraovarian-Associated Cancer The American College of Obstetricians and Gynecologists Vol. 100, No. 4, October 2002 788- 794

[25] Mc Meekin DS, Burger RA, Manetta A, Di Saia P, Barman ML. Endometrioid adenocarcinoma of the ovary and its relationship to endometriosis. Gynecol Oncol. 1995; 59:81-86

[26] M Takeuchi, K Matsuzaki, H. Uehara, H. Nishitani. Malignant transformation of Pelvic Endometriosis: MR Imaging findings and pathologic correlation. Radiographics 2006; 26:407-417

26

Pathophysiological Changes in Early Endometriosis

Tao Zhang, Gene Chi Wai Man and Chi Chiu Wang
Department of Obstetrics and Gynaecology, The Chinese University of Hong Kong, Prince of Wales Hospital, Shatin, New Territories, Hong Kong

1. Introduction

Endometriosis is a common but complex gynecological disorder of unknown pathogenesis. It is characterized by ectopic growth of endometrial tissues. Based on Sampson's classical implantation theory, retrograde menstruation, immune escape, adhesion, angiogenesis and growth of endometrial cells are essential milestones in the pathogenesis of endometriosis. The cellular communications of immune, endothelial and endometriotic cells during endometriosis development are mediated via cytokines and chemokines. Many specific cytokines in peritoneal fluid of patients with endometriosis are aberrant from normal women. However, it's not clear at which stage of endometriosis these aberrant cytokines begin to change and owing to the limitation with human study the functions of these cytokines were only investigated in vitro. On the other hand, the onset of angiogenesis is initiated by oxidative stress due to cellular and tissue hypoxia, which is mainly coordinated by the hypoxia-inducible factors (HIFs). HIFs stimulate VEGF transcription and activation in endometriosis lesions in acquiring new blood vessels for survival and growth. Monitoring inflammatory response, oxidative stress and angiogenesis in the endometriosis lesions is of vital importance in understanding the pathophysiological changes during early development of endometriosis.

In our studies, we investigated for the first time the dynamic changes of oxygen reactive species and angiogenesis in the endometriosis implants by in vivo imaging techniques and characterized regulation of cytokines, hypoxia and angiogenesis factors within the first 24 hour of experimental endometriosis in mice. We identified significant oxidative stress and hypoxia responses in the endometriosis implants in early phase only, but specific estrogen-dependent cytokine activations and angiogenesis signaling in late phase. In this chapter, we will describe the non-invasive in vivo imaging method as a valuable tool for monitoring oxidative stress and angiogenesis in endometriosis and to understand its role in the early development and growth of endometriosis. We will also demonstrate oxidative stress preceded hypoxia and cytokine activation and angiogenesis signaling in the pathogenesis of early endometriosis.

2. Development of endometriosis

2.1 Sampson's implantation theory

Endometriosis is one of most common gynecological disorder, but poorly understood condition. As early as in 1860, von Rokitansky (Rokitansky, 1860) is the first one to describe this disease in detail. Since then, several postulated theories explaining the pathogenesis of endometriosis were raised. The most popular theory is Sampson's classical implantation theory in 1921 (Sampson, 1921). He proposed that the endometrial fragments of uterine endometrium during menstruation can regurgitate through the fallopian tubes and survive in the peritoneal cavity, developing to endometriosis.

There have been numerous studies in human and primate support the implantation theory (Bartosik et al., 1986; Halme et al., 1984). However, this hypothesis cannot explain why only about 10% women suffer from endometriosis, but the incidence of retrograde menstruation should be much higher. What's more, the endometriotic lesion sometimes is present out of peritoneal cavity, such as lungs, brain and heart, instead of peritoneal cavity only (Felson et al., 1960; Joseph et al., 1994; Thibodeau et al., 1987). Besides, genetic, immunological factors and vascular and lymphatic spread are also essential for endometriosis development. Therefore, endometriosis is multifactorial and complicated condition. More studies are needed to explicitly understand the pathogenesis of endometriosis.

2.2 Pathophysiology

With numerous clinical and basic researches on endometriosis, especially peritoneal endometriosis, based on Sampson's retrograde menstruation theory, it's well accepted that the appearance of vital endometrial cells is the first step. Then immune escape, adhesion, implantation, angiogenesis and proliferation are all very important during the development of endometriosis (Fig. 1).

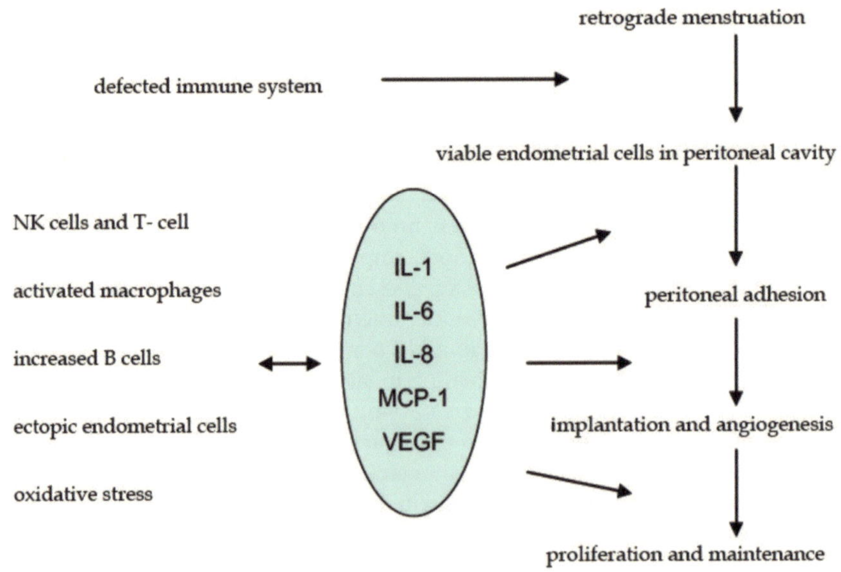

Fig. 1. Summary of the development of endometriosis

In healthy women, macrophages, lymphocytes, natural killer cells and leukocytes eliminate ectopic endometrial cells (Braun *et al.*, 1996). Though the number of immune cells in peritoneal fluid of women with endometriosis was significantly higher than women without this disease, the function of increased immune cells was decreased (Berkkanoglu *et al.*, 2003). Meanwhile, these defected immune cells may secrete some cytokines and growth factors, such as interleukin-1 (IL-1), interleukin-8 (IL-8), monocyte chemotactic protein 1 (MCP-1) and vascular endothelial growth factor (VEGF) etc., which may help the endometrial cells escape from immune surveillance to adhere to the peritoneum, establish microvessels and finally grow under the stimulation of estrogen cycle (Kyama *et al.*, 2003). However, the reasons causing impaired immune cells are not known. When and what kind of cells as well as molecules taking part in the process from survival to steady growth are still not clear.

2.3 Cellular communications

Endometrial cells have to contact with immune cells, peritoneal lining and vascular endothelial before final growth and maintenance in ectopic location. Cellular immune response is responsible for implantation of the retrograde and vital endometrial cells. The molecules secreted by immune cells would effect the reaction between endometrial cells and other cells.

2.3.1 Macrophages

Macrophages are the most abundant immune cells in peritoneal fluid and their main role is to phagocytose cellular debris and pathogens. They can also promote lymphocytes and other immune cells to respond to pathogens (Tariverdian *et al.*, 2009; van Furth *et al.*, 1979). It has been reported that the number and activity of macrophages in peritoneal fluid significantly increased. However they cannot clear the ectopic endometrial cells and inhibit the development of endometriosis. Modulators of activated macrophages for both immune and non-immune cells promote growth and maintenance of ectopic lesion (Lebovic *et al.*, 2001). There are several evidence to support the change of receptors expression on macrophages leads to impaired scavenger function, which might be caused by abnormal cytokines and growth factors in the peritoneal fluid of women with endometriosis (Berkkanoglu *et al.*, 2003).

2.3.2 Lymphocytes

The two main types of lymphocytes are: B cells accounting for humoral acquired response by secreting soluble antibodies into the body's fluids for eliminating foreign antigens, and T cells responsible for cellular responses. Both of which recognize specific antigen targets. T cells are mainly differentiated into helper T cells promoting antibody production secreted by B cells, regulatory T cells controlling immune response, and cytotoxic/suppressor T cells killing infected cells and cancer cells in the thymus. In endometriosis, it was reported that the proliferation and cytotoxic activity of lymphocytes in peripheral blood is decreased (Dmowski *et al.*, 1981; Steele *et al.*, 1984). Increased T cells, both helper and suppressor T cells, in peritoneal fluid and ectopic endometriotic tissue was observed in women with endometriosis (Dmowski *et al.*, 1994; Hill *et al.*, 1988; Mettler *et al.*, 1996). However, the changes are not consistent. Besides, the function and activity of peripheral T cells might be different from those in peritoneal fluid. In all, it's controversial if the alteration of lymphocytes in peripheral and peritoneal fluid play a role in the development of endometriosis.

2.3.3 Natural killer cells

Natural killer cells (NK cells) constitute a major component of the innate immune system. They have two ways to take part in host defense by expressing different receptors binding to target cells. One receptor type binds immunoglobulin G (IgG). The other includes killer-activating receptors promoting cytotoxic activity and killer-inhibitory receptors (KIR) suppressing cytotoxic activity (Moretta *et al.*, 1995). Oosterlynck and Wilson have found that the cytotoxic activity of peripheral and peritoneal fluid NK cells from women with endometriosis was obviously decreased with the severity of endometriosis (Oosterlynck *et al.*, 1991; Wilson *et al.*, 1994). The decreased NK-mediated cytotoxicity in the peritoneal fluid might contribute to the establishment of endometriosis. The mechanisms that cause aberrant NK cell cytotoxicity are unclear, but seem to be involved in KIR expression (Wu *et al.*, 2000). In a recent study, Maeda et al. reported KIR2DL1 as the subclass of KIR overexpressed on NK cells in peripheral and peritoneal fluid of patients with endometriosis.

2.3.4 Peritoneal cells

Several adhesion moleculars were found to be expressed in endometrium, which mediate the adhesion and invasion of endometrial cells to peritoneum. Koks found that endometrium preferentially adhere to the extracellular matrix (ECM) of the peritoneum mediated by integrin (Koks *et al.*, 2000). Endometrium expresses various integrins during menstruation shedding and the adhesion can be disrupted by blocking integrin. Integrins are cell-surface glycoproteins acting as receptors for ECM proteins. In normal eutopic endometrium, integrins are important in the interaction between glandular epithelial and stromal cells, and essential for implantation (Lessey *et al.*, 1992). After adherence of endometrial cells to the peritoneum, local degradation of the ECM is required for invasion and implantation. Metalloproteinases (MMPs) causing ECM breakdown, tissue collapse and menstruation was up-regulated in late secretory phase (Salamonsen *et al.*, 1996). This implies that the vital endometrial cells in peritoneal cavity during menstruation shedding already have the potential to invade into peritoneum. What's more, MMPs are present independent of the cycle phase in peritoneal and ovarian endometriosis (Salamonsen *et al.*, 1996), which promotes endometriotic cells to infiltrate into peritoneum further although endometriosis has been established.

2.3.5 Vascular endothelial cells

The ectopic endometrial cells require an accessible blood supply to proliferate and invade through the peritoneum after escaping immune surveillance. Greater angiogenic activity have been found in the peritoneal fluid of women with endometriosis, which are modulated by growth factors and cytokines such as VEGF & IL-8 secreted by ectopic endometrial cells and defected immune cells (Oosterlynck *et al.*, 1993). VEGF is a mitogen for endothelial cells and stimulates the proliferation of both vascular and lymphatic endothelial cells in vitro (Joukov *et al.*, 1997) and promotes angiogenesis or hyperplasia of lymphatic vessels in vivo (Jeltsch *et al.*, 1997). Increasing evidence indicate that VEGF plays an important role in the angiogenesis of peritoneal endometriosis (McLaren, 2000). VEGF is elevated in the peritoneal fluid and endometriotic lesion of women with endometriosis and correlated with the severity of this disease (McLaren *et al.*, 1996). Its expression is more pronounced around red endometriotic lesions as compared with the more inactive black implants (Donnez *et al.*, 1998).

2.4 Molecular modulations

Cellular communications in endometriosis mediated by inflammatory cytokines and growth factors is mainly regulated by nuclear factor-κB (NF-κB) signaling pathway (Fig. 2) (Gonzalez-Ramos *et al.*). NF-κB mediated gene transcription promoting inflammation, invasion, angiogenesis, and cell proliferation and inhibiting apoptosis of endometriotic cells through p50/p65 dimers and NF-κB inhibitor IκBα has been found *in vitro* and *in vivo* studies (Gonzalez-Ramos *et al.*, 2010). Constitutive activation of NF-κB has been demonstrated in endometriotic lesions and peritoneal macrophages of patients with endometriosis (Laird *et al.*, 2000). Some drugs such as GnRH blocking NF-κB have been proven efficient at reducing endometriosis-associated symptoms in women (Han *et al.*, 2003). Overload iron produced by erythrocytes from menstruation shedding and cytokines such as interleukin-1 (IL-1) and tumor necrosis factor-α (TNF-α) as well as oxidative stress stimulate NF-κB activation in macrophages and ectopic endometrial cells, which stimulates synthesis of proinflammatory cytokines, sending a positive feedback loop to the NF-κB signaling pathway. NF-κB activation enhances factors of anti-apoptosis, growth, invasion and angiogenesis as well as proinflammatory cytokines such as cyclooxygenase 2 (COX-2), vascular endothelial growth factor (VEGF), macrophage migration inhibitory factor (MIF), interleukin-1 (IL-1) and tumor necrosis factor-α (TNF-α), which promote the development of endometriosis. Intercellular adhesion molecule-1 (ICAM-1) and RANTES up-regulated by NF-κB activity could attract more macrophages to sites of inflammation.

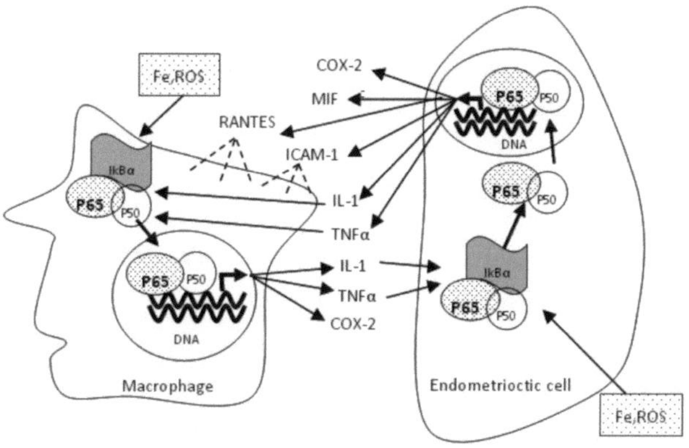

Fig. 2. NF-κB signaling pathway in endometriosis

3. Early pathogenesis

3.1 Oxidative stress

Oxidative stress has been proposed as a potential factor in the pathogenesis of endometriosis (Van Langendonckt *et al.*, 2002). Oxidative stress may occur when the balance of reactive oxygen species (ROS) and antioxidant is disturbed. Several studies have demonstrated that the oxidative stress is involved in endometriosis with increased concentration of ROS, enzymes producing ROS and lower concentration of antioxidant in peritoneal fluid and in the eutopic and ectopic endometrium of women with endometriosis (Ota *et al.*, 2001; Zeller *et al.*, 1987). It's postulated that oxidative stress is stimulated by erythrocytes (Brosens, 1994), apoptotic endometrial tissue, cell debris and macrophages (Murphy *et al.*, 1998). These inducers may cause activation and recruitment of mononuclear phagocytes which induce oxidative stress. Oxidative stress might lead to a localized pelvic inflammatory reaction with increased pro-inflammatory mediators, cytokines and growth factors (Gupta *et al.*, 2006). These cytokines and growth factors have been widely accepted to promote the immune modulation, adhesion, invasion and angiogenesis of endometriosis. Therefore, understanding of oxidative stress could give a light in the initiation and process of angiogenesis and inflammation during the development of endometriosis. However, two other studies could not find the imbalance between ROS and antioxidant in the peritoneal fluid of women with endometriosis (Ho *et al.*, 1997; Wang *et al.*, 1997). This discrepancy might be due to the use of markers of oxidative stress. Thus, further studies are needed to identify when and how oxidative stress play a role in the pathophysiology of endometriosis in particular during early development.

3.2 Proinflammatory responses

It's widely accepted that endometriosis is a pelvic inflammatory process with defected function of immune system and increased level of abnormal cytokines, chemokines and growth factors in the peritoneal fluid modulating the growth and inflammation of endometriosis. The proinflammatory cytokines and chemokines involved in development of endometriosis include IL-1, IL-6, IL-8, MCP-1 and RANTES (Table 1). These cytokines are mostly secreted by activated immune cells and endometrial cells. They act as paracrine and autocrine messengers in cellular communication. On the one hand, some of these cytokines mediate the adhesion of endometrial cells to peritoneum, such as ICAM-1 and TNF-α and promote proliferation of endometrial cells, such as IL8, as well as stimulate angiogenesis such as VEGF. On the other hand, some cytokines modulate immune cells function: transforming growth factor beta (TGF-β) inhibiting T and B lymphocytes and NK cells which may cause immune tolerance; MCP-1 activating macrophages. The imbalance and abnormal distribution of peritoneal fluid cytokines and their functions imply that inflammation plays a key role in the development of endometriosis.

Whether pelvic inflammation cause endometriosis or endometriosis results in pelvic inflammation is still not well defined. Due to the unsatisfactory diagnostic methods and the limitation of human researches, we are not able to answer this question in human because most patients have had endometriosis for an unknown disease course at the time of diagnosis. Studying endometriosis using animal models complement the understanding endometriosis in human. Chen et al. have found that the endometrial cells in the peritoneal fluid induced the production of IL-1β, TNF-α, VEGF and MCP-1 at 24 hours in the peritoneal fluid of mice. (Chen *et al.*). Similarly, IL-2, IL-4, IL-6, IL-10 and MCP-1, eosinophil chemotactic protein (eotaxin), macrophage inflammatory protein and RANTES as well as CC chemokine receptor (CCR1) were found remarkably expressed in endometriotic lesions on the 4th day in rat model by autologous transplantation of endometrial epithelial fragment to peritoneum (Umezawa *et al.*, 2008). These inflammation cytokines found in early endometriosis is consistent with those found in peritoneal fluid of women with endometriosis. Based on this finding, it can be supposed that endometrial cells in peritoneal cavity might cause inflammation mediating and promoting the development of endometriosis. More studies about early endometriosis are necessary to confirm this hypothesis.

Cytokines	Functions	References
IL-1	Activates T-lymphocytes	(Vigano *et al.*, 1998)
	Differentiates B cells	(Lebovic *et al.*, 2000)
	Increase IL-6, sICAM-1, IL-8 & VEGF	(Arici *et al.*, 1993)
IL-6	Stimulate B cell activity	(Le *et al.*, 1989)
	Differentiate T cells	(Giudice, 1994)
	Stimulate angiogenesis	(Lin *et al.*, 2006)
IL-8	Promote proliferation of endometrial and endometriotic stromal cells	(Iwabe *et al.*, 1998)
	Stimulate adhesion of endometrial cells to fibronectin	(Arici *et al.*, 1998)
	Recruit neutrophils and lymphocytes	(Garcia-Velasco *et al.*, 1999)
MCP-1	Activate macrophages	(Oral *et al.*, 1996)
	Stimulate endometrial cell proliferation	(Arici *et al.*, 1997)
RANTES	Attract macrophages and lymphcytes	(Khorram *et al.*, 1993)
ICAM-1	Mediate cell adhesion	(Oral *et al.*, 1996)
	Inhibit NK cells cytotoxicity	(Koninckx *et al.*, 1998)
TGF-β	Attract monocytes	(Oosterlynck *et al.*, 1994)
	Inhibit T and B lymphocytes and NK cell activity	
TNF-α	Initiate the cascade of cytokines and inflammatory response	(Laird *et al.*, 1996)
	Increase the adherence of cultured endometrial stromal cells	(Zhang *et al.*, 1993)
VEGF	Stimulate angiogenesis; Attract monocytes	(McLaren *et al.*, 1996)

Table 1. Functions of cytokines and growth factors involved in endometriosis

3.3 Angiogenesis

The establishment of new blood vessels is essential in growth and survival of endometriosis. Increased angiogenic activity has been demonstrated in peritoneal fluid of women with endometriosis and strong expression of angiogenic factors has been shown in active lesions (Donnez *et al.*, 1998; Nisolle *et al.*, 1993). Moreover, inhibition of endometrial implants by anti-angiogenic agents or VEGF receptors (VEGFR) blocker was observed in animal studies (Dabrosin *et al.*, 2002; Nap *et al.*, 2004). Many anti-angiogenic compounds are studied extensively in animal models of endometriosis. Vlahos stated that pentoxifylline used in the treatment of peripheral vascular disease for many years may cause suppression of endometriotic tissue by inhibiting angiogenesis through VEGF-C and VEGFR-2 expression in rat model (Vlahos *et al.*). Besides, progestins already used in the treatment of endometriosis inhibit human ectopic endometrial lesions in a mouse model by regulating cysteine-rich angiogenic inducer (CYR61), basic fibroblast growth factor (bFGF) and VEGFA (Monckedieck *et al.*, 2009). Endostain, a potent endogenous inhibitor of blood vessel growth, suppress angiogenesis by inhibiting endothelial migration without effecting normal estrous cycles (Becker *et al.*, 2006). What's more, either selective cyclooxygenase-2 (COX-2) inhibitor or immunoconjugate molecule (Icon) suppress angiogenesis in animal models by microvessels density assessment (Krikun *et al.*). However, there is no study to investigate the early process of angiogenesis in endometriosis, which makes new anti-angiogenesis therapy possible for prevention of reoccurrence after surgical treatment.

4. Experimental designs

Oxidative stress, proinflammatory responses and angiogenesis of endometriosis are important during early development of endometriosis. We postulate that the refluxed endometrial tissues in peritoneal cavity could stimulate oxidative stress and proinflammatory cytokines which promote the endometriotic adhesion, angiogenesis and implantation (Fig. 3). The methods we used are complementary to each other's insufficiency (Table 2).

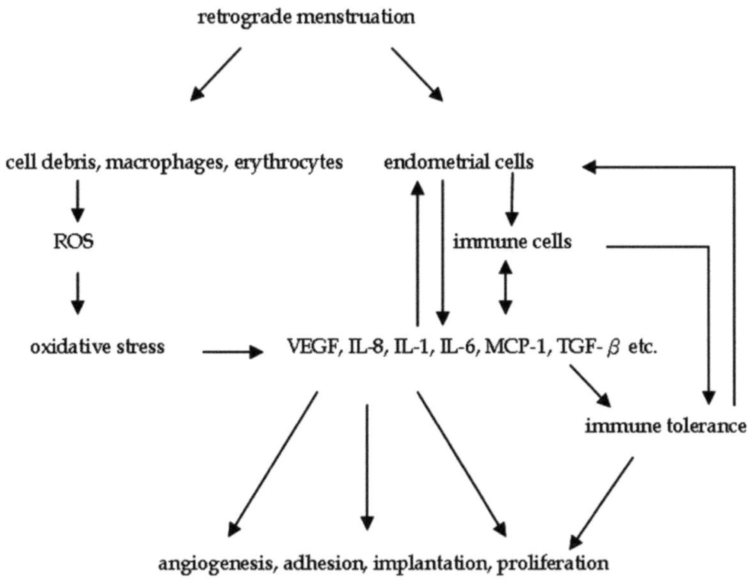

Fig. 3. Summary of early pathogenesis in endometriosis

	Method	Advantage	Disadvantage
Oxidative stress	IVIS	*in vivo*, longitudinal, semi-quantitative	Expensive
	ROS or RNS markers	*in vitro*, quantitative, sensitive	non-longitudinal, not stable
Angiogenesis	Cellvizio, IVIS	*in vivo*, longitudinal, semi-quantitative	expensive, superficial vessels
	Angiogenic markers	*in vitro*, quantitative	non-longitudinal
Cytokines	Antibody Array	small sample, all cytokines, semi-quantitative	expensive, non-longitudinal
	Multiplex	small sample, selected cytokines, quantitative	expensive, non-longitudinal
	ELISA	large sample, specific cytokines, quantitative, sensitive	non-longitudinal

Table 2. Comparison of available study methods

4.1 Oxidative stress in early endometriosis

In order to monitor the oxidative stress response in early development of endometriosis, an experimental endometriosis model in C57 mice was established by subcutaneous injection of mouse endometrium fragments. A chemiluminescent probe, L-012 (25mg/kg s.c.), was injected to the mice for the noninvasive *in vivo* oxidative stress imaging. L-012 is a new luminol derivative and sensitive chemiluminescence probe reacting with various types of ROS. ROS and reactive nitrogen species (RNS) production in the transplanted lesion can be monitored longitudinally by Xenogen IVIS 200 Imaging System. The results showed that *In vivo* imaging demonstrated significant increased bioluminescence signals for ROS/RNS from the transplanted lesions at the first hour interval. The signal reached a peak after 4 hours of transplantation. Then, the signal gradually decreased and maintained at minimal intensity in the rest of experiment. Immunohistochemistry showed positive lag correlation for the stained Hypoxia-inducible factors (HIF-1) in glandular epithelial cells and stromal tissue from the isolated lesions across the later time after transplantation. For angiogenesis, CD34, VEGF and Von Willebrand factor (vWF) signals were increased in parallel with HIF expression at 1 week thereafter. The non-invasive *in vivo* imaging method provides a valuable tool for monitoring oxidative stress in endometriosis and to understand its role in the early development and growth of endometriosis. The study indicated oxidative stress preceded HIF activation and VEGF angiogenesis in the pathogenesis of early endometriosis.

4.2 Cytokine profiling in early endometriosis

Both donor and recipient BALB/c mice at 7 weeks old were subjected to ovariectomy (OVX) and then were supplemented with 100ug/kg estradiol. Uterine horns from the donor mice were removed into F12 medium. Endometrium was punched into endometrial fragments after peeling off the serosa and myometrium under microscope. Fragments suspended in 0.3ml PBS were injected into peritoneal cavity of recipient mice. Peritoneal fluid was collected at experiment time intervals after transplantation. Cytokines profiles in peritoneal fluid were detected simultaneously. Differentially expressed cytokines were confirmed by ELISA quantification.

The results showed that the levels of CD30, CD36/SR-B3, Dickkopf-related protein (Dkk-1), epidermal growth factor (EGF), Eotaxin, IL-1 receptor antagonist (IL-1ra), IL-6 and Vascular cell adhesion protein 1 (VCAM-1) were significantly increased with the first hour of transplantation. This is the first report to analyze the peritoneal fluid cytokines profiles in experimental endometriosis in mice. The change pattern of cytokines could provide insights in understanding the early development of endometriosis. From the results, we can see that the oxidative stress and abnormal cytokine profiles might contribute to the early development of endometriosis.

4.3 Angiogenesis in early endometriosis

Mice were randomly treated with epigallocatchin-3-gallate (EGCG) extracted from green tea, Vitamin E (antioxidant controls) or vehicle (negative controls) for *in vivo* and *in vitro* microvessel imaging at the end of intervention. Microvascular networks in the endometriotic lesions *in vivo* were imaged by Cellvizio LAB LSU-488 with ProFlex Microprobe S1500. Microvessel length and area were measured using Cellvizio LAB Vessel Detection software and averaged from 4 perpendicular regions of the lesion in replicate.

Endometriotic implants were collected for angiogenesis microarray and pathway analysis after microvessel assessments *in vivo*. Differentially expressed angiogenesis molecules CD34, VEGFA, VEGFB, VEGFC, VEGFD, VEGFR1, VEGFR2 and VEGFR3 were confirmed by quantitative PCR, Western blot and immunhistochemistry. Effects of EGCG on angiogenesis signal transduction were further characterised in human endothelial cell line. Microvessel parameters and angiogenesis VEGFC/VEGFR2 signaling pathway including Jun proto-oncogene (cJUN), interferon-gamma (IFNG), matrix metallopeptidase-9 (MMP9) and chemokine (C-X-C motif) ligand-3 (CXCL3) in endometriotic implants and endothelial cells were studied. The results showed that EGCG, but not Vitamin E, inhibited microvessels in endometriotic implants. EGCG selectively suppressed VEGFC and tyrosine kinase receptor VEGFR2 expression. EGCG down regulated VEGFC/VEGFR2 signaling through cJUN, IFNG and MMP9/CXCL3 pathways for endothelial proliferation, inflammatory response and mobility. EGCG also suppressed VEGFC expression and reduced VEGFR2 and extracellular signal-regulated kinases (ERK) activation in endothelial cells. VEGFC supplementation attenuated the inhibitory effects by EGCG.

5. Prospective and proposal

5.1 Clinical significance and potential applications

Up to date, the only way to diagnose endometriosis is laparoscopy which is minimal invasive but expensive. Non-invasive and cheap diagnostic methods are urgent to be developed. CA-125 is a widely used serum marker for the diagnosis and evaluation of recurrent endometriosis or the success of a surgical treatment. A recent meta-analysis including twenty three studies and assessing the diagnostic performance of serum CA125 has shown that it's a poor diagnostic method with 90% specificity and 28% sensitivity (Mol *et al.*, 1998). One study has found serum IL-6 and peritoneal fluid TNF-α were able to discriminate between patients with and without endometriosis (Bedaiwy *et al.*, 2002). They stated the sensitivity and specificity of serum IL-6 reached 80% and 87% respectively, which is significantly higher than that of CA-125. It indicates that no inflammatory cytokine make a potential biomarker for diagnosis of endometriosis. Its predictive values in early endometriosis require further investigation.

In addition, the recognition of pathogenesis is able to provide new concept to the current unsatisfactory treatments. Hormone medicine is a commonly used drug for prevention of occurrence after surgical treatment. However, lots of patients are not sensitive to these medicines or cannot endure the side effects, such as vomiting and weight gain. New therapy with less adverse effects and more effective function needs to be developed. The study of oxidative stress, inflammation and angiogenesis in the pathogenesis of early endometriosis make it possible. For example, antioxidant therapy with 1200 IU of vitamin E and 1 g of vitamin C for a period of two months lead to a decrease in the inflammation cytokines such as MCP-1, RANTES and IL-6 in peritoneal fluid (Nalini Santanam, 2003). Another drug mifepristone with antioxidant effects was also found to exert an inhibitory effect on endometrial cell growth (Guo *et al.*). As angiogenesis, the VEGF inhibitor and anti-VEGF antibody have been demonstrated to be effective to control and inhibit implant lesion in mice model (Hull *et al.*, 2003). As process of endometriosis contains several steps, the ideal medicine has the potential to control the development of progression of endometrium in early pathophysiological stage (Fig. 4).

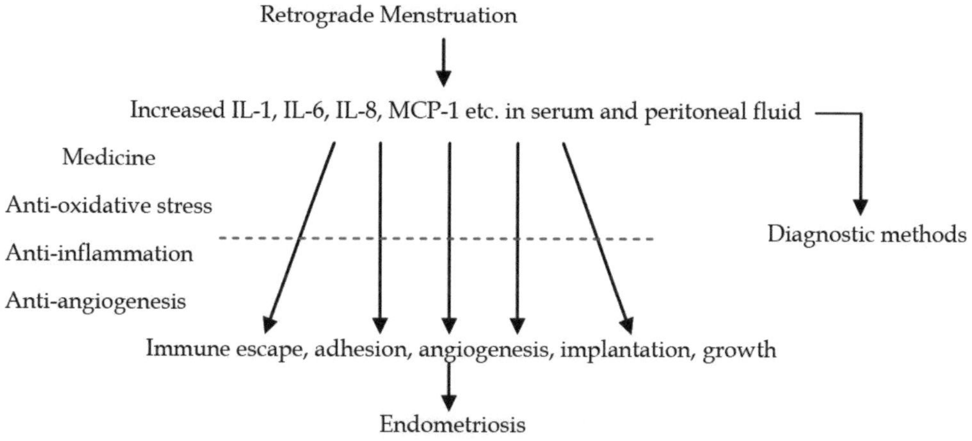

Fig. 4. Hypotheses and clinical potentials of endometriosis

5.2 Study limitations

Due to unavailable systematic studies, the understanding about this disease is still limited although endometriosis has been studied for many years. The limitations and difficulties are as below:

First, at the time of diagnosis endometriosis has already been established with unknown history. Hence, it's impossible to undertake clinical research from the onset to maintenance, which mainly makes the etiology still unknown. Second, it's difficult to have adequate control group. The control women involved in most studies are patients without endometriosis, which means they might have other disease, such as uterine myoma and benign ovarian tumor. The difference between normal eutopic and ectopic endometrium as well as normal pelvic environment and that with endometriosis is impossible to study in human. Third, we have already known genetic, immune system and peritoneal microenviroment are associated with endometriosis, which is supported by different curative effect with the same treatment for different patients and diverse symptoms. Therefore, the clinical treatment is individual and personal which increase the difficulty to observe and compare the different treatments. Fourth, only human and primates suffer from spontaneous endometriosis. The reproductive anatomy, physiology and estrogen cycle characteristics of monkeys are similar to human. Therefore, monkeys are the best animal model to do studies which can not carry out in humans. However, only few centers have the capacity to maintain this expensive animal. The most commonly used animal model is rodents, but there is an enormous phylogenetic gap between these animals and human. Hence, the question is how much data from these rodent models can be extrapolated to human situation. Fifth, primary endometrial and endometriotic epithelial cells cannot be passaged and fall into senescence within 2 weeks, but a stable cell line is necessary for the mechanism study. Until now, there are no stable and commercial normal endometrial and endometriotic glandular and stromal cells available for studying. Several researchers immortalized these cells by using human telomerase reverse transcriptase (hTERT) (Kyo *et al.*, 2003) or transfecting SV40 T-antigen vector (Zeitvogel *et al.*, 2001). However, how much characteristics these immortalized cells are similar to primary endometrial cells are needed to approve.

6. Conclusion

Endometriosis is a multifactorial disorder including retrograde menstruation, immune tolerance, adhesion, transplantation and proliferation modulated by abnormal inflammatory cytokines profile in peritoneal fluid. Future studies are necessary to focus on the whole picture of signaling pathway in early pathogenesis.

The current treatments mainly focus on inhibiting estrogen and its receptors which are not useful for every patient with endometriosis because estrogen is only one factor in the development of endometriosis. The signaling pathway is essential and makes it possible to develop an effective medication which could not only decrease estrogen level but also inhibit inflammation cytokines, ROS and angiogenesis. On the other hand, complete understanding of pathogenesis of endometriosis such as cytokines could provide a new way to diagnose and even to divide the disease into different stages according to pathophysiolocal characteristics, which makes the treatment individual and personal.

What's more, prevention of endometriosis after surgery is also very important. The current medicines used for prevention of recurrence are not very effective and have various side effects. The understanding of pathogenesis of early endometriosis may produce a better therapy to prevent recurrence. Ultimately, more clinical and basic researches should be carried out to overcome the complicated disease.

7. References

Arici, A, Head, JR, MacDonald, PC & Casey, ML (1993). Regulation of interleukin-8 gene expression in human endometrial cells in culture, *Mol Cell Endocrinol* 94(2): 195-204.

Arici, A, Oral, E, Attar, E, Tazuke, SI & Olive, DL (1997). Monocyte chemotactic protein-1 concentration in peritoneal fluid of women with endometriosis and its modulation of expression in mesothelial cells, *Fertil Steril* 67(6): 1065-72.

Arici, A, Seli, E, Zeyneloglu, HB, Senturk, LM, Oral, E & Olive, DL (1998). Interleukin-8 induces proliferation of endometrial stromal cells: a potential autocrine growth factor, *J Clin Endocrinol Metab* 83(4): 1201-5.

Bartosik, D, Jacobs, SL & Kelly, LJ (1986). Endometrial tissue in peritoneal fluid, *Fertil Steril* 46(5): 796-800.

Becker, CM, Sampson, DA, Short, SM, Javaherian, K, Folkman, J & D'Amato, RJ (2006). Short synthetic endostatin peptides inhibit endothelial migration in vitro and endometriosis in a mouse model, *Fertil Steril* 85(1): 71-7.

Bedaiwy, MA, Falcone, T, Sharma, RK, Goldberg, JM, Attaran, M, Nelson, DR & Agarwal, A (2002). Prediction of endometriosis with serum and peritoneal fluid markers: a prospective controlled trial, *Hum Reprod* 17(2): 426-31.

Berkkanoglu, M & Arici, A (2003). Immunology and endometriosis, *Am J Reprod Immunol* 50(1): 48-59.

Braun, DP, Gebel, H, House, R, Rana, N & Dmowski, NP (1996). Spontaneous and induced synthesis of cytokines by peripheral blood monocytes in patients with endometriosis, *Fertil Steril* 65(6): 1125-9.

Brosens, IA (1994). New principles in the management of endometriosis, *Acta Obstet Gynecol Scand Suppl* 159: 18-21.

Chen, QH, Zhou, WD, Su, ZY, Huang, QS, Jiang, JN & Chen, QX Change of proinflammatory cytokines follows certain patterns after induction of endometriosis in a mouse model, *Fertil Steril* 93(5): 1448-54.

Dabrosin, C, Gyorffy, S, Margetts, P, Ross, C & Gauldie, J (2002). Therapeutic effect of angiostatin gene transfer in a murine model of endometriosis, *Am J Pathol* 161(3): 909-18.

Dmowski, WP, Steele, RW & Baker, GF (1981). Deficient cellular immunity in endometriosis, *Am J Obstet Gynecol* 141(4): 377-83.

Dmowski, WP, Gebel, HM & Braun, DP (1994). The role of cell-mediated immunity in pathogenesis of endometriosis, *Acta Obstet Gynecol Scand Suppl* 159: 7-14.

Donnez, J, Smoes, P, Gillerot, S, Casanas-Roux, F & Nisolle, M (1998). Vascular endothelial growth factor (VEGF) in endometriosis, *Hum Reprod* 13(6): 1686-90.

Felson, H, Mc, GJ & Wasserman, P (1960). Stromal endometriosis involving the heart, *Am J Med* 29: 1072-6.

Garcia-Velasco, JA & Arici, A (1999). Interleukin-8 stimulates the adhesion of endometrial stromal cells to fibronectin, *Fertil Steril* 72(2): 336-40.

Giudice, LC (1994). Growth factors and growth modulators in human uterine endometrium: their potential relevance to reproductive medicine, *Fertil Steril* 61(1): 1-17.

Gonzalez-Ramos, R, Van Langendonckt, A, Defrere, S, Lousse, JC, Colette, S, Devoto, L & Donnez, J Involvement of the nuclear factor-kappaB pathway in the pathogenesis of endometriosis, *Fertil Steril* 94(6): 1985-94.

Gonzalez-Ramos, R, Van Langendonckt, A, Defrere, S, Lousse, JC, Colette, S, Devoto, L & Donnez, J (2010). Involvement of the nuclear factor-kappaB pathway in the pathogenesis of endometriosis, *Fertil Steril* 94(6): 1985-94.

Guo, SW, Liu, M, Shen, F & Liu, X Use of mifepristone to treat endometriosis: a review of clinical trials and trial-like studies conducted in China, *Womens Health (Lond Engl)* 7(1): 51-70.

Gupta, S, Agarwal, A, Krajcir, N & Alvarez, JG (2006). Role of oxidative stress in endometriosis, *Reprod Biomed Online* 13(1): 126-34.

Halme, J, Hammond, MG, Hulka, JF, Raj, SG & Talbert, LM (1984). Retrograde menstruation in healthy women and in patients with endometriosis, *Obstet Gynecol* 64(2): 151-4.

Han, S & Sidell, N (2003). RU486-induced growth inhibition of human endometrial cells involves the nuclear factor-kappa B signaling pathway, *J Clin Endocrinol Metab* 88(2): 713-9.

Hill, JA, Faris, HM, Schiff, I & Anderson, DJ (1988). Characterization of leukocyte subpopulations in the peritoneal fluid of women with endometriosis, *Fertil Steril* 50(2): 216-22.

Ho, HN, Wu, MY, Chen, SU, Chao, KH, Chen, CD & Yang, YS (1997). Total antioxidant status and nitric oxide do not increase in peritoneal fluids from women with endometriosis, *Hum Reprod* 12(12): 2810-5.

Hull, ML, Charnock-Jones, DS, Chan, CL, Bruner-Tran, KL, Osteen, KG, Tom, BD, Fan, TP & Smith, SK (2003). Antiangiogenic agents are effective inhibitors of endometriosis, *J Clin Endocrinol Metab* 88(6): 2889-99.

Iwabe, T, Harada, T, Tsudo, T, Tanikawa, M, Onohara, Y & Terakawa, N (1998). Pathogenetic significance of increased levels of interleukin-8 in the peritoneal fluid of patients with endometriosis, *Fertil Steril* 69(5): 924-30.

Jeltsch, M, Kaipainen, A, Joukov, V, Meng, X, Lakso, M, Rauvala, H, Swartz, M, Fukumura, D, Jain, RK & Alitalo, K (1997). Hyperplasia of lymphatic vessels in VEGF-C transgenic mice, *Science* 276(5317): 1423-5.

Jenkins, S, Olive, DL & Haney, AF (1986). Endometriosis: pathogenetic implications of the anatomic distribution, *Obstet Gynecol* 67(3): 335-8.

Joseph, J, Reed, CE & Sahn, SA (1994). Thoracic endometriosis. Recurrence following hysterectomy with bilateral salpingo-oophorectomy and successful treatment with talc pleurodesis, *Chest* 106(6): 1894-6.

Joukov, V, Sorsa, T, Kumar, V, Jeltsch, M, Claesson-Welsh, L, Cao, Y, Saksela, O, Kalkkinen, N & Alitalo, K (1997). Proteolytic processing regulates receptor specificity and activity of VEGF-C, *Embo J* 16(13): 3898-911.

Khorram, O, Taylor, RN, Ryan, IP, Schall, TJ & Landers, DV (1993). Peritoneal fluid concentrations of the cytokine RANTES correlate with the severity of endometriosis, *Am J Obstet Gynecol* 169(6): 1545-9.

Koks, CA, Groothuis, PG, Dunselman, GA, de Goeij, AF & Evers, JL (2000). Adhesion of menstrual endometrium to extracellular matrix: the possible role of integrin alpha(6)beta(1) and laminin interaction, *Mol Hum Reprod* 6(2): 170-7.

Koninckx, PR, Kennedy, SH & Barlow, DH (1998). Endometriotic disease: the role of peritoneal fluid, *Hum Reprod Update* 4(5): 741-51.

Koninckx, PR, Barlow, D & Kennedy, S (1999). Implantation versus infiltration: the Sampson versus the endometriotic disease theory, *Gynecol Obstet Invest* 47 Suppl 1: 3-9; discussion 9-10.

Krikun, G, Hu, Z, Osteen, K, Bruner-Tran, KL, Schatz, F, Taylor, HS, Toti, P, Arcuri, F, Konigsberg, W, Garen, A, Booth, CJ & Lockwood, CJ The immunoconjugate "icon" targets aberrantly expressed endothelial tissue factor causing regression of endometriosis, *Am J Pathol* 176(2): 1050-6.

Kyama, CM, Debrock, S, Mwenda, JM & D'Hooghe, TM (2003). Potential involvement of the immune system in the development of endometriosis, *Reprod Biol Endocrinol* 1: 123.

Kyo, S, Nakamura, M, Kiyono, T, Maida, Y, Kanaya, T, Tanaka, M, Yatabe, N & Inoue, M (2003). Successful immortalization of endometrial glandular cells with normal structural and functional characteristics, *Am J Pathol* 163(6): 2259-69.

Laird, SM, Tuckerman, EM, Saravelos, H & Li, TC (1996). The production of tumour necrosis factor alpha (TNF-alpha) by human endometrial cells in culture, *Hum Reprod* 11(6): 1318-23.

Laird, SM, Tuckerman, EM, Cork, BA & Li, TC (2000). Expression of nuclear factor kappa B in human endometrium; role in the control of interleukin 6 and leukaemia inhibitory factor production, *Mol Hum Reprod* 6(1): 34-40.

Le, JM & Vilcek, J (1989). Interleukin 6: a multifunctional cytokine regulating immune reactions and the acute phase protein response, *Lab Invest* 61(6): 588-602.

Lebovic, DI, Bentzien, F, Chao, VA, Garrett, EN, Meng, YG & Taylor, RN (2000). Induction of an angiogenic phenotype in endometriotic stromal cell cultures by interleukin-1beta, *Mol Hum Reprod* 6(3): 269-75.

Lebovic, DI, Mueller, MD & Taylor, RN (2001). Immunobiology of endometriosis, *Fertil Steril* 75(1): 1-10.

Lessey, BA, Damjanovich, L, Coutifaris, C, Castelbaum, A, Albelda, SM & Buck, CA (1992). Integrin adhesion molecules in the human endometrium. Correlation with the normal and abnormal menstrual cycle, *J Clin Invest* 90(1): 188-95.

Lin, YJ, Lai, MD, Lei, HY & Wing, LY (2006). Neutrophils and macrophages promote angiogenesis in the early stage of endometriosis in a mouse model, *Endocrinology* 147(3): 1278-86.

McLaren, J, Prentice, A, Charnock-Jones, DS, Millican, SA, Muller, KH, Sharkey, AM & Smith, SK (1996). Vascular endothelial growth factor is produced by peritoneal fluid macrophages in endometriosis and is regulated by ovarian steroids, *J Clin Invest* 98(2): 482-9.

McLaren, J, Prentice, A, Charnock-Jones, DS & Smith, SK (1996). Vascular endothelial growth factor (VEGF) concentrations are elevated in peritoneal fluid of women with endometriosis, *Hum Reprod* 11(1): 220-3.

McLaren, J (2000). Vascular endothelial growth factor and endometriotic angiogenesis, *Hum Reprod Update* 6(1): 45-55.

Mettler, L, Volkov, NI, Kulakov, VI, Jurgensen, A & Parwaresch, MR (1996). Lymphocyte subsets in the endometrium of patients with endometriosis throughout the menstrual cycle, *Am J Reprod Immunol* 36(6): 342-8.

Mol, BW, Bayram, N, Lijmer, JG, Wiegerinck, MA, Bongers, MY, van der Veen, F & Bossuyt, PM (1998). The performance of CA-125 measurement in the detection of endometriosis: a meta-analysis, *Fertil Steril* 70(6): 1101-8.

Monckedieck, V, Sannecke, C, Husen, B, Kumbartski, M, Kimmig, R, Totsch, M, Winterhager, E & Grummer, R (2009). Progestins inhibit expression of MMPs and of angiogenic factors in human ectopic endometrial lesions in a mouse model, *Mol Hum Reprod* 15(10): 633-43.

Moretta, A, Sivori, S, Vitale, M, Pende, D, Morelli, L, Augugliaro, R, Bottino, C & Moretta, L (1995). Existence of both inhibitory (p58) and activatory (p50) receptors for HLA-C molecules in human natural killer cells, *J Exp Med* 182(3): 875-84.

Murphy, AA, Palinski, W, Rankin, S, Morales, AJ & Parthasarathy, S (1998). Macrophage scavenger receptor(s) and oxidatively modified proteins in endometriosis, *Fertil Steril* 69(6): 1085-91.

Nalini Santanam, NK, Celia Dominguez, John A. Rock, Sampath Parthasarathy, Ana A. Murphy (2003). Antioxidant supplementation reduces total chemokines and inflammatory cytokines in women with enodmetriosis, *Fertility and Sterility* 80: s32-s33.

Nap, AW, Griffioen, AW, Dunselman, GA, Bouma-Ter Steege, JC, Thijssen, VL, Evers, JL & Groothuis, PG (2004). Antiangiogenesis therapy for endometriosis, *J Clin Endocrinol Metab* 89(3): 1089-95.

Nisolle, M, Casanas-Roux, F, Anaf, V, Mine, JM & Donnez, J (1993). Morphometric study of the stromal vascularization in peritoneal endometriosis, *Fertil Steril* 59(3): 681-4.

Oosterlynck, DJ, Cornillie, FJ, Waer, M, Vandeputte, M & Koninckx, PR (1991). Women with endometriosis show a defect in natural killer activity resulting in a decreased cytotoxicity to autologous endometrium, *Fertil Steril* 56(1): 45-51.

Oosterlynck, DJ, Meuleman, C, Sobis, H, Vandeputte, M & Koninckx, PR (1993). Angiogenic activity of peritoneal fluid from women with endometriosis, *Fertil Steril* 59(4): 778-82.

Oosterlynck, DJ, Meuleman, C, Waer, M & Koninckx, PR (1994). Transforming growth factor-beta activity is increased in peritoneal fluid from women with endometriosis, *Obstet Gynecol* 83(2): 287-92.

Oral, E, Olive, DL & Arici, A (1996). The peritoneal environment in endometriosis, *Hum Reprod Update* 2(5): 385-98.

Ota, H, Igarashi, S & Tanaka, T (2001). Xanthine oxidase in eutopic and ectopic endometrium in endometriosis and adenomyosis, *Fertil Steril* 75(4): 785-90.

Robert, M (1919). Uber den staud der frage der adenomyosites adenomyoma in allemeinen und adenomyonetitis sarcomatosa, *Zentralbl Gynakol* 36: 745-59

Rokitansky, CV (1860). Ueber Uterusdrusen-Neubildung in Uterus- und Ovarial-Sarcomen, *Ztschr kk Gesselsh Aerzte Wien* 16: 577.

Salamonsen, LA & Woolley, DE (1996). Matrix metalloproteinases in normal menstruation, *Hum Reprod* 11 Suppl 2: 124-33.

Sampson, J (1921). Perforating hemorrhagic (chocolate) cysts of the ovary, *Arch Surg* (3): 245-323.

Steele, RW, Dmowski, WP & Marmer, DJ (1984). Immunologic aspects of human endometriosis, *Am J Reprod Immunol* 6(1): 33-6.

Tariverdian, N, Siedentopf, F, Rucke, M, Blois, SM, Klapp, BF, Kentenich, H & Arck, PC (2009). Intraperitoneal immune cell status in infertile women with and without endometriosis, *J Reprod Immunol* 80(1-2): 80-90.

Thibodeau, LL, Prioleau, GR, Manuelidis, EE, Merino, MJ & Heafner, MD (1987). Cerebral endometriosis. Case report, *J Neurosurg* 66(4): 609-10.

Umezawa, M, Sakata, C, Tanaka, N, Kudo, S, Tabata, M, Takeda, K, Ihara, T & Sugamata, M (2008). Cytokine and chemokine expression in a rat endometriosis is similar to that in human endometriosis, *Cytokine* 43(2): 105-9.

van Furth, R, Raeburn, JA & van Zwet, TL (1979). Characteristics of human mononuclear phagocytes, *Blood* 54(2): 485-500.

Van Langendonckt, A, Casanas-Roux, F & Donnez, J (2002). Oxidative stress and peritoneal endometriosis, *Fertil Steril* 77(5): 861-70.

Vigano, P, Gaffuri, B, Somigliana, E, Busacca, M, Di Blasio, AM & Vignali, M (1998). Expression of intercellular adhesion molecule (ICAM)-1 mRNA and protein is enhanced in endometriosis versus endometrial stromal cells in culture, *Mol Hum Reprod* 4(12): 1150-6.

Vlahos, NF, Gregoriou, O, Deliveliotou, A, Perrea, D, Vlachos, A, Zhao, Y, Lai, J & Creatsas, G Effect of pentoxifylline on vascular endothelial growth factor C and flk-1 expression on endometrial implants in the rat endometriosis model, *Fertil Steril* 93(4): 1316-23.

Wang, Y, Sharma, RK, Falcone, T, Goldberg, J & Agarwal, A (1997). Importance of reactive oxygen species in the peritoneal fluid of women with endometriosis or idiopathic infertility, *Fertil Steril* 68(5): 826-30.

Wilson, TJ, Hertzog, PJ, Angus, D, Munnery, L, Wood, EC & Kola, I (1994). Decreased natural killer cell activity in endometriosis patients: relationship to disease pathogenesis, *Fertil Steril* 62(5): 1086-8.

Wu, MY, Yang, JH, Chao, KH, Hwang, JL, Yang, YS & Ho, HN (2000). Increase in the expression of killer cell inhibitory receptors on peritoneal natural killer cells in women with endometriosis, *Fertil Steril* 74(6): 1187-91.

Zeitvogel, A, Baumann, R & Starzinski-Powitz, A (2001). Identification of an invasive, N-cadherin-expressing epithelial cell type in endometriosis using a new cell culture model, *Am J Pathol* 159(5): 1839-52.

Zeller, JM, Henig, I, Radwanska, E & Dmowski, WP (1987). Enhancement of human monocyte and peritoneal macrophage chemiluminescence activities in women with endometriosis, *Am J Reprod Immunol Microbiol* 13(3): 78-82.

Zhang, RJ, Wild, RA & Ojago, JM (1993). Effect of tumor necrosis factor-alpha on adhesion of human endometrial stromal cells to peritoneal mesothelial cells: an in vitro system, *Fertil Steril* 59(6): 1196-201.

27

Medical Treatment in Endometriosis

Elham Pourmatroud
Ahvaz Jundishapur University of Medical Science (AJUMS), Iran

1. Introduction

Two important targets from medical treatment are: pain control and suppression of disease progress. Most of the time, the effectiveness is temporary and lasted while these drugs have been used, which is expected from the nature of endometriosis disease .Of course, there are some debts about the usefulness of pain relief agents, because 30-50% of patients feel better with placebo administration.

It must to keep in mind that those common administrated drugs couldn't help to restore the fertility potentials and in fact during their usage pregnancy cannot or should not be happened, regarding to inhibition of ovulation or teratogenic effects; of course by their administration with remission of disease (suppress the growth and activity of previous endometriotic implants) and reducing the chance of new peritoneal seeding, fertility may be preserved better; but at the end for achieving pregnancy other ways should be used.

Medical therapeutic drugs divided in two categories:

a. Non hormonal medical therapy.
b. Hormonal medical therapy.

Non hormonal therapeutic options, mainly work on inflammatory and immunologic aspect of endometriosis and hormonal attempts basically deprived endometriotic implants from their nutritive substance: estrogen.

2. Non hormonal medical therapy

2.1 Non-steroidal anti- inflammatory agents

With attention to inflammatory nature of endometriosis, for decades non- steroidal anti-inflammatory agents (NSAIDs) such as naproxen and ibuprofen have been administrated for pain control, in endometriosis. These drugs have been reduced prostaglandins (PGs) production, the main stimulator factor in peritoneal nerves and decrease the nociceptor input messenger from the peritoneal endometriotic implants into central nervous system. Their gastrointestinal upsets and inhibition of ovulation (Duffy &Stouffer,2002) against low cost and easy availability, always puts NSAIDs in a challenging situation; rather than, new NSAIDs as a selective cyclooxygenase (COX)-2 inhibitors like celecoxib without any effect on PG pathway, could induce apoptosis in endometriotic implants (Seo etal,2010). However the latest Cochrane review doesn't show significant effective role of these drugs in patients with endometriosis (Davis etal, 2007).

2.2 Cytokines inhibitors

Research in this field is still in primary stages. In animal experiments, cytokines antagonist agents like recombinant human tumor necrotizing factor alpha (TNF-α) binding protein could inhibit the progress of endometriotic implants and formation of their adhesion (Barrier etal,2004;D'Hooghe etal,2006). Etanercept (ETA) as a TNF antagonist could decrease the volume of peritoneal fluid and proliferation of lesions in endometriotic rats (Zulfikaroglu etal,2011). In a novel study, has been found that TNF could activate estrogen receptor α (ERα); therefore co-administration of a pure ER antagonist with TNF inhibitor could be a more efficacious therapeutic method than usage of one agent, separately (Gori etal,2011).

2.3 New anti inflammatores

In cases with persistent non responsive symptom to NSAIDs, other inflammatores like leukotrienes could be inhibited (Abu etal, 2000). In one new study, leukotriene receptor antagonist has been shown to have a significant effect in reduction of stromal proliferation in endometriotic implants (Ihara etal, 2004).

2.4 Immuno modulators

Pentoxiphylline administration in human, like a leukotriene receptor antagonist, had promising results in patients with endometriosis. Although it is famous as a vasodilator agent and increase tissue oxygenation in some disease; but could change the immune cell function by inhibition of cytokine and TNF-α secretion. Although in a Cochran review in year 2009, there were not shown enough evidence to support any differences in pregnancy rate in treated patients in comparison with placebo (Lu etal,2009); but in a new report, Vascular endothelial growth factor (VEGF)-C suggested to be an effective factor for significant reduction in endometriotic implants after Pentoxiphylline administration (Vlahos etal,2010).

Also, other immuno modulators like etanercept (ETA) had promising reductive effect equally to letrozole in early investigation (Ceyhan etal ,2011).

2.5 Alternative medicine

In a 16 weeks prospective clinical trial, Chinese herbal medicine (CHM) decoctions have been disclosed hopeful reduction in patient's symptoms especially with dysmenorrhea complaint rather than placebo (Flower etal, 2011). According to Cochrane review, CHM have been shown equal results in comparison with gestrinone with lesser side effects; beside that, the combination of oral CMH administration with a CMH enema appear better clinical outcomes (Flower etal, 2009).

As well, there are some published studies about the effectiveness of acupuncture in abdominal pain and significantly in dysmenorrhea relief (M.Chen etal ,2010 ; Rubi-Klein etal,2010). In another clinical trial, abdominal acupuncture causing decrease in CA125 level in endometriotic patients (Xiang etal, 2011).

3. Hormonal medical therapy

3.1 Oral contraceptive pill (OCP)

Oral combined contraceptive pills induce atrophy in peritoneal endometriotic implants by initial decidualization effect like a pseudo pregnancy situation; perhaps they could increase the apoptosis in endometriotic implants (Meresman etal , 2000). OCPs are the most prescripted drugs in endometriosis, especially in minimal and mild stages of disease for pain control ; although there is a new report about the effectiveness of OCPs usage in patients with deep endometriotic nodules (advance stage) (Mabrouk etal,2011) ,which eliminate the effectiveness of OCPs administration only in early stages of disease. In addition, there is not any differences between various available formulations in pain relief potency and any kind of OCPs which had 30-35μg of ethinyl estradiol could be used and there is no necessity for high dose (HD) contraceptive administration (with 50 μg of ethinyl estradiol) (Davis etal,2007) . About the usage methods has been shown that, continues usage had better clinical results rather than cyclic administration (Harada etal,2008). In cases of sever atrophy of endometrium and break through bleeding, supplemental estrogen for 7-10 days could be advised.

3.2 Progestins

Progestins at the first stage of administration induce decidualization in endometriotic tissues and at the second phase by proliferation inhibition makes atrophia. Also, progestins make depletion in estrogen receptors and inhibit their activation (Kirkland etal, 1992). Progestins could induce transformation of potent form of estrogens (estradiol) to weaker product (estrone) (Tseng etal, 1981) .In recent studies discover that there are two important catalyzer enzymes which metabolize progesterone in endometriotic implants. Aldo-Keto reductase 1C1 and 1C3 (AKR1C1 & AKR1C3) had significant up-regulation expression in ovarian endometriosis which interfere with inhibitory effects of human progesterone (Hevir etal, 2011). It found that exogenous progestins administration could inhibit their activity (Beranic etal, 2011).Various available progestins could be used: oral, parenteral, intrauterine device and implants. With higher dosage of administrated progestins, another effective role of them could be achieved: inhibition of matrix metalloproteinase (Osteen etal , 2003). Most of the time the clinical response to progestins are like the oral contraceptive pills (Schlaff etal,2006), without significant side effects except breakthrough bleeding which can be managed with short time, low dose estrogen administration. Also, the probably bone loss effect is reversible (Cundy etal,1996).The levonorgestrel releasing intrauterine device (LNG-IUS) is a valuable therapeutic option especially for women with deep infiltrative endometriotic implants (Lochat etal,2005).About the pain relief efficacy of progestin subdermal implants (Implanon) evidences are limited than other therapeutic modalities (Yisa etal,2005).

3.3 Gonadotropin-releasing hormone agonists

Gonadotropin -releasing hormone (GnRH) agonists are synthetic drugs which are resistant to degeneration in body and are produced by some variation in amino acids consequent in natural GnRH agonists. Their resistance to degeneration makes the pituitary gland into down regulation state and after suppression of FSH and LH production, menstruation and ovulation had been stopped and therefore, low estrogenic environment achieved which inhibits the proliferation in endometriotic implants. Beside initial flare effect, pseudo menopausal situation produce minor side effects like hot flashes, vaginal atrophia and dryness, headache and other vasomotor signs and symptoms (Dlugi etal,1990) which could be managed by add-back therapy, but after 6 or more continues cycles of drug administration, bone mineral density is going to be reduced sometimes in an irreversible manner (Taga etal,1996); but there is an interesting report about ten years usage of GnRH agonist with add-back therapy without any bone mineral loss (Bedaiwy etal,2006). Unlike the progestins and danazole, GnRH agonists had not adverse effects on lipid profile (Burry etal,1989).Several kinds of injectable GnRH agonists and nasal spray form are available with equal efficacy (Prentice etal,2000).

3.4 Gonadotropin-releasing hormone antagonists

Regarding to initial flare effect of GnRH agonist administration and probably exacerbation effect on endometriosis and a delay between their administration and real hypo estrogenic state and their intolerable side effects in some patients, GnRH antagonists became an suitable substitute for GnRH agonists. Weekly subcutaneous 3-mg cetrotide (GnRH antagonist) injection had been shown clinical efficacy without pseudo menopausal side effects (Finas etal, 2006; Kupker etal, 2002).There are some published advances in oral GnRH antagonist production: Elagolix (C.Chen et al, 2008). In a double blind study in 55 patients, weekly usage of this drug , results effective suppression of gonadal hormonal production (Struthers etal,2009), which could be a promising development in endometriosis treatments modalities instated of injectable options.

3.5 Androgens

Danazol is a derivation from testosterone which effect on endometriosis from several ways. Danazol inhibit some steroidogenic enzymes and elevate free testosterone and reduce estrogen level (Barbieri etal, 1981). Also, danazol inhibit mid cycle LH surge (Tamura etal, 1991) and PG F2α production in ovary (Kogo etal,1992),which both of them result chronic anovulation and decrease the chance of new peritoneal seeding.Danazol with 400-800 mg/daily recommended dosage regress the endometriotic implants (Telimaa etal,1987), but severe side effects prevent such dosage administration for an effective period (6 months) (Miller etal,1998).Oily skin, acne, hirsutism, irreversible voice deepness, variation in lipid profile, vaginal atrophia and hot flash limited it's prescription (Hayashi etal,2001).

3.6 Aromatase inhibitors

In opposition to other hormonal therapeutic options which reduce ovarian estrogenic production, aromatase inhibitors act not only locally on endometriotic implants, but also on all of estrogenic producers: ovary, brain, adipose tissues (Attar&Bulun, 2006). Anastrazole 1mg or letrozole 2.5mg daily could be effective in pain relief associated with endometriosis (Nothnick, 2011; Shippen&West, 2004). Because of stimulatory action of aromatase inhibitors in FSH secretion, in premenopausal women they could cause ovarian cysts;

therefore they administrate with GnRH agonist or OCPs or progestins. This method could reduce the concern about their disadvantage in prolong usage: bone loss (Ferrero etal ,2009).

3.7 Prolactin secretion inhibitors

Suppression of cellular immunity and NK cell activity in endometriotic patients has been well known. Also, in stressful situations inhibition of NK cell had been found (Chrousos etal, 2000). Prolactin and cortisol levels in serum are stress indicators. Of course the mechanism of hyper prolactinemia in response to stress isn't so clear, elevated level of serum prolactin had been found in endometriosis like other stressful conditions (Lima etal, 2006, Wang etal, 2009). Interestingly the mean serum prolactin levels are higher in advance stages in endometriotic patients (Gregoriou etal ,1999). Quinagolide as a dopamine receptor 2 agonist by reduction in VEGF receptor (a main factor for angiogenesis) could decrease the size of peritoneal lesions and in some cases could eradicate all of endometriotic implants (Gomez etal, 2011). From another aspect quinagolide, is a valuable option for hyper prolactinemia like other dopamine agonists (bromocriptine or caberguline) (Barlier&Jaquet,2006); therefore this drug could be effectively administrated in endometriosis.

4. References

Abu JI, Konje JC (2000). Leukotrienes in gynecology: the hypothetical value of anti-leukotriene therapy in dysmenorrhea and endometriosis. Hum Reprod Update, Vol. 6, PP.200-205

Attar E, Bulun S (2006). Aromatase inhibitors: the next generation of therapeutics for endometriosis? Fertil Steril, Vol. 85, PP.1307-18

Barbieri RL, Osathanondh R& Ryan KJ (1981). Danazol inhibition of steroidogenesis in the human corpus luteum .ObstetGynecol,Vol. 57, P. 722

Barlier A, Jaquet P (2006). Quinagolide a valuable treatment option for hyper prolactinemia. Eur J Endocrinol,Vol.154, No.2, PP.187-95

Barrier BF, Bates WB, Leland MM, et al (2004).Efficacy of anti-tumor necrosis factor therapy in the treatment of spontaneous endometriosis in baboons.FertilSteril, Vol.81, PP.775-79

Bedaiwy MA, Casper RF (2006).Treatment with leuprolide acetate and hormonal add-back for up to 10 years in stage 4 endometriosis patients with chronic pelvic pain.FertilSteril, Vol.86, PP.220-222

BeranicN,Gobec S&Rizner TL (2011).Progestins as inhibitors of the human 20-Ketosteroid reductase, AKR1C1 and AKR1C3.ChemBiol Interact, Vol.191,No.1-3,PP.227-33

Burry KA, Patton PE& Illingworth DR (1989). Metabolic changes during medical treatment of endometriosis: nafarelin acetate versus danazol, Am J ObstetGynecol , Vol.160, P.1454

Ceyhan ST, Onguru O, Fidan U, et al (2011).Comparison of aromatase inhibitor (letrozole) and immuno modulators (infliximab and etanercept) on regression of endometriotic implants in a rat model.Eur J ObstetGynecolReprodBiol , Vol.154, No.1, PP.100-4

Chen C, WU D, Guo Z, et al (2008). Discovery of R-(+)-4-{2-[5-(2- fluoro-3-methyl-2,6-dioxo-3,6-dihdro-2H-pyrimidin-1-yI]-1- phenylethylamino} butyrate (elgolix), a potent and orally available nonpeptide antagonist of the human gonadotropin releasing hormone receptor. J Med Chem, Vol.51,No.23, PP.7478-85

Chen M, Zhang H, Li J, et al (2010). Clinical observation on acupuncture combined with acupoint sticking therapy for treatment of dysmenorrhea caused by endometriosis. Zhongguo Zhen Jiu,Vol.30,No.9,PP.725-8

Chrousos GP, Elenkov IJ (2000).Interactions of the endocrine and immune systems. In: DeGroot LJ, Jameson JL (Editors), Endocrinology. New York: Academic Press ,PP. 571-586

Cundy T, Farquhar CM, Cornish J, etal (1996). Short-term effects of high dose oral medroxyprogesterone acetate on bone density in premenopausal women. J ClinEndocrinolMetab, Vol.81,P.1014

Davis L, Kennedy SS, Moore J, etal (2007). Modern combined oral contraceptives for pain associated with endometriosis. Cochrane Database Syst Rev.CD001019

D'Hooghe TM, Nugent N, Cuneo S, et al (2006). Recombinant human TNF binding protein (r-hTBP-1) inhibits the development of endometriosis in baboons: a prospective, randomized, placebo- and drug-controlled study. Biology of Reproduction. Vol.74, PP.131-36

Dlugi AM, Miller JD&Knittle J (1990). Lupron depot (leuprolide acetate for depot suspension) in the treatment of endometriosis: a randomized, placebo-controlled, double-blind study. Lupron Study Group, Fertil *Steril* . *Vol.*54,P.419

Duffy DM, Stouffer R .(2002). Follicular administration of a cyclooxygenase inhibitor can prevent oocyte release without alteration of normal luteal function in rhesus monkeys. HUM Reprod.V01.17, PP.2825-31

Ferrero S, Camerini G, Seracchioli R, et al (2009). Letrozole combined with norethisterone acetate compared With norethisterone acetate alone in the treatment of pain symptoms caused by endometriosis. Hum Reprod. *Vol.*24,PP.3033

Flower A, Liu JP, Chen S, etal (2009).Chinese herbal medicine for endometriosis. Cochrane Database Syst Rev .Vol.8, No.3,CD006568

Flower A, Lewith GT& Little P (2011).A feasibility study exploring the role of Chinese herbal medicine in the treatment of endometriosis. J Altern Complement Med. Vol.17, No.8,PP.691-9

Finas D, Hornung D, DiedrichK,etal (2006).Cetrolix in the treatment of female infertility and endometriosis. Expert OpinPhamacother . Vol.7, No.15, PP.2155-68

Gomez R, Abad A, Delgado F, et al (2011). Quinagolide on endometriotic lesions in patients with endometriosis associated hyper prolactinemia. FertilSteril, Vol.95,N0.3,PP.882-88

Gori I, Pellegrini C, Staedler D, et al (2011). Tumor necrosis factor-α activates estrogen signaling pathways in endometrial epithelial cells via estrogen receptor α. Mol Cell Endocrinol,Vol.345,No.1-2,PP:27-37

Gregoriou G, Bakas P, Vitoratos N, et al (1999). Evaluation of serum prolactin levels in patients with endometriosis and infertility. Gynecol Obstet Invest , Vol.48, PP.48-51

Harada T, Momoeda M, Taketani Y, etal (2008). Low-dose oral contraceptive pill for dysmenorrhea associated with endometriosis: a placebo-controlled, double-blind, randomized trial,FertilSteril.Vol.90,P.1583

Hayashi T, Takahashi T, Minami T, et al (2001). Fatal acute hepatic failure induced by danazol in a patient with endometriosis and aplastic anemia. J Gastroenterol. Vol.36,PP. 783-86

Hevir N, Vouk K, Sinkovec J, etal (2011). Aldo-KetoReductases AKR1C1, AkR1C2 and AKR1C3 may enhance progesterone metabolism in ovarian endometriosis. ChemBiol Interact .Vol.191,No.1-3,PP.217-26

Ihara T, Uchiide I&Sugamata M (2004).Light and electron microscopic evaluation of antileukotriene therapy for experimental rat endometriosis.FertilSteril .Vol.81, suppl.1,PP.819-23

Kirkland JL, Murthy L&Stancel GM (1992).Progesterone inhibits the estrogen-induced expression of*c-fos* messenger ribonucleic acid inthe uterus, Endocrinology .Vol.130,P.3223

Kogo H, Takasaki K, Yatabe Y, etal (1992). Inhibitory and stimulatory actions of danazol in rat ovarian and uterine tissues. Eur J Pharmacol, Vol.211, No.1,PP.69-73

Kupker W, Felberbaum RE, Krapp M, etal (2002).Use of GnRH antagonists in the treatment of endometriosis.Reprod Biomed Online, Vol.5,No.1, PP.12-16

Lima A.P, Rosa e Silva A.A.M (2006).Prolactin and cortisol levels in women with endometriosis. Brazilian J of Med BiolRes ,Vol.39, PP.1121-27

Lochat FB, Emembolu JO&Konje JC (2005).The efficacy, side effects and continuation rates in women with symptomatic endometriosis undergoing treatment with an intrauterine administered progesterone (levonorgestrone) :a 3 -year follow -up. Hum Reprod, Vol.20, PP.789-793

LU D, Song H, Li Y, etal (2009).Pentoxiphylline versus medical therapies for sub fertile women with endometriosis. Cochrane Database Of Systemic Reviews .Issue 3.Art. No:CD007677

Mabrouk M, Frasca C, Geraci E, et al (2011).Combined oral contraceptive therapy in women with posterior deep infiltrating endometriosis. J Minim Invasive Gynecol, Vol.18, No.4,PP.470-4

Meresman GF, Vighi S, Buquet RA, etal (2000). Apoptosis and expression of Bcl-2 and Bax in eutopic endometrium from women with endometriosis. FertilSteril. Vol.74,P.*760*

Miller JD, Shaw RW, Casper RF, et al (1998). Historical prospective cohort study of the recurrence of pain after discontinuation of treatment with danazol or a gonadotropin-releasing hormone agonist.FertilSteril. Vol.70,P.293

Nothnick WB (2011).The emerging use of aromatase inhibitors for endometriosis treatment.ReprodBiolEnocrinol,Vol.9,P.87

Osteen KG, Igarashi TM& Bruner-Tran KL (2003). Progesterone action in the human endometrium: induction of a unique tissue environment which limits matrix metalloproteinase (MMP) expression, Front Biosci, *Vol*.8,P.d78

Prentice A, Deary AJ, Goldbeck-Wood S, etal (2000). Gonadotropin- releasing hormone analogues for pain associated with endometriosis, Cochrane Database Syst Rev .CD000346

Rubi-Klein K, Kucera-Sliutz E, Nissel H, et al (2010). Is acupuncture in addition to conventional medicine effective as pain treatment for endometriosis? A randomized controlled cross-over trial.Eur J ObstetGynecolReprodBiol,Vol.153, No.1,PP.90-3

Schlaff WD, Carson SA, Luciano A, et al (2006). Subcutaneous injection of depot medroxyprogesterone acetate compared with leuprolide acetate in the treatment of endometriosis -associated pain. Hum Reprod,Vol. 21,PP.248-256

SeoSk, Nam A, Jeon YE, et al (2010).Expression and possible role of non-steroidal anti-inflammatory drug-activated gene-1 (NAG-1) in the human endometrium and endometriosis. Hum Reprod,Vol.25, N0.12, PP. 3043-9

Shippen ER, West WJ, Jr (2004).Successful treatment of severe endometriosis in two premenopausal women with an aromatase inhibitor.FertilSteril, *Vol.*81,P.1395

Struthers RS, Nicholls AJ, Grundy J, et al (2009).Suppression of gonadotropins and estradiol in premenopausal women by oral administration of the nonpeptide gonadotropin releasing hormone antagonist elagolix. J ClinEndocrinolMetab, Vol.94, No.2,PP.545-51

Taga M, Minaguchi H (1996). Reduction of bone mineral density by gonadotropin-releasing hormone agonist, nafarelin, is not completely reversible at 6 months after the cessation of administration. Acta Obstet Gynecol Scand, *Vol.*75,P.162

Tamura K, Okamoto R, Takeo S, etal (1991).Inhibition of the first ovulation and ovarian prostaglandin F2 alpha metabolism by danazol in rats.Eur JPharmacol, Vol.202,No.3,PP.317-22

Telimaa S, Puolakka J, RonnbergL,etal (1987). Placebo controlled Comparison of danazol and high-dose medroxyprogesterone acetate in the treatment of endometriosis, GynecolEndocrinol , Vol.1, *P.13*

Tseng L, Lui HC (1981). Stimulation of arylsulfotransferase activity by progestins in human endometrium in vitro, J ClinEndocrinolMetab, Vol.53,P.418

Vlahos NF, Grogoriou O, Deliveliotou A, et al (2010).Effect of Pentoxiphylline on vascular endothelial growth factor c and flk-1 expression on endometrial implants in the rat endometriosis model.FertilSteril,vol.93,No.4,PP.1316-23

Wang H, GorpudoloN&Behr B (2009).The role of prolactin and endometriosis associated infertility. ObstetGynecolSurv,Vol.64, No.8,PP.542-7

Xiang DF, Sun QZ &Liang XF (2011). Effect of abdominal acupuncture on pain of pelvic cavity in patients with endometriosis . Zhongguo Zhen Jiu,Vol.31,No.2, PP.113-6

Yisa SB, Okenwa AA &Husemeyer RP (2005).Treatment of pelvic endometriosis with etonogestrel subdermal implant (Implanon). J FamPlannReprod Health Care ,vol.31,PP.67-70

Zulfikaroglu E, Kilic S, Islimye M, et al (2011).Efficacy of anti-tumor necrosis factor therapy on endometriosis in an experimental rat model.RchGynecolObstet,Vol.283, No.4, PP.799-804

28

Sequential Management with Gonadotropin-Releasing Hormone Agonist and Dienogest of Endometriosis-Associated Uterine Myoma and Adenomyosis

Atsushi Imai*, Hiroshi Takagi, Kazutoshi Matsunami and Satoshi Ichigo
Institute of Endocrine-Related Cancer, Matsunami General Hospital, Japan

1. Introduction

Uterine leiomyoma and adenomyosis represent the most common benign tumors of the female reproductive system (Levy, 2008; Parker, 2007; Sankaran & Manyonda, 2008). These tumors are estrogen dependent, develop during the reproductive period, and are suppressed with menopause. Traditional treatments for myomas and adenomyosis have been various types of surgical techniques. Medical management of these tumors is an approach that has been used recently and is attractive for many gynecologists because of its relative ease and lack of complications (pelvic organ adhesion) compared with surgery. Indications for therapy are similar to those for surgical removal of these tumors and focus on preserving fertility and/or the patient's desire to maintain her uterus. Medications used include androgens, antiprogestogens (mifepristone), raloxifen, and gonadotropin-releasing hormone agonist (GnRHa) (Levy, 2008; Parker, 2007; Sankaran & Manyonda, 2008; Schweppe, 1999). At present, considering efficiency and safety issues, none of the above agents obtained adequate popularity except for GnRHa. However, GnRHa also have disadvantages including bone loss and menopausal symptoms. The effect of GnRHa is transient and reversal of estrogen deprivation occurs soon after discontinuation of the GnRHa and most myoma and adenomyosis returns to their initial size within several months after discontinuation.

Dienogest is a selective progestin that combines the pharmacologic properties of 19-norprogestins and progesterone derivatives, offering potent progestogenic effects without androgenic, mineral corticoid, or glucocorticoid activity (Harada & Taniguchi, 2010; Sasagawa *et al*, 2008; Sitruk-Ware, 2006). Previous trials demonstrated that dienogest provides effective reductions in endometriosis-associated pelvic pain and laparoscopic measures of pathology (Harada *et al*, 2009; Köhler *et al*, 2010; Schindler *et al*, 2006; Strowitzki *et al*, 2010b). Recently, the new progesterone 2 mg daily demonstrated equivalent efficacy to GnRHa (e.g. buserelin acetate and leuprolide acetate) for relieving the pain of endometriosis in two 24-week, randomized studies (Harada *et al*, 2009; Strowitzki *et al*, 2010a; Strowitzki *et al*, 2010b). Because uterine myoma/adenomyosis and endometriosis have many common

* Corresponding author: Institute of Endocrine-Related Cancer, Matsunami General Hospital, Kasamatsu, Japan.

features (Huang *et al*, 2010), these successful trials on endometriosis support that the use of dienogest inhibits myoma and adenomyosis growth. While evaluating superiority of dienogest in women with endometriosis, we have found significant shrinkage of myoma nodes coexisted with endometriosis over several months during an administration of dienogest (Ichigo *et al*, 2011). In this paper, we attempted to prevent their regrowth after discontinuation of GnRHa using dienogest. This retrospective study may be the first study that examined the efficacy and safety of dienogest following GnRHa therapy in perimenopausal women until leading to a natural menopause.

2. Materials and methods

2.1 Reproductive chart review

The data were collected from 13 perimenopausal patients sequentially treated with leuprolide acetate (1.88mg monthly, Takeda Pharmaceutical, Japan) for 6 months and dienogest (2mg/day, Mochida Pharmaceutical, Japan) for 6 months against endometriosis in our patient clinic from January 2008 to May 2011. In this retrospective chart review, we included all perimenopausal patients complicated with a myoma node measuring > 4cm or with adenomyosis measuring >10 cm at the age 46-52 years. Measurements of nodes or total uterine volume using MRI were performed at baseline and during treatment at months 6 and 12. For tecknical reasons, leuprolide acetate was supplied in vials and dienogest in tablets.

Size of myoma or overall uterine was measured at three diameters (transverse, vertical and anterior-posterior) with MRI. Half of multiplied three diameters was accepted as size of myomas and uterus. These measurements were repeated 6 and 12 months after starting the therapy.

2.2 Statistics

Pared t-*t*ests were used to analyze in each size change from baseline. Statitstical significance was defined as $P < 0.05$.

Case No.	Age (years)	Myoma type	Total myoma volume (cm^3) (% of baseline)		
			Baseline	After GnRHa treatment	After dienogest treatment
1	48	Intramural	108.6	78.6 (72.2)	80.6 (74.0)
2	49	Intramural	72.8	61.9 (85.0)	58.6 (80.5)
3	46	Intramural (multiple)	45.6	33.6 (73.7)	36.9 (80.9)
4	52	Intramural (multiple)	89.3	42.7 (47.8)	50.9 (57.0)
5#	52	Adenomyosis	117.5	56.3 (47.8)	50.3 (42.8)
6	50	Subserosal	88.7	85.6 (96.5)	81.7 (92.1)
7##	52	Subserosal (multiple)	87.2	43.6 (50.0)	45.2 (51.8)
Average		49.9 ± 2.3	87.1 ± 23.5	57.5 ± 19.3* (67.6 ± 19.5)	57.7 ± 17.3* (68.4 ± 18.1)

Table 1. Myoma volume change during sequential treatment with GnRHa and dienogest

The patients were sequentially treated with leuprolide acetate (1.88mg monthly) for 6 months and dienogest (2mg daily) for 6months. Measurements of nodes using MRI were performed at baseline, during treatment at months 6 (after GnRHa therapy) and 12 (after dienogest therapy).

MRI changes of case 5 are presented as a representative prolile in Fig.1.

Case 7 was submitted to laparotomy at month 8 because of bilateral ovarian abscess. See Fig. 2.

* $P < 0.01$ versus baseline.

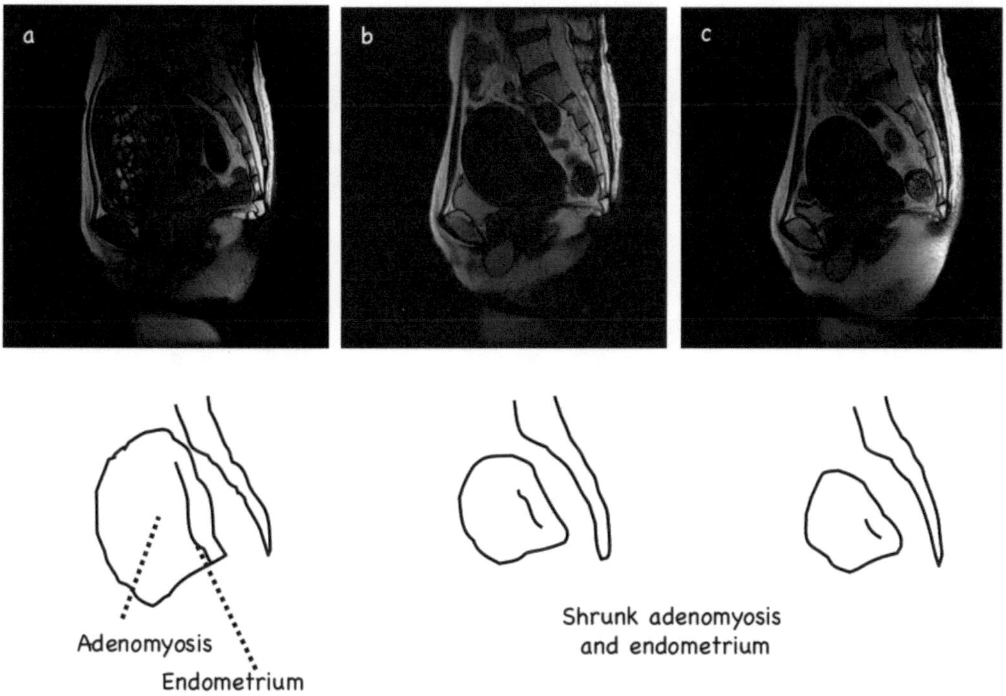

Fig. 1. Total uterine volume change in the patient with myoma during sequential treatment with GnRHa and dienogest (case 6 of Table 1).

The patient was sequentially treated with leuprolide acetate (1.88mg monthly) for 6 months and dienogest (2mg daily) for 6months. Sagittal T2-weighed MR imagings before (a), months 6 (after GnRHa therapy) (b) and 12 (after dienogest therapy)(c)

3. Results

Of 13 endometriosis patients sequentially treated with GnRHa and dienogest, 7 were associated with coexistent myoma node and adenomyosis; 4 intramural and 2 subserosal types and 1 of adenomyosis. Mean age was 49.9 ± 2.3 (46-52)(Table 1). Volume changes of total myoma and adenomyosis are presented as the percentage change from baseline in Table 1. A remarkable reduction in myoma / adenomyosis volume from baseline was noted:

the total volume of myoma/adenomyosis declined to 67.6 ± 19.5 % after GnRHa treatment table 1). During the dienogest-period, myoma volume remained as they shrunk; no regrowth occurred. Fig. 1 showed as a representative profile (case 6 of Table 1). One patient (case 7) discontinued therapy because of an unexpected event, onset on ovarian abscess developed in the endometrioma (see Fig.2).

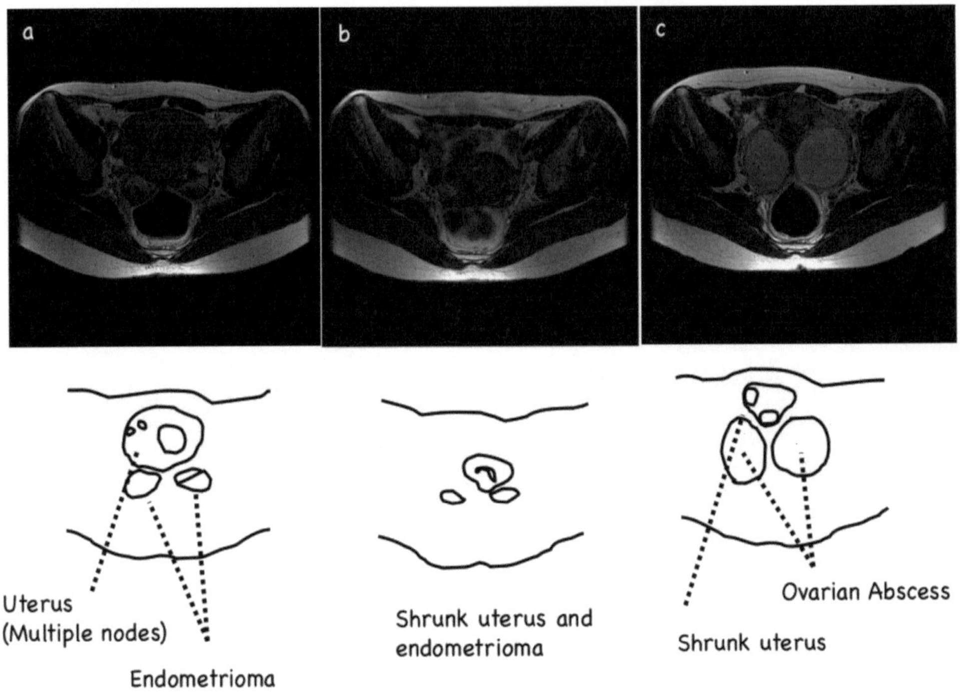

Fig. 2. Bilateral *de novo* ovarian abscesses in a 52-year-old woman with multilobular uterine myoma and bilateral ovarian endometriomas (case 7, table 1).

The patient was treated with leuprolide acetate (1.88mg monthly, Takeda Pharmaceutical, Japan) for 6 months. Axial T2-weighed MR imagings before (a) and after (b) GnRHa treatment showed remarkable shrinkage of uterine myoma and bilateral endometriomas. An attempt to prevent the recurrence submitted the patient to dienogest therapy (2mg daily, Mochida Pharmaceutical, Japan). After two months, she complaint a one-week history of increasing abdominal girth and a two-day history of fever. Axial T2-weighed MR imaging (c) showed two enlarged cystic lesions, one in the left adnexa and the other in the right adnexa. Both lesions were superimposed on the endometrioma with inhomogenous content and the thick wall, while shrunk uterine myoma was detected. There was no history of gynecological interventions including endometrioma aspiration, no had she ever used an intra-uterine device. The clinical and imaging findings and unresponsive to antibiotic therapy proposed the ovarian abscess developed in the endometriomas. At laparotomy, both ovarian cysts were markedly distended and filled with yellow-brown pus, and both ovaries were destroyed by multiple abscess pockets. Histology of the abscess wall confirmed endometriotic nature of the cyst.

4. Discussion

Uterine myoma/adenomyosis and endometriosis have many common features. Both are estrogen-dependent conditions that can often be the source of pelvic pain and menstrual abnormalities. In addition, both have range of symptom severity that is often poorly correlated to preoperative or operative findings, making surgical planning a challenge (Huang et al, 2010). Recently we found significant shrinkage of myoma nodes coexisted with endometriosis over several months during an administration of dienogest (Ichigo et al, 2011). To our knowledge this retrospective study may be the first study that examined the efficacy and safety of sequential management with dienogest following GnRHa therapy in perimenopausal women until leading to a natural menopause.

Many studies have reported the potential usefulness of the hypoestrogenic state induced by GnRHa for treatment of uterine myoma (Levy, 2008; Parker, 2007; Sankaran & Manyonda, 2008). A GnRHa down-regulates the pituitary-ovarian-gonadal axis, leading to suppression of ovarian steroidogenesis. In the present study our patients revealed an average reduction of 57.5 % in myoma volume in response to leuprolide acetae (1.8mg/month). The results are in agreement with those of previous studies (Levy, 2008; Parker, 2007; Parsanezhad *et al*, 2010; Sankaran & Manyonda, 2008). The GnRHa treatment is often associated with so-called ovarian defect symptoms, including vasomotor instability, vaginal dryness, and significant bone loss, which preclude the long-term use of this compound (Levy, 2008; Parker, 2007; Sankaran & Manyonda, 2008). These limit the standard use of GnRHa to 6 months. The regression of uterine or endometriosis volume is not permanent, with returning to their original size or even enlarging more rapidly upon cessation of GnRHa administration. GnRHa, therefore, can only be used in the short term, as temporizing measures in the perimenopausal woman, or pre-operatively to reduce myoma size, influence the type of surgery, restore hemoglobin levels and apparently reduce blood loss at operation (Sankaran & Manyonda, 2008).

There may be profound differences among the available progestins according to their structure, metabolites and pharmacodynamic actions (Harada & Taniguchi, 2010; Sasagawa *et al*, 2008; Sitruk-Ware, 2006). It is therefore inappropriate to consider the various effects of the older and newer progestins as class effects. While it has long been established that estrogen promotes myoma growth, many biochemical and clinical studies suggested that older progestins, without an estrogen component, may be effective in the treatment of endometriosis, but not adenomyosis or myomas (Levy, 2008; Parker, 2007; Sankaran & Manyonda, 2008). The newer progestin dienogest demonstrates a modest suppression of estradiol, representing a potential advantage over other therapies, such as GnRHa, which require estrogen add-back if used longer than 6 months (Harada & Taniguchi, 2010; Strowitzki *et al*, 2010a). Also in contrast to GnRHa, dienogest is not associated with an increased incidence of hot flashes (Strowitzki *et al*, 2010a; Strowitzki *et al*, 2010b). More recently the efficacy and safety of long-term usage of dienogest have been demonstrated in previous controlled studies in a large number of patients with endometriosis (Endrikat *et al*, 2007; Momoeda *et al*, 2009; Schindler *et al*, 2010; Sitruk-Ware, 2006). Our previous paper demonstrated that the use of dienogest have several advantages over GnRHa therapy to manage uterine myoma (Ichigo *et al*, 2011). Management of uterine myoma using dienogest is useful in women for whom temporary reduction in myoma volume is aimed and no surgical intervention is planned for any reason. Women with uterine myoma who have pain, pressure effect, hypermenorrhea, or other types of abnormal uterine bleeding who wish to retain the option of childbirth; women who wish to save their uterus; women who are not fit for surgical intervention; and young women with infertility can take advantage of this type of treatment. However, the total decline in myoma volume and controlling symptoms are greater in GnRHa protocol (Ichigo *et al*, 2011). The benefit of dienogest in controlling symptoms may persist after therapy of GnRHa in perimenopausal women.

In the previous study (Imai *et al*, 2003), because rapid regrowth frequently occurs after the therapy is stopped. we attempted to determine whether GnRHa therapy could lead perimenopausal women carrying symptomatic myomas to the natural onset of the menopause. A retrospective analysis of 145 patients who received GnRHa for 24 weeks demonstrated that after cessation of therapy no menstruation occurred over 25 weeks in women aged over 45 years, with elevated levels of follicle-stimulating hormone (FSH) and luteinising hormone (LH). To extend this observation, we studied prospectively 21 women, aged 45 years and older who had regular menstruation with symptoms attributed to myomas and elevated days 3 - 5 FSH and days 3 - 5 LH levels (> 25 mIU/ml). After discontinuation of GnRHa (leuprorelin acetate, 1.88 mg) therapy for 6 months, menstruation occurred in only two of 21 individuals but the remaining 19 cases had no menstrual bleeding. It is suggested that the rise in early follicular phase serum gonadotrophins, in particular FSH (> 25 mIU/ml), may precede the natural menopause following (or during) GnRHa therapy in older women. Measuring days 3 to 5 serum FSH concentrations may make it easier to decide on the optimal duration of therapy for symptomatic uterine fibroids in perimenopausal women aged > 45 years. However, in other words, approximately 10 % of women failed to become natural menopause.

Regarding an unexpected event of case 7 of table 1, she has no known previous history of pelvic inflammatory disease, IUD, or any surgical intervention, so she was very unlikely to present with ovarian abscess. It shows that an isolated ovarian abscess can develop in an endometrioma without any recognized risk factor. There are different theories about developing an abscess in the endometrioma (Hameed *et al*, 2010; Kavoussi *et al*, 2006). It may be due to an altered immune environment within endometrial glands and stroma. Recent studies have shown that progesterone-like substances enhance the sexual transmission of various pathogens, including bacteria (Huber & Gruber, 2001; Vassiliadou *et al*, 1999). Collection of altered menstrual type of blood in a cystic space in the ovary and can be a suitable culture medium for pathogens. Cystic wall of endometrioma is theoretically weak as compared to normal ovarian epithelium, so it is susceptible to bacterial invasion.

Lastly, we reported successful management of a series of patients with uterine myoma associated with endometriosis by sequential therapy with GnRHa and a progestine dienogest, although based on the finding in patients associated with endometriosis. The follow-up period of our study was too short to consider the recurrence rate of myomas after discontinuation of treatment in all subjects. Although prospective controlled study should be addressed, the use of dienogest treatment following GnRHa discontinuation for perimenopausal women with symptomatic uterine myoma or adenomyosis should be considered before choosing a more invasive interventions.

5. Conclusion

High recurrence rate rapidly after finishing GnRHa leads us to examine the efficacy of sequential management with GnRHa and dienogest in perimenopausal women with endometrisosis-associated uterine myoma. Consideration of GnRHa advantages on myoma shrinkage and low incidence of dienogest-induced adverse events may lead to long-term management of perimenopausal women with myoma and adenomyosis.

6. Conflict of interest

The authors declare that they have no conflict of interest.

7. References

Endrikat, J.; Graeser, T., Mellinger, U., Ertan, K. & Holz, C. (2007) A multicenter, prospective, randomized, double-blind, placebo-controlled study to investigate the efficacy of a continuous-combined hormone therapy preparation containing 1mg estradiol valerate/2mg dienogest on hot flushes in postmenopausal women. *Maturitas* Vol.58, pp. 201-201, ISSN 0378-5122

Hameed, A.; Mehta, V. & Sinha, P. (2010) A rare case of de novo gigantic ovarian abscess within an endometrioma. *Yale Journal of Biology and Medicine* Vol.83, pp. 73-75, ISSN 0044-0086

Harada, T.; Momoeda, M., Taketani, Y., Aso, T., Fukunaga, M., Hagino, H. & Terakawa, N. (2009) Dienogest is as effective as intranasal buserelin acetate for the relief of pain symptoms associated with endometriosis--a randomized, double-blind, multicenter, controlled trial. *Fertility and Sterility* Vol.91, pp. 675-681, ISSN 0015-0282

Harada, T. & Taniguchi, F. (2010) Dienogest: a new therapeutic agent for the treatment of endometriosis. *Women's Health* Vol.6, pp. 27-35, ISSN 1745-5057

Huang, J.; Lathi, R., Lemyre, M., Rodriguez, H., Nezhat, C. & Nezhat, C. (2010) Coexistence of endometriosis in women with symptomatic leiomyomas. *Fertility and Sterility* Vol.94, pp. 720-723, ISSN 0015-0282

Huber, J. & Gruber, C. (2001) Immunological and dermatological impact of progesterone. *Gynecological Endocrinology* Vol.15 (Suppl 6), pp. 18-212, ISSN 0951-3590

Ichigo, S.; Takagi, H., Matsunami, K., Suzuki, N. & Imai, A. (2011) Beneficial effects of dienogest on uterine myoma volume: a retrospective controlled study comparing with gonadotropin-releasing hormone agonist. *Archives of Gynecology and Obstetrics* Vol.Epub ahead of print, ISSN 0932-0067

Imai, A.; Sugiyama, M., Furui, T. & Tamaya, T. (2003) Treatment of perimenopausal women with uterine myoma: successful use of a depot GnRH agonist leading to a natural menopause. Journal of Obstetrics and Gynaecology Vol.23, pp 518-520, ISSN 0144-3615

Kavoussi, S.; Pearlman, M., Burke, W. & Lebovic, D. (2006) Endometrioma complicated by tubo-ovarian abscess in a woman with bacterial vaginosis. *Infectious Disease in Obstetrics and Gynecology* Vol.2006, pp. 1-3,

Köhler, G.; Faustmann, T., Gerlinger, C., Seitz, C. & Mueck, A. (2010) A dose-ranging study to determine the efficacy and safety of 1, 2, and 4mg of dienogest daily for endometriosis. *International Journal of Gynaecology and Obstetrics* Vol.108, pp. 21-25, ISSN: 0020-7292

Levy, B. (2008) Modern management of uterine fibroids. *Acta Obstetricia et Gynecologica Scandinavica* Vol.87, pp. 812-823, ISSN 1600-0412

Momoeda, M.; Harada, T., Terakawa, N., Aso, T., Fukunaga, M., Hagino, H. & Taketani, Y. (2009) Long-term use of dienogest for the treatment of endometriosis. *Journal of Obstetric and Gynaecological Research* Vol.35, pp. 1069-1076, ISSN 13418076

Parker, W. (2007) Uterine myomas: management. *Fertility and Sterility* Vol.88, pp. 255-271, ISSN 0015-0282

Parsanezhad, M.; Azmoon, M., Alborzi, S., Rajaeefard, A., Zarei, A., Kazerooni, T., Frank, V. & Schmidt, E. (2010) A randomized, controlled clinical trial comparing the effects of aromatase inhibitor (letrozole) and gonadotropin-releasing hormone agonist (triptorelin) on uterine leiomyoma volume and hormonal status. *Fertility and Sterility* Vol.93, pp. 192-198, ISSN 0015-0282

Sankaran, S. & Manyonda, I. (2008) Medical management of fibroids. *Best Practice & Research Clinical Obstetrics & Gynaecology* Vol.22, pp. 655-676, ISSN 1521-6934

Sasagawa, S.; Shimizu, Y., Kami, H., Takeuchi, T., Mita, S., Imada, K., Kato, S. & Mizuguchi, K. (2008) Dienogest is a selective progesterone receptor agonist in transactivation analysis with potent oral endometrial activity due to its efficient pharmacokinetic profile. *Steroids* Vol.73, pp. 222-231, ISSN 0039-128X

Schindler, A.; Christensen, B., Henkel, A., Oettel, M. & Moore, C. (2006) High-dose pilot study with the novel progestogen dienogestin patients with endometriosis. *Gynecolical Endocrinology* Vol.22, pp. 9-17, ISSN 0951-3590

Schindler, A.; Henkel, A., Moore, C. & Oettel, M. (2010) Effect and safety of high-dose dienogest (20 mg/day) in the treatment of women with endometriosis. *Archives of Gynecology and Obstetrics* Vol.282, pp. 507-514, ISSN 0932-0067

Schweppe, K. (1999) Progestins and uterine leiomyoma. *Gynecologycal Endocrinology* Vol.13 Suppl 4, pp. 21-24, ISSN 0951-3590

Sitruk-Ware, R. (2006) New progestagens for contraceptive use. *Human Reproduction Update* Vol.12, pp. 169-178, ISSN 1355-4786

Strowitzki, T.; Faustmann, T., Gerlinger, C. & Seitz, C. (2010a) Dienogest in the treatment of endometriosis-associated pelvic pain: a 12-week, randomized, double-blind, placebo-controlled study. *European Journal of Obstetrics & Gynecology and Reproductive Biology* Vol.151, pp. 193-198, ISSN 0301-2115

Strowitzki, T.; Marr, J., Gerlinger, C., Faustmann, T. & Seitz, C. (2010b) Dienogest is as effective as leuprolide acetate in treating the painful symptoms of endometriosis: a 24-week, randomized, multicentre, open-label trial. *Human Reproduction Update* Vol.25, pp. 633-641, ISSN 1355-4786

Vassiliadou, N.; Tucker, L. & Anderson, D. (1999) Progesterone-induced inhibition of chemokine receptor expression on peripheral blood mononuclear cells correlates with reduced HIV-1 infectability in vitro. *Journal of Immunology* Vol.162, pp. 7510-7518, ISSN 0022-1767